Advances in Clinical Pharmacology

Drugs and the Lung

Advances in Clinical Pharmacology

Series Editor : Sir John Vane

Drugs and the Lung, edited by Clive P. Page and W. James Metzger, 624 pages, 1994.

Advances in Clinical Pharmacology

Drugs and the Lung

Editors

Clive P. Page, Ph.D.

Reader in Pharmacology
King's College London
University of London, and
Co-Director
Sackler Institute of Pulmonary Pharmacology, and
Department of Thoracic Medicine
King's College Hospital Medical School
London, United Kingdom

W. James Metzger, M.D.

Professor and Chief
Section of Allergy/Immunology
Department of Medicine
East Carolina University
Greenville, North Carolina

Raven Press **New York**

Raven Press Ltd., 1185 Avenue of the Americas, New York, New York 10036

Made in the United States of America

Library of Congress Cataloging-in-Publication Data

Drugs and the lung / editors, Clive P. Page, W. James Metzger.
    p.   cm.
  Includes bibliographical references and index.
  ISBN 0-7817-0135-X
  1. Pulmonary pharmacology. 2. Respiratory agents. I. Page, C. P.
II. Metzger, W. James
  [DNLM: 1. Lung Diseases—drug therapy. WF 600 D794 1994]
  RM388.D784 1994
  615'.72—dc20
  DNLM/DLC
  for Library of Congress   93-42148
                                    CIP

9 8 7 6 5 4 3 2 1

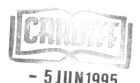

Contents

Contributing Authors

Jonathan R. S. Arch, Ph.D.
Department of Cellular Biochemistry
SmithKline Beecham Pharmaceuticals
Welwyn, Herts AL6 9AR
United Kingdom

Philip G. Bardin, M.B., Ch.B.,
F.C.P. (SA)
M.R.C. Post-Doctoral Senior
* Research Fellow*
University Medicine
Southampton General Hospital
Tremona Road
Southampton SO9 4XY
United Kingdom

Peter J. Barnes, M.A., D.M.,
D.Sc., F.R.C.P.
Chairman, Department of Thoracic
* Medicine*
National Heart and Lung Institute and
Honorary Consultant Physician
Royal Brompton Hospital
Dovehouse Street
London SW3 6LY
United Kingdom

Jonathan W. Becker, M.D.
Senior Research Fellow
Departments of Pediatrics and
* Medicine*
University of Washington
4540 Sand Point Way Northeast
Seattle, Washington 98195

C. Warren Bierman, M.D.
Clinical Professor of Pediatrics
Department of Pediatrics
University of Washington
4540 Sand Point Way Northeast
Seattle, Washington 98195

Ralph L. Brattsand, Ph.D.
Associate Professor of Experimental
* Pharmacology*
Research and Development,
* Pharmacology 1*
Astra Draco AB
Scheelevägen 2
S-221 00 Lund
Sweden

William W. Busse, M.D.
Professor of Medicine
Departments of Medicine, Head, and
* Allergy/Clinical Immunology*
University of Wisconsin Medical
* School*
600 Highland Avenue
Madison, Wisconsin 53792

Franklin Cerasoli, Jr., Ph.D.
Principal Research Scientist
Head of Pharmacology
Preclinical Development
Ariad Pharmaceuticals, Inc.
26 Landsdowne Street
Cambridge, Massachusetts 02139

John F. Costello, M.D., F.R.C.P.
Director
Department of Thoracic Medicine
King's College School of Medicine
Denmark Hill
London SE5 9RS
United Kingdom

Stephen G. Farmer, Ph.D.
Senior Research Pharmacologist
Department of Pulmonary
* Pharmacology*
Zeneca Pharmaceuticals Group
1800 Concord Pike
Wilmington, Delaware 19897-2300

Dean A. Handley, Ph.D.
Fellow
Atherosclerosis and Vascular Diseases
Preclinical Research Department
Sandoz Research Institute
Route 10
East Hanover, New Jersey 07936

Stephen T. Holgate, M.D.,
F.R.C.P., M.R.C.P.
MRC Clinical Professor of
*   Immunopharmacology*
University Medicine
Southampton General Hospital
Tremona Road
Southampton S09 4XY
United Kingdom

Michael J. Holtzman, M.D.
Associate Professor of Medicine
Division of Pulmonary and Critical
*   Care Medicine*
Department of Internal Medicine
Washington University School of
*   Medicine*
Barnes Hospital
660 South Euclid Avenue
St. Louis, Missouri 63110

Jutta C. Joseph, Pharm.D.
Assistant Professor of Pharmacy
*   Practice*
Department of Pharmacy Practice
Washington State University
West 601 First Avenue
Spokane, Washington 99204-0399

Dwight C. Look, M.D.
Instructor of Medicine
Division of Pulmonary and Critical
*   Care Medicine*
Department of Internal Medicine
Washington University School of
*   Medicine*
660 South Euclid Avenue
St. Louis, Missouri 63110

Carlo Alberto Maggi, M.D.
Department of Pharmacology
Menarini Pharmaceuticals
Via Sette Santi 3
50131 Florence
Italy

Stefano Manzini, Ph.D.
Department of Pharmacology
Menarini Ricerche Sud SpA
Via Tito Speri 10
00040 Pomezia, Rome
Italy

A. M. Masi, M.D.
Division of Pulmonary and Critical
*   Care Medicine*
Department of Internal Medicine
Washington University School of
*   Medicine*
660 South Euclid Avenue
St. Louis, Missouri 63110

John Morley, Ph.D., F.R.C.P.
Haldane Research, Ltd.
Kenmore Close
Kent Road
Kew TW9 5JG
United Kingdom

Kenneth J. Murray, Ph.D.
Doctor
Department of Cellular Biochemistry
SmithKline Beecham Pharmaceuticals
The Frythe
Welwyn, Herts AL6 9AR
United Kingdom

Clive P. Page, Ph.D.
Department of Thoracic Medicine
Sackler Institute of Pulmonary
*   Pharmacology*
King's College Hospital Medical
*   School*
University of London
Manresa Road
London SW3 6LX
United Kingdom

Jonathan D. Plitman, M.D.
Assistant Professor of Medicine
Department of Pulmonary and Critical
  Care Medicine
Vanderbilt University School of
  Medicine
B-1308 Medical Center North
Nashville, Tennessee 37232-2650

Charlotte Rayner, M.B.B.S.,
  M.R.C.P.
Medical Registrar
Royal Brompton National Heart and
  Lung Hospital
London SW3 6LR
United Kingdom

Olof B. N. Selroos, M.D., Ph.D.
Associate Professor of Pulmonary
  Medicine
Research and Development
Astra Draco AB
Scheelevägen 2
S-221 00 Lund
Sweden; and Mjölbolsta Hospital
SF-10350
Finland

Vickie R. Shannon, M.D.
Instructor of Medicine
Division of Pulmonary and Critical
  Care Medicine
Department of Internal Medicine
Washington University School of
  Medicine
660 South Euclid Avenue
St. Louis, Missouri 63110

James R. Snapper, M.D.
Professor of Medicine and Senior
  Investigator
Department of Pulmonary and Critical
  Care Medicine
Center for Lung Research
Vanderbilt University School of
  Medicine
1161 21st Avenue South
Nashville, Tennessee 37232-2650

Christine A. Sorkness, Pharm.D.
Professor of Pharmacy and Medicine
  (CHS)
School of Pharmacy
University of Wisconsin-Madison
425 North Charter Street
Madison, Wisconsin 53706

Domenico Spina, Ph.D.
C. J. Martin Research Fellow
Department of Pharmacology
University of Western Australia
Nedlands 6009
Western Australia

Stephen G. Spiro, M.D., F.R.C.P.
Consultant Physician
Department of Thoracic Medicine
University College Hospital
Middlesex Hospital
London WIN 8AA
United Kingdom

Paul Sullivan, M.R.C.P.
Research Fellow
Department of Thoracic Medicine
King's College School of Medicine
  and Dentistry
Bessemer Road
London SE5 9PJ
United Kingdom

Theodore J. Torphy, Ph.D.
Director of Inflammation and
  Respiratory Pharmacology
Department of Inflammation and
  Respiratory Pharmacology
SmithKline Beecham Pharmaceuticals
709 Swedeland Road
King of Prussia, Pennsylvania 19406-0939

**Kenneth W. T. Tsang, M.B.,
  Ch.B., M.R.C.P.**
Research Registrar
Host Defence Unit
Department of Thoracic Medicine
*Royal Brompton National Heart and
  Lung Institute*
Emmanuel Kay Building
Manresa Road
London SW3 6LR
United Kingdom

Robert Wilson, M.D., M.R.C.P.
Consultant Physician
Senior Lecturer
Host Defence Unit
Department of Thoracic Medicine
*Royal Brompton National Heart and
  Lung Institute*
Emmanuel Kaye Building
Manresa Road
London SW3 6LR
United Kingdom

Preface

Lung diseases now represent a considerable burden to health systems and economies around the world. For example, the incidence of asthma has risen dramatically and the morbidity associated with a variety of other lung diseases such as cancer is far from disappearing, while the prevalence of tuberculosis is resurging. Not surprisingly, therefore, there continues to be considerable interest in the development of novel research strategies for the treatment of lung diseases. Perhaps just as important, reappraisal of existing treatment regimes continues. This book represents a comprehensive collection of articles reviewing the current status of a range of drugs in use for the treatment of lung diseases, as well as providing chapters on many new classes of drugs being developed for the treatment of various lung diseases. We have deliberately made the chapters biased towards the clinical action of the various drugs where the information is available, but drawing on information from experimental studies when appropriate.

This book will be of interest to clinicians, scientists, and students as a reference source for each of the major drug classes in use or under investigation for the treatment of immunologic lung diseases.

Clive P. Page
W. James Metzger

Advances in Clinical Pharmacology

Drugs and the Lung

Drugs and the Lung,
edited by C.P. Page and W.J. Metzger.
Raven Press, Ltd., New York © 1994

1

β₂-Agonists

Domenico Spina

Department of Pharmacology, University of Western Australia,
Nedlands 6009, Western Australia

β-Adrenoceptor agonists afford symptomatic bronchodilator relief against a number of bronchospastic stimuli, including antigen, exercise, and chemical irritants, and are the agents of first choice in the treatment of asthma. The major action attributed to β-adrenoceptor agonists in asthma, and its beneficial effect, is the functional antagonism of airway smooth muscle contraction. It is apparent, however, that β-adrenoceptor agonists act on a number of different cell types within the lung, including mast cells and endothelial cells. Hence, the pharmacological action of β-adrenoceptor agonists on these other cell types might also contribute toward the symptomatic relief in asthma.

The relatively short duration of action of β-adrenoceptor agonists particularly against bronchospastic stimuli has led to the development of longer acting β-adrenoceptor agonists including salmeterol and formoterol. These agents have durations of activity that are at least twice those of the current short-acting β-adrenoceptor agonists. This increased duration of activity may be advantageous in the treatment of nocturnal asthma.

There is no doubt that β-adrenoceptor agonists are efficacious against acute exacerbations in asthma. However, a number of studies have again raised the possibility that regular chronic treatment with β-adrenoceptor agonists may be responsible for the increase in asthma mortality and morbidity, a controversy that has intensified following the introduction of the longer-acting β-adrenoceptor agonists.

A number of reviews have been written with regard to the use of β-adrenoceptor agonists in asthma (1,2). This chapter highlights more recent data concerning the use of both short- and longer-acting β-adrenoceptor agonists in asthma.

STRUCTURE AND METABOLISM

The majority of the β-adrenoceptor agonists currently used in treating asthma are derived from the known structure of adrenaline. Thus, β-adrenoceptor agonists share a phenylethylamine structure, with a catechol, resorcinol, or related moiety, which confers potency, and an ethanolamine side chain, which confers selectivity to the molecule. A number of structures of the currently available β-adrenoceptor agonists and the new generation of long-acting β-adrenoceptor agonists are illustrated in Fig. 1.

Adrenaline

Adrenaline possesses a benzene ring structure that is hydroxylated in the 3 and 4 position (catechol). It also contains a methyl ethanolamine side chain. Hence, adrenaline possesses activity at both α- and β-adrenoceptors, with the latter effect of greater importance in the clinical efficacy of this drug in asthma. The pharmacological action of adrenaline is predominantly terminated by tissue uptake (extraneuronal uptake) in airway smooth muscle, gut, and liver. However, adrenaline is also sequestered into storage vesicles of nerve endings (neuronal uptake), although this is the smaller of the two uptake compartments (3). Following uptake into sympathetic nerve terminals, adrenaline is metabolized by deamination and oxidation by monoamine oxidase (MAO) to 3,4-dihydroxymandelic acid (3). Following uptake into extraneuronal sites, adrenaline is predominantly metabolized by catechol-O-methyl transferase (COMT), resulting in the formation of 3-O-methyl adrenaline (metanephrine). Thus, the combined effects of the two metabolic pathways result in the secretion of 3-methoxy-4-hydroxy mandelic acid (vanillylmandelic acid) (3).

Adrenaline is a short-acting but potent bronchodilator that is active following inhaled and parenteral, but not oral, administration.

Isoprenaline

Isoprenaline was developed in an attempt to increase agonist selectivity for β-adrenoceptors. Significantly greater β-adrenergic selectivity was achieved with isoprenaline by the incorporation of an isopropyl ethanolamine side chain. Following oral administration, large doses of isoprenaline are required to produce pharmacological effects, since isoprenaline undergoes sulfate conjugation in the gut and liver (4,5). In contrast, following intravenous administration, mainly unchanged drug is excreted in the urine (5). However, the powerful cardiovascular stimulatory effect of isoprenaline can preclude its intravenous use. Isoprenaline also undergoes significant 3-O-methylation when administered intrabronchially or by inhalation in man

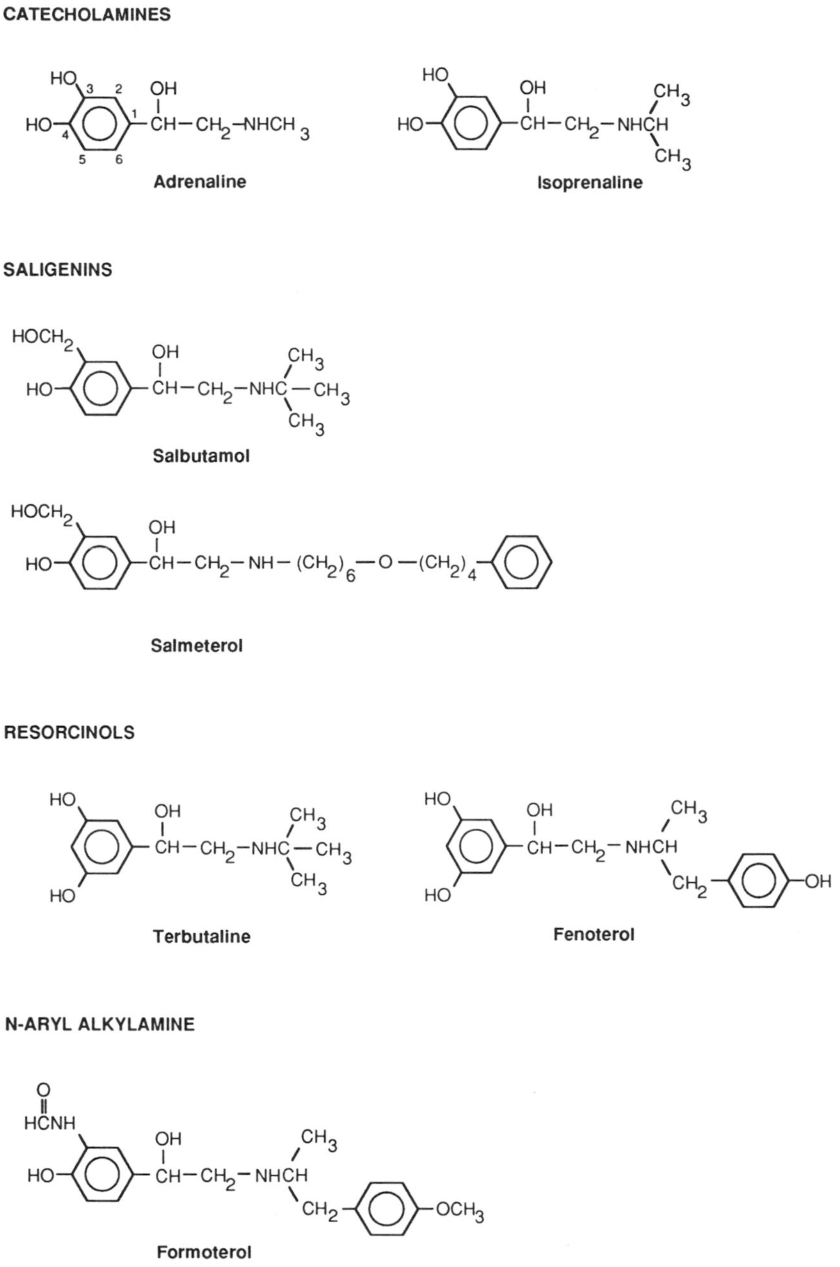

CATECHOLAMINES

Adrenaline

Isoprenaline

SALIGENINS

Salbutamol

Salmeterol

RESORCINOLS

Terbutaline

Fenoterol

N-ARYL ALKYLAMINE

Formoterol

FIG. 1. Chemical structures of some β-adrenoceptor agonist bronchodilators.

(5,6). Only approximately 10% of a conventionally delivered metered inhaled dose (MDI) of isoprenaline is deposited into the lungs, while the remainder is swallowed and largely inactivated by sulfate conjugation (5). Hence, a greater airway selectivity for pulmonary β-adrenoceptors is achieved when the agonist is given by the inhaled route.

Salbutamol

In an attempt to minimize enzymatic degradation, a number of modifications were made to the basic structure of the catecholamines. Resistance to COMT degradation was achieved by the addition of a methyl group to the 3-hydroxyl group, forming a saligen derivative (e.g., salbutamol). Furthermore, greater selectivity for β_2- over β_1-adrenoceptors was achieved following the addition of a tertiary butyl group to the ethanolamine side chain (7).

Salbutamol is orally active although it remains susceptible to 4-O'-sulfate conjugation in the intestinal wall and liver in man (8,9). Following intrabronchial administration of salbutamol, there is rapid clearance with no metabolism across the airway wall (10). Both the free drug and sulfate metabolite appear in the urine following aerosol administration, indicating that much of the aerosol dose is swallowed (8,9). Salbutamol is also active following intravenous administration of this drug, with lesser amounts of the sulfate conjugate appearing in the urine compared with the inhaled and oral route (8,9).

Terbutaline

Another method employed to confer resistance to metabolism by COMT led to the synthesis of terbutaline, a β-adrenoceptor agonist that possesses a resorcinol ring structure (11). Its β_2-selectivity is defined by the tertiary butyl group on the N-terminal, as for salbutamol. Terbutaline is also susceptible to sulfate conjugation when given by the oral route in man (12,13). Predominantly unchanged drug is detected in plasma following intratracheal administration of terbutaline in rats, indicating the absence of metabolism across the airway wall (14,15). Thus, terbutaline is effective when given by the inhaled, oral, or intravenous route (16).

Fenoterol

Fenoterol has a resorcinol ring structure and thus, like terbutaline, is also resistant to metabolism via COMT. Fenoterol has increased selectivity for β_2- over β_1-adrenoceptors by virtue of a large cyclic structure attached to the N-terminal. However, fenoterol appears to be less selective for β_2-adrenoceptors than salbutamol and terbutaline (7). Fenoterol is effective orally although it is susceptible to 5-O'-sulfation (17,18). Fenoterol is also effective by intravenous injection and by inhalation and is excreted in the urine relatively slowly, with 12% of a inhaled dose excreted after 24 h (17,18).

Salmeterol

Salmeterol is derived from salbutamol and consists of a phenylethanolamine head and a long nonpolar N-substituent (Fig. 1). The long nonpolar region confers a substantial increase in duration of activity of this molecule (19). The pharmacokinetic properties of salmeterol have recently been reviewed (20). Salmeterol is significantly bound to plasma protein *in vitro,* and is extensively metabolized by hydroxylation and slowly eliminated in urine and feces (20).

Formoterol

Formoterol contains a formamide group in the 3 position on the benzene ring and an N-aralkyl side chain (Fig. 1). Formoterol is active by both the oral and inhaled routes and the pharmacokinetic properties of this drug have recently been reviewed (21). The elimination half-life of formoterol after inhalation was calculated to be 1.7 to 2.3 h (22), similar to that observed for salbutamol (23). Only 10% and 24% of an oral and inhaled dose, respectively, of formoterol was recovered in the urine after 24 h (21,24). Following oral administration of formoterol (80 μg), 6% and 8% of the dose was recovered over a 10-h period, as the unchanged and glucuronide conjugate, respectively (21). It is not known whether formoterol is present in a compartment with a prolonged half-life that would account for the very low levels of excreted drug. Detection of this compartment is difficult given the low dose of formoterol that is required for therapeutic activity (21).

ROUTE OF ADMINISTRATION

Maximal bronchodilator activity can be achieved when β-adrenoceptor agonists are given by either the oral or intravenous route. When given systemically a dose-dependent fall in forced expiratory volume in 1 sec (FEV_1) is observed with isoprenaline and salbutamol (25), terbutaline (26), fenoterol (18), and formoterol (27). The increases in heart rate observed with maximal bronchodilator doses of the noncatecholamine β-adrenoceptor agonists are considerably lower than those achieved for isoprenaline. However, to achieve maximal bronchodilation by the systemic route, cardiac stimulation is unavoidable as a consequence of a reduction in total peripheral resistance resulting in reflex activation of cardiac $β_1$-adrenoceptors (28). Furthermore, because a significant population of β_2-adrenoceptors exists in the human heart (29–31), some cardiac activation is to be expected for even very selective β_2-adrenoceptor agonists.

The inhaled route offers a number of advantages over the systemic route, including direct access to the lung and rapid onset of action with considerably lower systemic activity. Comparison of the dose-effect curves for terbutaline (26), salbutamol (32), and formoterol (27), given systemically or by inhalation, demonstrate that at maximal levels of bronchodilation the systemic side effects are considerably less significant by the inhaled than by the systemic route.

In mild asthmatics, inhaled salbutamol was shown to provide better bronchodilator relief than intravenous salbutamol (33). In contrast, patients with acute, severe asthma who responded poorly to inhaled salbutamol responded favorably to intravenous salbutamol (34,35). The diminished bronchodilator efficacy observed in severe asthma is possibly a consequence of reduced penetration of the bronchodilator due to mucus plugging and edema in severe asthma (36). In contrast, a number of studies have shown the inhaled route to be as effective as the intravenous route in acute severe or moderately severe asthma (37–39). The difference in the results may be related to the severity of the disease and the size of the population studied. Recently, a large multicenter study demonstrated that in severe acute asthma, salbutamol was more efficacious by the inhaled route than by the intravenous route. Consequently, it has been recommended that a nebulized bronchodilator should be used in the treatment of severe acute asthma (40).

DURATION OF ACTION BY INHALED ROUTE

Baseline FEV₁

Catecholamine β-adrenoceptor agonists including isoprenaline and isoetharine exert their maximal bronchodilator effect within 5 min. In contrast, the noncatecholamines including salbutamol, terbutaline, and fenoterol induced 80% maximal bronchodilation within 5 min, with maximal bronchodilation between 15 and 60 min (3). The duration of bronchodilation for equieffective doses of the noncatecholamine β-adrenoceptor agonists is sustained for approximately 3 to 6 h (18,41–49).

In contrast to the short-acting β-adrenoceptor agonists, both formoterol (50) and salmeterol (50,51) have a considerably longer onset time as assessed *in vitro*. Clinical data also suggest that both formoterol (27,52) and salmeterol (53) are slower in onset than salbutamol in their ability to reduce baseline FEV_1. Furthermore, salmeterol is slower in onset than salbutamol in providing relief against acute bronchoconstriction in asthma (54).

Significantly longer duration of action is observed with the new generation of β-adrenoceptor agonists. Both formoterol (27,52,55–57) and salmeterol

(49,53,58) provide sustained bronchodilation for 6 to 12 h in asthmatic adults. Formoterol also provides sustained bronchodilation in asthmatic children for a similar length of time (59–61). Since the duration of drug activity is dependent on the dose (62), it is possible that the long duration of action of these drugs *in vivo* might be attributed to the use of maximal doses of bronchodilator. However, it has been shown that formoterol produces sustained bronchodilation for 8 to 12 h compared with 2 to 6 h for an equieffective dose of salbutamol (27,59).

The reason for the long duration of action of salmeterol and formoterol is not fully understood. *In vitro* studies demonstrate that both formoterol and salmeterol have similar affinity for β-adrenoceptors (63). In contrast, *in vitro* studies indicate that salmeterol, a lipophilic molecule, appears to have a significantly longer duration of action and is retained within the vicinity of the β-adrenoceptor for considerably longer than formoterol and salbutamol (50,63–65). When delivered intratracheally, lipophilic molecules such as glucocorticoids, theophylline, and long-acting β-adrenoceptor agonists pass readily through the airway wall (14,15,50,64,66–68). However, unlike theophylline, glucocorticoids and long-acting β-adrenoceptor agonists are significantly retained within the lung, which may be attributed to high-affinity binding to receptors and/or retention within lipid membranes (50,64,66,68). This may explain the long duration of action of both salmeterol and formoterol. Indeed it is believed that the nonpolar N-substituent of salmeterol is embedded within the lipophilic regions of the β-adrenoceptor (19), although this does not apply for formoterol, as it lacks the nonpolar N-substituent (50). In contrast, short-acting hydrophilic β-adrenoceptor agonists are retained within the airway wall to a lesser extent compared with lipophilic agonists (14,15). Furthermore, their passage across the airway epithelium is significantly retarded compared with more lipophilic agonists (50,64,67).

Hence, the prolonged duration of activity observed for long-acting β-adrenoceptor agonists appears to be due to retention within the lung. Interestingly, the duration of bronchodilation for equieffective doses of orally administered salbutamol and formoterol was found to be similar (27). The reason for this is not clear, but systemic factors do not appear to play a role since the plasma half-lives for salbutamol and formoterol are similar (27).

Bronchospasm

Very few studies have assessed the duration of action of β-adrenoceptor agonists following spasmogen-induced bronchoconstriction. This is of considerable importance given that most asthmatics tend to take β-adrenoceptor agonists during exacerbations of asthma. The duration of action of a number of noncatecholamine β-adrenoceptor agonists at clinically relevant doses against histamine- (48,49,69), exercise- (70), and eucapnic and isocapnic hyperventilation–induced (71,72) bronchospasm peaks between 1 and 2 h and resolves by 4 h. Thus, β-adrenoceptor agonists provide less protection against spasmogen-induced bronchoconstriction than with their effects on baseline FEV_1. This presumably reflects the inability of β-adrenoceptor agonists to functionally antagonize bronchospastic agonists at a time when the concentration of β-adrenoceptor agonist at effector sites is reduced, although high enough to induce a maximal reduction of baseline FEV_1 (48). In contrast, both salmeterol (49,58) and formoterol (59,73,74) functionally antagonize histamine- and methacholine-induced bronchospasm respectively, for 5 to 12 h. Furthermore, significant protection against exercise-induced bronchospasm was afforded for up to 6.5 h by salmeterol (70) and for between 4 and 8 h by formoterol (75,76). In contrast, the protection afforded by salbutamol was considerably less, resolving after 4 h. Similarly, formoterol afforded protection against cold air hyperventilation-induced bronchospasm for 8 h, while the beneficial effect of salbutamol had resolved after 4 h (77). This substantially longer duration of action of salmeterol and formoterol against bronchospasm induced by provoking stimuli is obviously of clinical importance in providing symptomatic relief over a prolonged period of time.

β-ADRENOCEPTOR AGONIST SELECTIVITY AND EFFICACY

Selectivity

Isoprenaline provides fast bronchodilator relief, although it possesses powerful cardiac stimulatory activity. It was subsequently shown that the rise in asthma deaths during the 1960s was correlated with the consumption of isoprenaline (78,79). It was suggested that overreliance on the use of isoprenaline, which provides short-term bronchodilator relief, contributed to the delay in the introduction of corticosteroid therapy in patients whose asthma was deteriorating because of worsening inflammation or tolerance (78,79). It was also thought that the powerful cardiac stimulatory effects may have been a contributing factor (80). The demonstration of β-adrenoceptor subtypes (81) prompted the development of more $β_2$-selective bronchodilators such as salbutamol, fenoterol, and terbutaline.

Studies in the guinea pig have demonstrated that these are selective and potent $β_2$-adrenoceptor agonists at guinea pig tracheal $β_2$-adrenoceptors, although fenoterol is a full agonist compared with salbutamol and terbutaline, which demonstrate partial agonist activity at cardiac $β_1$-adrenoceptors (7). These studies demonstrate that fenoterol is less $β_2$-selective than salbutamol. However, it should be recognized that $β_2$-adrenoceptors are present on human cardiac muscle and are responsible for mediating inotrophic effects (82,83). Thus, $β_2$-adrenoceptor agonists can have both direct and indirect cardiac effects. A number of studies have shown that fenoterol has greater inotrophic, chronotropic, electrocardiographic, and hypokalemic effects than salbutamol and terbutaline in both healthy individuals (84–87) and asthmatics (88–90). Fenoterol is approximately twofold more potent than salbutamol with regard to increasing heart rate and reducing plasma levels of potassium (84,86,90).

The cardiostimulatory and hypokalemic effects of β_2-selective agonists observed in the studies cited above occur at doses that are not recommended by the manufacturers. However, under conditions of severe exacerbation of asthma, large doses of β_2-adrenoceptor agonist may be consumed, which might result in cardiostimulatory and hypokalemic side effects (86,87,89,90). This is particularly relevant for fenoterol since it is marketed at a higher equivalent dose than salbutamol and as a consequence, side effects are more likely to be manifested in asthmatics who undergo acute exacerbations of asthma (90). However, it is important to recognize that tolerance to these extrapulmonary effects occurs following chronic β-adrenoceptor agonist therapy (83,91).

Unlike the β-adrenoceptor agonists currently used in asthma, formoterol and salmeterol are considerably more potent and have greater β_2-selectivity. Formoterol is approximately 80 to 144 times more potent than salbutamol in relaxing isolated guinea pig trachea *in vitro* (50,92) and 204-fold more β_2-selective than salbutamol, although it is a full agonist in guinea pig atria (92). Similarly, in guinea pig trachea and human bronchus, salmeterol is twofold to eightfold and 16-fold more potent, respectively, as a relaxant agonist than salbutamol (51). Furthermore, salmeterol is at least 2000 times more β_2-selective than salbutamol and is a weak partial agonist in rat atria (51). Accordingly, therapeutic doses of inhaled formoterol (21) and salmeterol (20) produce minimal systemic side effects.

Efficacy

Efficacy is a dimensionless proportionality factor that describes the ability of an agonist to induce a response in a particular tissue (93). Hence, an agonist with high efficacy can elicit a maximal response by occupying relatively fewer receptors (greater proportion of spare receptors) than an agonist with low efficacy.

A number of *in vitro* studies with airway smooth muscle have demonstrated an inverse relationship between the level of contraction induced by a spasmogen and the potency and maximum degree of relaxation induced by β-adrenoceptor agonists (94–97). Thus, under normal contractile conditions, β-adrenoceptor agonists may induce maximal relaxation, but the capacity of these agonists to induce relaxation of highly contracted muscle may differ (96). The ability of β-adrenoceptor agonists to induce maximal relaxation was significantly reduced in maximally contracted preparations of human bronchus (98), guinea pig trachea (96,99), bovine trachea (95), and canine trachea (97).

The contractile response induced by methacholine was antagonized by isoprenaline in bovine trachea (95) and by salbutamol and fenoterol (99) but not terbutaline (100) in guinea pig tracheal tissue. The reasons for the failure of Gustafsson and Persson (100) to observe a similar phenomenon with terbutaline is puzzling, but may be due to the use of low concentrations of this β-adrenoceptor agonist. These studies indicate that β-adrenoceptor agonists are effective at inhibiting the development of contraction. Furthermore, the ability of β-adrenoceptor agonists to functionally antagonize spasmogen-induced contractile responses is also dependent on the contractile agonist used as demonstrated both *in vitro* (94,95,101,102) and *in vivo* (103).

Very few studies have compared the efficacies of the different β-adrenoceptor agonists. The efficacy of fenoterol was shown to be twice that of salbutamol in guinea pig trachea (99). No study has compared the efficacy of these agonists *in vivo*. Many studies have demonstrated that all three agonists are indistinguishable with respect to their ability to reduce baseline FEV_1 at equieffective doses (46,104,105). However, one study has demonstrated that at equieffective doses, salbutamol and fenoterol were more potent than terbutaline in antagonizing histamine-induced bronchospasm in asthmatics (90). Hence, in severe asthma, the ability of a β-adrenoceptor agonist to reverse bronchospasm will be dependent on its efficacy. Thus, it would seem advantageous to develop β-adrenoceptors with high efficacy (106).

Little is known of the relative efficacy of salmeterol and formoterol. It was shown that unlike isoprenaline and salbutamol, which are full agonists at human bronchial smooth muscle β-adrenoceptors, salmeterol appeared to behave as a partial agonist (51). Furthermore, both salbutamol and formoterol demonstrate greater efficacy than salmeterol, but only in tissue precontracted with supramaximal doses of spasmogen (107,108).

Clearly, more data are needed to assess the clinical importance of high β_2-adrenoceptor efficacy in the treatment of asthma. Furthermore, the potential disadvantage of a high-efficacy β_2-adrenoceptor agonist requires evaluation, given that fenoterol, at doses equieffective with doses of salbutamol and terbutaline, has the potential to produce greater cardiovascular side effects (90).

MECHANISM OF ACTION

For more detailed explanation the reader is referred to a number of reviews (2,109). Briefly, β-adrenoceptor agonists mediate their effects by binding to cell surface glycoproteins, which belong to the family of guanyl nucleotide binding protein (G protein) coupled receptors that are characterized by seven transmembrane spanning regions. The agonist/β-adrenoceptor complex activates membrane-bound adenylate cyclase through stimulatory G proteins (Gs). The activation of adenylate cyclase results in the production of the second messenger substance adenosine $3',5'$-cyclic monophosphate (cAMP). This second messenger can activate various cAMP-dependent protein kinases. Protein kinases activated in this manner then mediate effects including the relaxation of airway smooth muscle by phosphorylating myosin light chain kinase (MLCK) and inhibition of mediator release from inflammatory cells.

SITES OF ACTION

Airway Smooth Muscle

A number of functional and biochemical studies, together with radioligand binding and autoradiographic techniques, have demonstrated that airway smooth muscle from nondiseased and asthmatic lung contains β_2-adrenoceptors. Functional studies indicate that β_2-adrenoceptor agonists mediate relaxation of human airway smooth muscle (106).

Mast Cells

In 1968, it was shown that isoprenaline inhibited histamine release from leukocytes isolated from allergic individuals (110). It was subsequently demonstrated that β-adrenoceptor agonists inhibit histamine release from passively sensitized chopped human lung (111–113) and human dispersed mast cells *in vitro* (114,115). This effect is mediated by activation of β_2-adrenoceptors present on mast cells in human lung (116). Activation of these receptors inhibits not only the release of histamine, but also slow reacting substance of anaphylaxis (SRS-A), prostaglandin D_2, leukotriene C_4, and leukotriene D_4 (112,116). Similarly, it has been demonstrated that salmeterol inhibits immunoglobin E (IgE)-dependent release of histamine, prostaglandin D_2, and sulfidopeptide leukotrienes from human lung fragments *in vitro* (117). Furthermore, β-adrenoceptor agonists are potent mast cell stabilizers, approximately 2,000 to 30,000 times more potent than the putative mast cell stabilizer disodium cromoglycate with respect to inhibiting mediator release from human lung mast cells *in vitro* (112,113,115). Similarly, formoterol was shown to be approximately 12,000 times more potent than disodium cromoglycate with respect to inhibiting IgE-dependent release of SRS-A from rat peritoneal mast cells (118).

Following acute allergen provocation in asthmatics, a rise in circulating plasma levels of histamine and neutrophil chemotactic factor (119,120) and a rise in the level of histamine, prostaglandin D_2, and sulfidopeptide leukotrienes in bronchoalveolar lavage fluid have been documented (121–123). In asthmatics, salbutamol inhibits the allergen-induced rise in plasma histamine and neutrophil chemotactic factor (119,121). Furthermore, salbutamol was two orders of magnitude more effective than disodium cromoglycate in inhibiting allergen-induced mediator release *in vivo* (121). In contrast, both salbutamol and salmeterol failed to attenuate the allergen-induced rise in urinary excreted leukotriene E_4, which suggests that β-adrenoceptor agonists have little effect on mast cell mediator release *in vivo* (124). However, a number of cells, including airway epithelial cells, macrophages, and eosinophils, secrete sulfidopeptide leukotrienes (125). The percentage of the total leukotriene E_4 secreted in the urine, which is mast cell derived, is difficult to assess. Furthermore, it has previously been shown that the exercise-induced rise in plasma histamine is increased in patients exposed to terbutaline (126). It was suggested that inhalation of β-adrenoceptor agonist may increase blood flow to poorly perfused regions of the lung. Thus, any histamine released within these regions will now become accessible to the plasma, resulting in an artifactual rise in plasma histamine (126). This is a potential confounding factor in assessing the effect of β-adrenoceptor agonists on mediator concentrations in body fluids not taken from lung.

It would appear that β-adrenoceptor agonists are capable of inhibiting IgE-dependent release of mediators from mast cells, and this is another potential site at which this class of drug can modulate the acute bronchoconstrictor response to allergen. Recently, it has been documented that mast cells are capable of generating various cytokines (127,128). The effect of β-adrenoceptor activation on the release of cytokines from human lung mast cells is not known.

Endothelial Cells

Local instillation of allergen onto the bronchial mucosa of asthmatic subjects causes acute swelling and narrowing of the airways as visualized through a bronchoscope (123,129,130). It appears that this response is mediated by smooth muscle constriction and bronchial wall edema. A number of pharmacological agonists, including histamine, bradykinin, sulfidopeptide leukotrienes, and capsaicin or activation of IgE-bearing cells, are capable of increasing plasma protein extravasation and edema within the bronchial wall, as documented in animal studies (131,132). Systemic administration of terbutaline attenuated topically applied histamine-, bradykinin-, and capsaicin-induced plasma protein extravasation and/or edema in bronchial wall or lumen (131,133,134). Thus, vascular leakage is a result of endothelial cell contraction, which promotes gap formation between endothelial cells in pulmonary venules. It is presumed that the "antiedema" property of β-adrenoceptor agonists is a consequence of functional antagonism of endothelial cell contraction (135).

Several studies have failed to demonstrate the anti-edema property of β-adrenoceptor agonists. Intravenously administered salbutamol failed to attenuate intravenously administered platelet activating factor (PAF)- (136) or topically applied leukotriene D_4- (137) induced airway edema in guinea pigs. However, the bronchospasm mediated by intravenously administered leukotriene D_4 was inhibited. A number of factors, including hemodynamic changes mediated by the intravenous administration of β-adrenoceptor agonists and the failure to take into account residual blood volume remaining within the pulmonary vasculature, may confound analysis (134). Such methodological problems can be minimized by measuring plasma protein extravasation and edema within the bronchial lumen and/or introducing β-adrenoceptor agonist directly into the lung (132,138). It has subsequently been demonstrated that formoterol inhibits allergen- and bradykinin-induced luminal edema (139) and histamine-induced (140) plasma protein extravasation and edema. The anti-edema effect of formoterol was greater than that of salbutamol in terms of potency and duration of activity (139). Similarly, salmeterol was also effective against histamine-induced plasma protein extravasation in guinea pigs (141).

The effect of β-adrenoceptor agonists on bronchial edema in asthma has yet to be established, although a number of studies have been performed in the skin. In healthy individuals, the wheal response to intradermal injection of bradykinin (142) and histamine (143), and both the wheal and flare response to intradermal injection of anti-IgE (144–146) are attenuated by prior injection of β-adrenoceptor agonists. The allergen-induced early cutaneous response is also attenuated in atopic patients by β-adrenoceptor agonists (147,148). Furthermore, formoterol produces longer-lasting protection against anti-IgE–induced wheal and to a lesser extent on flare responses than terbutaline in healthy individuals (145,146). Together these data indicate that both mediator- and IgE-dependent increases in the early cutaneous response is attenuated by β-adrenoceptor agonists as a result of inhibition of mast cell degranulation and/or direct effect on endothelial cells. Circumstantial evidence to support the latter was demonstrated by Gronneberg and Zetterstrom (149), who showed that formoterol is effective against anti-IgE–induced wheal responses when injected 30 min after exposure to anti-IgE.

Thus, conclusive evidence for an anti-edema effect by β-adrenoceptor agonists in asthma is presently not available. There is no doubt concerning the efficacy of β-adrenoceptor agonists against the acute inflammatory response (inhibition of mast cell degranulation and edema). However, the anti-edema property of β-adrenoceptor agonists appears to be less effective in chronic inflammation (150,151) and markedly less effective than glucocorticosteroids (144).

Inflammatory Cells

A number of inflammatory cells are thought to play a central role in the pathogenesis of asthma, including eosinophils (152), lymphocytes (153,154), platelets (155,156), and macrophages (157). Increasing the intracellular level of cAMP inhibits the function of many inflammatory cells (158). Hence, the effects of β-adrenoceptor agonists in modulating the function of inflammatory cells has been investigated.

Platelets

Human platelets contain β_2-adrenoceptors that appear to be poorly coupled to adenylate cyclase (159). Thus, it seems unlikely that β_2-adrenoceptor agonists modulate platelet function directly. It is therefore of interest that salbutamol inhibited exercise-induced platelet activation (160). Whether β-adrenoceptor agonists can indirectly influence platelet function in asthma is not known.

Eosinophils

The effect of β-adrenoceptor agonists on eosinophil function remains the subject of much debate. Human eosinophils from individuals with blood eosinophilia contain β_2-adrenoceptors that are coupled to adenylate cyclase (161). However, activation of these receptors by salbutamol failed to inhibit zymosan-induced superoxide generation and the release of eosinophil peroxidase (161). Similarly, isoprenaline, formoterol, and salmeterol failed to inhibit N-formyl-methionyl-leucyl-phenylalanine (FMLP)–induced eosinophil-derived cationic protein (ECP) release and zymosan-treated serum-induced migration of eosinophils from healthy individuals *in vitro* (162). Furthermore, the cytokine-induced enhancement of FMLP-mediated ECP release was also not affected by β-adrenoceptor agonists. In contrast, the cytokine-induced enhancement of FMLP-mediated chemotaxis of eosinophils was inhibited by salbutamol, formoterol, and salmeterol *in vitro* (163). The reasons for the discrepancies in the literature are not clear. However, it would appear that cAMP may modulate only some aspects of eosinophil function. The type IV selective phosphodiesterase inhibitor rolipram inhibits respiratory burst in guinea pig eosinophils (164), yet is ineffective against FMLP-mediated ECP release from human eosinophils (162).

Few studies have assessed the effect of β-adrenoceptor agonist therapy on pulmonary eosinophil number and activation in asthma. Regular 4-week treatment with inhaled terbutaline (500 μg, q.i.d) failed to alter the number of circulating eosinophils (165) or to significantly reduce the levels of ECP recovered in bronchoalveolar lavage fluid in mild asymptomatic asthmatics (166). Quantitative light and electron microscopic analysis of bronchial biopsies from these patients revealed that terbutaline failed to alter the number of eosinophils or foci of eosinophil-derived granules (167). In contrast, anti-inflammatory agents including budesonide and disodium cromoglycate reduced the levels of ECP (166) and the number of eosinophils (168) in asthmatics as assessed from bronchoalveolar lavage fluid. Furthermore, budesonide was also effective in reducing the number of eosinophils and foci of eosinophil-derived granules in bronchial biopsies (167). More recently, it was shown that following 6-week treatment with salmeterol in allergic asthmatics, the improvement in symptoms, peak flow, and bronchial reactivity was not associated with changes in eosinophil activation (169), nor in the number of eosinophils (170), as assessed from bronchoalveolar lavage fluid and bronchial biopsies, respectively.

Thus, β-adrenoceptor agonists are likely to have little effect on eosinophil function in chronic inflammation. Clearly more data are required before β-adrenoceptor agonists are attributed "anti-eosinophilic" properties. The effect of β-adrenoceptor agonists on pulmonary recruitment and the activation status of eosinophils following acute exacerbations in asthma is not known. Furthermore, the effect of β-adrenoceptor agonists on the expression of adhesion molecules on endothelial cells and eosinophils warrants investigation.

Macrophages

Human alveolar macrophages may play a role in asthma, as they contain low-affinity IgE receptors (171). The role of β-adrenoceptors in human alveolar macrophages is controversial. Radioligand-binding studies indicate that a small population of β_2-adrenoceptors reside on human alveolar macrophages (172). Activation of these receptors result in a two- to sixfold (172,173) increase in cAMP. However, the presence of contaminating cells may be responsible for the elevation in cAMP (173). Furthermore, isoprenaline and salbutamol failed to inhibit zymosan- or IgE-induced release of mediators or superoxide anions by human alveolar macrophages (173,174). More recently it was shown that salmeterol inhibited the release of thromboxane from human alveolar macrophages (175). However, large concentrations of salmeterol were used and the inhibitory effect was propranolol-insensitive. Hence, convincing evidence for an effect of β-adrenoceptor agonists in modulating mediator release by macrophages in asthma is lacking.

Lymphocytes

There is increasing evidence that lymphocytes play an important role in asthma (153,154). Human lymphocytes contain β-adrenoceptors that are coupled to adenylate cyclase and are susceptible to β-adrenoceptor desensitization (176–178). The role of β-adrenoceptors on lymphocytes is not known, although β-adrenoceptor stimulation inhibits lymphocyte proliferation, cytokine generation, expression of cytokine receptors, and antibody production *in vitro* (179,180). In asthma, lymphocyte β-adrenoceptor density and function are reduced as a consequence of disease (181–183) and following regular treatment with β-adrenoceptor agonists (176–178). The consequences of these changes in asthma are not known.

Lymphocytes are a heterogeneous population of cells including B and T cells. The latter group may be further subdivided into T-helper (CD4+), T-suppressor/cytotoxic (CD8+), and natural killer (NKA) cells (153,154). Radioligand binding studies demonstrate that B cells contain a large number of β-adrenoceptors that are poorly coupled to adenylate cyclase. In contrast, T-cell subsets possess β-adrenoceptors that are functionally linked to adenylate cyclase (184). In healthy individuals, 7-day treatment with terbutaline (500 μg, t.i.d) resulted in a greater reduction in cell number, β-adrenoceptor density, and adenylate cyclase activity in circulating CD8+ than CD4+ cells, and an increase in the CD4+/CD8+ ratio (184,185). These data suggest that there is differential regulation of T-cell subsets following β-adrenoceptor stimulation. Hence, the antiproliferative potential of β-adrenoceptor agonists demonstrated *in vivo* appears to be less in CD4+ than in CD8+ T-cells (186). These changes observed following β-adrenoceptor agonist therapy is interesting given that an increase in CD4+ cells with a concomitant reduction in CD8+ cells is thought to participate in the exacerbation of asthma (153,154). The effect of regular treatment with β-adrenoceptor agonists on T-cell activation, cytokine generation, and the immune response in asthma is not known. Recently, it was demonstrated that following 6-week regular treatment with salmeterol compared with placebo, there was no change in the percentage of CD4+ and CD8+ cells, as assessed by flow cytometric analysis of bronchoalveolar lavage fluid (187).

Neutrophils

A role for neutrophils in the pathophysiology of asthma appears to be less likely as illustrated by studies showing no difference in the number of neutrophils in bronchial biopsies between atopic asthmatics and healthy individuals (188–191). Nonetheless, human neutrophils possess β$_2$-adrenoceptors (192) that are linked to adenylate cyclase (193–195). β-Adrenoceptor agonists inhibit the release of lysosomal β-glucuronidase and inhibit the generation of superoxide anions and inflammatory mediators from human neutrophils activated by zymosan-treated serum and by calcium ionophore A23187 (195–197).

BENEFICIAL CLINICAL EFFECTS OF β-ADRENOCEPTOR AGONISTS

Acute Bronchospasm

Acute administration of β-adrenoceptor agonists in patients with asthma results in a significant loss in airway sensitivity to spasmogens. The β-adrenoceptor agonist-induced reduction in airway sensitivity to histamine is both dose- (48,69,198,199) and time-dependent (48,49,69) with no change in the slope of the spasmogen dose-response curve (48,69,103,200). In contrast, some studies have shown an increase in the slope of the histamine dose-response curve following inhalation of β-adrenoceptor agonist (199,201). In susceptible individuals, β-adrenoceptor agonists also afford protection against bronchospasm induced by a wide range of provocative stimuli including allergen (119,121,176,202,203), eucapnic and isocapnic hyperventilation (71,72,204), exercise (126,205,206), and hypo-osmolar (207) and hyperosmolar stimuli (208).

Both salmeterol and formoterol can reduce bronchial responsiveness to histamine and methacholine, respectively (49,57,58,59). Similarly, the longer-acting β-adrenoceptor agonists including salmeterol and formoterol are efficacious as inhibitors of allergen- (57,58), cold air hyperventilation- (77), and exercise-induced bronchospasm (70,75,76). This antagonism persists well after the effects of shorter-acting β-adrenoceptor agonists have resolved. This is most likely a reflection of the increased retention of salmeterol and formoterol within the lung compared with salbutamol (50,51,64).

A number of studies have shown that there is apparently no direct relationship between the ability of β-adrenoceptor agonists to induce a fall in baseline FEV_1 and their ability to reduce the potency of bronchoconstrictor agents (69,103,199,209–211). However, the inability to obtain a direct relationship might be attributed to the use of maximal bronchodilator doses of β-adrenoceptor agonist (69,199). In a recent study, a direct relationship between reduction in baseline FEV_1 and the decrease in spasmogen potency was found when submaximal doses of β-adrenoceptor agonist was used (198). However, the muscarinic receptor antagonist ipratropium bromide failed to alter airway sensitivity to histamine despite causing a fall in baseline FEV_1 (198). These studies, together with the demonstration of a difference in the effectiveness of β-adrenoceptor agonists against changes in FEV_1 and spasmogen potency in time course studies (48,69), illustrate that bronchodilation per se is not necessary for the changes in spasmogen-induced reactivity. It is therefore the ability of β-adrenoceptor agonists to functionally antagonize the response to spasmogens that is important.

Late Asthmatic Response

Clinical Studies

A characteristic feature of some asthmatics is the development of a late phase airway obstruction 4 to 10 h following exposure to allergen. This phenomenon, which can be modeled under controlled laboratory conditions, is associated with pulmonary recruitment of eosinophils (212) and increased bronchial responsiveness to spasmogens (202). β-Adrenoceptor agonists do not inhibit the development of the allergen-induced late asthmatic response (202,213). In contrast, glucocorticosteroids, disodium cromoglycate (202), theophylline (214,215), and the sulfidopeptide leukotriene receptor antagonist ICI 204.219 (216) inhibit the development of the late asthmatic response via mechanisms unrelated to bronchodilation. Due to the relatively short duration of action of the current β-adrenoceptor agonists, it is generally assumed that β-adrenoceptor agonists, while providing symptomatic relief, have minimal effect on the underlying inflammatory process (217,218). However, a number of recent studies have shown that β-adrenoceptor agonists can attenuate the late asthmatic response. Both fenoterol and salbutamol were shown to reverse the fall in baseline FEV_1 during the late asthmatic response to house dust mite or occupational sensitizing agents (219,220). This appears most likely to be due to a direct action on bronchial smooth muscle (219,220). The duration of this effect was not assessed.

The failure of salbutamol to attenuate the late asthmatic response (202) could be attributed to the use of doses of salbutamol that were too low, since duration of action is dose-dependent (62). Inhalation of high-dose nebulized terbutaline (5 mg) (221) and salbutamol (2.5 mg) (222) or a high-dose salbutamol by MDI (500 μg) (223) prior to allergen challenge appears to attenuate the development of the late asthmatic response. More recently it has been shown that at clinically relevant doses both salmeterol (58) and formoterol (57,223) inhibit the late asthmatic response when given prior to allergen inhalation. It has been suggested that the attenuation of the late response by high-dose salbutamol and salmeterol is due to a putative anti-inflammatory effect based on the diminished bronchodilator activity of β-adrenoceptor agonists at the time of the late response (58,222). However, these data only provide circumstantial evidence of anti-inflammatory activity, since the effect of β-adrenoceptor agonists on the recruitment of inflammatory cells, notably lymphocytes and eosinophils, was not assessed during the late response. An alternative explanation of the data is that β-adrenoceptor agonists mask the expression of the late response due to functional antagonism of the allergen-induced changes in FEV_1 (57,224).

Only a few studies have investigated the effect of β-adrenoceptor agonists on the cutaneous late response. In atopic patients, the cutaneous late phase response is characterized by an influx of inflammatory cells, including $CD4^+$ T lymphocytes and activated eosinophils (153,225,226). Intradermal injection of terbutaline was shown to either inhibit (147) or to have no effect (227) against allergen-induced infiltration of eosinophils. The discrepancy between these studies may be a consequence of the use of a tenfold higher concentration of allergen in the latter study. Similarly, repeated injections of terbutaline or a single injection of formoterol attenuated the late cutaneous response, as assessed by changes in wheal volume (149). The effect on inflammatory cells was not assessed. Given the ineffectiveness of β-adrenoceptor agonists on eosinophil function per se, it has been suggested that the inhibition of cellular recruitment at sites of inflammation by β-adrenoceptor agonists might be attributable to reducing gap junction formation (149,228). Indeed, various vasoactive amines, including histamine, increase polymorphonuclear cell diapedesis across arterial endothelial cells, while noradrenaline decreased polymorphonuclear leukocyte diapedesis by a propranolol-sensitive mechanism (229). However, whether β-adrenoceptor agonists can influence inflammatory cell recruitment in this way is controversial, given that inflammatory cell diapedesis and edema occur via different mechanisms (135,230,231). Furthermore, salmeterol at doses that attenuated zymosan-induced plasma protein extravasation by 50%, had no effect on neutrophil accumulation at skin sites (141).

Animal Studies

In experimental animals, exposure to PAF resulted in increased airway responsiveness to spasmogens and pulmonary recruitment of inflammatory cells, features that are characteristic of asthma (232). The β-adrenoceptor agonist isoprenaline failed to inhibit PAF-induced pulmonary recruitment of inflammatory cells and bronchial hyperresponsiveness (233,234). Similarly, salbutamol failed to inhibit PAF-induced pulmonary eosinophilia in guinea pigs (141). In contrast, disodium cromoglycate, ketotifen, glucocorticosteroid, and theophylline effectively inhibited PAF-induced bronchial hyperresponsiveness and pulmonary recruitment of inflammatory cells (233,234). However, salmeterol, but not salbutamol, was shown to attenuate both PAF-(141) and allergen- (235) induced pulmonary eosinophilia in guinea pigs, an effect that was sensitive to β-adrenoceptor blockade. In contrast, both salmeterol and formoterol were ineffective against allergen-induced pulmonary eosinophilia (236). The discrepancy in the results from these animal studies might be attributable to the use of different allergen concentrations.

Bronchial Hyperresponsiveness

The allergen-induced increase in airway responsiveness that commonly accompanies the late response is not modified by inhaled salbutamol. In contrast, both glucocorticosteroids and disodium cromoglycate attenuate the increase in airway responsiveness (202). These data suggest that β-adrenoceptor agonists fail to modify the underlying inflammatory process presumably responsible for the exacerbation of bronchial hyperresponsiveness. However, inhalation of nebulized salbutamol (2.5 mg) significantly attenuated the allergen-induced increase in airway responsiveness to histamine over a 3.5- to 7.5-h period (222). Similarly, salmeterol and formoterol have both been demonstrated to attenuate the allergen-induced exacerbation of bronchial hyperresponsiveness observed during and 24 to 32 h following inhalation of allergen (57,58). However, contradictory conclusions have been drawn from these studies. The inhibitory effect of high-dose salbutamol (222) and salmeterol (58) on exacerbation of bronchial hyperresponsiveness was attributed to the possible anti-inflammatory properties of β-adrenoceptor agonists. This conclusion was based on the fact that the bronchodilator effect of high-dose salbutamol during the late asthmatic response and of salmeterol 32 h after allergen inhalation was minimal (58). In contrast, the beneficial effect afforded by formoterol at 24 h could be explained in terms of functional antagonism of the changes in airway tone (57).

In studies where dose-response curves to spasmogens have been completed, such curves generated in asthmatics tend to be positioned to the left and describe an increased maximum response compared with healthy individuals (237,238). The excessive airway narrowing observed in asthma, which is reflected by an increase in the maximum response to spasmogens, is a consequence of the inflammatory process (238). It is therefore of interest that 4-week regular treatment with budesonide in mild asthmatics resulted in a small decrease in airway sensitivity to methacholine, but more importantly was associated with a significant reduction in the level of maximal airway narrowing (239). In contrast, 8-week regular treatment with salmeterol caused a substantial decrease in airway sensitivity to methacholine, but had no effect on the level of maximal airway narrowing (240). These data also suggest that salmeterol lacks anti-inflammatory activity and illustrate the effectiveness of glucocorticosteroids in this regard.

Nocturnal Asthma

In normal individuals lung function varies in a circadian rhythm with slight bronchoconstriction occurring during the night. This is significantly exaggerated in most asthmatics (241–243). Most patients are awoken at least occasionally by nocturnal wheeze and cough (244), the frequency increasing in more severe asthma. It has been demonstrated that clinically stable patients with nocturnal asthma become hypoxemic during the night (245,246) and have poorer daytime cognitive performance and poorer subjective and objective sleep quality than normal subjects (247). A decrement in sleep quality leads to muscle fatigue, and hypoxemia can develop during bronchoconstriction. These events can be fatal in patients with severe acute exacerbations (242).

A number of mechanisms have been proposed to account for nocturnal wheezing (242,243). Both sleep and nocturnal bronchoconstriction are often in phase (248) and nocturnal bronchoconstriction is triggered by different stages of sleep (249). However, significant bronchoconstriction can still be observed in asthmatics kept awake during the night (250,251). Hence, the role of sleep per se in the pathogenesis of nocturnal asthma is not understood. Posture does not appear to be important (252), while the diurnal variation in plasma adrenaline and cortisol levels (253) have been suggested as important trigger factors. More recent data suggest that neither plasma corticosteroid (254) nor adrenaline levels (255) influence nocturnal wheeze. However, vagal activity is increased during the night and the fall in lung function is attenuated by muscarinic antagonists (256–258). The possible role of the inhibitory, nonadrenergic, noncholinergic nervous system in nocturnal asthma has also been suggested (259). Furthermore, the role of platelet activation in nocturnal asthma requires further investigation (260). Together these studies indicate that a number of trigger factors exist that are influenced by circadian rhythm. These factors impinge on the existing baseline airway reactivity and induce an exaggerated bronchoconstriction. Hence, treatment of the underlying disease will effectively reduce nocturnal asthma (241–243).

The exaggerated bronchoconstriction observed in nocturnal asthma can be attenuated by β_2-adrenoceptor agonists, ipratropium bromide (242), theophylline (243,261), glucocorticosteroids (262), and the potassium channel activator, cromakalim (263). However, the choice of drug is determined by the patients ability to tolerate side effects. The efficacy of β_2-adrenoceptor agonists is dependent on the duration of action of these drugs. Slow release (264) and maintenance salbutamol (261) were not entirely effective against nocturnal asthma, presumably due to a decline in clinically effective levels of salbutamol in the airways. In contrast, oral terbutaline significantly protected asthmatics against nocturnal asthma (265–267), which was associated with a marginal reduction in nocturnal inhaler use (265,266). Comparisons between different bronchodilators is futile unless equieffective doses are used. However, the protective effect of terbutaline was associated with no improvement in the quality of sleep, as assessed by electroencephalography (266). These studies demonstrate that protection against nocturnal asthma can be afforded if high concentrations of β-adrenoceptor agonist are tolerated. However, the effect on sleep quality requires further study.

Formoterol provided significant protection against nocturnal bronchoconstriction following a single inhalation (268) and significantly reduced the frequency of sleep disturbances during 1-month (269) and 3-month treatment periods (270). Similarly, 2-week treatment with salmeterol provided better subjective sleep quality than treatment with salbutamol in asthmatics without nocturnal asthma (271). It was also shown that treatment with salmeterol for 1 week provided significant protection against the fall in lung function during the night and improved objective sleep quality (272), although the latter effect has been disputed (273). These studies indicate that symptoms of nocturnal asthma may be reduced with long-acting bronchodilator drugs.

Since nocturnal asthma can be exacerbated following exposure to allergens, therapy designed to inhibit the inflammatory response is more desirable (241–253). The role of long-acting β-adrenoceptors in this regard remains controversial.

CHRONIC β-ADRENOCEPTOR AGONIST THERAPY

With the finding that asthma mortality and morbidity are increasing, the question of whether this is a consequence of the increased use of β_2-adrenoceptor agonists has been raised (274). This hypothesis is highly controversial, yet few studies have investigated the effect of long-term treatment with β-adrenoceptor agonists in asthma.

Tolerance

Baseline FEV₁

The clinical response to inhaled β-adrenoceptor agonists has been shown to diminish as the severity of the disease increases (275). A number of factors may account for this, including reduced penetration of β-adrenoceptor agonist to the airways as lung function deteriorates (36), the increasing influence of inflammation and mucus plugging in affecting airway caliber, which is not modified by β-adrenoceptor agonist (275), and loss of bronchodilator function due to increased severity of bronchospasm (275). Alternatively, prolonged use of β-adrenoceptor agonist therapy results in β-adrenoceptor down-regulation (276). Subsequently it was demonstrated that healthy individuals continually exposed to β-adrenoceptor agonists become refractory to β-adrenoceptor stimulation (277,278). In contrast, asthmatic individuals chronically treated with salbutamol (91,176,278,279), terbutaline (280), or the long-acting β-adrenoceptor agonists formoterol (269,281) and salmeterol (240,271) do not develop tolerance to the bronchodilator activity of these agonists as assessed by measurements of changes in FEV_1 and airways conductance. Interestingly, β-adrenoceptor desensitization was observed in leukocytes taken from asthmatics following regular β-adrenoceptor agonist therapy (176). Thus, asthmatics are resistant to desensitization possibly because there is a relatively large population of "spare" β-adrenoceptors in airway smooth muscle. This contrasts with responses mediated via "extrapulmonary" β-adrenoceptors for which tolerance can be demonstrated in asthmatics (91,176,280).

Bronchospasm

Some studies have assessed the effect of regular β-adrenoceptor agonist therapy on the protection afforded by β-adrenoceptor agonists against bronchospasm. A slight reduction in the effectiveness of β-adrenoceptor agonists to protect against exercise- (282) and allergen-induced bronchospasm (176), with a loss in the ability of β-adrenoceptor agonists to protect against histamine-induced bronchospasm, was observed in asthmatics treated regularly with β-adrenoceptor agonist (283,284). This latter finding was not confirmed by others (176,278,279). Similarly, it has recently been demonstrated that the extent of protection afforded by salmeterol against methacholine-induced bronchospasm was reduced after 4 to 8 weeks of regular treatment (240). In contrast, no development of tolerance to the bronchodilator effects of salmeterol was observed (240). Since the loss of protection afforded by β-adrenoceptor agonists is manifested under conditions of elevated basal tone, asthmatics might be susceptible to β-adrenoceptor desensitization during regular β-adrenoceptor agonist therapy. Alternatively, the loss in protection against bronchospastic stimuli following regular β-adrenoceptor agonist therapy might be a consequence of the inability of β-adrenoceptor agonists to control the inflammatory process (285).

Bronchial Hyperresponsiveness

The apparent lack of protection afforded by regular β-adrenoceptor agonist therapy against bronchospastic stimuli was investigated further in studies assessing the effect of long-term treatment with β-adrenoceptor agonists on bronchial hyperresponsiveness. No change in bronchial responsiveness was seen following regular 4-week treatment with salbutamol (100–500 μg, q.i.d.) (278,279) or terbutaline (300 μg, t.i.d.) (176) and following regular 2-year treatment with terbutaline (375 μg, b.i.d.) (286). In contrast, regular administration of terbutaline (750 μg, t.i.d.) for 2 weeks followed by cessation of administration for 23 h resulted in a rebound increase in bronchial responsiveness to histamine (284). This effect was attributed to β-adrenoceptor agonist-induced desensitization, which was not sufficient to reduce the response to inhaled β-adrenoceptor agonists. However, it was sufficient to reduce the protective effect of endogenous catecholamines in the lung and thus cause rebound bronchial hyperresponsiveness (284). In other chronic studies, a small increase in bronchial responsiveness was observed following regular 2-week (500 μg, q.i.d.) (165) and 6-month treatment with terbutaline (500 μg, q.i.d.) (287) and regular 2-month treatment with fenoterol (200 μg, t.i.d.) (288). Similarly, a small increase in airway responsiveness to histamine was observed following regular 1-year treatment with salbutamol (400 μg, q.i.d.) (285). It is interesting to note that the small increase in bronchial hyperresponsiveness to histamine was not attributable to β-adrenoceptor desensitization (as reflected by changes in baseline lung function to salbutamol) and was not observed following regular treatment with ipratropium bromide (285).

The effect of regular treatment with β-adrenoceptor agonists on bronchial hyperresponsiveness is conflicting, possibly due to patient selection, number, and/or the doses of β-adrenoceptor agonist used. One criticism of some of these studies is the absence of a control group and the clinical significance of these small changes. The increase in bronchial hyperresponsiveness following regular β-adrenoceptor agonist treatment might simply reflect a deterioration of the disease over time. Interestingly, bronchial hyperresponsiveness to histamine was significantly reduced when the same patients (166,289) or a parallel group of patients (286,287) were treated with glucocorticosteroid. Furthermore, the changes in bronchial hyperresponsiveness in response to glucocorticosteroids were of similar magnitude to those observed for β-adrenoceptor agonists but in the opposite direction (165, 287,289). These changes produced by glucocorticosteroids have often been used to argue the beneficial anti-inflammatory nature of this class of drug (218).

The magnitude of the changes in bronchial hyperresponsiveness produced by regular treatment with β-adrenoceptor agonists is small, ranging from 0.6 to 1.5 doubling dose of spasmogen (165,284,286–288). The clinical significance of these small changes is not known, although it is of a similar order to that observed during the pollen season, which is also associated with exacerbation of symptoms (290,291). Furthermore, a small change in bronchial hyperresponsiveness in the population may significantly increase the proportion of patients with severe asthma (292).

Regular β-adrenoceptor agonist therapy may increase or not affect bronchial hyperresponsiveness, although a deterioration in lung function (293) and an increase in asthma symptoms (286) is observed. In contrast, regular treatment with glucocorticosteroids not only significantly improves bronchial hyperresponsiveness but also improves lung function and reduces symptoms (286,289). Together these studies indicate that, unlike glucocorticosteroids, regular treatment with β-adrenoceptor agonists fails to control the disease.

Regular Versus Symptomatic Therapy

Regular 2-week treatment with inhaled salbutamol provided better control of asthma than symptomatic use of salbutamol (294). However, closer examination of the results demonstrates that for a similar degree of control of asthma symptoms, the total aerosol consumption per day was 10.8 and 5.7 puffs in the prophylactic and intermittent group, respectively. These findings indicate that there was no advantage in taking regular salbutamol over symptomatic use. Similarly, better control of symptoms and lung function was apparently observed in asthmatics taking salbutamol regularly compared with the symptomatic use of salbutamol for 1 year, although none of the data was analyzed statistically (295). However, the apparent beneficial effect afforded with regular treatment with salbutamol was at the expense of more bronchodilator: 5.0 and 1.7 doses of salbutamol in the prophylactic and the symptomatic group, respectively. Furthermore, the FEV_1 values in the intermittent group tended to fall, together with an increase in the consumption of rescue β-adrenoceptor agonist medication, when this group of patients were crossed over to regular bronchodilator use. Conversely, the regularly treated group demonstrated improved FEV_1 with less consumption of β-adrenoceptor agonist when crossed over to the intermittent arm of the experiment (295). Finally, a recent study demonstrated that in patients treated with theophylline, regular but not symptomatic administration of terbutaline significantly improved asthma symptoms and pulmonary function in asthmatics (296), an effect that was not confirmed by others (261). Neither study was designed to compare the relative effectiveness of regular and symptomatic β-adrenoceptor agonist therapy. The difference in the two studies may be due to patient selection, differences in protocols, or the use of different β-adrenoceptor agonists.

A number of studies have demonstrated that regular β-adrenoceptor therapy is no better or worse than symptomatic treatment. No significant difference in symptoms was observed in asthmatics taking regular or symptomatic salbutamol for 2 weeks (297) or 1 month (298). However, to achieve comparable control of symptoms and lung function, less bronchodilator was consumed when asthmatics were taking salbutamol symptomatically rather than regularly (297,298). More recently, the effect of 6-month dry-powder inhaled fenoterol taken either regularly (200 µg, q.i.d.) or symptomatically in a double-blind, placebo-controlled, randomized crossover study was investigated. It was shown that asthmatics taking prophylactic compared with symptomatic β-adrenoceptor agonist treatment had improved daytime measurements of lung function. However, this was at the expense of poorer control of their asthma as assessed by a number of variables and a 3.4-fold increase in total daily bronchodilator use (299). More importantly, these findings were also observed in asthmatics who were taking glucocorticosteroid or disodium cromoglycate and bronchial hyperresponsiveness was higher in 34% of the patients taking regular compared with symptomatic fenoterol (299). A criticism of this study is the absence of quantitative data. All comparisons are in terms of the percent of patients showing better control during each of the two treatment arms. No indication of the magnitude of the differences or their possible clinical significance is made. Furthermore, it has been suggested that since the patients in the study did not require frequent β-adrenoceptor agonist medication at the start of the trial, these patients would be susceptible to β-adrenoceptor agonist-induced desensitization, which might account for the observed results (300). However, this seems unlikely given that a deterioration in asthma was observed following regular treatment with terbutaline for 2 years, in the absence of β-adrenoceptor desensitization (286).

In a further study comparing regular and symptomatic use of bronchodilators, a three to four times greater annual decline in FEV_1 was observed in asthmatics treated regularly than in patients treated on demand with salbutamol (400 µg, q.i.d.) for 2 years (293). Interestingly, the perception of quality of life and the number and duration of exacerbations was similar in the two groups of patients, despite the fall in FEV_1. This suggests that patients taking regular β-adrenoceptor agonist treatment may be unaware of a true deterioration of disease (293). A similar finding was observed with ipratropium bromide, suggesting that the decline in FEV_1 is a feature common to bronchodilators. Interestingly, patients preferred salbutamol treatment, indicating that β-adrenoceptor agonists are better at masking a deterioration in asthma (293).

In contrast to the poor clinical efficacy of regular short-acting β-adrenoceptor agonists in asthma observed in chronic studies, it has been demonstrated that regular treatment with salmeterol for 4 weeks (12.5, 50, 100 μg, b.i.d.) (301) and regular 3-month (12 μg, b.i.d.) (302) or 12-month (12 μg, b.i.d.) (281) treatment with formoterol results in greater increases in spirometry and/or peak flow than placebo or salbutamol. Asthma symptoms were reduced (301) and the number of episodes of asthma and sleep disruption were less with formoterol than with salbutamol (302). The question of whether persistent functional antagonism of airway bronchoconstriction masks the disease process has not been resolved with these studies.

More crossover-designed studies comparing regular with symptomatic β-adrenoceptor agonist therapy with large sample sizes are needed to answer the question of whether regular β-adrenoceptor therapy is detrimental to disease. The obvious symptomatic beneficial effect of β-adrenoceptor agonists may be accompanied by a worsening of symptoms when these agents are taken regularly over a long period of time, as a result of a failure to treat the inflammatory process in asthma. It is therefore prudent to consider β-adrenoceptor agonists for symptomatic use and the early introduction of anti-inflammatory drugs such as glucocorticosteroids, xanthines, and disodium cromoglycate in the treatment of asthma.

Asthma Deaths

Case Control Studies

During the 1960s an increase in asthma mortality was correlated with the consumption of isoprenaline. An overreliance on the use of isoprenaline contributing to a delay in the use of glucocorticosteroids has been suggested as a possible cause (78,79). A similar rise in asthma deaths was also observed during the 1970s in New Zealand, which was correlated with the sale of fenoterol (303,304). A number of explanations were forwarded to account for the deaths, including the combined use of β-adrenoceptor agonists and theophylline replacing inhaled glucocorticosteroid and disodium cromoglycate (305), overreliance on domiciliary nebulizers (306,307), underestimation of the severity of the disease, poor compliance, and the number but not the choice of drugs used (308–310). A large case-control study was performed to determine the contribution of drug therapy in asthma deaths in New Zealand. It was subsequently demonstrated that in 117 fatal cases of asthma, there was a 1.55-fold increased risk of death in patients taking fenoterol by MDI (304). Patients taking salbutamol by MDI, corticosteroids, or theophylline were not at risk of death in any of these groups of patients. Further analysis of subgroups defining markers of asthma severity revealed that the risk of death in patients prescribed fenoterol was twofold higher in patients taking drugs in three or more categories of asthma therapy or with a previous hospital admission. Furthermore, the association between risk of death and the use of fenoterol was 6- or 13-fold higher in patients prescribed oral corticosteroid alone or together with a recent hospital admission, respectively (304). The authors suggested that the use of fenoterol by MDI in severe asthma increased the risk of death. However, the nature of the experimental design raises a number of criticisms. These include the inappropriate use of controls from a less severe patient category, the inability to determine which bronchodilator drug was used near or at death and the use of markers of asthma for chronic rather than for severe acute illness (311–313). An alternative conclusion from this study is that fenoterol is prescribed for patients with severe asthma and thus is a marker of disease severity (311–313). To answer these criticisms, another case-control study was performed in which information relating to drug prescription was obtained from prior hospital admission for both cases and controls, and the severity of controls and cases were more closely matched. As with the previous study, there was a twofold increase in the risk of death in patients prescribed fenoterol. The risk factor was increased by six- or tenfold in patients taking fenoterol and who were also prescribed oral corticosteroid or together with a recent hospital admission, respectively (314). Interestingly, in contrast to their previous study (304), oral corticosteroids and theophylline (prescribed at discharge) were associated with an increased risk of death in some subgroups defined by markers of asthma severity. However, when the influence of fenoterol was removed from the analysis, the increased risk of death in patients prescribed these drugs was also removed in these subgroups. A further case-control study assessing different methods of matching cases and controls also showed that severe asthmatics taking fenoterol were at a greater risk of death (315).

Similar findings were reported recently in a large case-control study in Canada. The use of inhaled fenoterol and salbutamol, and oral but not inhaled corticosteroids and theophylline, was also associated with an increased risk of death and near-death from asthma (316). In this study it was demonstrated that case patients tended to have more severe asthma than the controls. On this basis alone, the data would suggest that β-adrenoceptor agonists are not a risk factor and that the extent of their use is more likely to be a marker of severity. However, when the data were adjusted for exposure to other anti-asthma drugs and the number of hospitalizations, the use of fenoterol and salbutamol was associated with increased risk in morbidity and mortality. In contrast, following adjustment, oral corticosteroids were confined to a small increased risk in morbidity (316). An interesting finding from this study was that on a microgram equivalent basis, the risk factor for asthma death was similar for both fenoterol and salbutamol (316).

Together these studies demonstrate an association between the regular consumption of β-adrenoceptor agonists and risk of death in asthma. Because of the design of these studies it is difficult to determine whether there is a causal relationship between β-adrenoceptor agonist consumption and increased asthma mortality/morbidity. However, it does seem reasonable to suggest that the sole reliance on β-adrenoceptor agonist therapy may delay the introduction of anti-inflammatory drugs, which might place patients at risk. The suggestion that β-adrenoceptor agonists per se are responsible for placing patients at risk is highly controversial, and without the proper experimental design the issue will be difficult to resolve.

Mechanisms

A number of mechanism(s) by which β-adrenoceptor agonists could lead to a worsening of asthma have been proposed. It has been hypothesized that β-adrenoceptor agonists may increase the penetration of allergen into the airways by virtue of their ability to dilate the airways (299,317). However, bronchodilation induced by ipratropium bromide was not associated with an increase in airway hyperresponsiveness in asthmatics (285). Thus, it is more likely that individuals taking β-adrenoceptor agonists are able to tolerate greater antigen loads and/or remain exposed to low levels of allergen for greater periods (119,203,299,317), which may lead to an exacerbation of asthma (203). The effect of regular treatment with β-adrenoceptor agonists on the ability of asthmatics to tolerate environments that contain sensitizing agents and, moreover, whether this leads to increased penetration and/or concentration of sensitizing agents within the lung, are yet to be established.

It has also been suggested that mast cell degranulation is a normal defense mechanism. The release of bronchospastic mediators following antigen challenge, may limit the further penetration of allergen down the bronchial tree. Furthermore, mast cells release heparin, a molecule that possesses anti-inflammatory properties. Inhibition of this normal defense mechanism by β-adrenoceptor agonists may contribute to the detrimental effects associated with β-adrenoceptor agonist therapy, as this interferes with the normal defense and repair mechanisms of the lung (318).

In animal studies, it has been demonstrated that the intravenous administration of (±) isoprenaline can induce nerve-mediated bronchial hyperresponsiveness to histamine in guinea pigs (319). Furthermore, this effect is observed with the dextro isomer of isoprenaline and is propranolol-insensitive. It has subsequently been suggested that the dextro isomer present in racemic mixtures of the currently used β-adrenoceptor agonists may be harmful in asthma (317,320). This is supported by data showing that intra-tracheal administration of dextro isomers of β-adrenoceptor agonists is associated with increased bronchial responsiveness to histamine in guinea pigs (320). This hypothesis is of particular interest, since toxic effects of various molecules including thalidomide and penicillamine reside specifically with particular enantiomers of these drugs (321). The extent to which the dextro isomers of β-adrenoceptor agonists have detrimental effects in asthma is not known.

ADVERSE SIDE EFFECTS WITH THERAPEUTIC DOSES

Skeletal Muscle Tremor

Activation of β_2-adrenoceptors in skeletal muscle results in tremor (79). Thus, skeletal muscle tremor is the most common immediate adverse reaction to the β_2-adrenoceptor agonists. However, tolerance usually develops following chronic β_2-adrenoceptor therapy (91,280,322).

Cardiovascular System

When given by inhalation at therapeutic doses, the incidence of tachycardia is minimized (80). In contrast, when given by the systemic route, significant changes in heart rate and blood pressure can be observed (25). Furthermore, high inhaled doses of β_2-adrenoceptor agonists can also lead to a dose-dependent increase in heart rate and fall in diastolic blood pressure (86,90,91). Tolerance develops to the changes in heart rate following chronic therapy (91). Untoward cardiovascular effects are more likely to be manifested in patients with serious cardiac problems (322).

Metabolic Changes

Hypokalemia

Hypokalemia is observed following inhaled and systemic administration of β_2-adrenoceptor agonists (322). The change in plasma concentration of potassium ions is minimal in response to normal therapeutic doses, although a dose-dependent decrease in the plasma level of potassium ions is observed with increasing dose of β_2-adrenoceptor agonists (90). Hypokalemia is mediated by β_2-adrenoceptor–induced uptake of potassium ions in skeletal muscle (31,323,324). Tolerance to this effect is observed following chronic therapy (91). The effect of lowering plasma potassium ions and cardiac stimulation may become significant in patients with heart disease (322).

Glyconeolysis

β$_2$-Adrenoceptor activation also can result in glyconeolysis (325). Ketoacidosis may occur in diabetic patients prescribed β$_2$-adrenoceptor agonists, which depends on the degree of tolerance that has developed to the metabolic effects of β$_2$-adrenoceptor agonists (322).

Lipolysis

β$_2$-Adrenoceptor agonists mobilize free fatty acids from adipose tissue, a response mediated via β$_1$-adrenoceptors (80). These changes are relevant in asthmatics who are diabetic (322).

Arterial Oxygen Tension

β$_2$-Adrenoceptor agonists may reduce arterial oxygen tension as a consequence of ventilation/perfusion mismatching (326). Such effects may present problems in individuals who are severely hypoxemic to begin with and who may therefore require oxygen supplementation (322).

CONCLUSION

β-Adrenoceptor agonists provide effective bronchodilator relief in asthmatics undergoing acute bronchospasm. Thus, they are the drug of choice in the symptomatic relief of asthma. Their major influence is the functional antagonism of spasmogen-induced contraction of airway smooth muscle. However, because β-adrenoceptors are widely distributed throughout the lung, the beneficial therapeutic effect of β-adrenoceptor agonists may also be mediated at sites other than airway smooth muscle, including mast cells and endothelial cells. The effect of β-adrenoceptor agonists on mast cells and endothelial cells has been cited by many authors as evidence for an acute anti-inflammatory property. However, evidence for anti-inflammatory activity in chronic inflammation is lacking.

More recently, β-adrenoceptor agonists, including salmeterol and formoterol, have been developed that provide significantly longer protection against bronchospasm than currently available shorter-acting β-adrenoceptor agonists. In particular, these drugs offer significant protection in nocturnal asthma. Some studies have suggested that long-acting β-adrenoceptor agonists possess acute anti-inflammatory properties. However, evidence for such an effect is controversial and no evidence for an anti-inflammatory effect in chronic asthma has been documented.

Considerable controversy has been raised concerning the regular use of β-adrenoceptor agonists in asthma and the possibility that the regular consumption of these drugs may place patients at risk. Although a causal relationship has not been established, a number of studies have observed an association between regular β-adrenoceptor agonist consumption and increased asthma mortality/morbidity. More controlled studies are required to clearly establish such a relationship. However, it is clear that relying solely on β-adrenoceptor agonist therapy alone, which provides excellent symptomatic relief, can result in patients perceiving that their asthma is improving, when in reality the delay in their receiving anti-inflammatory medication may place them at risk.

It would seem prudent to suggest that in patients with mild to moderate asthma, β-adrenoceptor agonists should be used only for symptomatic relief. The role of β-adrenoceptor agonists in chronic severe asthma is more controversial. Given that no randomized placebo controlled study has been performed that investigates the effect of regular β-adrenoceptor agonist treatment with this group of patients, the suggestion from case controlled studies of the possible risk factors posed by β-adrenoceptor agonist treatment should be tempered. However, what these studies do clearly suggest is that in this group of patients, it is imperative that therapeutic strategies should be directed to the more frequent and early use of anti-inflammatory drugs, with β-adrenoceptor agonists taken as needed.

ACKNOWLEDGMENTS

This work was supported by the National Health and Medical Research Council of Australia.

REFERENCES

1. Kerribijn KF. Beta agonists. In: Kaliner MA, Barnes PJ, Persson CGA, eds. *Asthma: its pathology and treatment,* vol 49. New York: Marcel Dekker, 1991;523–559.
2. Goldie RG, Paterson JW, Lulich KM. Pharmacology and therapeutics of β-adrenoceptor agonists. In: Page CP, Barnes PJ, eds. *Pharmacology of asthma.* Berlin: Springer-Verlag, 1991;167–205.
3. Reed CE. Beta agonists. Adrenergic bronchodilators: pharmacology and toxicology. *J Allergy Clin Immunol* 1985;76:335–341.
4. George CF, Blackwell EW, Davis DS. Metabolism of isoprenaline in the intestine. *J Pharm Pharmacol* 1974;26:265–267.
5. Davies DS. Pharmacokinetics of inhaled substances. *Postgrad Med J* 1975;51(suppl 7):69–75.
6. Blackwell EW, Briant RH, Conolly ME, Davies DS, Dollery CT. Metabolism of isoprenaline after aerosol and direct intrabronchial administration in man and dog. *Br J Pharmacol* 1974;50:587–591.
7. Brittain RT, Dean CM, Jack D. Sympathomimetic bronchodilator drugs. *Pharmacol Ther* 1976;2:423–462.
8. Evans ME, Walker SR, Brittain RT, Paterson JW. The metabolism of salbutamol in man. *Xenobiotica* 1973;3:113–120.
9. Morgan DJ, Paull JD, Richmond BH, Wison-Evered E, Ziccone SP. Pharmacokinetics of intravenous and oral salbutamol and its sulphate conjugate. *Br J Clin Pharmacol* 1986;22:587–593.

10. Shenfield GM, Evans ME, Paterson JW. Absorption of drugs by the lung. *Br J Clin Pharmacol* 1976;3:583–589.
11. Bergman J, Persson H, Wetterlin K. Two new groups of selective stimulants of adrenergic β-receptors. *Experentia* 1969;25:899–901.
12. Nilsson HT, Persson K, Tegner K. The metabolism of terbutaline in man. *Xenobiotica* 1972;2:363–375.
13. Davies DS, George CF, Blackwell E, Conolly ME, Dollery CT. Metabolism of terbutaline in man and dog. *Br J Clin Pharmacol* 1974;1:129–136.
14. Ryrfeldt A, Nilsson E. Physiological disposition of ibuterol and terbutaline in the isolated perfused rat lung. *Acta Pharmacol Toxicol* 1976;39:39–45.
15. Ryrfeldt A, Nilsson E. Uptake and biotransformation of ibuterol and terbutaline in isolated perfused rat and guinea pig lungs. *Biochem Pharmacol* 1978;27:301–305.
16. Leifer KN, Wittig HJ. The beta-2 sympathomimetic aerosols in the treatment of asthma. *Ann Allergy* 1975;35:69–80.
17. Heel RC, Brogden RN, Speight TM, Avery GS. Fenoterol: a review of its pharmacological properties and therapeutic efficacy in asthma. *Drugs* 1978;15:3–32.
18. Svedmyr N. Fenoterol: A beta2-adrenergic agonist for use in asthma. Pharmacology, pharmacokinetics, clinical efficacy and adverse effects. *Pharmacotherapy* 1985;5:109–126.
19. Jack D. A way of looking at agonism and antagonism: lessons from salbutamol, salmeterol and other β-adrenoceptor agonists. *Br J Clin Pharmacol* 1991;31:501–514.
20. Brogden RN, Faulds D. Salmeterol xinafoate. A review of its pharmacological properties and therapeutic potential in reversible obstructive airways disease. *Drugs* 1991;42:893–912.
21. Faulds D, Hollingshead LM, Goa KL. Formoterol. A review of its pharmacological properties and therapeutic potential in reversible obstructive disease. *Drugs* 1991;42:115–137.
22. Maesen FPV, Smeets JJ, Gubbelmans HLL, Zweers PGMA. Bronchodilator effect of inhaled formoterol vs salbutamol over 12 hours. *Chest* 1990;97:590–594.
23. Price AH, Clissold SP. Salbutamol in the 1980s. A reappraisal of its clinical efficacy. *Drugs* 1989;38:77–122.
24. Yokoi K, Murase K, Shiobara Y. The development of a radioimmunoassay for formoterol. *Life Sci* 1983;33:1665–1672.
25. Svedmyr N, Thiringer G. The effects of salbutamol and isoprenaline on beta-receptors in patients with chronic obstructive lung disease. *Br Med J* 1971;47(suppl):44–46.
26. Thiringer G, Svedmyr N. Comparison of infused and inhaled terbutaline in patients with asthma. *Scand J Respir* 1976;57:17–24.
27. Lofdahl C-G, Svedmyr N. Formoterol fumarate, a new β$_2$-adrenoceptor agonist. *Allergy* 1989;44:264–271.
28. Gibson D, Coltart DJ. Haemodynamic effects of intravenous salbutamol in patients with mitral valve disease: comparison with isoprenaline and atropine. *Postgrad Med J* 1971;47(suppl):40–44.
29. Heitz A, Schwartz J, Velly J. β-adrenoceptors of the human myocardium: determination of β$_1$ and β$_2$ subtypes by radioligand binding. *Br J Pharmacol* 1983;80:711–717.
30. Robberecht P, Delhaye M, Taton G, et al. The human heart beta-adrenergic receptors. I. Heterogeneity of the binding sites: presence of 50% beta$_1$- and 50% beta$_2$- adrenergic receptors. *Mol Pharmacol* 1983;24:169–173.
31. Corea L, Bentivoglio M, Verdecchia P, et al. Noninvasive assessment of chronotropic and inotropic response to preferential beta-1 and beta-2 adrenoceptor stimulation. *Clin Pharmacol Ther* 1984;35:776–781.
32. Larsson S, Svedmyr N. Bronchodilating effect and side effects of beta2-adrenoceptor stimulants by different modes of administration (tablets, metered aerosol, and combinations thereof). A study with salbutamol in asthmatics. *Am Rev Respir Dis* 1977;116:861–869.
33. Hertzel MR, Clark TJH. Comparison of intravenous and aerosol salbutamol. *Br Med J* 1976;ii:919–919.
34. Williams S, Seaton A. Intravenous or inhaled salbutamol in severe asthma? *Thorax* 1977;32:555–558.
35. Cheong B, Reynolds SR, Rajan G, Ward MJ. Intravenous β agonist in severe acute asthma. *Br Med J* 1988;297:448–450.

36. Barnes PJ, Pride NB. Dose-response curves to inhaled β-adrenoceptor agonists in normal and asthmatic subjects. *Br J Clin Pharmacol* 1983;15:677–682.
37. Bloomfield P, Carmichael J, Petrie GR, Jewell NP, Crompton GK. Comparison of salbutamol given intravenously and by intermittent positive-pressure breathing in life-threatening asthma. *Br Med J* 1979;1:848–850.
38. Pierce RJ, Payne CR, Williams SJ, Denison DM, Clark TJH. Comparison of intravenous and inhaled terbutaline in the treatment of asthma. *Chest* 1981;79:506–511.
39. Williams SJ, Winner SJ, Clark TJH. Comparison of inhaled and intravenous terbutaline in acute severe asthma. *Thorax* 1981;36:629–631.
40. Swedish Society of Chest Medicine. High-inhaled versus intravenous salbutamol combined with theophylline in severe acute asthma. *Eur Respir J* 1990;3:163–170.
41. Freedman BJ. Trial of a terbutaline aerosol in the treatment of asthma and a comparison of its effects with those of a salbutamol aerosol. *Br J Dis Chest* 1972;66:222–229.
42. Choo-Kang YFJ, MacDonald HL, Horne NW. A comparison of salbutamol and terbutaline aerosols in bronchial asthma. *Practitioner* 1973;211:801–813.
43. Hartnett BJS, Marlin GE. Comparison of terbutaline and salbutamol aerosols. *Aust NZ J Med* 1977;7:13–15.
44. Ruffin RE, Montgomery JM, Newhouse MT. Site of beta-adrenergic receptors in the respiratory tract. Use of fenoterol administered by two methods. *Chest* 1978;74:256–260.
45. Fairshter RD, Novey HS, Wilson AR. Site and duration of bronchodilation in asthmatic patients after oral administration of terbutaline. *Chest* 1981;79:50–57.
46. Gray BJ, Frame MH, Costello JF. A comparative double-blind study of the bronchodilator effects and side effects of inhaled fenoterol and terbutaline administered in equipotent doses. *Br J Dis Chest* 1982;76:341–350.
47. Webb J, Rees J, Clark TJH. A comparison of the effects of different methods of administration of β-2-sympathomimetics in patients with asthma. *Br J Dis Chest* 1982;76:351–357.
48. Ahrens RC, Harris JB, Milavetz G, Annis L, Ries R. Use of bronchial provocation with histamine to compare the pharmacodynamics of inhaled albuterol and metaproterenol in patients with asthma. *J Allergy Clin Immunol* 1987;79:876–882.
49. Gongora HC, Wisniewski AFZ, Tattersfield AE. A single-dose comparison of inhaled albuterol and two formulations of salmeterol on airway reactivity in asthmatic subjects. *Am Rev Respir Dis* 1991;144:626–629.
50. Jeppsson A-B, Lofdahl C-G, Waldeck B, Widmark E. On the predictive value of experiments in vitro in the evaluation of the effect duration of bronchodilator drugs for local administration. *Pulmon Pharmacol* 1989;2:81–85.
51. Ball DI, Brittain RT, Coleman RA, et al. Salmeterol, a novel, long-acting β$_2$-adrenoceptor agonist: characterization of pharmacological activity in vitro and in vivo. *Br J Pharmacol* 1991;104:665–671.
52. Derom EY, Pauwels RA. Time course of bronchodilating effect of inhaled formoterol, a potent and long acting sympathomimetic. *Thorax* 1992;47:30–33.
53. Ullman A, Svedmyr N. Salmeterol, a new long acting inhaled β$_2$ adrenoceptor agonist: comparison with salbutamol in adult asthmatic patients. *Thorax* 1988;43:674–678.
54. Beach JR, Young CL, Stenton SC, et al. A comparison of the speeds of action of salmeterol and salbutamol in reversing methacholine-induced bronchoconstriction. *Pulmon Pharmacol* 1992;5:133–135.
55. Sykes AP, Ayres JG. A study of the duration of the bronchodilator effect of 12 μg and 24 μg of inhaled formoterol and 200 μg inhaled salbutamol in asthma. *Respir Med* 1990;84:135–138.
56. Maesen FPV, Smeets JJ, Gubbelmans HLL, Zweers PGMA. Bronchodilator effect of inhaled formoterol vs salbutamol over 12 hours. *Chest* 1990;97:590–594.
57. Wong BJO, Kamada DH, Ramsdale EH. Effect of formoterol compared with beclomethasone and placebo on allergen induced airway responses. *Thorax* 1991;46:770P (abstract).
58. Twentyman OP, Finnerly JP, Harris A, Palmer J, Holgate ST. Protection against allergen-induced asthma by salmeterol. *Lancet* 1990;336:1338–1342.
59. Becker AB, Simmons FER. Formoterol, a new long-acting selective β$_2$-adrenergic receptor agonist: double-blind comparison with salbutamol and placebo in children with asthma. *J Allergy Clin Immunol* 1989;84:891–895.

60. von Berg A, Berdel D. Formoterol and salbutamol metered aerosols: comparison of a new and an established beta-2-agonist for their bronchodilating efficacy in the treatment of childhood bronchial asthma. *Pediatr Pulmonol* 1989;7:89–93.
61. Graff-Lonnevig V, Browaldh L. Twelve hours' bronchodilating effect of inhaled formoterol in children with asthma: a double-blind cross-over study versus salbutamol. *Clin Exp Allergy* 1990;20:429–432.
62. Ruffin RE, Obminski G, Newhouse MT. Aerosol salbutamol administration by IPPB: lowest effective dose. *Thorax* 1978;33:689–693.
63. Coleman RA, Johnson M, Nials AT, Summer MJ. Salmeterol, but not formoterol, persists at β₂-adrenoceptors *in vitro*. *Br J Pharmacol* 1990;99:121P (abstract).
64. Jeppsson A-B, Roos C, Waldeck B, Widmark E. Pharmacodynamic and pharmacokinetic aspects on the transport of bronchodilator drugs through the tracheal epithelium of the guinea-pig. *Pharmacol Toxicol* 1989;64:58–63.
65. Nials AT, Butchers PR, Coleman RA, Johnson M, Vardey CJ. Salmeterol and formoterol: Are they both long-acting β₂-adrenoceptor agonists? *Br J Pharmacol* 1990; 99:120P (abstract).
66. Ryrfeldt A, Persson G, Nilsson E. Pulmonary disposition of the potent glucocorticoid budesonide, evaluated in an isolated perfused rat lung model. *Biochem Pharmacol* 1989;38:17–22.
67. Yang J, Mitzner W, Hirshman C. Role of the epithelium in airway smooth muscle responses to relaxant agonists. *J Appl Physiol* 1991;71:1434–1440.
68. Kroll F, Karlsson J-A, Nilsson E, Ryrfeldt A, Persson CGA. Rapid clearance of xanthines from airway and pulmonary tissues. *Am Rev Respir Dis* 1990;141:1167–1171.
69. Salome CM, Schoeffel RE, Woolcock AJ. Effect of aerosol fenoterol on the severity of bronchial hyperreactivity in patients with asthma. *Thorax* 1983;38:854–858.
70. Anderson AD, Rodwell LT, Du Toit J, Young IH. Duration of protection by inhaled salmeterol in exercise-induced asthma. *Chest* 1991;100:1254–1260.
71. Smith CM, Anderson SD, Seale JP. The duration of action of the combination of fenoterol hydrobromide and ipratropium bromide in protecting against asthma provoked by hyperpnea. *Chest* 1988;94:709–717.
72. Malo J-L, Ghezzo H, Trudeau C, Cartier A, Morris J. Duration of action of inhaled terbutaline at two different doses and of albuterol in protecting against bronchoconstriction induced by hyperventilation of dry cold air in asthmatic subjects. *Am Rev Respir Dis* 1989;140:817–821.
73. Nix A, Nichol GM, Robson A, Barnes PJ, Chung KF. Effect of formoterol, a long-lasting β₂-adrenoceptor agonist, against methacholine-induced bronchoconstriction. *Br J Clin Pharmacol* 1990;29:321–324.
74. Ramsdale EH, Otis J, Kline PA, Gontovnick LS, Hargreave FE, O'Byrne PM. Prolonged protection against methacholine-induced bronchoconstriction by the inhaled β₂-agonist formoterol. *Am Rev Respir Dis* 1991;143:998–1000.
75. McAlpine LG, Thomson NC. Prophylaxis of exercise-induced asthma with inhaled formoterol, a long-acting β₂-adrenergic agonist. *Respir Med* 1990;84:293–295.
76. Patessio A, Podda A, Carone M, Trombetta N, Donner CF. Protective effect and duration of action of formoterol aerosol on exercise-induced asthma. *Eur Respir J* 1991;4:296–300.
77. Malo J-L, Cartier A, Trudeau C, Ghezzo H, Gontovnick L. Formoterol, a new inhaled beta-2 adrenergic agonist, has a longer blocking effect than albuterol on hyperventilation-induced bronchoconstriction. *Am Rev Respir Dis* 1990;142:1147–1152.
78. Sly RM, Anderson JA, Bierman CW, et al. Position statement. Adverse effects and complications of treatment with beta-adrenergic agonist drugs. *J Allergy Clin Immunol* 1985;75:443–449.
79. Sly RM. Mortality from asthma, 1979–1984. *J Allergy Clin Immunol* 1988;82:705–717.
80. Paterson JW, Lulich KM, Goldie RG. A comment on β₂-agonists and their use in asthma. *Trends Pharmacol Sci* 1983;4:67–69.
81. Lands AM, Arnold A, McAullif JP, Luduena FS, Brown TG. Differentiation of receptor systems activated by sympathomimetic amines. *Nature* 1967;597–598.
82. Lipworth BJ. The β-agonist controversy: fact or fiction? *Clin Exp Allergy* 1992;22:659–664.
83. Lipworth BJ, McDevitt DG. Inhaled β₂-adrenoceptor agonists in asthma: help or hindrance? *Br J Clin Pharmacol* 1992;33:129–138.

84. Scheinin M, Koulu M, Laurikainen E, Alonen H. Hypokalaemia and other nonbronchial effects of inhaled fenoterol and salbutamol: a placebo-controlled dose-response study in healthy volunteers. *Br J Clin Pharmacol* 1987;24:645–653.
85. Deenstra M, Haalboom JRE, Struyvenberg A. Decrease of plasma potassium due to inhalation of beta-2-agonists: absence of an additional effect of intravenous theophylline. *Eur J Clin Invest* 1988;18:162–165.
86. Crane J, Burgess C, Beasley R. Cardiovascular and hypokalaemic effects of inhaled salbutamol, fenoterol, and isoprenaline. *Thorax* 1989;44:136–140.
87. Flatt A, Crane J, Purdie G, Kwong T, Beasley R, Burgess C. The cardiovascular effects of beta adrenergic agonist drugs administered by nebulisation. *Postgrad Med J* 1990;66:98–101.
88. Tandon MK. Cardiopulmonary effects of fenoterol and salbutamol aerosols. *Chest* 1980;77:429–431.
89. Bellamy D, Penketh A. A cumulative dose comparison between salbutamol and fenoterol metered dose aerosols in asthmatic patients. *Postgrad Med J* 1987;63:459–461.
90. Wong CS, Pavord ID, Williams J, Britton JR, Tattersfield AE. Bronchodilator, cardiovascular, and hypokalaemic effects of fenoterol, salbutamol and terbutaline in asthma. *Lancet* 1990;336:1396–1399.
91. Lipworth BJ, Struthers AD, McDevitt DG. Tachyphylaxis to systemic but not to airway responses during prolonged therapy with high dose inhaled salbutamol in asthmatics. *Am Rev Respir Dis* 1989;140:586–592.
92. Decker N, Quennedey MC, Rouot B, Schwartz J, Velly J. Effects of N-aralkyl substitution of β agonists on α- and β-adrenoceptor subtypes: pharmacological studies and binding assays. *J Pharm Pharmacol* 1982;34:107–112.
93. Stephenson RP. A modification of receptor theory. *Br J Pharmacol* 1956;11:379–393.
94. Van den Brink FG. The model of functional interaction. I. Development and first check of a new model of functional synergism and antagonism. *Eur J Pharmacol* 1973;22:270–278.
95. Van den Brink FG. The model of functional interaction. II. Experimental verification of a new model: the antagonism of β-adrenoceptor stimulants and other agonists. *Eur J Pharmacol* 1973;22:279–286.
96. Buckner CK, Saini RK. On the use of functional antagonism to estimate dissociation constants for β-adrenoceptor agonists in isolated guinea-pig trachea. *J Pharmacol Exp Ther* 1975;194:565–574.
97. Torphy TJ, Rinard GA, Rietow MG, Mayer SE. Functional antagonism in canine tracheal smooth muscle: inhibition by methacholine of the mechanical and biochemical responses to isoproterenol. *J Pharmacol Exp Ther* 1983;227:694–699.
98. Advenier C, Naline E, Matran R, et al. Interaction between fenoterol, ipratropium bromide, and acetylcholine on human isolated bronchus. *J Allergy Clin Immunol* 1988;82:40–46.
99. O'Donnell SR, Wanstall JC. Evidence that the efficacy (intrinsic activity) of fenoterol is higher than that of salbutamol on β-adrenoceptors in guinea-pig trachea. *Eur J Pharmacol* 1978;47:333–340.
100. Gustafsson B, Persson CGA. Effect of different bronchodilators on airway smooth muscle responsiveness to contractile agents. *Thorax* 1991;46:360–365.
101. Farmer JB, Leher DN. The effect of isoprenaline on the contraction of smooth muscle produced by histamine, acetylcholine or other agents. *J Pharm Pharmacol* 1966;18:649–656.
102. Mitchell HW, Denborough MA. Drug interactions in cat isolated tracheal smooth muscle. *Clin Exp Pharmacol Physiol* 1979;6:249–257.
103. Phillips GD, Finnerty JP, Holgate ST. Comparative protective effect of the inhaled β_2-agonist salbutamol (albuterol) on bronchoconstriction by histamine, methacholine, and adenosine 5'-monophosphate in asthma. *J Allergy Clin Immunol* 1990;85:755–762.
104. Madsen BW, Tandon MK, Paterson JW. Crossover study of the efficacy of four beta-2 sympathomimetic bronchodilator aerosols. *Br J Clin Pharmacol* 1979;8:75–82.
105. Hockley B, Johnson NMcI. Fenoterol versus salbutamol nebulisation in asthma. *Postgrad Med J* 1983;59:504–505.
106. Goldie RG, Paterson JW, Lulich KM. Adrenoceptors in airway smooth muscle. *Pharmacol Ther* 1990;48:295–322.
107. Dougall IG, Harper D, Jackson DM, Leff P. Estimation of the efficacy and affinity of

the β₂-adrenoceptor agonist salmeterol in guinea pig trachea. *Br J Pharmacol* 1991;104:1057–1061.

108. Linden A, Bergendal A, Ullman A, Skoogh B-E, Lofdhal, C-G. Long- and short-acting β₂-agonists in the isolated guinea-pig trachea—efficacy, potency and functional antagonism. *Eur Respir J* 1991;4 (suppl 14):199s (abstract).

109. Tota MR, Candelore MR, Dixon RAF, Strader CD. Biophysical and genetic analysis of the ligand binding site of the β-adrenoceptor. *Trends Pharmacol Sci* 1991;12:4–6.

110. Lichtenstein LM, Margolis S. Histamine release in vitro: inhibition by catecholamines and methylxanthines. *Science* 1968;161:902–903.

111. Assem ESK, Schild HO. Inhibition by sympathomimetic amines of histamine release induced by antigen in passively sensitized human lung. *Nature* 1969;224:1028–1029.

112. Butchers PR, Fullerton JR, Skidmore IF, Thompson LE, Vardey CE, Wheeldon A. A comparison of the anti-anaphylactic actions of salbutamol and disodium cromoglycate in the rat, the rat mast cell and human lung tissue. *Br J Pharmacol* 1979;67:23–32.

113. Church MK, Young KD. The characteristics of inhibition of histamine release from human lung fragments by sodium cromoglycate, salbutamol and chlorpromazine. *Br J Pharmacol* 1983;78:671–679.

114. Peters SP, Schulman ES, Schleimer RP, MacGlashan Jr DW, Newball HH, Lichtenstein LM. Dispersed human lung mast cells. Pharmacological aspects and comparison with human lung tissue fragments. *Am Rev Respir Dis* 1982;126:1034–1039.

115. Church MK, Hiroi J. Inhibition of IgE dependent histamine release from human dispersed mast cells by antiallergic drugs and salbutamol. *Br J Pharmacol* 1987;90:421–429.

116. Butchers PR, Skidmore IF, Vardey CJ, Wheeldon A. Characterization of the receptor mediating the anti-anaphylactic effects of β-adrenoceptor agonists in human lung tissue in vitro. *Br J Pharmacol* 1980;71:663–667.

117. Butchers PR, Vardey CJ, Johnson M. Salmeterol: a potent and long-acting inhibitor of inflammatory mediator release from human lung. *Br J Pharmacol* 1991;104:672–676.

118. Tomioka K, Yamada T, Tachikawa S. Effects of formoterol (BD 40A), a β-adrenoceptor stimulant, on isolated guinea-pig lung parenchymal strips and antigen-induced SRS-A release in rats. *Arch Int Pharmacodyn* 1984;267:91–102.

119. Martin GL, Atkins PC, Dunsky EH, Zweiman B. Effects of theophylline, terbutaline and prednisone on antigen-induced bronchospasm and mediator release. *J Allergy Clin Immunol* 1980;66:204–212.

120. Nagy L, Lee TH, Kay AB. Neutrophil chemotactic activity in antigen-induced late asthmatic reactions. *N Engl J Med* 1982;306:498–501.

121. Howarth PH, Durham SR, Lee TH, et al. Influence of albuterol, cromolyn sodium and ipratropium bromide on the airway and circulatory mediator responses to allergen bronchial provocation in asthma. *Am Rev Respir Dis* 1985;132:986–992.

122. Murray JJ, Tonnel AB, Brash AR, et al. Release of prostaglandin D₂ into human airways during acute antigen challenge. *N Engl J Med* 1986;315:800–804.

123. Miadonna A, Tedeschi A, Brasca C, Folco G, Sala A, Murphy RC. Mediator release after endobronchial antigen challenge in patients with respiratory allergy. *J Allergy Clin Immunol* 1990;85:906–913.

124. Taylor IK, O'Shaughnessy KM, Choudry NB, et al. A comparative study in atopic subjects with asthma of the effects of salmeterol and salbutamol on allergen-induced bronchoconstriction, increase in airway reactivity, and increase in urinary leukotriene E₄ excretion. *J Allergy Clin Immunol* 1992;89:575–583.

125. Holtzman MJ. Arachidonic acid metabolism. Implications of biological chemistry for lung function and disease. *Am Rev Respir Dis* 1991;143:188–203.

126. Anderson SD, Bye PTP, Schoeffel RE, Seale JP, Taylor KM, Ferris L. Arterial plasma histamine levels at rest, and during and after exercise in patients with asthma: effects of terbutaline aerosol. *Thorax* 1981;36:259–267.

127. Wodnar-Filipowicz A, Heusser CH, Moroni C. Production of the haemopoietic growth factors GM-CSF and interleukin-3 by mast cells in response to IgE receptor-mediated activation. *Nature* 1989;339:150–152.

128. Plaut M, Pierce JH, Watson CJ, et al. Mast cell lines produce lymphokines in response to cross-linkage of FcεRI or to calcium ionophore. *Nature* 1989;339:64–67.

129. Fick RB Jr, Metzger WJ, Richerson HB, et al. Increased bronchovascular perme-

ability after allergen exposure in sensitive asthmatics. *J Appl Physiol* 1987;63:1147–1155.

130. Metzger WJ, Zavala D, Richerson HB, et al. Local allergen challenge and bronchoalveolar lavage of allergic asthmatic lungs. Description of the model and local airway inflammation. *Am Rev Respir Dis* 1987;135:433–440.

131. Persson CGA. Role of plasma exudation in the asthmatic airways. *Lancet* 1986;2:1126–1129.

132. Erjefalt I, Persson CGA. Allergen, bradykinin, and capsaicin increase outward but not inward macromolecular permeability of guinea-pig tracheobronchial mucosa. *Clin Exp Allergy* 1991;21:217–224.

133. Persson CGA, Erjefalt I. Terbutaline and adrenaline inhibit leakage of fluid and protein in guinea pig lung. *Eur J Pharmacol* 1979;55:199–201.

134. Erjefalt I, Persson CGA. Pharmacological control of plasma exudation into tracheobronchial airways. *Am Rev Respir Dis* 1991;143:1008–1014.

135. Grega GJ. Contractile elements in endothelial cells as potential targets for drug action. *Trends Pharmacol Sci* 1986;8:452–457.

136. Boschetto P, Roberts NM, Rogers DF, Barnes P. Effect of antiasthma drugs on microvascular leakage in guinea-pig airways. *Am Rev Respir Dis* 1989;139:416–421.

137. Woodward DF, Weichman BM, Wasserman MA. Differential inhibition of LTD_4-mediated bronchopulmonary effects by salbutamol. *Eur J Pharmacol* 1984;100:219–222.

138. Erjefalt I, Persson CGA. Inflammatory passage of plasma macromolecules into airway wall and lumen. *Pulmon Pharmacol* 1989;2:93–102.

139. Erjefalt I, Persson CGA. Long duration and high potency of antiexudative effects of formoterol in guinea-pig tracheobronchial airways. *Am Rev Respir Dis* 1991;144:788–791.

140. Tokuyama K, Lotvall JO, Lofdahl C-G, Barnes PJ, Chung KF. Inhaled formoterol inhibits histamine-induced airflow obstruction and airway microvascular leakage. *Eur J Pharmacol* 1991;193:35–39.

141. Whelan CJ, Johnson M. Inhibition by salmeterol of increased vascular permeability and granulocyte accumulation in guinea-pig lung and skin. *Br J Pharmacol* 1992;105:831–838.

142. Basran GS, Paul W, Morley J, Turner-Warick M. Evidence in man of synergistic interaction between putative mediators of acute inflammation and asthma. *Lancet* 1982;1:935–937.

143. Basran GS, Paul W, Morley J, Turner-Warwick M. Adrenoceptor-agonist inhibition of the histamine-induced cutaneous response in man. *Br J Dermatol* 1982;107(suppl 23):140–142.

144. Gronneberg R, Strandberg K, Stalenheim G, Zetterstrom O. Effect in man of antiallergic drugs on the immediate and late phase cutaneous allergic reactions induced by anti-IgE. *Allergy* 1981;36:201–208.

145. Gronneberg R, Zetterstrom O. Inhibition of anti-IgE induced skin response in normals by formoterol, a new β_2-adrenoceptor agonist, and terbutaline. 1. Dose response relation and duration of effect on the early wheal and flare response. *Allergy* 1990;45:334–339.

146. Gronneberg R, Strandberg K, Hagermark O. Effect of terbutaline, a β-adrenergic receptor stimulating compound, on cutaneous responses to histamine, allergen, compound 48/80 and trypsin. *Allergy* 1979;34:303–309.

147. Ting S, Zweiman B, Lavker R. Terbutaline modulation of human allergic skin reactions. *J Allergy Clin Immunol* 1983;71:437–441.

148. Gronneberg R, Zetterstrom O. Inhibition of anti-IgE induced skin response in normals by formoterol, a new β_2-adrenoceptor agonist, and terbutaline. 2. Effect on the late phase reaction. *Allergy* 1990;45:340–346.

149. Gronneberg R, Zetterstrom O. Inhibitory effects of formoterol and terbutaline on the development of late phase skin reactions. *Clin Exp Allergy* 1992;22:257–263.

150. Erjefalt IAL, G-Wagner Z, Strand SE, Persson CGA. A method for studies of tracheobronchial microvascular permeability to macromolecules. *J Pharmacol Meth* 1985;14:275–283.

151. Archer CB, MacDonald DM. Treatment of atopic dermatitis with salbutamol. *Clin Exp Dermatol* 1987;12:323–325.

152. Frigas E, Gleich GJ. The eosinophil and the pathophysiology of asthma. *J Allergy Clin Immunol* 1986;77:527–537.
153. Frew AJ, Kay AB. Eosinophils and T-lymphocytes in late-phase allergic reactions. *J Allergy Clin Immunol* 1990;85:533–539.
154. Kay AB. Asthma and inflammation. *J Allergy Clin Immunol* 1991;87:893–910.
155. Morley J, Sanjar S, Page CP. The platelet in asthma. *Lancet* 1984;2:1142–1144.
156. Page CP. Platelets as inflammatory cells. *Immunopharmacology* 1989;17:51–59.
157. Fuller RW. Pharmacological regulation of airway macrophage function. *Clin Exp Allergy* 1991;21:651–654.
158. Torphy TJ, Undem BJ. Phosphodiesterase inhibitors: new opportunities for the treatment of asthma. *Thorax* 1991;46:512–524.
159. Cook N, Nahorski SR, Barnett DB. Human platelet β$_2$-adrenoceptors: agonist-induced internalisation and down-regulation in intact cells. *Br J Pharmacol* 1987;92:587–596.
160. Johnson CE, Belfield PW, Davis S, Cooke NJ, Spencer A, Davies JA. Platelet activation during exercise-induced asthma. Effect of prophylaxis with salbutamol. *Thorax* 1986;42:290–294.
161. Yukawa T, Ukena D, Krogel C, et al. Beta2-adrenergic receptors on eosinophils. Binding and functional studies. *Am Rev Respir Dis* 1990;141:1446–1452.
162. Butchers PR, Reynolds LH. The effect of β-adrenoceptor agonists on the degranulation and migration of human eosinophils in vitro. *Am Rev Respir Dis* 1992;145:A695 (abstract).
163. Koenderman L, Maikoe T, Warringa R, Raaijmakers J. Salmeterol is a potent inhibitor of cytokine-primed eosinophil chemotaxis. *Am Rev Respir Dis* 1992;145:A421. (abstract).
164. Dent G, Giembycz MA, Rabe KF, Barnes PJ. Inhibition of eosinophil cyclic nucleotide PDE activity and opsonised zymosan-stimulated respiratory burst by "type IV"-selective PDE inhibitors. *Br J Pharmacol* 1991;103:1339–1346.
165. Kraan J, Koeter GH, van der Mark ThW, Sluiter HJ, De Vries K. Changes in bronchial hyperreactivity induced by 4 weeks of treatment with antiasthmatic drugs in patients with allergic asthma: a comparison between budesonide and terbutaline. *J Allergy Clin Immunol* 1985;76:628–636.
166. Adelroth E, Rosenhall L, Johansson S-A, Linden M, Venge P. Inflammatory cells and eosinophilic activity in asthmatics investigated by bronchoalveolar lavage. The effects of antiasthmatic treatment with budesonide or terbutaline. *Am Rev Respir Dis* 1990;142:91–99.
167. Jeffery PK, Godfrey RW, Adelroth E, et al. Effects of treatment on airway inflammation and thickening of basement membrane reticular collagen in asthma. A quantitative light and electron microscopic study. *Am Rev Respir Dis* 1992;145:890–899.
168. Diaz P, Galleguillos FR, Gonzalez MC, Pantin CFA, Kay AB. Bronchoalveolar lavage in asthma: the effect of disodium cromoglycate (cromolyn) on leukocyte counts, immunoglobulins, and complement. *J Allergy Clin Immunol* 1984;74:41–48.
169. Roberts JA, Bradding P, Walls AF, Hogate ST, Howarth PH. The effect of salmeterol xinafoate therapy on lavage findings in asthma. *Am Rev Respir Dis* 1992;145:A418 (abstract).
170. Roberts JA, Bradding P, Walls AF, et al. The influence of salmeterol xinafoate on mucosal inflammation in asthma. *Am Rev Respir Dis* 1992;145:A418 (abstract).
171. Capron M, Jouault T, Prin L, et al. Functional study of a monoclonal antibody to IgE Fc receptor (FcεR2) of eosinophils, platelets and macrophages. *J Exp Med* 1986;164:72–89.
172. Liggett SB. Identification and characterization of a homogenous population of β$_2$-adrenergic receptors on human alveolar macrophages. *Am Rev Respir Dis* 1989;139:552–555.
173. Fuller RW, O'Malley G, Baker AJ, MacDermot J. Human alveolar macrophage activation: inhibition by forskolin but not β-adrenoceptor stimulation or phosphodiesterase inhibition. *Pulmon Pharmacol* 1988;1:101–106.
174. Calhoun WJ, Stevens CA, Lambert SB. Modulation of superoxide production of alveolar macrophages and peripheral blood mononuclear cells by β-agonists and theophylline. *J Lab Clin Med* 1991;117:514–522.
175. Baker AJ, Fuller RW. Comparison of the anti-inflammatory effects of salmeterol on

human airway macrophages with those on peripheral monocytes. *Eur Respir J* 1991;4(suppl 14):426s (abstract).

176. Tashkin DP, Conolly ME, Deutsch RI, et al. Subsensitization of beta-adrenoceptors in airways and lymphocytes of healthy and asthmatic subjects. *Am Rev Respir Dis* 1982;125:185–193.

177. Sano Y, Watt G, Townley RG. Decreased mononuclear cell beta-adrenergic receptors in bronchial asthma: parallel studies of lymphocytes and granulocyte desensitization. *J Allergy Clin Immunol* 1983;72:495–503.

178. Motojima S, Fukuda T, Makino S. Measurement of β-adrenergic receptors on lymphoctes in normal subjects and asthmatics in relation to β-adrenergic hyperglycaemic response and bronchial responsiveness. *Allergy* 1983;38:331–337.

179. Bourne HR, Lichtenstein LM, Melmon KL, Henney CS, Weinstein Y, Shearer GM. Modulation of inflammation and immunity by cyclic AMP. *Science* 1974;184:19–28.

180. Kammer GM. The adenylate cyclase-cAMP-protein kinase A pathway and regulation of immune response. *Immunol Today* 1988;9:222–228.

181. Brooks SM, McGowan K, Bernstein IL, et al. Relationship between numbers of beta-adrenergic receptors in lymphocytes and disease severity in asthma. *J Allergy Clin Immunol* 1979;63:401–406.

182. Koeter GH, Meurs H, Kauffman HF, et al. The role of the adrenergic system in allergy and bronchial hyperreactivity. *Eur J Respir Dis* 1982;62(suppl 121):72–78.

183. Meurs H, Koeter GH, De Vries K, et al. The beta-adrenergic system and allergic bronchial asthma: changes in lymphocyte beta-adrenergic receptor number and adenylate cyclase activity after an allergen induced asthmatic attack. *J Allergy Clin Immunol* 1982;70:272–280.

184. Maisel AS, Fowler P, Rearden A, Motulsky HJ, Michel MC. A new method for isolation of human lymphocyte subsets reveals differential regulation of β-adrenergic receptors by terbutaline treatment. *Clin Pharmacol Ther* 1989;46:429–439.

185. Maisel AS, Knowlton KU, Fowler P, et al. Adrenergic control of circulating lymphocyte subpopulations. Effects of congestive heart failure, dynamic exercise, and terbutaline treatment. *J Clin Invest* 1990;85:462–467.

186. Maisel AS, Michel MC. β-adrenoceptor control of immune function in congestive heart failure. *Br J Clin Pharmacol* 1990;30:49S–53S.

187. Gratziou C, Roberts JA, Bradding P, Holgate ST, Howarth PH. The influence of the long acting β-agonist, salmeterol xinafoate, on T-lymphocyte lavage pouplations and activation status in asthma. *Am Rev Respir Dis* 1992;145:A67 (abstract).

188. Beasley R, Roche WR, Roberts JA, Holgate ST. Cellular events in the bronchi in mild asthma and after bronchial provocation. *Am Rev Respir Dis* 1989;139:806–817.

189. Jeffery PK, Wardlaw AJ, Nelson FC, Collins JV, Kay AB. Bronchial biopsies in asthma: an ultrastructural, quantitative study and correlation with hyperreactivity. *Am Rev Respir Dis* 1989;140:1745–1753.

190. Azzawi W, Bradley B, Jeffery PK, et al. Identification of activated T lymphocytes and eosinophils in bronchial biopsies in stable atopic asthma. *Am Rev Respir Dis* 1990;142:1407–1413.

191. Bradley BL, Azzawi M, Jacobson M, et al. Eosinophils, T-lymphocytes, mast cells, neutrophils, and macrophages in bronchial biopsy specimens from atopic subjects with asthma: comparison with biopsy specimens from atopic subjects without asthma and normal control subjects and relationship to bronchial hyperresponsiveness. *J Allergy Clin Immunol* 1991;88:661–674.

192. Galant SP, Underwood S, Duriseti L, et al. Characterization of high affinity beta$_2$-adrenergic receptor binding of (−)-[3H] dihydroalprenolol to human polymorphonuclear cell particulates. *J Lab Clin Med* 1978;92:613–618.

193. Galant SP, Duriseti L, Underwood S, et al. Beta-adrenergic receptors of polymorphonuclear particulates in bronchial asthma. *J Clin Invest* 1980;65:577–585.

194. Davis PB, Simpson DM, Paget GL, et al. β-adrenergic responses in drug-free subjects with asthma. *J Allergy Clin Immunol* 1986;77:871–879.

195. Nielson CP. β-adrenergic modulation of the polymorphonuclear leukocyte respiratory burst is dependent upon the mechanism of cell activation. *J Immunol* 1987;139:2392–2397.

196. Busse WW, Sosman JM. Isoproterenol inhibition of isolated human neutrophil function. *J Allergy Clin Immunol* 1984;73:404–410.
197. Mack JA, Nielson CP, Stevens CP, et al. β-adrenoceptor-mediated modulation of calcium ionophore activated polymorphonuclear leucocytes. *Br J Pharmacol* 1986;88: 417–423.
198. Britton J, Hanley SP, Garrett HV, Hadfield JW, Tattersfield AE. Dose related effects of salbutamol and ipratropium bromide on airway calibre and reactivity in subjects with asthma. *Thorax* 1988;43:300–305.
199. Bel EH, Zwinderman AH, Timmers MC, Dijkman JH, Sterk PJ. The protective effect of a beta2 agonist against excessive airway narrowing in response to bronchoconstrictor stimuli in asthma and chronic obstructive lung disease. *Thorax* 1991;46:9–11.
200. Salome CM, Schoeffel RE, Woolcock AJ. Effect of aerosol and oral fenoterol on histamine and methacholine challenge in asthmatic subjects. *Thorax* 1981;36:580–584.
201. Chung KF, Morgan B, Keyes SJ, Snashall PD. Histamine dose-response relationships in normal and asthmatic subjects. The importance of starting airway calibre. *Am Rev Respir Dis* 1982;126:849–854.
202. Cockcroft DW, Murdock KY. Comparative effects of inhaled salbutamol, sodium cromoglycate, and beclomethasone dipropionate on allergen-induced early asthmatic responses, late asthmatic responses, and increased bronchial hyperresponsiveness to histamine. *J Allergy Clin Immunol* 1987;79:734–740.
203. Lai CKW, Twentyman OP, Holgate ST. The effect of an increase in inhaled allergen dose after rimiterol hydrobromide on the occurrence and magnitude of the late asthmatic response and the associated change in non-specific bronchial hyperresponsiveness. *Am Rev Respir Dis* 1989;140:917–923.
204. Latimer KM, O'Byrne PM, Morris MM, Roberts R, Hargreave FE. Bronchoconstriction stimulated by airway cooling. Better protection with combined inhalation of terbutaline sulphate and cromolyn sodium than either alone. *Am Rev Respir Dis* 1983;128:440–443.
205. Neijens HJ, Kerrebijn KF. Variation with time in bronchial responsiveness to histamine and to specific allergen provocation. *Eur J Respir Dis* 1983;64:591–597.
206. Morton AR, Scott CA, Fitch KD. Rimiterol and the prevention of exercise-induced asthma. *J Allergy Clin Immunol* 1989;83:61–65.
207. Moscato G, Rampulla C, Dellabianca A, Zanotti E, Candura S. Effect of salbutamol and inhaled sodium cromoglycate on the airway and neutrophil chemotactic activity in "fog"-induced bronchospasm. *J Allergy Clin Immunol* 1988;82:382–388.
208. Boulet L-P, Turcotte H, Tennina S. Comparative efficacy of salbutamol, ipratropium, and cromoglycate in the prevention of bronchospasm induced by exercise and hyperosmolar challenges. *J Allergy Clin Immunol* 1989;83:882–887.
209. Casterline CL, Evans R, Ward GW. The effect of atropine and albuterol aerosols on the human bronchial response to histamine. *J Allergy Clin Immunol* 1976;58:607–613.
210. Cockcroft DW, Killian DN, Mellon JJA, Hargreave FE. Protective effect of drugs on histamine induced asthma. *Thorax* 1977;32:429–437.
211. Bandouvakis J, Cartier A, Roberts R, Ryan G, Hargreave FE. The effect of ipratropium and fenoterol on methacholine- and histamine-induced bronchoconstriction. *Br J Dis Chest* 1981;75:295–305.
212. De Monchey JGR, Kauffman HF, Venge P, et al. Bronchoalveolar eosinophilia during allergen-induced late asthmatic reactions. *Am Rev Respir Dis* 1985;131:373–376.
213. Booij-Noord H, De Vries K, Sluiter HJ, Orie NGM. Late bronchial obstructive reaction to experimental inhalation of house dust extract. *Clin Allergy* 1972;2:43–61.
214. Pauwels R, Van Renterghem D, Van Der Straeten M, Johannesson N, Persson CGA. The effect of theophylline and enprofylline on allergen-induced bronchoconstriction. *J Allergy Clin Immunol* 1985;76:583–590.
215. Ward AJM, McKenniff MG, Evans JM, Page CP, Costello JF. Suppression of the late asthmatic response (LAR) with subbronchodilator concentrations of theophylline. *Am Rev Respir Dis* 1992;145:A740 (abstract).
216. Taylor IK, O'Shaughnessy KM, Fuller RW, Dollery CT. Effect of cysteinyl-leukotriene receptor antagonist ICI 204.219 on allergen-induced bronchoconstriction and airway hyperreactivity in atopic subjects. *Lancet* 1991;337:690–694.

217. Abbott A. New directions in asthma: some cause for concern. *Trends Pharmacol Sci* 1988;9:149–151.
218. Barnes PJ. A new approach to the treatment of asthma. *N Engl J Med* 1989;321:1517–1527.
219. Van Bever HP, Desager KN, Stevens WJ. The effect of inhaled fenoterol, administered during the late asthmatic reaction to house dust mite (Dermatophagoides pternoyssinus). *J Allergy Clin Immunol* 1990;85:700–703.
220. Malo J-L, Ghezzo H, L'Archeveque J, Cartier A. Late asthmatic reactions to occupational sensitizing agents: frequency of changes in nonspecific bronchial hyperresponsiveness to inhaled β₂-adrenergic agonists. *J Allergy Clin Immunol* 1990;85:834–842.
221. Hegardt B, Pauwels R, Van Der Straeten M. Inhibitory effect of KWD 2131, terbutaline and DSCG on the immediate and late allergen-induced bronchoconstriction. *Allergy* 1981;36:115–122.
222. Twentyman OP, Finnerty JP, Holgate ST. The inhibitory effect of nebulized albuterol on the early and late asthmatic reactions and increase in airway responsiveness provoked by inhaled allergen in asthma. *Am Rev Respir Dis* 1991;144:782–787.
223. Palmquist M, Balder B, Lowhagen O, Melander B, Svedmyr N, Wahlander L. Late asthmatic reaction decreased after pretreatment with salbutamol and formoterol, a new long-acting β₂-agonist. *J Allergy Clin Immunol* 1992;89:844–849.
224. Britton J, Pavord I, Wong C, Tattersfield AE. β₂-agonists in asthma. *Lancet* 1991; 337:300 (letter).
225. Henocq E, Vargaftig BB. Skin eosinophilia in atopic patients. *J Allergy Clin Immunol* 1988;41:691–695.
226. Hammarlund A, Pipkorn U, Enerback L. Mast cells, tissue histamine and eosinophils in early- and late-phase skin reactions: effects of a single dose of prednisolone. *Int Arch Allergy Appl Immunol* 1990;93:171–177.
227. Imbeau SA, Harruff R, Hirscher M, Reed CE. Terbutaline's effects on the allergy skin test. *J Allergy Clin Immunol* 1978;62:193–196.
228. Johnson M, Vardey CJ, Whelan CJ. The therapeutic potential of long acting β₂-adrenoceptor agonists in allergic inflammation. *Clin Exp Allergy* 1992;22:177–181.
229. Doukas J, Shepro D, Hechtman HB. Vasoactive amines directly modify endothelial cells to affect polymorphonuclear leukocyte diapedesis in vitro. *Blood* 1987;69:1563–1569.
230. Gundel RH, Wegner CD, Torcellini CA, Letts LG. The role of intercellular adhesion molecule-1 in chronic airway inflammation. *Clin Exp Allergy* 1992;22:569–575.
231. Hansel TT, Walker C. The migration of eosinophils into the sputum of asthmatics: the role of adhesion molecules. *Clin Exp Allergy* 1992;22:345–356.
232. Page CP. The role of platelet activating factor in asthma. *J Allergy Clin Immunol* 1988;81:144–152.
233. Mazzoni L, Morley J, Page CP, Sanjar S. The induction of airway hyperresponsiveness by platelet activating factor in the guinea pig. *J Physiol* 1988;368:107P (abstract).
234. Sanjar S, Aoki S, Boubeckeur K, Chapman ID, Smith D, King MA, Morley J. Eosinophil accumulation in pulmonary airways of guinea-pigs induced by exposure to an aerosol of platelet-activating factor: effect of anti-asthma drugs. *Br J Pharmacol* 1990;99:267–272.
235. Sanjar S, McCabe PJ, Reynolds LH. Salmeterol, a long-acting β₂-agonist inhibits antigen-induced bronchial eosinophil accumulation. *Am Rev Respir Dis* 1991;143:A755 (abstract).
236. Boubecker K, Marguin V, Bouhelal R, Morley J. Failure of long-acting beta-adrenoceptor agonists to diminish allergic eosinophilia of the airways in guinea pigs. *Fundam Clin Pharmacol* 1991;5:402 (abstract).
237. Woolcock AJ, Salome CM, Yan K. The shape of the dose-response curve to histamine in asthmatic and normal subjects. *Am Rev Respir Dis* 1984;130:71–75.
238. Sterk PJ, Bel EH. In vivo challenge. The shape of the dose-response curve to inhaled bronchoconstrictor agents in asthma and in chronic obstructive pulmonary disease. *Am Rev Respir Dis* 1991;143:1433–1437.
239. Bel EH, Timmers MC, Zwinderman AH, Dijkman JH, Sterk PJ. The effect of inhaled

corticosteroids on the maximal degree of airway narrowing to methacholine in asthmatic subjects. *Am Rev Respir Dis* 1991;143:109–113.
240. Cheung D, Timmers MC, Zwinderman AH, Bel EH, Dijkman JH, Sterk PJ. The prolonged effects of salmeterol on airway hyperresponsiveness in asthma. *Am Rev Respir Dis* 1992;145:A59.
241. Clark TJH. Diurnal rhythm of asthma. *Chest* 1987;91:137S–141S.
242. Douglas NJ. Nocturnal asthma. *Q J Med* 1989;71:279–289.
243. Bush RK. Nocturnal asthma: mechanisms and the role of theophylline in treatment. *Postgrad Med J* 1991;67(suppl 4):S20–S24.
244. Turner-Warwick M. Epidemiology of nocturnal asthma. *Am J Med* 1988;85(suppl 1B):6–8.
245. Catterall JR, Douglas NJ, Calverley PMA, et al. Irregular breathing and hypoxaemia during sleep in chronic stable asthma. *Lancet* 1982;1:301–304.
246. Montplaisir J, Walsh J, Malo JL. Nocturnal asthma: features of attacks, sleep and breathing patterns. *Am Rev Respir Dis* 1982;125:18–22.
247. Fitzpatrick MF, Engleman H, Whyte KF, Deary IJ, Shapiro CM, Douglas NJ. Morbidity in nocturnal asthma: sleep quality and daytime cognitive performance. *Thorax* 1991;46:569–573.
248. Clark TJH, Hetzel MR. Diurnal variation of asthma. *Br J Dis Chest* 1977;71:87–92.
249. Bellia V, Cuttitta G, Insalaco G, Visconti A, Bonsignore G. Relationship of nocturnal bronchoconstriction to sleep stages. *Am Rev Respir Dis* 1989;140:363–367.
250. Hetzel MR, Clark TJH. Does sleep cause nocturnal asthma? *Thorax* 1979;34:749–754.
251. Catterall JR, Rhind GB, Stewart IC, Whyte KF, Shapiro CM, Douglas NJ. Effect of sleep deprivation on overnight bronchoconstriction in nocturnal asthma. *Thorax* 1986;41:676–680.
252. Whyte KF, Douglas NJ. Posture and nocturnal asthma. *Thorax* 1989;44:579–581.
253. Barnes P, Fitzgerald M, Brown M, Dollery C. Nocturnal asthma and changes in circulating epinephrine, histamine and cortisol. *N Engl J Med* 1980;303:263–267.
254. Soutar CA, Costello J, Ijaduola O, Turner-Warwick M. Nocturnal and morning asthma. Relationship to plasma corticosteroids and response to cortisol infusion. *Thorax* 1975;30:436–440.
255. Morrison JFJ, Teale C, Pearson SB, et al. Adrenaline and nocturnal asthma. *Br Med J* 1990;301:199–203.
256. Coe CI, Barnes PJ. Reduction of nocturnal asthma by an inhaled anticholinergic drug. *Chest* 1986;90:485–488.
257. Morrison JFJ, Pearson SB, Dean HG. Parasympathetic nervous system in nocturnal asthma. *Br Med J* 1988;296:1427–1429.
258. Morrison JFJ, Pearson SB. The effect of circadian rhythm of vagal activity on bronchomotor tone in asthma. *Br J Clin Pharmacol* 1989;28:545–549.
259. Mackay TW, Fitzpatrick MF, Douglas NJ. Non-adrenergic, non-cholinergic nervous system and overnight airway calibre in asthmatic and normal subjects. *Lancet* 1991;338:1289–1292.
260. Morrison JFJ, Pearson SB, Dean HG, Craig IR, Bramley PN. Platelet activation in nocturnal asthma. *Thorax* 1991;46:197–200.
261. Joad JP, Ahrens RC, Lindgren SD, Weinberger MM. Relative efficacy of maintenance therapy with theophylline, inhaled albuterol, and the combination for chronic asthma. *J Allergy Clin Immunol* 1987;79:78–85.
262. Dahl R, Pedersen B, Hagglof B. Nocturnal asthma: effect of treatment with oral sustained-release terbutaline, inhaled budesonide, and the two in combination. *J Allergy Clin Immunol* 1989;83:811–815.
263. Williams AJ, Lee TH, Cochrane GM, et al. Attenuation of nocturnal asthma by cromakalim. *Lancet* 1990;336:334–336.
264. Fairfax AJ, McNabb WR, Davies HJ, Spiro SG. Slow-release oral salbutamol and aminophylline in nocturnal asthma: relation of overnight changes in lung function and plasma drug levels. *Thorax* 1980;35:526–530.
265. Westermann CJJ, Van Weelden BM, Laros CD. Sustained-release terbutaline in nocturnal asthma. *Allergy* 1986;41:308–310.
266. Stewart IC, Rhind GB, Power JT, Flenley DC, Douglas NJ. Effect of sustained release

terbutaline on symptoms and sleep quality in patients with nocturnal asthma. *Thorax* 1987;42:797–800.

267. Postma DS, Koeter GH, Keyzer JJ, Meurs M. Influence of slow-release terbutaline on the circadian variation of catecholamines, histamine, and lung function in nonallergic patients with partly reversible airflow obstruction. *J Allergy Clin Immunol* 1986; 77:471–477.

268. Maesen FPV, Smeets JJ, Gubbelmans HLL, Zweers PGMA. Formoterol in the treatment of nocturnal asthma. *Chest* 1990;98:866–870.

269. Wallin A, Melander B, Rosenhall L, Sandsrtom T, Wahlander L. Formoterol, a new long acting beta2 agonist for inhalation twice daily, compared with salbutamol in the treatment of asthma. *Thorax* 1990;45:259–261.

270. Kesten S, Chapman KR, Broder I, et al. A three-month comparison of twice daily inhaled formoterol versus four daily inhaled albuterol in the management of asthma. *Am Rev Respir Dis* 1991;144:622–625.

271. Ullman A, Hedner J, Svedmyr N. Inhaled salmeterol and salbutamol in asthmatic patients. An evaluation of asthma symptoms and the possible development of tachyphylaxis. *Am Rev Respir Dis* 1990;142:571–575.

272. Fitzpatrick MF, Mackay T, Driver H, Douglas NJ. Salmeterol in nocturnal asthma: a double blind, placebo controlled trial of a long acting β_2 agonist. *Br Med J* 1990; 301:1365–1368.

273. Sarin S, Shami S, Cheatle T. Salmeterol in nocturnal asthma. *Br Med J* 1991;302:347 (letter).

274. Costello J. Asthma—the problem and the paradox. *Postgrad Med J* 1991;67 (suppl 4):S1–S5.

275. Paterson JW, Lulich KM, Goldie RG. Drug effects on beta-adrenoceptor function in asthma. In: Morley J ed. *Perspectives in asthma: beta-adrenoceptors in asthma,* vol 2. New York: Academic Press, 1984;245–268.

276. Conolly ME, Davies DS, Dollery CT, George CF. Resistance to β-adrenoceptor stimulants, a possible explanation for the rise in asthma deaths. *Br J Pharmacol* 1971; 43:389–402.

277. Holgate ST, Baldwin CJ, Tattersfield AF. β-adrenergic agonist resistance in normal human airways. *Lancet* 1977;2:375–377.

278. Harvey JE, Tattersfield AE. Airway response to salbutamol: effect of regular salbutamol inhalations in normal, atopic, and asthmatic subjects. *Thorax* 1982;37:280–287.

279. Peel ET, Gibson GJ. Effects of long-term inhaled salbutamol therapy on the provocation of asthma by histamine. *Am Rev Respir Dis* 1980;121:973–978.

280. Larsson S, Svedmyr N, Thiringer G. Lack of bronchial beta adrenoceptor resistance in asthmatics during long-term treatment with terbutaline. *J Allergy Clin Immunol* 1977;59:93–100.

281. Arvidsson P, Larsson S, Lofdahl C-G, et al. Inhaled formoterol during one year in asthma: a comparison with salbutamol. *Eur Respir J* 1991;4:1168–1173.

282. Gibson GJ, Greenacre JK, Konig P, Conolly ME, Pride NB. Use of exercise challenge to investigate possible tolerance to beta-adrenoceptor stimulation in asthma. *Br J Dis Chest* 1978;72:199–206.

283. Conolly ME, Tashkin DP, Hui KKP, Littner MR, Wolfe R. Selective subsensitization of beta-adrenergic receptors in central airways of asthmatics and normal subjects during long-term therapy with inhaled salbutamol. *J Allergy Clin Immunol* 1982;70:423–431.

284. Vathenen AS, Knox AJ, Higgins BG, et al. Rebound increase in bronchial responsiveness after treatment with inhaled terbutaline. *Lancet* 1988;1:554–558.

285. van Schayck CP, Graafsma SJ, Visch MB, Dompeling E, van Weel C, van Herwaarden CLA. Increased bronchial hyperresponsiveness after inhaling salbutamol during 1 year is not caused by subsensitization to salbutamol. *J Allergy Clin Immunol* 1990;86:793–800.

286. Haahtela T, Jarvinen M, Kava T, et al. Comparison of a β_2-agonist, terbutaline, with an inhaled corticosteroid, budesonide, in newly detected asthma. *N Engl J Med* 1991;325:388–392.

287. Kerribijn FF, Van Essen-Zandvliet EEM, Neijens JH. Effect of long term treatment

with inhaled corticosteroids and beta-agonists on the bronchial responsiveness in children with asthma. *J Allergy Clin Immunol* 1987;79:653–659.
288. Raes M, Mulder P, Kerrebijn KF. Long-term effect of ipratropium bromide and fenoterol on the bronchial hyperresponsiveness to asthma in children with asthma. *J Allergy Clin Immunol* 1989;84:874–879.
289. Waalkens HJ, Gerritsen J, Koeter GH, Krouwels FH, van Aalderen WMC, Knol K. Budesonide and terbutaline or terbutaline alone in children with mild asthma: effects on bronchial hyperresponsiveness and diurnal variation in peak flow. *Thorax* 1991; 46:499–503.
290. Boulet L-P, Cartier A, Thomson NC, Roberts RS, Dolovich J, Hargreave FE. Asthma and increases in nonallergic bronchial responsiveness from seasonal pollen exposure. *J Allergy Clin Immunol* 1983;71:399–406.
291. Sotomayor H, Badier M, Vervloet D, Orehek J. Seasonal increase of carbachol airway responsiveness in patients allergic to grass pollen. Reversal by corticosteroids. *Am Rev Respir Dis* 1984;130:56–58.
292. Mitchell EA. Is current treatment increasing asthma mortality and morbidity? *Thorax* 1989;44:81–84.
293. van Schayck CP, Dompeling E, van Herwaarden CLA, et al. Bronchodilator treatment in moderate asthma or chronic bronchitis: continuous or on demand? A randomised controlled study. *Br Med J* 1991;303:1426–1431.
294. Shepherd GL, Hetzel MR, Clark TJH. Regular versus symptomatic aerosol bronchodilator treatment of asthma. *Br J Dis Chest* 1981;75:215–217.
295. Beswick KBJ, Pover GM, Sampson S. Long term regularly inhaled salbutamol. *Curr Med Res Opin* 1986;10:228–234.
296. Vandewalker ML, Kray KT, Weber RW, Nelson HS. Addition of terbutaline to optimal theophylline therapy. Double blind crossover study in asthmatic patients. *Chest* 1986;90:198–203.
297. Marin JM, Carrizo S, Ejea MV. Effects of beta$_2$-agonist in asthma prescribed in "a fixed" regimen or "as needed." *Eur Respir J* 1991;4 (suppl 14):198s (abstract).
298. Patakas D, Maniki E, Tsara V, Daskalopoulou E. Intermittent and continuous salbutamol rotacaps inhalation in asthmatic patients. *Respiration* 1988;54:174–178.
299. Sears MR, Taylor DR, Print GG, et al. Regular inhaled beta agonist treatment in bronchial asthma. *Lancet* 1990;336:1391–1396.
300. Nelson HS, Szefler SJ, Martins RJ. Regular inhaled beta-adrenergic agonists in the treatment of bronchial asthma: beneficial or detrimental? *Am Rev Respir Dis* 1991; 144:249–250.
301. Dahl R, Earnshaw JS, Palmer JBD. Salmeterol: a four week study of a long-acting beta-adrenoceptor agonist for the treatment of reversible airways disease. *Eur Respir J* 1991;4:1178–1184.
302. Kesten S, Chapman KR, Broder I, et al. A three-month comparison of twice daily inhaled formoterol versus four daily inhaled albuterol in the management of asthma. *Am Rev Respir Dis* 1991;144:622–625.
303. Jackson RT, Beaglehole R, Rea HH, Sutherland DC. Mortality from asthma: a new epidemic in New Zealand. *Br Med J* 1982;285:771–774.
304. Crane S, Pearce N, Flatt A, et al. Prescribed fenoterol and death from asthma in New Zealand 1981–1983: case controlled study. *Lancet* 1989;1:917–922.
305. Wilson JD, Sutherland DC, Thomas AC. Has the change to beta-agonists combined with oral theophylline increased cases of fatal asthma? *Lancet* 1981;2:1235–1237.
306. Grant IWB. Asthma in New Zealand. *Br Med J* 1983;286:374–377.
307. Sears MR, Rea HH, Fenwick J, et al. 75 deaths in asthmatics prescribed home nebulisers. *Br Med J* 1987;294:477–480.
308. Sears MR, Rea HH, Beaglehole R, et al. Asthma mortality in New Zealand: a two year national study. *N Z Med J* 1985;98:271–275.
309. Sears MR, Rea HH, Rothwell RPG, et al. Asthma mortality: comparison between New Zealand and England. *Br Med J* 1986;293:1342–1345.
310. Rea HH, Scragg R, Jackson R, Beaglehole R, Fenwick J, Sutherland DC. A case-controlled study of deaths from asthma. *Thorax* 1986;41:833–839.
311. O'Donnell TV, Rea HH, Holst PE, Sears MR. Fenoterol and fatal asthma. *Lancet* 1989;1:1070–1071 (letter).

312. Buist AS, Burney PGJ, Feinstein AR, et al. Fenoterol and fatal asthma. *Lancet* 1989;1:1071 (letter).
313. Poole C, Lanes SF, Walker AM. Fenoterol and fatal asthma. *Lancet* 1990;335:920 (letter).
314. Pearce N, Grainger J, Atkinson M, et al. Case-control study of prescribed fenoterol and death from asthma in New Zealand, 1977–81. *Thorax* 1990;45:170–175.
315. Grainger J, Woodman K, Pearce N, et al. Prescribed fenoterol and death from asthma in New Zealand, 1981–7: a further case-control study. *Thorax* 1991;46:105–111.
316. Spitzer WO, Suissa S, Ernst P, et al. A nested case-control of the relation between beta-agonists and death and near-death from asthma. *N Engl J Med* 1992;326:501–506.
317. Morley J, Sanjar S, Newth C. Viewpoint: untoward effects of beta-adrenoceptor agonists in asthma. *Eur Respir J* 1990;3:228–233.
318. Page CP. One explanation of the asthma paradox: inhibition of natural anti-inflammatory mechanism by β_2-agonists. *Lancet* 1991;337:717–720.
319. Sanjar S, Kristersson A, Mazzoni L, Morley J, Schaeublin E. Increased airway reactivity in the guinea pig follows exposure to intravenous isoprenaline. *J Physiol* 1990;425:43–54.
320. Chapman ID, Buchheit KH, Manley P, Morley J. Active enantiomers may cause adverse effects in asthma. *Trends Pharmacol Sci* 1992;13:231–232 (letter).
321. Kean WF, Lock CJL, Howard-Lock HE. Chirality in antirheumatic drugs. *Lancet* 1991;338:1565–1568.
322. Lulich KM, Goldie RG, Ryan G, Paterson JW. Adverse reactions to β_2-agonist bronchodilators. *Med Toxicol* 1986;1:286–299.
323. Vick RL, Todd EP, Luedke DW. Epinephrine-induced hypokalaemia: relation to liver and skeletal muscle. *J Pharmacol Exp Ther* 1972;181:139–146.
324. Buur T, Clausen T, Holmberg E, et al. Desensitization by terbutaline of beta-adrenoceptors in the guinea-pig soleus muscle: biochemical alterations associated with functional change. *Br J Pharmacol* 1982;76:313–317.
325. Smith SR, Kendall MJ. Metabolic responses to beta2 stimulants. *J R Coll Physicians Lond* 1984;18:190–194.
326. Paterson JW, Woolcock AJ, Shenfield GM. Bronchodilator drugs. *Am Rev Respir Dis* 1979;120:1149–1188.

Drugs and the Lung,
edited by C.P. Page and W.J. Metzger.
Raven Press, Ltd., New York © 1994

2

Anticholinergic Therapy

Peter J. Barnes

Department of Thoracic Medicine, National Heart and Lung Institute,
Royal Brompton Hospital, London SW3 6LY, United Kingdom

Cholinergic antagonists are now widely used in the treatment of chronic obstructive pulmonary disease (COPD) and have proved to be useful additional bronchodilators in the management of asthma. The theoretical rationale for their use is discussed and some of the new developments in cholinergic pharmacology that may throw new light on understanding the pathophysiology of obstructive airway disease are described in this chapter.

CHOLINERGIC CONTROL OF AIRWAYS

Cholinergic nerve fibers arise in the nucleus ambiguus and dorsal motor nucleus of the vagus of the brain stem (1) and travel down the vagus nerve to relay in parasympathetic ganglia that are located within the airway wall (2–4). From these ganglia short postganglionic fibers travel to airway smooth muscle and submucosal glands (Fig. 1). In animals, electrical stimulation of the vagus nerve causes release of acetylcholine from cholinergic nerve terminals, with activation of muscarinic cholinergic receptors on smooth muscle and gland cells, which results in bronchoconstriction and mucus secretion (5). Prior administration of a muscarinic receptor antagonist, such as atropine, prevents vagally induced bronchoconstriction.

Cholinergic innervation is greatest in large airways and diminishes peripherally (6,7). Studies in animals have demonstrated that cholinergic nerve effects are greatest in large airways and minimal in small airways. Receptor mapping studies have demonstrated a high density of muscarinic receptors in smooth muscle of large airways, but few in peripheral airways of ferrets (8,9), although in human airways muscarinic receptors are also seen in peripheral airways (10). In humans, studies that have tried to distinguish large and small airway effects have shown that cholinergic bronchoconstriction predominantly involves larger airways, whereas β-agonists are equally effective in large and small airways (11). This relative diminution of cholin-

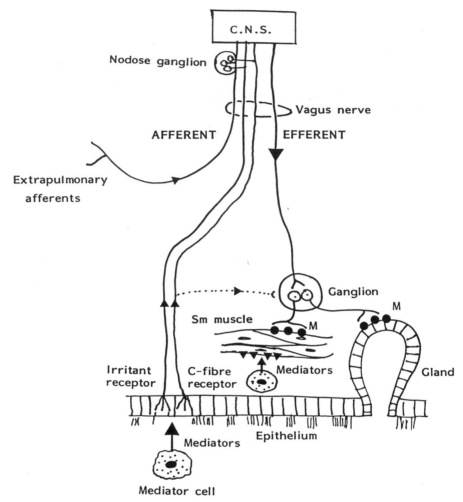

FIG. 1. Cholinergic neural pathways. Efferent cholinergic nerves arise in the brain stem and synapse in ganglia situated in the airway wall itself. Short postganglionic nerve fibers innervate target cells in the airways via activation of muscarinic receptors. Cholinergic nerves may be activated via reflex mechanisms triggered from afferent nerves in the airway.

ergic control in small airways may have important clinical implications, since anticholinergic drugs are likely to be less useful than β-agonists when bronchoconstriction involves small airways.

In animals, there is a certain degree of resting bronchomotor tone caused by tonic parasympathetic activity (5). This tone can be reversed by atropine and enhanced by administration of an inhibitor of acetylcholinesterase (which normally rapidly inactivates acetylcholine released from nerve terminals). Normal human subjects also have resting bronchomotor tone, since atropine causes bronchodilatation (12) and inhalation of the acetylcholines-terase inhibitor edrophonium results in bronchoconstriction (13).

MUSCARINIC RECEPTORS

Cholinergic effects on the airways are mediated by muscarinic receptors on target cells in the airways (14,15). More is now known about muscarinic receptor structure, and muscarinic receptors have now been cloned (16,17). Recently, several different subtypes of muscarinic receptor have been distin-guished, raising the possibility of developing more selective acetylcholi-nergic agents (see below). In the airways, smooth muscle muscarinic recep-tor activation results in rapid phosphoinositide hydrolysis (18–21) and the formation of inositol 1,4,5-trisphosphate, which releases calcium ions from intracellular stores. Muscarinic receptor activation also inhibits adenylyl cy-clase and therefore reduces adenosine $3',5'$-cyclic monophosphate (cAMP) in airway smooth muscle (22), which may therefore counteract the broncho-dilator effects of β-agonists (Fig. 2).

Muscarinic receptors mediate the mucus secretory response to vagus nerve stimulation. Cholinergic agonists are potent secretagogues and stim-

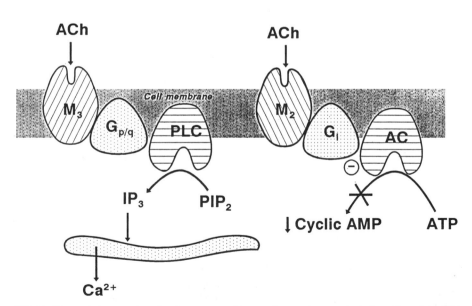

FIG. 2. Muscarinic receptors in airway smooth muscle may be coupled via a G-protein (G_q) to phosphoinositide hydrolysis to intracellular calcium ion release (M_3-receptor) or via G_i to inhibition of adenylyl cyclase (M_2-receptor).

ulate mucus secretion from submucosal glands (23) and also from goblet cells in the epithelium, which are the major source of mucus in peripheral airways (24).

REFLEX BRONCHOCONSTRICTION

A wide variety of stimuli are able to elicit reflex cholinergic bronchoconstriction (25). Sensory afferent endings, which include irritant receptors and unmyelinated nerve endings (C fibers), are found in airway epithelium, larynx, and nasopharynx (26,27). Sensory receptors may be triggered by many stimuli, including dust, cigarette smoke, mechanical stimulation, and chemical mediators such as histamine, prostaglandins, and bradykinin, which will lead to reflex bronchoconstriction. Reflex bronchoconstriction may be inhibited by anticholinergic drugs. These drugs may therefore have a variable effect on airway obstruction, which will be dependent on the degree of cholinergic reflex bronchoconstriction.

CHOLINERGIC MECHANISMS IN AIRWAY DISEASE

Since cholinergic nerves are the predominant neural bronchoconstrictor mechanism, it is not surprising that they are involved in obstructive diseases of the airways.

Asthma

Because many of the stimuli that produce bronchospasm in asthma are known to activate sensory receptors and reflex bronchoconstriction in animals, it was logical to suggest that asthma may be due to exaggerated cholinergic reflex mechanisms (5). There are several mechanisms by which cholinergic tone might be increased in asthma. An increase in cholinergic tone could arise because of increased afferent receptor stimulation by inflammatory mediators, such as histamine or prostaglandins, which may be released from mast cells and other inflammatory cells in the asthmatic airway or from bradykinin formed from precursors in exuded plasma. Mediators may also increase the release of acetylcholine from cholinergic nerve terminals by an action on cholinergic nerve endings themselves, or by an increase in nerve traffic through cholinergic ganglia (28). Theoretically cholinergic nerve contraction may be increased if bronchodilator neural mechanisms are diminished in asthma as a result of inflammation. Nitric oxide (NO) is the major transmitter of bronchodilator nerves in human airways (29,30) and inhibition of NO synthesis results in exaggerated cholinergic neural responses in both animal and human airways (31–33). NO may be degraded more rapidly in asthma by the effects of superoxide anions released from inflammatory cells in the airways, thus resulting in exaggerated cholinergic bronchoconstriction.

The effect of acetylcholine on asthmatic airways is also exaggerated, as a manifestation of nonspecific hyperresponsiveness of the airways, which is so characteristic of asthma. All these considerations suggest that cholinergic mechanisms may contribute to bronchospasm of asthmatic airways, and this would imply that acetylcholinergic drugs would be valuable in treating asthma. However, asthmatic airways are hyperresponsive to many spasmogens in addition to acetylcholine; mediators such as histamine, leukotrienes, and prostaglandins have a direct contractile effect on bronchial smooth muscle, which is not blocked by anticholinergic drugs. Anticholinergic agents will only counteract the cholinergic reflex component of bronchoconstriction, which may be less prominent in human airways than animal studies had indicated. By contrast, β_2-agonists reverse bronchoconstriction irrespective of the mechanism, since they act as functional antagonists.

Airway obstruction in asthma may be due to more than spasm of airway smooth muscle. In severe asthma there may be edema of the airway wall and extravasation of plasma into the airway lumen as a result of increased permeability of bronchial vessels (34). It is unlikely that anticholinergic agents could have any effect on this leakiness and therefore would not have the capacity to reverse this element of bronchial obstruction.

Although anticholinergics are less effective than β_2-agonists as bronchodilators in chronic asthma, several studies suggest that they may be almost as effective in acute exacerbations (35–37), indicating that cholinergic bronchoconstriction is the major component of airway narrowing in asthma attacks (and, by implication, in fatal asthma). In patients with chronic asthma that has been poorly controlled, there is a progressive decline in lung function over the years (38,39), which presumably results from chronic inflammation. Vagal tone increases the airway narrowing further, and for the reasons discussed below, will have a greater effect on airway resistance in narrowed airways. This may explain why anticholinergics are often of greater use in chronic asthmatics with a major element of fixed airway obstruction.

Chronic Obstructive Pulmonary Disease

In COPD there is irreversible structural narrowing of airways. In chronic obstructive bronchitis this appears to be a combination of fibrosis, particularly in peripheral airways and mucus hyperplasia, whereas in emphysema it is due to closure of peripheral airways due to loss of elastic recoil provided by the alveolar wall attachments. In addition, there is a degree of vagal bronchomotor tone. While in normal airways this tone has little effect on airway caliber, when the airways are narrowed the same degree of tone will have a much more marked effect on airway resistance (which is proportional to the fourth power on the radius). Reversing this tone by anticholinergic drugs will, therefore, have a significant beneficial effect (Fig. 3). The relative benefit of anticholinergic drugs is likely to be greater in COPD than in asthma, in which additional factors (such as direct effects of mediators and mucosal edema) are likely to be operative. There is some variability in airway function in patients with COPD, and there is evidence that anticholinergics reduce this variability, which may suggest that changes in vagal cholinergic tone are the major determinant of this variability (40). Anticholinergics are as effective as β_2-agonists in exacerbations of COPD, indicating that, as in asthmatic patients, the major component of increased airway obstruction is due to an increase in cholinergic tone (41).

Anticholinergic drugs usually cause bronchodilatation in normal subjects, asthmatics, and COPD patients. The extent of bronchodilatation is variable

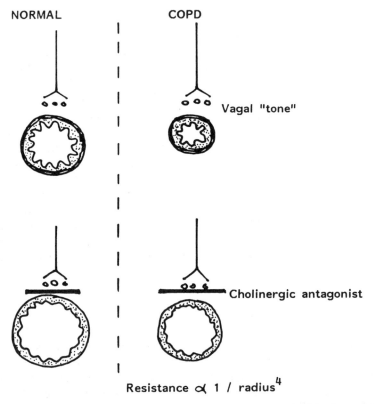

FIG. 3. Normal airways have a certain amount of cholinergic tone, resulting in a small degree of airway narrowing, which is revealed by a small bronchodilator response to anticholinergics. In COPD, in which there is fixed narrowing of the airways, the same amount of cholinergic tone will have a greater effect on airway resistance for geometric reasons. Conversely anticholinergics will have a relatively greater bronchodilator effect. In COPD, cholinergic tone may be the only reversible component of airway narrowing.

between individuals, which presumably reflects the degree of vagal tone. Anticholinergic drugs are competitive antagonists of acetylcholine, so the bronchodilator effect is related to the dose given until maximal blockade of endogenous acetylcholine is obtained. In asthmatic patients the degree of bronchodilatation seen in anticholinergic drugs is less marked than with β-agonists (which will relax airway smooth muscle irrespective of the constrictor stimuli). This may demonstrate that airway narrowing in asthma is due to more factors than vagal tone alone. In COPD, however, anticholinergics may produce equivalent or even greater bronchodilatation than β-agonists, since vagal tone is the major reversible element in such patients (42). Although the onset of bronchodilatation after ancicholinergic drugs may be slower than after a β-agonist, the duration of bronchodilatation may be greater than 8 h and therefore significantly longer than conventional inhaled $β_2$-agonists such as salbutamol (43). This may be used to advantage when the two drugs are used in combination.

Anticholinergics appear to be at least as effective as β-agonists in COPD patients (44), and often a greater improvement has been reported with anticholinergics (45,46), although very few studies have investigated dose-response relationships. The mechanisms by which anticholinergics may have a greater effect on airway function in COPD is uncertain, since if cholinergic tone were the only reversible component it may be predicted that $β_2$-agonists would be equally effective in inhibiting cholinergic tone. Perhaps anticholinergics might have a greater effect than β-agonists in COPD because of some additional effect on mucus secretion. Cholinergic agonists are potent stimulants of mucus secretion in human airways *in vitro* (43,47), and act predominantly on submucosal glands, which are the major source of mucus in proximal airways. In more peripheral airways the only source of airway mucus is epithelial goblet cells, and there is evidence in animals that these are under cholinergic control (24). In addition cigarette smoke is a potent stimulus to goblet cell discharge in animals and the effects of the particulate phase are mediated by a cholinergic reflex (48). If the same applies to human airways, it is possible that inhaled anticholinergics reduce goblet cell secretions and thereby improve the airway obstruction in peripheral airways.

The prolonged duration of bronchodilatation compared with β-agonists may be of advantage in these patients. It is likely that the fall in lung function that occurs at night in patients with COPD (49) may also benefit from high-dose anticholinergic drugs given at night, since an increase in vagal tone is the most likely mechanism for the increased nocturnal bronchoconstriction (50,51).

MUSCARINIC RECEPTOR SUBTYPES

With the development of selective drugs, subclasses of muscarinic receptors have now been demonstrated in many tissues (52,53). Receptor subtypes have now been cloned and expressed, and at least five distinct receptor proteins have now been recognized in animal and human tissues (52).

Three distinct subtypes of receptor have now been recognized pharmacologically. M_1-receptors are pirenzepine-sensitive and are usually localized to neuronal structures. M_2-receptors are present in atrium and mediate the heart-rate slowing with cholinergic stimulation. M_2-receptors are selectively blocked by AF-DX 116, methoctramine, or gallamine, and are different from muscarinic receptors on smooth muscle (M_3-receptors), which are sensitive to 4-diphenylocetoxy-*N*-methyl-piperidine methiodide (4-DAMP) and hexahydro-siladifenidol. All three muscarinic receptor subtypes have now been described in airways (15,54–56), but their precise relevance to airway disease and therapy is not yet certain (Fig. 4).

M_1-Receptors

The discovery that the muscarinic antagonist pirenzepine was able to discriminate between high- and low-affinity muscarinic receptor binding sites (57) supported previous suggestions that subtypes of muscarinic receptor might exist. Receptors with a high affinity for pirenzepine, which are designated M_1-receptors, are found in cerebral cortex and autonomic ganglia, in contrast to lower-affinity receptors, which predominate in heart and smooth muscle (M_2-receptors). Pirenzepine is used clinically to reduce gastric acid secretion and, while it was previously believed to act directly on acid-secreting cells, it is now clear that it acts predominantly on ganglia in the stom-

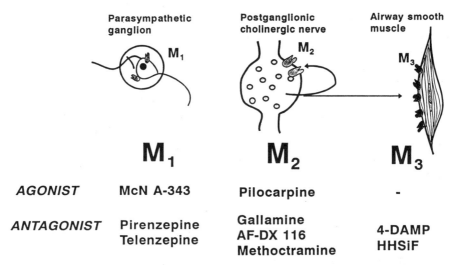

FIG. 4. Muscarinic receptor subtypes.

ach to inhibit neurally mediated gastric secretion (58). Since the innervation of the airways is derived embryologically from that of the gut, it seems likely that excitatory M_1-receptors might also exist in airway ganglia. There appear to be considerable species differences in the location of muscarinic receptors in pulmonary nerves, however. *In vitro,* pirenzepine has a low affinity for acetylcholine-induced contraction of rabbit airways (59) and for binding of the nonselective antagonist [³H]quinuclidinyl benzilate (QNB) to bovine airways (18,60), suggesting that M_1-receptors are not present in airway smooth muscle. Similarly, pirenzepine is only weakly effective in inhibiting cholinergic agonist-stimulated phosphoinositide turnover in bovine airway smooth muscle (18,60).

Pirenzepine is a bronchodilator when given intravenously to human subjects (61), although at the dose used it might be acting nonselectively and blocking smooth muscle muscarinic receptors. A recent study has shown that lower doses of intravenous pirenzepine, while having no effect on forced expiratory volume in 1 sec (FEV_1), increases expired flow at low lung volumes, suggesting an effect on more peripheral airways (62). This might be consistent with the existence of M_1-receptors in peripheral but not central human airways.

Recent evidence suggests that M_1-receptors may also be present in human airway cholinergic nerves. The effects of inhaled pirenzepine and ipratropium bromide were studied on cholinergic reflex bronchoconstriction triggered by the inhalation of the irritant gas, sulfur dioxide, in allergic volunteers (63). A dose of inhaled pirenzepine was found that did not inhibit bronchoconstriction due to an inhaled cholinergic agonist (methacholine), whereas ipratropium bromide was able to block the bronchoconstrictor effect. The same dose of pirenzepine, however, was as effective as ipratropium bromide in blocking cholinergic reflex bronchoconstriction and, since it could not be acting directly on airway smooth muscle receptors, it might be acting on some peripheral part of the cholinergic pathway, which is most likely to be parasympathetic ganglia in the airways (Fig. 5). In support of this possibility, pirenzepine has been shown to depress cholinergic ganglionic neurotransmission in rabbit bronchi *in vitro* (64).

The physiological role of the M_1-receptors in ganglia is still not certain. Classically, ganglionic transmission is via nicotinic cholinergic receptors, which are blocked by hexamethonium. It is possible that excitatory M_1-receptors are facilitatory to nicotinic receptors and may be involved in "setting" the efficacy of ganglionic transmission. Activation of these receptors probably closes K^+ channels, resulting in a slow depolarization of the ganglion cell (65). Perhaps they might be involved in the chronic regulation of cholinergic tone, whereas nicotinic receptors (which act as "fast" receptors and open ion channels) are more important in rapid signaling, such as occurs during reflex activation of the cholinergic pathway. If so, then M_1-antagonists such as pirenzepine and telenzepine might have a useful therapeutic role in asthma and COPD, since they may reduce vagal tone. Since increased

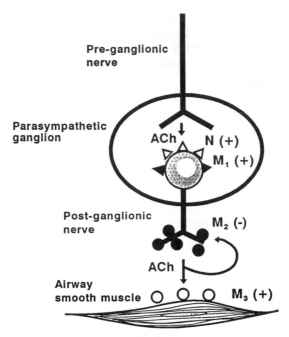

FIG. 5. Muscarinic receptor subtypes in airways. Ganglionic transmission is mediated via nicotinic receptors (N), but M_1-receptors may play a facilitatory role. M_2-receptors at the post-ganglionic terminal may inhibit the release of acetylcholine (ACh), which acts on M_3-receptors on airway smooth muscle.

vagal tone may play a crucial role in nocturnal exacerbations of asthma, pirenzepine might prove to be efficacious in preventing nocturnal wheeze.

The results of binding studies in lung are unexpected. Binding of [³H]QNB to both rabbit and human peripheral lung membranes is displaced by pirenzepine with a shallow inhibitory curve, suggesting the presence of high- and low-affinity sites (66–68). The high-affinity binding site has the characteristic expected of a M_1-receptor and this is confirmed by the use of [³H]pirenzepine to label the receptors (68). M_1-receptors make up more than half of the binding sites in lung of both species, which cannot be accounted for by receptors on airway ganglia or nerves, as they would make up only a small fraction of the membranes. Autoradiographic mapping studies suggest that M_1-receptors in human airways are present on submucosal glands, and are also seen in alveolar walls (10). These autoradiographic studies have recently been supported by *in situ* hybridization studies using complementary deoxyribonucleic acid (cDNA) and oligonucleotide probes, which hybridize to the specific messenger RNA (mRNA) encoded by the genes for the different muscarinic receptor subtypes (69). In human lung M_1-receptor mRNA is localized to submucosal glands and to alveolar walls, whereas in rabbit lung the muscarinic receptors localized to the peripheral lung appear to belong to the M_4-receptor subtype (70), which corresponds with recent functional data in this species (71).

M_2-Receptors

Muscarinic receptors, which inhibit the release of acetylcholine from cholinergic nerves, have been described in the gut (72). Such muscarinic autoreceptors have also been described in the airways, which are inhibited by gallamine and are therefore classified as M_2-receptors, thus differing from the muscarinic receptor subtypes on airway smooth muscle (M_3-receptors) (28). These muscarinic receptors appear to be located prejunctionally on postganglionic parasympathetic nerves (73) and have a powerful inhibitory influence on acetylcholine release (Fig. 5). Muscarinic autoreceptors have been demonstrated in guinea pig (74–76), cat (77), rat (78), and dog (79,80). The presence of prejunctional M_2-receptors on airway cholinergic nerves has recently been confirmed in guinea pig trachea by direct measurement of acetylcholine release (72,81).

Recently, similar feedback inhibitory receptors have also been localized to postganglionic cholinergic nerves in human airways *in vitro* (75). In normal subjects pilocarpine, which selectively stimulates the prejunctional receptors, has an inhibitory effect on cholinergic reflex bronchoconstriction induced by sulfur dioxide (SO_2), suggesting that these inhibitory receptors are present *in vivo,* and presumably serve to limit cholinergic bronchoconstriction (82). Other evidence now also supports this observation (83). In asthmatic patients pilocarpine has no such inhibitory action, indicating that there might be some dysfunction of the autoreceptor that would result in exaggerated cholinergic reflex bronchoconstriction (82,84) (Fig. 5). A functional defect in muscarinic autoreceptors may also explain why β-blockers produce such marked bronchoconstriction in asthmatic patients, since any increase in cholinergic tone due to blockade of inhibitory β-receptors on cholinergic nerves would normally be switched off by M_2-receptors in the nerves, and a lack of such receptors may lead to increased acetylcholine release, resulting in exaggerated bronchoconstriction (85). Support for this idea is provided by the protective effect of oxitropium bromide against propranolol-induced bronchoconstriction in asthmatic patients (86).

The mechanism by which M_2-autoreceptors on cholinergic nerves may become dysfunctional is not certain. It is possible that chronic inflammation in airways may lead to down-regulation of M_2-receptors, which may have an important functional effect if the density of prejunctional muscarinic receptors is relatively low. Recently experimental studies have demonstrated that influenza virus may inactivate M_2- rather than M_3-receptors (87,88). This finding may be related to the action of viral neuraminidase on sialic acid residues of M_2-receptors (89), and provides a possible explanation for increased airway reactivity after influenza infections. There is also evidence that the eosinophil cationic major basic protein may selectively impair M_2-receptor function through an allosteric effect (90). Reactive oxygen species released in the acute inflammatory reaction may also result in impaired M_2-receptor function, and this could be important in acute exacerbations of asthma, when cholinergic bronchoconstriction apparently increases (Fig. 6).

Although the bronchoconstrictor responses to cholinergic agonists appear to involve the activation of M_3-receptors leading to phosphoinositide hydrolysis, binding studies have indicated a high proportion of M_2-receptors in airway smooth muscle (91). This has been confirmed in cultured human airway smooth muscle cells using cDNA probes to the human M_2-receptor (69). Recently it has been established that these M_2-receptors have a functional role in counteracting the bronchodilator response to β-agonists, both *in vitro* (92) and *in vivo* (93). These M_2-receptors may be coupled to a large conductance potassium channel (K_{Ca}) via G_1, resulting in closure of the channel (94). In this way M_2-receptor activation may lead to functional antagonism of β-agonist–induced opening of the same channel (95) (Fig. 2).

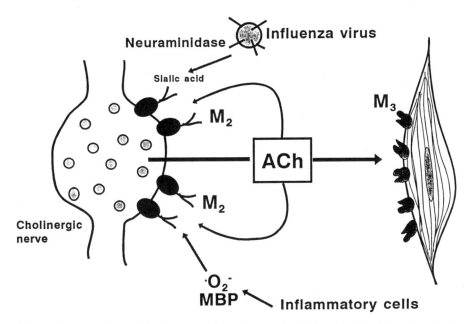

FIG. 6. There may be a defect in muscarinic autoreceptors in bronchoconstriction. This may be due to impaired function of M_2-receptors in response to neuraminidase from viruses, superoxide anions from inflammatory cells, or from eosinophil basic proteins, such as major basic protein (MBP).

M_3-Receptors

Muscarinic receptors on airway smooth muscle are sensitive to 4-DAMP and hexahydro-siladifenidol and are therefore classified as M_3-receptors. Binding studies in guinea pig and human lung membranes indicate the presence of M_3-receptors (68). Autoradiographic studies have demonstrated M_3-receptors in airway smooth muscle of large and small human airways (10), and this has been confirmed by *in situ* hybridization studies with M_3-selective cDNA probes (69).

M_3-receptors are also localized to submucosal glands in human airways, which appear to have a mixed population of M_1- and M_3-receptors in a proportion of 1:2 (10). This is consistent with functional studies that have demonstrated a secretory response to cholinergic agonists that is intermediate between an M_1- and M_3-receptor–mediated response (96,97).

M_4- and M_5-Receptors

In rabbit lung there is evidence from binding studies for the existence of an M_4-receptor and this has been confirmed by the presence of m_4-receptor mRNA on Northern blotting (71). *In situ* hybridization has demonstrated that this m_4-receptor mRNA is localized to alveolar walls, and vascular and airway smooth muscle (70). There is preliminary evidence that the muscarinic autoreceptor on guinea pig airway cholinergic nerves belongs to the M_4-receptor subtype (98). In human lung Northern analysis has not revealed any evidence of either m_4- or m_5-receptor mRNA and *in situ* hybridization has not revealed any evidence for expression of these receptor subtypes (69).

Clinical Relevance of Receptor Subtypes

The discovery of at least three muscarinic subtypes in lung has important clinical implications, since it raises the possibility of more selective anticholinergic therapy in the future. Atropine, ipratropium bromide, and oxitropium bromide are nonselective as anticholinergic drugs and therefore block prejunctional (M_2) and postjunctional (M_3) receptors. Inhibition of the autoreceptor means that more acetylcholine will be released during cholinergic nerve stimulation and this may overcome postjunctional blockade, thus making these nonselective antagonists less efficient than a selective antagonist of M_3-receptors. Direct evidence for this is the increase in acetylcholine release on nerve stimulation, which occurs in the presence of atropine (99,100), and the fact that ipratropium bromide in low doses causes an increase in vagally mediated bronchoconstriction (74). A similar analogy exists with α-adrenoceptors and the nonselective antagonist phentolamine, by acting on a prejunctional α_2-receptor, increases noradrenaline release and is thus far less effective in the treatment of high blood pressure than a selective α_1-antagonist such as prazosin, which acts only on the postjunctional receptor. Unfortunately, muscarinic drugs with the high selectivity shown by prazosin for postjunctional receptors are not yet available for clinical use.

Blockade of muscarinic autoreceptors by drugs such as ipratropium bromide might account for some of the cases of paradoxical bronchoconstriction after inhaled anticholinergic drugs in patients with COPD (101). Presumably anticholinergic drugs selective for M_3-receptors may be more effective and should not have the same risk of precipitating paradoxical bronchoconstriction.

The demonstration of different muscarinic receptor subtypes in airways may have important clinical implications. Further elucidation of the physiological role for these receptor subtypes will depend on the development of more selective antagonists. Drugs such as methoctramine that have a high degree of selectivity for M_2-receptors are promising tools for elucidation of the role of muscarinic receptor subtypes, but drugs with a higher selectivity for M_3-receptors are likely to be most useful clinically in airway disease. Active efforts are under way to develop such selective drugs, but it has proved difficult to develop highly selective drugs, and this may be related to the fact that the binding site for acetylcholine is highly conserved between the different subtypes of muscarinic receptor (53). The most selective muscarinic antagonists, such as gallamine and methoctramine, appear to interact noncompetitively, possibly due to interaction with an allosteric site.

CLINICAL USE

Datura plants, which contain the muscarinic antagonist stramonium, were smoked for relief of asthma two centuries ago. Atropine, a related naturally occurring compound, was also introduced for treating asthma but, because these compounds had side effects, particularly drying of secretions, less soluble quaternary compounds, such as atropine methylnitrate and ipratropium bromide, were introduced. These compounds are topically active and are not significantly absorbed from the respiratory tract or from the gastrointestinal tract.

Clinical Application

In asthmatic subjects anticholinergic drugs are less effective as bronchodilators than β-agonists (42,43) and offer less efficient protection against various bronchial challenges, although their duration of action is significantly longer. These drugs may be more effective in older patients with asthma in whom there is an element of fixed airway obstruction. Nebulized anticholinergic drugs are effective in acute severe asthma, although they are less effective than β-agonists in this situation. Nevertheless, in the acute and chronic treatment of asthma anticholinergic drugs may have an additive effect with β-agonists and should therefore be considered when control of asthma is not adequate with β-agonists (35–37), particularly if there are problems with theophylline, or inhaled β-agonists give troublesome tremor in elderly patients. The time course of bronchodilatation with anticholinergic drugs is slower than with β-agonists, reaching a peak only 1 h after inhalation, but persisting for over 6 h.

In COPD anticholinergic drugs may be as effective as, or even superior to, β-agonists (44,45). Their relatively greater effect in chronic obstructive airways disease than in asthma may be explained by an inhibitory effect on vagal tone that, while not necessarily being increased in COPD, may be the only reversible element of airway obstruction that is exaggerated by geometric factors in a narrowed airway.

Ipratropium Bromide

Ipratropium bromide is the most widely used anticholinergic inhaler and is available as a metered dose inhaler (MDI) and nebulized preparation (102). The onset of bronchodilatation is relatively slow and is usually maximal 30 to 60 min after inhalation, but may persist for up to 8 h. It is usually given by MDI four times daily on a regular basis, rather than intermittently for symptom relief, in view of its slow onset of action.

Oxitropium Bromide

Oxitropium bromide is a new quaternary anticholinergic bronchodilator that is similar to ipratropium bromide in terms of receptor blockade (103). It is available in higher doses by inhalation and may therefore have a more prolonged effect. Thus, it may be useful in some patients with nocturnal asthma (50).

New Developments

For the reasons discussed above, there is now a search for more selective anticholinergics that block M_3-receptors or block M_3- and M_1-receptors (104). An M_1-receptor selective antagonist telenzepine, which has a longer duration of action than pirenzepine, has no useful effect on airway function in patients with COPD at doses that cause significant side effects such as dry mouth (105). Recently a novel anticholinergic tiotropium bromide (Ba 679) that has M_1- and M_3-selectivity by a more rapid off-rate from M_2-receptors has been described (106). Tiotropium has the particular advantage of a very long duration of action and in animal studies its bronchodilator effect persists for over 24 h. In preliminary clinical studies tiotropium also has a long duration of bronchodilatation in patients with COPD (107) and therefore represents an important advance in this class of drug.

SIDE EFFECTS

Inhaled anticholinergic drugs are usually well tolerated and there is no evidence for any decline in responsiveness with continued use. On stopping inhaled anticholinergics a small rebound increase in responsiveness has been described (108), but the clinical relevance of this is uncertain. Atropine has side effects that are dose related and are due to cholinergic antagonism in other systems, which may lead to dryness of the mouth, blurred vision, and urinary retention. Systemic side effects after ipratropium bromide are very uncommon because there is virtually no systemic absorption (43).

Effects on Mucus Secretion

Because cholinergic agonists stimulate mucus secretion there have been several studies of mucus secretion with anticholinergic drugs, as there has been concern that they may reduce secretion and lead to more viscous mucus. Atropine reduces mucociliary clearance in normal subjects and in patients with asthma and chronic bronchitis, but ipratropium bromide, even in high doses, has no detectable effect in either normal subjects or in patients with airway disease (109).

Taste

A significant unwanted effect is the unpleasant bitter taste of inhaled ipratropium, which may contribute to poor compliance with this drug.

Glaucoma

Nebulized ipratropium bromide may precipitate glaucoma in elderly patients due to a direct effect of the nebulized drug on the eye. This may be prevented by nebulization with a mouthpiece rather than a face mask.

Paradoxical Bronchoconstriction

There are several reports of paradoxical bronchoconstriction with ipratropium bromide, particularly when given nebulized. This is largely explained by the hypotonicity of the nebulized solution and by antibacterial additives, such as benzalkonium chloride and ethylenediamine-tetraacetic acid

(EDTA). Nebulized solutions free of these problems are less likely to cause bronchoconstriction (110). Occasionally, bronchoconstriction may occur with ipratropium bromide given by MDI. It is possible that this is due to blockade of prejunctional M_2-receptors on airway cholinergic nerves, which normally inhibit acetylcholine release.

CONCLUSIONS

Cholinergic tone is the only major reversible component of airway narrowing in patients with COPD, in whom anticholinergics are the most useful bronchodilators, since they have a long duration of action and are relatively free of side effects. The demonstration that anticholinergics are sometimes more effective than β_2-agonists suggests that they may have some additional effect other than on airway smooth muscle. This may be an effect on airway mucus secretion, particularly on goblet cell secretion in peripheral airways. In chronic asthma, anticholinergics are of less use since airway narrowing is also due to the direct effects of inflammatory mediators on airway smooth muscle, although they may be useful in chronic asthmatic patients who develop fixed airway obstruction. Anticholinergics are very effective in acute exacerbations of asthma and COPD, suggesting that an increase in cholinergic tone is a major mechanism for the worsening of airway function. The recognition that there are several subtypes of muscarinic receptor has important clinical implications, and more selective antagonists that inhibit the M_3-subtype of receptor on airway smooth muscle and glands are now under development.

REFERENCES

1. Kalia M, Mesulam M-M. Brain stem projections of sensory and motor components of the vagus in the cat. II. Laryngeal, tracheobronchial, pulmonary, cardiac and gastrointestinal branches. *J Comp Neurol* 1980;193:467–508.
2. Barnes PJ. Neural control of human airways in health and disease. *Am Rev Respir Dis* 1986;134:1289–1314.
3. Widdicombe JG, Karlsson J-A, Barnes PJ. Cholinergic mechanisms in bronchial hyperresponsiveness and asthma. In: Kaliner MA, Barnes PJ, Persson CGA, eds. *Asthma, Its pathology and treatment.* New York: Marcel Dekker, 1991;327–356.
4. Barnes PJ. Neural control of airway function: new perspectives. *Molec Aspects Med* 1990;11:351–423.
5. Nadel JA, Barnes PJ, Holtzman MJ. Autonomic factors in the hyperreactivity of airway smooth muscle. In: *Handbook of physiology: the respiratory system,* III. Bethesda: American Physiological Society 1986;693–702.
6. Richardson JB. Nerve supply to the lung. *Am Rev Respir Dis* 1979;119:785–802.
7. Barnes PJ. Cholinergic control of airway smooth muscle. *Am Rev Respir Dis* 1987;136:S42–S45.
8. Barnes PJ, Nadel JA, Roberts JM, Basbaum CB. Muscarinic receptors in lung and trachea: autoradiographic localization using [³]quinuclidinyl benzilate. *Eur J Pharmacol* 1982;86:103–106.
9. Barnes PJ, Basbaum CB, Nadel JA. Autoradiographic localization of autonomic recep-

tors in airway smooth muscle: marked differences between large and small airways. *Am Rev Respir Dis* 1983;127:758–762.

10. Mak JCW, Barnes PJ. Autoradiographic visualization of muscarinic receptor subtypes in human and guinea pig lung. *Am Rev Respir Dis* 1990;141:1559–1568.

11. Ingram RH, Wellman JJ, McFadden ER Jr, Mead J. Relative contribution of large and small airways to flow limitation in normal subjects before and after atropine and iso-proterenol. *J Clin Invest* 1977;59:696–703.

12. Vincent NJ, Knudson R, Leith DF, Macklem PT, Mead J. Factors influencing pulmonary resistance. *J Appl Physiol* 1970;29:236–243.

13. Quigley C, Fuller RW, Dixon CMS, Barnes PJ. Inhaled acetylcholinesterase inhibitors cause dose-related bronchoconstriction in asthmatic and normal subjects. *Am Rev Respir Dis* 1985;131:A283.

14. Barnes PJ. Muscarinic receptors in lung. *Postgrad Med J* 1987;63(suppl):13–19.

15. Barnes PJ. Muscarinic receptors in airways: recent developments. *J Appl Physiol* 1990;68:1777–1785.

16. Bonner TI, Buckley NJ, Young AC, Brann MR. Identification of a family of muscarinic acetylcholine receptor genes. *Science* 1987;237:527–532.

17. Buckley NJ, Bonner TI, Buckley CM, Brann MR. Antagonist binding properties of five cloned muscarinic receptors expressed in CHO-K1 cells. *Mol Pharmacol* 1989; 35:469–476.

18. Grandordy BM, Cuss FM Sampson AS, Palmer JB, Barnes PJ. Phosphatidylinositol response to cholinergic agonists in airway smooth muscle: relationship to contraction and muscarinic receptor occupancy. *J Pharmacol Exp Ther* 1986;238:273–279.

19. Chilvers EF, Challiss RAJ, Barnes PJ, Nahorski SR. Mass changes of inositol (1,4,5)trisphosphate in trachealis muscle following agonist stimulation. *Eur J Pharmacol* 1989;164:587–590.

20. Chilvers ER, Batty IH, Barnes PJ, Nahorski SR. Formation of inositol polyphosphates in airway smooth muscle after muscarinic receptor stimulation. *J Pharmacol Exp Ther* 1990;252:786–789.

21. Roffel AF, Elzinga CRS, Zaagsma J. Muscarinic M_3-receptors mediate contraction of human central and peripheral airway smooth muscle. *Pulmon Pharmacol* 1990;3:47–51.

22. Jones CA, Madison JM, Tom-Moy M, Brown JK. Muscarinic cholinergic inhibition of adenylate cyclase in airway smooth muscle. *Am J Physiol* 1987;253:C90–104.

23. Ueki I, German V, Nadel J. Micropipette measurement of airway submucosal gland secretion: autonomic effects. *Am Rev Respir Dis* 1980;121:351–357.

24. Tokuyama K, Kuo H-P, Rohde JAL, Barnes PJ, Rogers DF. Neural control of goblet cell secretion in guinea pig airways. *Am J Physiol* 1990;259:L108–L115.

25. Nadel JA, Barnes PJ. Autonomic regulation of the airways. *Annu Rev Med* 1984; 35:451–467.

26. Sant'Ambrogio G. Information arising from the tracheobronchial tree of mammals. *Physiol Rev* 1982;62:531–569.

27. Karlsson J-A, Sant'Ambrogio G, Widdicombe JG. Afferent neural pathways in cough and reflex bronchoconstriction. *J Appl Physiol* 1988;65:1007–1023.

28. Barnes PJ. Modulation of neurotransmission in airways. *Physiol Rev* 1992;72:699–729.

29. Belvisi MG, Stretton CD, Barnes PJ. Nitric oxide is the endogenous neurotransmitter of bronchodilator nerves in human airways. *Eur J Pharmacol* 1992;210:221–222.

30. Belvisi MG, Stretton CD, Miura M, Verleden GM, Tadjarimi S, Yacoub MH, Barnes PJ. Inhibitory NANC nerves in human tracheal smooth muscle: a quest for the neurotransmitter. *J Appl Physiol* 1992;73:2505–2510.

31. Belvisi MG, Stretton CD, Barnes PJ. Nitric oxide as an endogenous modulator of cholinergic neurotransmission in guinea pig airways. *Eur J Pharmacol* 1991;198:219–221.

32. Belvisi MG, Miura M, Stretton CD, Barnes PJ. Endogenous vasoactive intestinal peptide and nitric oxide modulate cholinergic neurotransmission in guinea pig trachea. *Eur J Pharmacol* 1992;231:97–102.

33. Ward JR, Belvisi MG, Fox AJ, Miura M, Tadjirarimi S, Yacoub MH, Barnes PJ. Modulation of cholinergic neurotransmission by nitric oxide in human airway smooth muscle. *J Clin Invest* 1993; 92:736–742.

34. Chung KF, Rogers DF, Barnes PJ, Evans TW. The role of increased airway microvascular permeability and plasma exudation in asthma. *Eur Respir J* 1990;3:329–337.
35. Ward MJ, Macfarlane JT, Davies D. A place for ipratropium bromide in the treatment of severe acute asthma. *Br J Dis Chest* 1985;79:374–378.
36. Rebuck AS, Chapman KR, Abboud R, Pare PD, Kreishman H, Wolkove N, Vickerson P. Nebulized anticholinergic and sympathomimetic treatment of asthma and chronic obstructive airways disease in the emergency room. *Am J Med* 1987;82:59–64.
37. O'Driscoll BR, Taylor RJ, Horsley MG, Chambers DU, Bernstein A. Nebulised salbumatol with and without ipratropium bromide in acute airflow obstruction. *Lancet* 1989;1:1418–1420.
38. Brown JP, Greville WH, Finucane KE. Asthma and irreversible airflow obstruction. *Thorax* 1984;39:131–136.
39. Peat JK, Woolcock AJ, Cullen K. Rate of decline of lung function in subjects with asthma. *Eur J Respir Dis* 1987;70:171–179.
40. Gross NJ, Co E, Skorodin MS. Cholinergic bronchomotor tone in COPD: estimates of its amount in comparison with that in normal subjects. *Chest* 1989;96:984–987.
41. Patrick DM, Dales RE, Stark RM, Laliberte G, Dickinson G. Severe exacerbations of COPD and asthma: incremental benefit of adding ipratropium to usual therapy. *Chest* 1990;98:295–297.
42. Lefcoe NM, Toogood JH, Blennerhassett G, Baskerville J, Patterson NAM. The addition of an aerosol anticholinergic to an oral beta agonist plus theophylline in asthma and bronchitis. *Chest* 1982;82:300–305.
43. Gross NJ, Skorodin MS. Anticholinergic, antimuscarinic bronchodilators. *Am Rev Respir Dis* 1984;129:856–870.
44. Chapman KR. The role of anticholinergic bronchodilators in adult asthma and COPD. *Lung* 1990;168(suppl):295–303.
45. Gross NJ, Skorodin MS. Role of the parasympathetic system in airway obstruction due to emphysema. *N Engl J Med* 1984;311:321–325.
46. Braun SR, McKenzie WN, Copeland C, Knight L, Ellersieck M. A comparison of the effect of ipratropium and albuterol in the treatment of chronic obstructive airway disease. *Arch Intern Med* 1989;149:544–547.
47. Rogers DF, Aursudkij B, Barnes PJ. Effects of tachykinins on mucus secretion on human bronchi *in vitro*. *Eur J Pharmacol* 1989;174:283–286.
48. Kuo H-P, Rohde JAL, Barnes PJ, Rogers DF. Cigarette smoke induced goblet cell secretion: dose-dependent differential nerve activation. *Am J Physiol* 1992;215:297–300.
49. Connolly CK. Diurnal rhythms in airway obstruction. *Br J Dis Chest* 1979;73:357–366.
50. Coe CI, Barnes PJ. Reduction of nocturnal asthma by an inhaled anticholinergic drug. *Chest* 1986;90:485–488.
51. Morrison JFJ, Pearson SB, Dean HG. Parasympathetic nervous system in nocturnal asthma. *Br Med J* 1988;296:1427–1429.
52. Hulme EC, Birdsall NJM, Buckley NJ. Muscarinic receptor subtypes. *Annu Rev Pharmacol* 1990;30:633–673.
53. Kurtenbach E, Curtis CAM, Pedder EK, Aiken A, Harris ACM, Hulme EC. Muscarinic acetylcholine receptors. *J Biol Chem* 1990;265:13702–13708.
54. Minette PA, Barnes PJ. Muscarinic receptor subtypes in airways: function and clinical significance. *Am Rev Respir Dis* 1990;141:S162–S165.
55. Maclagan J, Barnes PJ. Muscarinic pharmacology of the airways. *Trends Pharmacol Sci* 1989;10(suppl):88–92.
56. Barnes PJ. Muscarinic receptor subtypes in airways. *Life Sci* 1993;52:521–528.
57. Hammer R, Berrie CP, Birdsall NJM, Burgen AS, Hulme EC. Pirenzipine distinguishes between different subclasses of muscarinic receptors. *Nature* 1980;283:90–92.
58. Hirschowitz BI, Fong J, Molina E. Effects of pirenzepine and atropine on vagal and cholinergic gastric secretion and gastric release and on heart rate in the dog. *J Pharmacol Exp Ther* 1983;225:263–268.
59. Bloom JW, Yamamura HI, Baumgartner C, Halonen M. A muscarinic receptor with high affinity for pirenzepine mediates vagally induced bronchoconstriction. *Eur J Pharmacol* 1987;133:21–27.

60. Madison JM, Jones CA, Tom-Moy M, Brown JR. Affinities of pirenzepine for muscarinic cholinergic receptors in membranes isolated from bovine tracheal mucosa and smooth muscle. *Am Rev Respir Dis* 1987;135:719–724.
61. Sertl K, Meryn S, Graninger W, Lagnner A, Schlick W, Ramers H. Acute effects of pirenzepine on bronchospasm. *Int J Clin Pharmacol Ther Toxicol* 1986;24:655–657.
62. Cazzola M, Rano S, de Santis D, Principe PJ, Marmo E. Respiratory responses to pirenzepine in healthy subjects. *Int J Clin Pharmacol Ther Toxicol* 1987;25(2):105–109.
63. Lammers J-WJ, Minette P, McCusker M, Barnes PJ. The role of pirenzepine-sensitive (M_1) muscarinic receptors in vagally mediated bronchoconstriction in humans. *Am Rev Respir Dis* 1989;139:446–449.
64. Bloom JW, Baumgartener-Folkerts C, Palmer JD, Yamamura HI, Halonen M. A muscarinic receptor subtype modulates vagally stimulated bronchial contraction. *J Appl Physiol* 1988;65:2144–2150.
65. Ashe JH, Yarosh CA. Differential and selective antagonism of the slow-inhibitory postsynaptic potential and slow-excitatory postsynaptic potential by gallanin and pirenzepine in the superior cervical ganglion of the rabbit. *Neuropharmacology* 1984;23:1321–1329.
66. Bloom JW, Halonen M, Lawrence LJ, Rould E, Seaver NA, Yamamura HI. Characterization of high affinity [^{3}] pirenzepine and ($-$)[^{3}]quinuclidinyl benzilate binding to muscarinic receptors in rabbit peripheral lung. *J Pharmacol Exp Ther* 1987;240:51–58.
67. Casale TB, Ecklund P. Characterization of muscarinic receptor subtypes in human peripheral lung. *J Appl Physiol* 1988;65:594–600.
68. Mak JCW, Barnes PJ. Muscarinic receptor subtypes in human and guinea pig lung. *Eur J Pharmacol* 1989;164:223–230.
69. Mak JCW, Baraniuk JN, Barnes PJ. Localization of muscarinic receptor subtype mRNAs in human lung. *Am J Respir Cell Mol Biol* 1992;7:344–348.
70. Mak JCW, Buckley NJ, Barnes PJ. Visualization of muscarinic m_4 mRNA by in situ hybridization in rabbit lung. *Life Sci* 1993;53:1501–1508.
71. Lazareno S, Buckley NJ, Roberts FF. Characterization of muscarinic M_4 binding sites in rabbit lung, chicken heart and NG 108-15 cells. *Mol Pharmacol* 1990;38:805–815.
72. Kilbinger H, Wessler T. Inhibition by acetylcholine of the stimulation-evoked release of [^3H]acetylcholine from the guinea-pig myenteric plexus. *Neuroscience* 1980;5:1331–1340.
73. Faulkner D, Fryer AD, Maclagan J. Post-ganglionic muscarinic inhibitory receptors in pulmonary parasympathetic nerves in guinea-pig. *Br J Pharmacol* 1986;88:181–187.
74. Fryer AD, Maclagan J. Muscarinic inhibitory receptors in pulmonary parasympathetic nerves in the guinea-pig. *Br J Pharmacol* 1984;83:973–978.
75. Minette PA, Barnes PJ. Prejunctional inhibitory muscarinic receptors on cholinergic nerves in human and guinea-pig airways. *J Appl Physiol* 1988;64:2532–2537.
76. Watson N, Barnes PJ, Maclagan J. Action of methoctramine, a muscarinic M_2-receptor antagonist on muscarinic and nicotine cholinoceptors in guinea pig airways *in vivo* and *in vitro*. *Br J Pharmacol* 1992;105:107–112.
77. Blaber LC, Fryer AD, Maclagan J. Neuronal muscarinic receptors attenuate vagally-induced contraction of feline bronchial smooth muscle. *Br J Pharmacol* 1985;86:723–728.
78. Aas P, Maclagan J. Evidence for prejunctional M_{X2X} muscarinic receptors in pulmonary cholinergic nerves in the rat. *Br J Pharmacol* 1990;101:73–76.
79. Ito Y, Yoshitomi T. Autoregulation of acetylcholine release from vagus nerve terminals through activation of muscarinic receptors in the dog trachea. *Br J Pharmacol* 1988;93:636–646.
80. Janssen LJ, Daniel EE. Characterization of the prejunctional β-adrenoceptors in canine bronchial smooth muscle. *J Pharmacol Exp Ther* 1991;254:741–749.
81. Del Monte M, Omini C, Subissi A. Mechanism of the potentiation of neurally-induced bronchoconstriction by gallamine in the guinea pig. *Br J Pharmacol* 1990;99:582–588.
82. Minette PAH, Lammers J, Dixon CMS, McCusker MT, Barnes PJ. A muscarinic agonist inhibits reflex bronchoconstriction in normal but not in asthmatic subjects. *J Appl Physiol* 1989;67:2461–2465.

83. Ayala LE, Ahmed T. Is there a loss of a protective muscarinic receptor mechanism in asthma? *Chest* 1991;96:1285–1291.
84. Barnes PJ. Muscarinic autoreceptors in airways: their possible role in airway disease. *Chest* 1989;96:1220–1221.
85. Barnes PJ. Muscarinic receptor subtypes: implications for lung disease. *Thorax* 1989;44:161–167.
86. Ind PW, Dixon CMS, Fuller RW, Barnes PJ. Anticholinergic blockade of beta-blocker induced bronchoconstriction. *Am Rev Respir Dis* 1989;139:1390–1394.
87. Fryer AD, Fakahany EE, Jacoby DB. Parainfluenza virus type I reduces the affinity of agonists for muscarinic receptors in guinea-pig lung and heart. *Eur J Pharmacol* 1990;181:51–58.
88. Fryer AD, Jacoby DB. Parainfluenza virus infection damages inhibitory M_2-muscarinic receptors on pulmonary parasympathetic nerves in the guinea pig. *Br J Pharmacol* 1991;102:267–271.
89. Gies J-P, Landry Y. Sialic acid is selectively involved in the interaction of agonists M_2-muscarinic acetylcholine receptors. *Biochem Biophys Res Commun* 1988;150:673–680.
90. Jacoby DB, Gleich GJ, Fryer AD. Human eosinophil major basic protein is an endogenous allosteric antagonist at the inhibitory muscarinic M_2 receptor. *J Clin Invest* 1993;91:1314–1318.
91. Roffel AF, Elzinga CRS, van Amsterdam RGM, de Zeeuw RA, Zaagsma J. Muscarinic M_2-receptors in bovine tracheal smooth muscle: discrepancies between binding and function. *Eur J Pharmacol* 1988;153:73–82.
92. Yang CM, Chow S-P, Sung T-C. Muscarinic receptor subtypes coupled to generation of different second messengers in isolated tracheal smooth muscle cells. *Br J Pharmacol* 1991;104:613–618.
93. Fernandes LB, Fryer AD, Hirschman CA. M_2 muscarinic receptors inhibit isoproterenol-induced relaxation of canine airway smooth muscle. *J Pharmacol Exp Ther* 1992;262:119–126.
94. Kume H, Kotlikoff MI. Muscarinic inhibition of single K_{Ca} channels in smooth muscle cells by a pertussis-sensitive G protein. *Am J Physiol* 1991;261:C1204–12049.
95. Kume H, Graziano MP, Kotlikoff MI. Stimulatory and inhibitory regulation of calcium-activation potassium channels by guanine nucleotide binding proteins. *Proc Natl Acad Sci USA* 1992;89:11051–11055.
96. Gater P, Alabaster VA, Piper I. Characterization of the muscarinic receptor subtype mediating mucus secretion in the cat trachea *in vitro*. Pulmon Pharmacol 1989;2:87–92.
97. Yang CM, Farley JM, Dwyer TM. Muscarinic stimulation of submucosal glands in swine trachea. *J Appl Physiol* 1988;64:200–209.
98. Kilbinger M, van Barbeleben RS, Siefken H. Is the presynaptic muscarinic receptor in guinea-pig trachea an M_2-receptor? *Life Sci* 1993;52:577.
99. D'Agostino G, Chiari MC, Grana E, Kilbinger H. Muscarinic inhibition of acetylcholine release from a novel *in vitro* preparation of the guinea pig trachea. *Naunyn-Schmiedebergs Arch Pharmacol* 1990;342:141–145.
100. Kilbinger H, Schoreider R, Siefken H, Wolf D, D'Argostino G. Characterization of prejunctional muscarinic autoreceptors in guinea pig trachea. *Br J Pharmacol* 1991; 103:1757–1763.
101. Connolly CK. Adverse reaction to ipratropium bromide. *Br Med J* 1982;285:934–935.
102. Gross NJ. Ipratropium bromide. *N Engl J Med* 1988;319:486–494.
103. Frith PA, Jenner B, Dangerfield R, Atkinson J, Drennan C. Oxitropium bromide. Dose response and time-response study of a new anticholinergic drug. *Chest* 1986;89:249–253.
104. Barnes PJ. New drugs for asthma. *Eur Respir J* 1992;5:1126–1136.
105. Ukena D, Wehinger C, Engelstatter R, Steinijans V, Sybrecht GW. The muscarinic M_1-receptor selective antagonist telenzepine has no bronchodilator effects in patients with chronic obstructive airways disease. *Eur Respir J* 1993; in press.
106. Disse B, Reichal R, Speck G, Travnecker W, Rominger KL, Hammer R. Ba679BR, a novel anticholinergic bronchodilator: preclinical and clinical aspects. *Life Sci* 1993; 52:537–544.
107. Maesen FPV, Smeets JJ, Costongs MAL, Cornelissen PJG, Wald FDM. BA 679 BR.

A new long-acting antimuscarinic bronchodilator. *Eur Resp J* 1992;5(suppl 15):211S.
108. Newcomb R, Tashkin DP, Hui KK, Connolly ME, Lee E, Dauphinee B. Rebound hyperresponsiveness to muscarinic stimulation after chronic therapy with an inhaled muscarinic antagonist. *Am Rev Respir Dis* 1985;132:12–15.
109. Pavia D, Bateman JRM, Clarke SW. Deposition and clearance of inhaled particles. *Clin Resp Physiol* 1980;16:335–366.
110. Raferty P, Beasley R, Holgate ST. Comparison of the efficacy of preservative from ipratropium bromide and Atrovent nebuliser solution. *Thorax* 1988;43:446–450.

Drugs and the Lung,
edited by C.P. Page and W.J. Metzger.
Raven Press, Ltd., New York © 1994

3

Xanthines

*Paul Sullivan, †Clive P. Page, and ‡John F. Costello

*†‡Department of Thoracic Medicine, *King's College School of Medicine and Dentistry, London SE5 9PJ, United Kingdom; †Sackler Institute of Pulmonary Pharmacology, King's College Hospital Medical School, London SW3 6LX, United Kingdom; ‡King's College School of Medicine, London SE5 9RS, United Kingdom

HISTORICAL BACKGROUND

In 1860 Henry Hyde Salter described the efficacious use of strong coffee taken on an empty stomach as a treatment for asthma (1); the recommended quantity, two breakfast cups, probably contained enough caffeine to produce significant bronchodilation (2). Theophylline and caffeine are similar; theophylline is a purine compound, one of the methyl xanthines, i.e., methyl groups attached to a basic xanthine structure. Caffeine is a similar molecule with three rather than theophylline's two methyl groups, and both can antagonize the action of adenosine, which is also a purine.

Theophylline was first isolated from tea in 1888, and it came into clinical use initially as a diuretic. *In vitro* and animal work early in this century revealed its effect of relaxing airway smooth muscle. This finding led to the first use of theophylline in the treatment of asthma in 1922, when theophylline and theobromine suppositories were tested and found to be effective in three asthmatic subjects (3). Theophylline, which is more effective as a bronchodilator than caffeine [approximately two and a half times as potent, milligram for milligram (4)], was first used clinically in the 1930s. In 1937 Herrman and Aynesworth demonstrated an increase in vital capacity following the intravenous administration of aminophylline (5). The ability of this drug to reverse severe bronchoconstriction was soon recognized (6) and the rapid onset of its action was noted (7). Oral preparations have been shown to produce an improvement in symptoms associated with an increased timed vital capacity during both acute exacerbations of asthma (8) and severe chronic disease (9).

CLINICAL USE

Stable Chronic Disease

There is impressive evidence that theophylline can offer additional benefit when it is used in conjunction with beta agonists and corticosteroids. When oral theophylline is added to a regimen of inhaled salbutamol, with or without corticosteroids, there is a significant increase in lung function and decrease in symptoms in asthmatic patients. Furthermore, the patients report a preference for the combination, even if the drugs are administered in a double-blind and placebo-controlled manner (10,11). If asthmatic subjects are given increasing doses of oral terbutaline until maximal benefit is achieved, the addition of oral theophylline induces further improvement (12). Similarly, when subjects were given different theophylline doses until no further improvement in forced expiratory volume in 1 sec (FEV_1) could be obtained, inhaled beta-agonist caused a further rise in FEV_1; the bronchodilator response to the beta-agonist was not affected by the serum theophylline concentration (13). The synergy between theophylline and beta-agonists is confirmed by the observation that a half dose of oral terbutaline plus a half dose of oral theophylline produces better results than a full dose of either drug alone (14). Theophylline is also beneficial when used alongside oral corticosteroids. When theophylline was replaced with placebo in asthmatics taking maintenance doses of 10 to 30 mg of prednisolone per day, there was a significant fall in FEV_1, a rise in symptom score, and a rise in the mean oral steroid requirement (15).

In patients with partially reversible airflow obstruction, theophylline also improves the FEV_1 both before and after inhaled salbutamol (16). In chronic obstructive pulmonary disease (COPD) long-term theophylline also increases minute volume, improves gas exchange, and reduces breathlessness. The subjective improvement in dyspnea occurs even in the absence of any change in spirometry, maximal oxygen uptake, or maximum achievable work load (17), and may be related to hemodynamic changes or to improvement of respiratory muscle power. Patients with COPD, like asthmatics, express a preference for theophylline plus salbutamol over salbutamol alone, and in patients with severe disease, as evidenced by a mean FEV_1 of 38% of the predicted value, theophylline scored better than salbutamol when assessed in terms of daily peak flows, patient preference, and treatment failures (18). In these patients theophylline is therefore of particular benefit.

Acute Asthma

A number of studies have examined the effects of intravenous aminophylline used in the emergency department as a treatment for acute asthma.

One study, involving 133 patients, compared intravenous aminophylline (as a bolus followed by an infusion) with placebo in patients who were also receiving nebulized beta-agonists and intravenous steroids. There were no significant differences between aminophylline and placebo treatment in terms of FEV_1, forced vital capacity (FVC), or peak expiratory flow rate (PEFR) at 1 and 2 h, and no difference in patient or physician satisfaction. However, a significantly greater number of the aminophylline-treated patients were discharged home directly from the emergency department, which is difficult to explain in view of the failure to demonstrate any objective or subjective improvement (19). A study of 44 emergency patients failed to show any objective improvement when intravenous aminophylline was added to inhaled beta-agonists and parenteral steroids (20). Much of the published data are derived from relatively small groups of patients. In an attempt to overcome this problem Littenberg (21) has performed a meta-analysis of 13 reports of controlled trials of intravenous aminophylline therapy in severe, acute asthma. The results of the pooled data for all the studies did not show any benefit from aminophylline treatment. However, the study designs were very variable and in some cases aminophylline was used as a single drug treatment, which does not reflect its use in current clinical practice. It was compared variously with placebo, inhaled bronchodilators, intravenous beta-agonists, and subcutaneous adrenaline. When the studies that examined the addition of aminophylline to beta-agonist therapy were examined as a group, there was a trend toward objective benefit in the treatment group although significance was not achieved. Littenberg points out that the combined patient number was still relatively small and the power of the meta-analysis to detect significant improvement was relatively low (21).

These data might be taken to suggest that the administration of intravenous aminophylline is of no benefit in the emergency treatment of asthma. There are, however, no data on the effect of aminophylline in the subgroup of patients with severe asthma who do not improve sufficiently after intravenous corticosteroids and inhaled beta-agonists. In these patients additional medical treatment is necessary since positive pressure ventilation, the only alternative, is associated with a high incidence of complications (22). Many physicians would add either intravenous aminophylline or an intravenous beta-agonist at this stage. In bronchi taken from patients who have died from asthma there is a decreased sensitivity to the bronchodilator action of beta-agonists when compared with bronchi from people who have died of other causes; this may be due to tachyphylaxis to endogenous and exogenous beta-agonists or it may be a feature of the disease itself. The response to theophylline remains intact (23,24). These findings suggest that intravenous aminophylline may be of benefit in severe, life-threatening disease when inhaled beta-agonists do not improve the patient's condition. In-hospital, asthma deaths are relatively infrequent and a very large number of patients may need to be included in a study if an effect on mortality is to be demonstrated. The results of studies that are currently available do not preclude a useful role for intravenous aminophylline as a treatment for severe asthma.

EFFECTS IN RESPIRATORY DISEASE

Bronchodilation

Oral sustained-release theophylline causes a significant increase in FEV_1 and in peak flow readings throughout the day in stable asthmatics (13,25,26), and the improvement persists during long-term treatment (27). Patients suffering with chronic bronchitis and chronic obstructive lung disease without beta-agonist reversibility also demonstrate significantly better FEV_1 values with oral theophylline (18).

When given as a single dose, xanthines produce acute bronchodilation. A single intravenous dose of aminophylline causes bronchodilation in stable asthmatics (28) and in patients with chronic obstructive lung disease (29), even if the patient is already taking inhaled beta-agonists and steroids.

Protection Against Bronchoconstriction

After inhaled allergen challenge, asthmatic subjects exhibit an immediate and transient period of bronchoconstriction, which is termed the early asthmatic response (EAR) and is followed in some cases by a second phase of constriction, the late asthmatic response (LAR). Theophylline produces a significant attenuation of the EAR after allergen challenge (30) but an even more significant reduction in the size of the LAR (31). Similar results are observed during oral theophylline therapy after challenge with toluene diisocyanate in sensitive asthmatics (32,33). Low serum concentrations of theophylline (mean 6.4 mg/L) reduce the response of asthmatic airways to inhaled histamine and methacholine (34,35), and in the past theophylline has been shown to protect against the effects of intravenous histamine and methacholine challenges (36) and against bronchoconstriction after cold air inhalation (37). In normal subjects methacholine sensitivity is also decreased by theophylline (38).

Effects on Exercise-Induced Asthma

Asthmatic patients with a history of exercise-induced bronchospasm were treated with intravenous theophylline immediately prior to a 6-min exercise provocation in a double-blind study. All of the subjects demonstrated a fall in PEFR of at least 20% after exercise when they had been given placebo. After theophylline administration there was a significant attenuation of the reduction in PEFR caused by exercise; the mean serum theophylline concentration after infusion was 13.2 mg/L. Another study has shown a similar effect with lower serum concentrations. Magnussen et al. (37) found that the protection against exercise-induced asthma produced by intravenous theophylline was dose dependent and that significant protection was afforded by a serum theophylline concentration of only 6 mg/L.

Effects on Smooth Muscle Tone In Vitro

At therapeutic concentrations, aminophylline induces a dose-dependent relaxation of the spontaneous tone of resting guinea pig trachealis muscle. Theophylline has also been reported to relax both large and small human airways *in vitro,* albeit at high concentrations (39,40). Results of experiments investigating the effect of theophylline on histamine-induced smooth muscle contraction are conflicting. Allen et al. (41) found that theophylline antagonized the smooth muscle response to histamine *in vitro* and Supinski et al. (42) abolished the contractile response to histamine by adding theophylline at a concentration of 100 mol/L, which is within the therapeutic range. Other investigators, however, have failed to show any effect on the histamine response, even at a concentration of 440 mol/L, although the effect on resting tone was demonstrated (43).

Effects on Mucociliary Clearance

The airways from the trachea to the terminal bronchioles are lined by ciliated epithelium. In airways proximal to the respiratory bronchioles the cilia are covered with a layer of mucus that is moved toward the upper trachea by ciliary beat activity; the efficiency of mucociliary transport depends not only upon the function of the cilia but also upon the composition and the viscosity of the mucus layer (44). Histological studies of bronchi from patients who died from severe asthma have shown destruction of the epithelium with a decrease in the number of ciliated cells (45), and there is often an excessive quantity of mucus within the airways. In less-severe disease there is evidence of impairment of mucus transport; antigen challenge is followed by a period of mucociliary paresis in sensitized sheep and in allergic asthmatics (46,47). The sulfidopeptide leukotrienes LTC_4, LTD_4, and LTE_4, which are present at increased concentrations in the airways of asthmatics, increase mucus production and increase its viscosity by altering the glycoprotein content (48). Platelet-activating factor (PAF) is also involved in the pathogenesis of asthma; this mediator increases mucus secretion and impairs mucociliary clearance in animals (49), as well as causing epithelial damage with an associated loss of cilia.

There is evidence that theophylline can increase mucociliary clearance and therefore mitigate these effects; this action may be important in the treatment of acute exacerbations of asthma, when mucus accumulation and plugging occurs. In a study of normal subjects, smokers, and patients with lung cancer, theophylline caused a dose-dependent increase in the rate of clearance of radioactivity after inhalation of a radiolabeled aerosol (50). Co-tromanes et al. (51) demonstrated an increased transit velocity in the small and medium-sized airways. Unfortunately the same effects are not found in patients with COPD and emphysema, in whom retention of mucus is an important problem. In a study of nine patients a single infusion of aminophylline did not significantly alter the rate of radioaerosol clearance (52).

Effects on Diaphragmatic Contractility

It has been suggested that theophylline increases the force of contraction of the diaphragm and abolishes diaphragmatic fatigue, and that this action contributes to the symptomatic improvement seen during treatment with this drug. *In vitro* aminophylline increases the force of contraction of rat dia-phragm strips and the effect persists after 2 weeks of exposure (53). In an-esthetized dogs aminophylline increases the force of diaphragmatic contrac-tion to low-frequency stimulation and increases the maximal twitch tension (54). *In vivo,* oral theophylline increases the ratio between transdiaphrag-matic pressure and the diaphragmatic electromyogram (EMG) activity in normal subjects (55) and increases the maximum sustainable ventilation in both normals and patients with COPD (56).

Evidence that theophylline affects diaphragmatic fatigue comes from work with resistive load breathing. In patients with COPD, theophylline at a se-rum level of 13 mg/L not only increased the transdiaphragmatic pressure (P_{di}) during maximal inspiration with a closed airway but also decreased respi-ratory muscle fatigue after resistive load breathing (57). In dogs diaphrag-matic fatigue is demonstrated by the decline in the response to phrenic nerve stimulation during resistive load breathing, and this fatigue is lessened by aminophylline, even if the animal is hypoxic and acidotic (58).

The effect of theophylline on muscle appears to be selective for the dia-phragm. Intravenous aminophylline has no effect on either the force of con-traction or the development of fatigue in the adductor pollicis muscle of nor-mal subjects (59), and theophylline does not effect either the development of fatigue or the speed of recovery when the sternocleidomastoid muscle is exercised to exhaustion (60).

The mechanism of increased contractility appears to be mediated by al-teration of the intracellular calcium concentration. In frog striated muscle, theophylline's effect on contraction is dependent upon the presence of cal-cium in the extracellular medium (61). In rat diaphragm theophylline in-creases intracellular calcium and causes an increase in contractility, which is blocked by verapamil, a calcium channel blocker (62), and in dogs aminophylline produces a dose-dependent increase in P_{di} during electrical stimulation that is reversed by verapamil (63). Aminophylline has been shown to enhance intracellular calcium accumulation in rat diaphragmatic muscle with a peak activity at 18.75 mg/L, which is within the therapeutic range (64). In frog striated muscle cells adenosine decreases calcium influx and it may be that theophylline affects calcium movement by acting as an adenosine antagonist (65).

Respiratory Drive

There is evidence that theophylline increases ventilatory drive and modifies the response to hypercapnia and hypoxia. When six normal volunteers were given aminophylline intravenously they exhibited a 19% increase in minute ventilation and a 47% increase to their ventilatory response to hypercapnia (66). During experimental hypoxia in untreated normal subjects there is an initial increase in minute volume. If hypoxia is prolonged, the minute ventilation declines and plateaus, although it remains higher than during normoxia. Theophylline increases the minute ventilation during the plateau phase in normal subjects, largely by increasing the respiratory rate (67). Predosing with theophylline does not, however, affect the initial peak response to acute hypoxia in normal subjects (68,69). Animal experiments have shown that the concentration of adenosine in the brain increases during sustained hypoxia and it has been suggested that this may cause the decline in ventilation that follows the acute hypoxic response and that theophylline may increase ventilation during sustained hypoxia by acting as an adenosine antagonist (70). This hypothesis is supported by the finding that administration of an adenosine analogue intravenously or directly into the cerebrospinal fluid (CSF) of an anesthetized cat produces inhibition of phrenic nerve activity and that theophylline blocks such an effect (71).

Sleep

Theophylline improves nocturnal blood gas tensions in patients with chronic pulmonary disease but it does not affect the number of hypopneic episodes. It does not affect oxygenation during REM sleep, when patients are most likely to become hypopneic, and it does not decrease the number of apneas or on the duration of REM (72). Patients with confirmed obstructive sleep apnea experience significantly fewer apneic and hypopneic episodes after a nocturnal dose of theophylline and fewer episodes of oxygen desaturation. However, the overall sleep quality is worse after theophylline, with a decrease in the total sleep time per hour, and a decrease in the period between going to sleep for the first time and final waking time the next day (73).

The Pulmonary Circulation

Theophylline produces hemodynamic changes that may have important clinical effects, particularly in patients suffering from COPD. These patients tend to have a chronically raised pulmonary vascular resistance and a high pulmonary artery pressure in response to chronic hypoxia. "Right-sided" heart failure may result, with the associated problems of edema and visceral congestion. There is evidence that treatment with theophylline reverses some of these changes and improves right-sided cardiac function. In patients with chronic obstructive pulmonary disease with cor pulmonale, an intravenous aminophylline infusion caused a 36% fall in mean pulmonary artery pressure and a 28% fall in pulmonary vascular resistance, which was accompanied by a rise in stroke work in both ventricles. In a similar group without cor pulmonale, there was a decrease in both right and left ventricular end diastolic pressure, which was accompanied by a rise in cardiac index, suggesting a positive inotropic action (74,75). Intravenous aminophylline increased the ejection fraction for both ventricles in a study of patients with COPD, restoring the value to normal for the right ventricle in six of eight patients (76). A fall in pulmonary vascular resistance and pulmonary artery pressure has also been seen during oral theophylline treatment in patients with COPD (77) and has been shown to produce an increased left and right ventricular ejection fraction after 72 h, which is sustained during chronic therapy (78). The combination of pulmonary vasodilation with lowered pulmonary arterial pressure, lower filling pressures, and increased cardiac output is of potential benefit in COPD, especially if cor pulmonale is present, and may account for the improvement in symptoms that can occur in the absence of improved lung function in some patients on theophylline.

The reduction of pulmonary vascular resistance may be due to theophylline's ability to attenuate hypoxic pulmonary vasoconstriction. In isolated pig and rat lungs aminophylline markedly reduces the pulmonary artery pressure during hypoxia but has little effect during normoxia. This result is unchanged if the lung is perfused with plasma instead of blood, indicating that the pressure changes are due to an action on vascular tone rather than blood cell deformability. In human subjects, when experimental regional hypoxia was induced by inflation of a balloon in a lobar bronchus, theophylline attenuated the subsequent fall in blood flow to the hypoxic area; the arterial Po_2 also fell (79), since local hypoxic vasoconstriction protects against V/Q mismatching and therefore against hypoxia. Theophylline may therefore, like the beta-agonists, theoretically worsen hypoxia in patients with asthma if ventilation is not uniform by increasing blood flow to underventilated alveoli. Clinicians should pay particular attention to the patient's oxygenation if intravenous aminophylline is used in the treatment of acute severe asthma.

EFFECTS OF THEOPHYLLINE ON THE IMMUNE SYSTEM

Recent attention has focused on the intriguing evidence that theophylline may have potent anti-inflammatory activity (80). The model of airway inflammation in asthma that is most commonly used for the evaluation of the anti-inflammatory response is the late asthmatic reaction (31). When a susceptible asthmatic inhales an antigen to which he or she is sensitive, there is a fall in lung function within a few minutes, which is called the early asthmatic response (EAR). The EAR is thought to be due in the main to the release of preformed mediators, such as histamine, from mast cells. This recovers but may be followed 4 to 6 h later by a delayed fall in lung function through recruitment and activation of inflammatory cells such as eosinophils and basophils and further release of preformed and newly formed mediators, termed the late asthmatic reaction (LAR). The LAR is therefore considered a useful model of airway inflammation in asthma and has been used to measure the anti-inflammatory effects of a wide variety of potential anti-asthmatic agents. Several studies of the effect of theophylline on the LAR have been reported: Pauwels et al. (81) showed a clear inhibitory effect of a single intravenous dose of aminophylline and enprofylline, but not placebo, on the LAR, but not the EAR, in a group of five asthmatics. Fabbri's group (82) evaluated the effect of theophylline, verapamil, cromoglycate, and beclomethasone on toluene diisocyanate induced EAR and LAR; theophylline, like the corticosteroids, had little effect of the EAR but significantly reduced the LAR (the other two drugs had little or no effect). Further studies from Cockcroft et al. (30) and Hendeles et al. (83) showed an attenuating effect of theophylline on the LAR, although its effects on other parameters, such as bronchial hyperreactivity, were variable.

We have recently completed a double-blind parallel-group comparison of 5 weeks of oral theophylline versus placebo in a group of 19 asthmatics (31). We measured a variety of lymphocyte markers in peripheral blood, blood theophylline levels, and the house dust mite antigen-induced EAR and LAR. The cellular data were inconclusive but the lung function data showed a highly significantly attenuating effect of theophylline, achieved at a low mean plasma level, in some individual cases as low as 3 mg/L. We conclude that theophylline, given over a 5-week period probably has important anti-inflammatory activity, and this can be achieved at relatively low and therefore nontoxic blood levels. These findings have been extended in a second study from our laboratory showing that 5 weeks of oral theophylline significantly reduces the number of EG2$^+$ eosinophils in bronchial biopsies obtained from allergic asthmatics.

Another manifestation of the immunomodulation that is associated with theophylline has been demonstrated by mouse experiments involving bronchial challenge with live bacteria. In untreated animals only 22% of *Staphylococcus aureus* bacteria were still alive after 4 h, whereas in animals treated with aminophylline 55% of *S. aureus* were viable at 4 h. The results were even more striking when gram negative organisms were used. Control animals killed 74% of *Proteus mirabilis* bacteria by 4 h. In contrast, after aminophylline treatment these bacteria were able to proliferate within the mouse lungs and their numbers more than doubled in 4 h (84).

Effects on Individual Cell Types

Mast Cells

In vitro theophylline reduces histamine release from rat peritoneal mast cells (i.e., connective tissue type mast cells similar to those found in the lungs) after stimulation by antigen or by anti-immunoglobulin E (IgE) receptor antibodies (85), and it reduces histamine release from human basophils and lung fragments but only at high concentration (86). An increase in intracellular adenosine 3′,5′-cyclic monophosphate (cAMP) after treatment of mast cells with forskolin causes a marked reduction of PGD_2, LTB_4, and LTC_4 release after antigen stimulation, and the addition of a phosphodiesterase inhibitor abolishes their release, lessens histamine release, and impairs ionophore-induced liberation of PAF and free arachidonic acid. These effects are seen after a cAMP elevation of less than 20% (87). The suppression of mast cell mediator release is also seen *in vivo;* there is a reduction in histamine release when subjects with allergic rhinitis are challenged with antigen after a 1-week course of theophylline (88). There is also a reduction in the early response to allergen in the skin during treatment with theophylline but no change in the skin's response to injected histamine, indicating that theophylline has an effect on endogenous histamine release (89). However, the effect of theophylline on acute allergic bronchoconstriction is minimal (31,81,83), suggesting that theophylline is unlikely to inhibit lung mast cells *in vivo* in any major way.

Eosinophils

Theophylline and cAMP analogues diminish immunoglobulin-induced eosinophil degranulation *in vitro*. Addition of cholera toxin to eosinophils causes a progressive rise in the intracellular cAMP concentration, which is accompanied by a reduction in degranulation (90), suggesting that phosphodiesterase inhibition might have the potential to suppress eosinophil function. However, at concentrations below 10 mol/L (therapeutic range 55–110 mol/L), theophylline increases eosinophil superoxide release *in vitro* and this effect is reversed by the addition of adenosine, suggesting that at lower concentrations theophylline acts predominantly by adenosine antagonism to increase eosinophil function (91), although there is no *in vivo* or clinical correlate of this phenomenon. A number of groups have observed an effect of theophylline and related molecules on eosinophil activation and recruitment *in vivo*. Theophylline administered acutely (92) or chronically (93) has been reported to reduce eosinophil infiltration induced by allergen challenge in actively sensitized guinea pigs. Theophylline and isbufylline have been shown to inhibit eosinophil recruitment into the airways after challenge with a range of stimuli (93,94).

Lymphocytes

If peripheral blood lymphocytes are incubated with theophylline they begin to suppress autologous cell responses (95), and this phenomenon can be shown to be due to the presence of a subgroup of T cells that is sensitive to *in vitro* stimulation by theophylline (96). When compared with asthmatics on other treatments, asthmatics on long-term theophylline have more peripheral T cells that are able to suppress plaque formation in lymphocyte culture and a reduced *in vitro* graft versus host (GVH) response; elimination of the putative T-suppressor cells restores the GVH response to normal (97). In other work, asthmatics have been shown to have abnormal T-suppressor function; concanavalin A (ConA) is a substance that enhances T-cell suppression of co-cultured lymphocytes from normal volunteers. This response to ConA is impaired in asthmatics and oral theophylline partially restores the response at serum levels above 5 g/L (98). Two studies in asthmatic children have reported a decrease in the number of peripheral blood T lymphocytes that express suppressor activity and one of these found a correlation between T-suppressor numbers and the severity of asthma. In both studies theophylline treatment led to a restoration of normal T-suppressor numbers (99,100).

The immunosuppressive action of theophylline has been reported to be of use in the treatment of renal transplant rejection. When aminophylline was added to conventional prophylactic drug therapy after renal transplant there was a decrease in the dose of steroid required to control rejection episodes. There was also a fall in the CD4/CD8 T-cell ratio (101). Of particular importance is the finding that theophylline has an immunosuppressive action that may be separate from and additional to that of glucocorticoids. In four patients with rejection episodes that were not responding to steroids the addition of aminophylline arrested the rejection and increased T-suppressor cell numbers (102). Theophylline also increases T-suppressor cell function during renal transplant rejection episodes, increasing the degree of inhibition of the GVH response (103). Rats, after heart transplant, also exhibit increased graft survival with theophylline treatment (104).

Natural Killer Cells

In vitro theophylline produces a dose-dependent reduction in natural killer cell activity. *In vivo,* one study has shown a significant loss of natural killer cell activity after 1 week of treatment (105), although other work has failed to confirm this finding (106).

Monocytes and Macrophages

Peripheral blood mononuclear cells and bronchoalveolar lavage alveolar macrophages from normal subjects secrete less superoxide anion after exposure to low therapeutic concentrations of theophylline (5 g/ml) *in vitro* (107) and alveolar macrophages have been shown to generate less superoxide *ex vivo* after *in vivo* theophylline treatment. Oral theophylline also reduces alveolar macrophage intracellular killing, bactericidal activity, and hydrogen peroxide release, and the degree of impairment correlates with bronchoalveolar lavage theophylline concentration (108). *In vitro* theophylline exposure leads to a blunting of the proliferation response to ConA in normal adult monocytes and an increase in the concentration of cAMP within the cells; in preterm human neonates the same effect is seen after *in vivo* aminophylline therapy (109). cAMP causes a reduction in mouse macrophage interleukin-1 (IL-1) production and a decrease in bone marrow macrophage proliferation and DNA synthesis (110,111). In asthmatic children theophylline treatment has also been shown to inhibit mononuclear cell chemotaxis *ex vivo* (112).

Neutrophils

Theophylline causes a dose-dependent reduction of polymorphonuclear cell superoxide production at concentrations above 1.8 g/ml and it is synergistic with isoprenaline in this respect. It also reduces neutrophil LTB_4 production by 90% at therapeutic concentration *in vitro*. *In vivo* theophylline has been shown to increase polymorph intracellular cAMP concentration in normal subjects (113) and to reduce the chemotaxis of neutrophils *ex vivo* obtained from asthmatic children treated for 10 days with theophylline (112).

MECHANISM OF ACTION

Phosphodiesterase Inhibition

It is still commonly believed that theophylline causes bronchodilation by inhibition of the enzyme phosphodiesterase (PDE), which breaks down cAMP, thereby increasing intracellular cAMP concentration. There is a reasonably good correlation between the potency of tracheal relaxation and the inhibition of PDE in lung homogenates; however, the degree of inhibition of this enzyme is only trivial at concentrations of theophylline that are therapeutically relevant (114). It could be argued that airway smooth muscle cells might concentrate theophylline so that higher intracellular concentrations are achieved, but studies of the distribution of infused theophylline provide no direct evidence for this. Furthermore, many other drugs that have a greater inhibitory effect on PDE, such as dipyridamole, cromoglycate, and papaverine, have no bronchodilator effect (115).

Also, theophylline relaxes airway smooth muscle *in vitro* without any detectable changes in cyclic nucleotides (116). If PDE inhibition were the major mode of action of theophylline, there should be synergy with beta-agonists, which also increase intracellular cAMP concentrations, but this has not been convincingly demonstrated in man (117). *In vitro* canine tracheal smooth muscle, however, shows synergy between the relaxant action of these two drugs (118).

Different types of PDE isotypes are now recognized. Theophylline is an inhibitor of cyclic guanosine monophosphate (cGMP)–PDE as well as of cAMP–PDE (119). However, nitroglycerine is a potent inhibitor of cGMP–PDE, yet has no bronchodilator effect (120). It is possible that PDE is compartmentalized within the cell and that theophylline inhibits a pool of PDE, which is important for interacting with the cAMP generated by bronchodilator receptor activation.

Adenosine Receptor Antagonism

Theophylline, at therapeutic concentrations, is a potent antagonist of adenosine receptors, suggesting a possible mechanism for its therapeutic effects. Adenosine is produced by several cell types in the lung under hypoxic conditions, and its plasma concentration increases after antigen challenge in asthmatic subjects (121). Adenosine has little or no effect on human airway smooth muscle *in vitro* (122), but when given by inhalation causes bronchoconstriction in asthmatic subjects (123), suggesting that it may have an indirect effect, although this does not appear to involve a cholinergic reflex and may be due to release of preformed mediators from airway mast cells. Adenosine has no effect on airway function in normal subjects, suggesting that asthmatic subjects are hyperresponsive to adenosine, as they are to other bronchoconstrictors. Theophylline appears to have a selective inhibitory effect against adenosine-induced bronchoconstriction (124), although this does not prove that adenosine inhibition is the mechanism of action of theophylline, but merely demonstrates that theophylline, in therapeutic concentrations, is able to antagonize the effects of adenosine on the airways. However, evidence is now accumulating that adenosine antagonism is not the mechanism of bronchodilation induced by theophylline, since enprofylline, which is some five times more potent than theophylline as a bronchodilator, has no significant effect on adenosine receptors (125). Thus, theophylline inhibits the cardiovascular and respiratory effects of infused adenosine in man, but enprofylline has no effect (126).

It is likely that the bronchodilator action of theophylline is unrelated to its antagonism of adenosine receptors, although many of the systemic side effects of theophylline may be explained by this mechanism, reflecting the ubiquitous actions of adenosine.

Endogenous Catecholamine Release

Endogenous catecholamines, particularly adrenaline, may be important in regulating bronchomotor tone in asthma (127). Theophylline increases the secretion of catecholamines from the adrenal medulla (128), although the increase in plasma catecholamine concentration is insufficient to account for any bronchodilator effect. In normal subjects in the upright posture the bronchodilator response to acute aminophylline infusion is blocked by propranolol, implying that endogenous stimulation of airway β-receptors, presumably by circulating adrenaline, may contribute to the bronchodilator effect in normal subjects (128). However, this catecholamine response is probably secondary to the cardiovascular effects of intravenous aminophylline (and bronchodilation is not seen in normal subjects when supine), and this is unlikely to be a prominent mode of action of theophylline in asthmatic subjects.

Prostaglandin Inhibition

Theophylline antagonizes some of the effects of prostaglandins on vascular smooth muscle *in vitro* (129). However, these effects are seen at concentrations of theophylline that are higher than those used therapeutically, and are likely to be a reflection of functional antagonism (see below), since theophylline inhibits smooth muscle induced by a range of spasmogens.

Effects on Calcium Mobilization

Another potential explanation for the bronchodilator effect of theophylline is that there is some interference with calcium mobilization in the target cell. Theophylline does not block entry of calcium ions via voltage-dependent channels, and drugs such as nifedipine, which do, are, in any case, not bronchodilators (130). However, in airway smooth muscle calcium ions also enter via receptor-operated channels and are released from intracellular stores. Recent studies have shown that theophylline does not appear to block calcium entry in animal airway smooth muscle, although there is some evidence that theophylline increases calcium uptake into mitochondria of airway smooth muscle (131), but again the concentrations required for this effect are higher than the therapeutic range. Release of calcium from intracellular stores is brought about by hydrolysis of membrane phosphoinositides (PIs), via the formation of inositol trisphosphate. Several spasmogens stimulate PI hydrolysis (132,133), and an attractive mechanism of action of theophylline might be that they inhibit PI hydrolysis.

However, in bovine airway smooth muscle concentrations of theophylline that relax the smooth muscle have no effect on either basal or stimulated PI turnover (134). It is possible that theophylline might have an effect on a product of PI hydrolysis, such as IP_3. Recent studies have demonstrated that removal of the cell membrane of airway smooth muscle by detergents prevents the bronchodilator effect of theophylline, suggesting that theophylline works on some surface membrane mechanism, rather than via an intracellular mechanism (132).

Functional Antagonism

Xanthines such as theophylline have traditionally been suggested to work in asthma through bronchodilation. While it remains clear that theophylline is a bronchodilator in asthmatic subjects, it remains somewhat of a puzzle why theophylline does not affect the lung function of normal subjects, in contrast to the actions of beta-agonists and muscarinic antagonists. *In vitro* theophylline relaxes both large and small human airways, an effect that may be enhanced by epithelial removal (135). However, theophylline only induces airway smooth muscle relaxation at high concentrations (above 100 M), suggesting that this action may not be important for the clinical benefit observed with this drug *in vivo*. However, theophylline will produce functional antagonism of the contraction of airway smooth muscle induced by a wide range of spasmogens. This functional antagonism is not equal for the airway smooth muscle contraction induced by all spasmogens, as, for example, it has been reported that theophylline can preferentially inhibit airway smooth muscle contraction induced by histamine when compared to acetylcholine (ACh)-induced contraction (43). Furthermore, it has been reported that theophylline will inhibit airway smooth muscle contraction induced by nerve stimulation concentrations far lower than the contraction induced by substances directly contracting muscle. This phenomenon has been observed also for the ability of theophylline to induce PAF-induced bronchoconstriction in comparison with 5-hydroxytryptamine (5-HT)–induced bronchoconstriction.

ADVERSE ACTIONS

Toxic serum concentrations of theophylline may occur as a cumulative effect during chronic stable dosing as well as after acute overdose. There is a poor correlation between the prescribed dose and the serum concentration in individual patients (136); furthermore, a number of factors affect the bio-

TABLE 1. *Conditions that affect theophylline pharmacokinetics*

Condition	Effect	Reference
Age	Decreased hepatic and renal clearance in the elderly	139
	Increased susceptibility to drug interaction in the elderly	140
Heart failure	Decreased clearance	141
Liver disease	Decreased clearance; serum albumin concentration is a useful predictor of impaired theophylline metabolism	142
Hypoxia	Experimental hypoxia in rats leads to decreased hepatic and renal clearance and an acute rise in serum theophylline concentration	143
Smoking	Increased clearance; therefore, potential increase in serum concentration upon cessation of smoking	144
Hypothyroidism	Decreased clearance	145
Hyperthyroidism	Increased clearance; therefore, potential increase in serum concentration if hyperthyroidism is treated	145
Pregnancy	Decreased clearance in third trimester	146

TABLE 2. *The effect of some common medications on serum theophylline clearance (137)*

Decrease	Increase
Erythromycin; ciprofloxacin	Isoprenaline
Cimetidine; propranolol	Terbatuline
Verapamil; diltiazem	Phenytoin
Nifedipine; frusemide	Barbiturates
Allopurinol; disulfiram	Bnezodiazepines
Interferon; influenza vaccine	

availability and clearance of theophylline and a change in circumstances may therefore lead to a sudden change in serum concentration (Table 1). Theophylline is particularly sensitive to pharmacological interactions (Table 2) (137). The effects of theophylline at high serum concentrations may be serious or fatal, but even when the serum level is within the accepted therapeutic range subjective side effects may be unpleasant and may affect compliance. In a study of patients in general practice 41% were not taking all of their theophylline medication and most of these had discontinued the use of the drug completely (138).

SIDE EFFECTS (AT THERAPEUTIC CONCENTRATION)

Subjective and Behavioral Effects

At serum concentrations below 20 mg/L theophylline may cause epigastric pain, nausea, tremor, sleep disturbances, and agitation. It has also been associated with increased depressive symptoms (147). In children it may cause behavioral and learning problems although the evidence for this is poor. Rachelefsky et al. (148) studied asthmatic children who were taking theophylline. Teachers were able to correctly identify seven out of the ten children on active treatment and their assessment revealed evidence of increased activity and decreased concentration. However, in the same study, the parents were unable to detect any differences due to treatment and formal psychometric testing showed no objective changes. Another study demonstrated that children already taking theophylline who had behavioral and learning difficulties improved if their treatment is changed to cromolyn in a blind crossover manner (149). Other studies have not confirmed these findings, and, in fact, in adolescents there is evidence of an improvement in memory on theophylline (150). A more recent study has shown that the long-term treatment of asthmatic children with theophylline does not alter overall performance in school (151).

Gastroesophageal Reflux (GOR)

It has been suggested that theophylline may increase GOR in susceptible individuals and may therefore worsen asthma if bronchoconstriction is triggered by aspiration of gastric acid. In a study of 25 asthmatics with symptoms of GOR, 24-h esophageal pH monitoring showed that the degree and duration of reflux increased during theophylline treatment, as did reflux symptoms. There was, however, no corresponding increase in the severity of asthma (152). In asthmatics without previous reflux symptoms chronic oral theophylline administration does not significantly alter esophageal pH at night (153). There is, then, no evidence that theophylline causes an increase in the severity of respiratory disease by this mechanism, although it may exacerbate existing upper gastrointestinal symptoms.

Cardiac Actions

Theophylline may cause tachycardias at concentrations that are within the therapeutic range. In a group of 16 patients with multifocal atrial tachycardia the arrhythmia resolved when theophylline was withdrawn and reappeared after challenge with a therapeutic theophylline level (154). Theophylline may also induce angina in susceptible individuals by a mechanism that is independent of the heart rate. Some subjects experience chest pain during rapid atrial pacing only if they have received theophylline (155).

Rare Side Effects

Urticaria has been described after theophylline administration and a number of cases of Stevens-Johnson syndrome have been reported (156–158).

There has been one case of severe painful ulceration at the lower end of the esophagus after the patient took a slow-release theophylline tablet.

TOXICITY (AT HIGH SERUM CONCENTRATION)

At higher serum concentrations the adverse actions of theophylline are serious and may be life threatening. The subjective symptoms include abdominal pain, nausea, tremor, headache, and hallucinations (159). In a series of patients who had taken theophylline in overdose, all had tachycardia, 80% had GI disturbances, 50% had hypotension, and 20% had seizures (160). The most dangerous features of toxicity are seizures, which may lead to neurological damage or death, ventricular tachycardia and fibrillation, and rhabdomyolysis with acute renal failure. There is no consistent relationship between the serum concentration and the occurrence of morbidity once in the toxic range (161), but there is a correlation between the age of the patient and the occurrence of life-threatening side effects (162).

Arrhythmias

The commonest arrhythmia after theophylline overdose is sinus tachycardia. Multifocal and unifocal atrial tachycardia, which responds to verapamil, may occur, as may supraventricular tachycardia responsive to both propranolol and verapamil (163,164). Ventricular arrhythmias are more dangerous and occur in up to 20% of cases of overdose; the probability of ventricular tachycardia is not related to the serum theophylline concentration once the maximum therapeutic level is exceeded (165). Ventricular tachycardia (VT) may be persistent (166), although in dogs VT responds to β-blockade and, remarkably, to verapamil (167). T-wave inversion in the absence of myocardial disease has also been reported during an episode of theophylline toxicity (168).

Seizures

The occurrence of seizures is associated with a poor prognosis, a 50% mortality, and a significant morbidity (169). They may occur even when the theophylline concentration is within the therapeutic range and are more common in older patients or when there is preexisting neurological abnormality or brain damage (170,171).

Metabolic Changes

After theophylline overdose hypokalemia, hypophosphatemia, and hypomagnesemia are common; it is important that these conditions are detected and treated since they may increase the likelihood of seizures (172). Blood glucose becomes elevated and may be above 20 mg/L, and there may be a mixed metabolic acidosis and respiratory alkalosis. These abnormalities are related to the serum theophylline level (173). The metabolic acidosis is due to lactate accumulation in most cases but one report describes severe ketoacidosis in a nondiabetic patient after prolonged overdose (174). Theophylline toxicity should be included alongside aspirin poisoning in the differential diagnosis of metabolic acidosis and mixed metabolic acidosis with respiratory alkalosis.

Rhabdomyolysis

There have been a number of reports of rhabdomyolysis after theophylline overdose. Seizures and defibrillation may be implicated and it is of note that severe widespread muscle damage has been seen postmortem after theophylline-induced fits (175). Rhabdomyolysis leads to myoglobinuria and acute renal failure (176,177). There is also one report of raised CK-MB of myocardial origin with no ECG evidence of infarction in an elderly patient with theophylline toxicity, suggesting diffuse myocardial muscle damage (178).

MECHANISMS OF ADVERSE ACTIONS

Cardiovascular

When isoprenaline is given at the same time as theophylline the chronotropic action of the two drugs is additive but theophylline does not affect the slope of the dose-response curve for isoprenaline, suggesting that phosphodiesterase inhibition is not the mechanism of the sinus tachycardia produced by theophylline (179). In dogs, adenosine causes the heart rate to fall and theophylline reverses the effect. The sinus tachycardia seen during theophylline treatment, then, may be partly due to antagonism of the negative chronotropic action of adenosine (180). Theophylline reduces forearm blood flow (and therefore systemic vascular resistance) and this may also play a part by inducing a reflex sinus tachycardia (181).

As well as sinus tachycardia, theophylline may produce a number of rhythm disturbances in man, including multifocal atrial tachycardia (MAT), supraventricular tachycardia (SVT), and ventricular tachycardia (VT). In isolated human atrial fibers theophylline increases the number of spontaneous action potentials and this is antagonized by diltiazem, a calcium channel blocker (182). Electrophysiological studies in young people and in patients with COPD revealed a decreased sinoatrial and atrioventricular node refractory period and an increased sinoatrial and His-Purkinje conduction velocity (154,183). These changes would be consistent with a tendency to cause MAT and reentrant SVT, although they do not account for ventricular arrhythmias, which tend to occur at higher, toxic levels, and may be due to separate mechanisms such as phosphodiesterase inhibition.

Central Nervous System

Theophylline stimulates the central nervous system in animals and in man, producing irritability and anxiety (184). It is a lipophilic drug and is therefore able to cross the blood-brain barrier, achieving a concentration in cerebrospinal fluid of 0.35 to 0.41 times that in the plasma (185,186). As well as acting specifically on ventilatory drive, theophylline leads to a global increase in central nervous system activity, which may account for its association with tremor and seizures and with improved verbal learning (147). Normal subjects receiving chronic oral theophylline with serum concentrations in the lower part of the therapeutic range have EEG evidence of increased electrical activity in the brain and the spinal cord but no change in the activity of peripheral nerves (187). Experiments in the rat show that an increased number of cells discharge after hippocampal stimuli during aminophylline treatment, electrically induced seizures are more severe and more prolonged (188), and theophylline potentiates the effect of kainic acid, a proconvulsant agent. *In vitro* theophylline is able to induce epileptiform activity in hippocampal slices at concentrations as low as 3 μM, and it induces burst firing in response to electrical stimulation (189).

Gamma aminobutyric acid (GABA) is an inhibitory neurotransmitter that potentiates the binding of benzodiazepines to their receptors in the CNS. There is no known endogenous ligand for the benzodiazepine receptor but it is thought that one must exist. Theophylline interferes with GABA's action on the benzodiazepine receptor, thereby decreasing the receptor's affinity for benzodiazepines. If an endogenous benzodiazepine exists, then, theophylline would antagonize its action and this would account for theophylline's action as a stimulant of the CNS. Adenosine agonists abolish these actions suggesting that theophylline's effect on the GABA/benzodiazepine receptor complex is mediated by antagonism at the adenosine receptor (184). Further evidence for the involvement of adenosine receptors comes from an experiment that shows up-regulation of adenosine A_1 receptors in rat cerebral cortex and cerebellum after chronic theophylline exposure and an associated decrease in sensitivity to convulsant agents after withdrawal of theophylline (190).

Theophylline and benzodiazepines antagonize each other *in vivo*. In mice aminophylline decreases the protection afforded by benzodiazepines against convulsions (191). In man aminophylline antagonizes the sedation produced by benzodiazepines. In three clinical studies aminophylline has been found to reverse sedation induced by diazepam; after a bolus dose of diazepam, intravenous aminophylline produced an immediate and sustained recovery of consciousness, whereas placebo-treated patients remained unconscious for 1 to 2 h and aminophylline also reversed the EEG changes induced by diazepam. After diazepam sedation for upper GI endoscopy, the number of patients fully conscious at 30 and 60 min was increased with aminophylline and reaction times and visual analogue alertness scores were improved. When enprofylline, a similar compound that does not act as an adenosine antagonist, was given, there was no effect, suggesting that in man theophylline stimulates the central nervous system by acting as an adenosine antagonist (192–194).

TREATMENT OF THEOPHYLLINE TOXICITY

In a 5-year retrospective analysis of 54 patients with theophylline toxicity the incidence of serious side effects was low despite very high serum concentrations in some patients (195). The blood level does not predict for life-threatening events such as seizures, and it has therefore been suggested that conservative management should be employed after theophylline overdose unless serious side effects occur (196). ECG monitoring is advisable in all patients as arrhythmias are common, even at lower toxic concentrations. Activated charcoal may be administered orally at 2-h intervals; this regimen enhances theophylline clearance, reducing the mean biological half-life from 10.2 to 4.6 h and producing a rapid clinical improvement after overdose (197). Unfortunately, persistent vomiting precludes this treatment option in many patients (198).

If a very rapid reduction of the theophylline concentration is required hemoperfusion or hemodialysis may be used. Hemodialysis removes 36% of plasma theophylline during each pass through the circuit, reducing the half-life by more than 50% (199). In severe toxicity theophylline clearance has been accelerated by using hemoperfusion and hemodialysis simultaneously (200).

There is evidence that theophylline induces seizures by an action that is antagonized by benzodiazepines and these drugs are recommended as first-time treatment (201). The occurrence of muscle damage with rhabdomyolysis of renal failure after theophylline-induced seizures emphasizes the need for urgent and adequate antiepileptic treatment. If arrhythmias occur after theophylline overdose the serum potassium and magnesium concentrations and the acid base status should be corrected by appropriate replacement. Hypokalemia may be severe and a high infusion rate may be required. Atrial and supraventricular tachycardias may respond to verapamil or propranolol; if the rhythm is resistant, intravenous adenosine may theoretically abolish the rhythm, since theophylline is a competitive antagonist of adenosine and adenosine decreases nodal conduction. It is of note that verapamil has been effective in experimental VT in animals given toxic doses of theophylline; however it is doubtful whether the use of this negative inotrope would be justified in cases of VT in man. Intravenous beta-blockers have been shown to abolish both supraventricular and ventricular tachycardias after theophylline overdose. These drugs also reverse the metabolic abnormalities (201). Propranolol decreases theophylline clearance, but sotalol has less effect in this respect (202) and it has additional class III antiarrhythmic activity; sotalol would therefore be preferable. Beta-blockers must be used cautiously unless it is clear that the patient is not asthmatic, since severe bronchospasm may result (203).

FUTURE DIRECTIONS

Traditionally the use of preparations containing xanthines has been governed by the perceived need to achieve plasma levels within a therapeutic window of 10 to 20 mg/ml. In fact many of the so-called advances in this area over the last decade have been related to the preparation of formulations of slow-release theophylline to maintain plasma levels of theophylline within the therapeutic window over a 24-h period in order to maximize therapeutic benefit and reduce the risk of toxicity. Nonetheless it remains clear that while the measurement of plasma levels is desirable under certain circumstances, in many situations where theophylline is administered chronically for maintenance therapy of asthma, plasma levels within the therapeutic window are rarely achieved. On the one hand this raises doubts about the need to routinely monitor plasma levels of theophylline, and on the other hand it raises the question as to whether plasma levels within the therapeutic window are actually necessary for maintenance therapy.

Certainly much of the early work with theophylline that determined the current therapeutic window revealed that much of the clinical benefit of theophylline was achieved at plasma levels less than 10 mg/ml. Furthermore, plasma levels of 5 mg/ml have been shown to be effective in preventing exercise-induced bronchoconstriction, and lower plasma levels of theophylline will provide protection against bronchoconstriction than are required to elicit bonchodilatation. Our own studies have revealed a clear effect of theophylline on the allergen-induced LAR at plasma levels less than 10 mg/ml. The possibility exists therefore that nonbronchodilator effects of theophylline may well occur at lower plasma concentrations. If this work can be substantiated further, then the therapeutic range may need to be redefined, allowing the use of theophylline to be broadened. At lower plasma levels there will be less risk from side effects, which at present are the main limiting factor to the wider use of theophylline, particularly in children. This recent evidence also raises the real possibility that the clinical use of theophylline should be altered, since it may be more appropriate to use the drug as a chronic orally active prophylactic agent rather than as a bronchodilator.

The recognition that there are now five distinct isozymes of PDE with relative anatomical specificity raises the real possibility that more potent theophylline-like drugs will appear as new medicines in the coming years.

The development of these drugs, many based on the xanthine structure, has been an important impetus for the development of an orally active prophylactic nonsteroidal anti-inflammatory drug. Clearly these agents have been demonstrated to have anti-inflammatory activity in experimental models and the recent arrival of the early examples of PDE selective inhibitors in clinical trials may herald a new era in the treatment of asthma.

REFERENCES

1. Salter HH. On asthma, its pathology and treatment. *J Churchill* 1860.
2. Becker AB, Simons KJ, Gillespie CA, Simons FE. The bronchodilator effects and pharmacokinetics of caffeine in asthma. *N Engl J Med* 1984;310(12):743–746.
3. Persson CG. Overview of effects of theophylline. *J Allergy Clin Immunol* 1986;78(4 Pt 2):780–787.
4. Gong H Jr, Simmons MS, Tashkin DP, Hui KK, Lee EY. Bronchodilator effects of caffeine in coffee. A dose-response study of asthmatic subjects. *Chest* 1986;89(3):335–342.
5. Herrman G, Aynesworth MB. Successful treatment of extreme dyspnea, "status asthmaticus" using theophylline ethylene diamine intravenously. *J Lab Clin Med* 1937;23:135.
6. Brown GT. Aminophylline in asthma. *J Allergy* 1938;10:64–65.
7. Carr HA. The treatment of acute attacks of bronchial asthma by intravenous injection of aminophylline. *J Lab Clin Med* 1940;25:1295–1299.
8. Turner-Warwick M. Study of theophylline plasma levels after oral administration of new theophylline compounds. *Br Med J* 1957;13:67–69.
9. Jackson RH, McHenry JI, Moreland FB, Raymer WJ, Etter RL. Clinical evaluation of elixophylline with correlation of pulmonary function studies and theophylline serum levels in acute and chronic asthmatic patients. *Dis Chest* 1964;45:75–85.
10. Eriksson NE, Haglind K, Ewald U. Combined theophylline/beta-agonists maintenance therapy in chronic asthma. *Eur J Respir Dis* 1983;64(3):172–177.
11. Sahay JN, Chatterjee SS. A 21-day double-blind study of the effect of adding sustained-release theophylline (Nuelin SA) to inhaled salbutamol in patients with asthma. *Br J Dis Chest* 1983;77(1):66–70.
12. Stalenheim G, Lindstrom B, Lonnerholm G. Oral terbutaline alone and in combination with theophylline: dose, plasma concentration, and effect in long-term treatment of bronchial asthma. *Eur Respir J* 1989;2(9):861–867.
13. Klein JJ, Lefkowitz MS, Spector SL, Cherniack RM. Relationship between serum theophylline levels and pulmonary function before and after inhaled beta-agonist in "stable" asthmatics. *Am Rev Respir Dis* 1983;127(4):413–416.
14. Laursen LC, Johannesson N, Weeke B. Effects of enprofylline and theophylline on exercise-induced asthma. *Allergy* 1985;40(7):506–509.
15. Brenner M, Berkowitz R, Marshall N, Strunk RC. Need for theophylline in severe steroid-requiring asthmatics. *Clin Allergy* 1988;18(2):143–150.
16. Myhre KI, Arnulf V, Walstad RA. Long-term therapy with sustained-release theophylline. *Pharmatherapeutica* 1985;4(2):92–97.
17. Vereen LE, Kinasewitz GT, George RB. Effect of aminophylline on exercise performance in patients with irreversible airway obstruction. *Arch Intern Med* 1986;146(7):1349–1351.
18. Taylor DR, Buick B, Kinney C, Lowry RC, McDevitt DG. The efficacy of orally administered theophylline, inhaled salbutamol, and a combination of the two as chronic therapy in the management of chronic bronchitis with reversible air-flow obstruction. *Am Rev Respir Dis* 1985;131(5):747–751.
19. Wrenn K, Slovis CM, Murphy F, Greenberg RS. Aminophylline therapy for acute bronchospastic disease in the emergency room. *Ann Intern Med* 1991;115(4):241–247.
20. Self TH, Abou-Shala N, Burns R, Stewart CF, Ellis RF, Tsiu SJ, Kellermann AL.

Inhaled albuterol and oral prednisone therapy in hospitalized adult asthmatics. Does aminophylline add any benefit? *Chest* 1990;98(6):1317–1321.

21. Littenberg B. Aminophylline treatment in severe, acute asthma. A meta-analysis. *JAMA* 1988;259(11):1678–1684.

22. Mansel JK, Stogner SW, Petrini MF, Norman JR. Mechanical ventilation in patients with acute severe asthma. *Am J Med* 1990;89(1):42–48.

23. Goldie RG, Spina D, Henry PJ, Lulich KM, Paterson JW. In vitro responsiveness of human asthmatic bronchus to carbachol, histamine, beta-adrenoceptor agonists and theophylline. *Br J Clin Pharmacol* 1986;22(6):669–676.

24. Bai TR. Abnormalities in airway smooth muscle in fatal asthma. A comparison between trachea and bronchus. *Am Rev Respir Dis* 1991;143(2):441–443.

25. Alanko K, Sahlstrom K. Comparison of bronchodilator effects of oral salbutamol and theophylline and their combination with hydroxyzine. *Ann Clin Res* 1983;15(1):10–14.

26. Barlow TJ, Graham P, Harris JM, Hartley JP, Turton CW. A double-blind, placebo-controlled comparison of the efficacy of standard and individually titrated doses of theophylline in patients with chronic asthma. *Br J Dis Chest* 1988;82(3):251–261.

27. Grassi V, Boschetti E, Tantucci C. Round table on antiasthmatic drugs; beta-agonists and theophylline. Workshop on pathogenesis and therapy of bronchial asthma Cortina d'Ampezzo/1–4 April, 1987. *Eur Respir J Suppl* 1989;6:551s–555s.

28. Magnussen H, Jorres R, Hartmann V. Bronchodilator effect of theophylline preparations and aerosol fenoterol in stable asthma. *Chest* 1986;90(5):722–725.

29. Georgopoulos D, Wong D, Anthonisen NR. Interactive effects of systemically administered salbutamol and aminophylline in patients with chronic obstructive pulmonary disease. *Am Rev Respir Dis* 1988;138(6):1499–1503.

30. Cockcroft DW, Murdock KY, Gore BP, O'Byrne PM, Manning P. Theophylline does not inhibit allergen-induced increase in airway responsiveness to methacholine. *J Allergy Clin Immunol* 1989;83(5):913–920.

31. Ward AJ, McKennif M, Page C, Costello J. The immunomodulator effect of theophylline on the late asthmatic response. *Am Rev Resp Dis* 1993;147:518–523.

32. Pauwels RA. New aspects of the therapeutic potential of theophylline in asthma. *J Allergy Clin Immunol* 1989;83(2 Pt 2):548–553.

33. Crescioli S, Spinazzi A, Plebani M, Pozzani M, Mapp CE, Boschetto P, Fabbri LM. Theophylline inhibits early and late asthmatic reactions induced by allergens in asthmatic subjects. *Ann Allergy* 1991;66(3):245–251.

34. Magnussen H, Reuss G, Jorres R. Theophylline has a dose-related effect on the airway response to inhaled histamine and methacholine in asthmatics. *Am Rev Respir Dis* 1987;136(5):1163–1167.

35. Levene S, McKenzie SA. Protective effect of theophylline on histamine-induced bronchoconstriction in asthmatic children. *Br J Clin Pharmacol* 1986;21(4):445–449.

36. Segal MS, Levinson L, Bresnick E, Beakey JF. Evaluation of therapeutic substances employed for the relief of bronchospasm. VI. Aminophylline. *J Clin Invest* 1949; 28:1190–1195.

37. Magnussen H, Reuss G, Jorres R. Methylxanthines inhibit exercise-induced bronchoconstriction at low serum theophylline concentration and in a dose-dependent fashion. *J Allergy Clin Immunol* 1988;81(3):531–537.

38. Seppala OP, Iisalo E. Measuring the bronchial effects of bronchodilating drugs in healthy subjects with methacholine provocations: theophylline protects against induced bronchoconstriction in a dose-dependent manner. *Int J Clin Pharmacol Ther Toxicol* 1990;28(9):380–386.

39. Guillot C, Fornaris M, Badier M, Orehek J. Spontaneous and provoked resistance to isoprotenerol in isolated human bronchi. *JACI* 1984;74:713–718.

40. Finney MJ, Karlsson JA, Persson CG. Effects of bronchoconstrictors and bronchodilators on a novel human small airway preparation. *Br J Pharmacol* 1985;85(1):29–36.

41. Allen SL, Cortijo J, Foster RW, Morgan GP, Small RC, Weston AH. Mechanical and electrical aspects of the relaxant action of aminophylline in guinea-pig isolated trachealis. *Br J Pharmacol* 1986;88(2):473–483.

42. Supinski GS, Deal EC Jr, Kelsen SG. Comparative effects of theophylline and adenosine on respiratory skeletal and smooth muscle. *Am Rev Respir Dis* 1986;133(5):809–813.

43. Gustafsson B, Persson C. Effect of different bronchodilators on airway smooth muscle responsiveness to contractile agents. *Thorax* 1991;46:360–365.
44. Wanner A. Effects of methylxanthines on airway mucocillary function. *Am J Med* 1985;79(suppl 6A):16–20.
45. Dunnil MS, Massarella GR, Anderson JA. A comparison of the quantitative anatomy of the bronchi in normal subjects, in status asthmaticus, in chronic bronchitis and in emphysema. *Thorax* 1969;24:176–179.
46. Allegra L, Abraham WM, Chapman GA, Wanner A. Duration of mucocilary clearance dysfunction following antigen challenge. *J Appl Physiol* 1983;55:726–730.
47. Mezey RJ, Cohn MA, Fernandez RJ, Januszkiewicz AJ, Wanner A. Mucociliary transport in allergic patients with antigen induced bronchospasm. *Am Rev Respir Dis* 1978;118(4):677–684.
48. Marom Z, Shelhammer JH, Bach MK, et al. Slow reacting substances, leukotrienes C4 and D4 increase the release of mucus from human airways in vitro. *Am Rev Respir Dis* 1982;126:449–451.
49. Smith LJ. The role of platelet activating factor in asthma. *Am Rev Respir Dis* 1991;143:S100–S102.
50. Matthys H, Vastag E, Daikeler G, et al. Mucocilary clearance in patients with chronic bronchitis and bronchial carcinoma. *Br J Clin Pract* 1983;suppl 23:10–15.
51. Cotromanes E, Gerrity TR, Garrard CS, Harshbarger RD, Yeates DB, Kendzierski DL, Lourenco RV. Aerosol penetration and mucociliary transport in the healthy human lung. Effect of low serum theophylline levels. *Chest* 1985;88(2):194–200.
52. Pearson MG, Ahmad D, Chamberlain MJ, Morgan WK, Vinitski S. Aminophylline and mucociliary clearance in patients with irreversible airflow limitation. *Br J Clin Pharmacol* 1985;20(6):688–690.
53. Kuei JH, Sieck GC. Chronic aminophylline administration. Effect on diaphragm contractility and fatigue resistance in vitro. *Am Rev Respir Dis* 1991;144(1):121–125.
54. Howell S, Roussos C. Isoproterenol and aminophylline improve contractility of fatigued canine diaphragm. *Am Rev Respir Dis* 1984;129(1):118–124.
55. Supinski GS, Deal EC Jr, Kelsen SG. The effects of caffeine and theophylline on diaphragm contractility. *Am Rev Respir Dis* 1984;130(3):429–433.
56. Belman MJ, Sieck GC, Mazar A. Aminophylline and its influence on ventilatory endurance in humans. *Am Rev Respir Dis* 1985;131(2):226–229.
57. Murciano D, Aubier M, Lecocguic Y, Pariente R. Effects of theophylline on diaphragmatic strength and fatigue in patients with chronic obstructive pulmonary disease. *N Engl J Med* 1984;311(6):349–353.
58. Vires N, Aubier M, Murciano D, Fleury B, Talamo C, Pariente R. Effects of aminophylline on diaphragmatic fatigue during acute respiratory failure. *Am Rev Respir Dis* 1984;129(3):396–402.
59. Wiles CM, Moxham J, Newham D, Edwards RH. Aminophylline and fatigue of adductor pollicis in man. *Clin Sci* 1983;64(5):547–550.
60. Efthimiou J, Felming J, Edwards RH, Spiro SG. Effect of aminophylline on fatigue of the sternomastoid muscle in man. *Thorax* 1986;41(2):122–127.
61. Ridings JW, Barry SR, Faulkner JA. Aminophylline enhances contractility of frog skeletal muscle: an effect dependent on extracellular calcium. *J Appl Physiol* 1989;67(2):671–676.
62. Kolbeck RC, Speir WA. Theophylline, fatigue, and diaphragm contractility: cellular levels of 45Ca and cAMP. *J Appl Physiol* 1991;70(5):1933–1937.
63. Dimarco AF, Nochomovitz M, DiMarco MS, Altose MD, Kelsen SG. Comparative effects of aminophylline on diaphragm and cardiac contractility. *Am Rev Respir Dis* 1985;132(4):800–805.
64. Saadeh GM, Ayash RE, Saadeh FM, Nassar CF. Effect of aminophylline on calcium transport across the rat diaphragm. *Gen Pharmacol* 1985;16(5):541–543.
65. Aubier M. Effect of theophylline on diaphragmatic and other skeletal muscle function. *J Allergy Clin Immunol* 1986;78(4 Pt 2):787–792.
66. Morice AH, Schofield P, Keal EE, Sever PS. A comparison of the ventilatory, cardiovascular and metabolic effects of salbutamol, aminophylline and vasoactive intestinal peptide in normal subjects. *Br J Clin Pharmacol* 1986;22(2):149–153.
67. Georgopoulos D, Holtby SG, Berezanski D, Anthonisen NR. Aminophylline effects on

ventilatory response to hypoxia and hyperoxia in normal adults. *J Appl Physiol* 1989;67(3):1150–1156.

68. Parsons ST, Griffiths TL, Christie JM, Holgate ST. Effect of theophylline and dipyridamole on the respiratory response to isocapnic hypoxia in normal human subjects. *Clin Sci* 1991;80(2):107–112.
69. Javaheri S, Guerra L. Lung function, hypoxic and hypercapnic ventilatory responses, and respiratory muscle strength in normal subjects taking oral theophylline. *Thorax* 1990;45(10):743–747.
70. Easton PA, Anthonisen NR. Ventilatory response to sustained hypoxia after pretreatment with aminophylline. *J Appl Physiol* 1988;64(4):1445–1450.
71. Eldridge FL, Millhorn DE, Kiley JP. Antagonism by theophylline of respiratory inhibition induced by adenosine. *J Appl Physiol* 1985;59(5):1428–1433.
72. Berry RB, Desa MM, Branum JP, Light RW. Effect of theophylline on sleep and sleep-disordered breathing in patients with chronic obstructive pulmonary disease. *Am Rev Respir Dis* 1991;143(2):245–250.
73. Mulloy E, McNicholas WT. Theophylline in obstructive sleep apnea. A double-blind evaluation. *Chest* 1992;101(3):753–757.
74. Parker J, Kelkar K, West R. Haemodynamic effects of aminophylline in cor pulmonale. *Circulation* 1966;33:17–25.
75. Parker J, Ashekiou PB, Di Giorgi S, West RJ. Haemodynamic effects of aminophylline in COPD. *Circulation* 1967;35:365–372.
76. Matthey RA, Berger HJ, Loke J, Gottschalk A. Effects of aminophylline on left and right ventricular performance in COPD; a non invasive assessment of radionuclide angiocardiography. *Am J Med* 1978;65:903–910.
77. Matthay RA. Favorable cardiovascular effects of theophylline in COPD. *Chest* 1987; 92(1 suppl):22S–26S.
78. Matthay RA. Effects of theophylline on cardiovascular performance in chronic obstructive pulmonary disease. *Chest* 1985;88(2 suppl):112S–117S.
79. Voelkel NF, Sill V. Effect of aminophylline on hypoxic pulmonary vasoconstriction [letter]. *Am Rev Respir Dis* 1983;128(2):328–329.
80. Pauwels R. The effects of theophylline on airway inflammation. *Chest* 1987;92(1 suppl):32S–37S.
81. Pauwels R, Van Renterghem D, Van der Straeten M, Johannesson N, Persson CG. The effect of theophylline and enprofylline on allergen-induced bronchoconstriction. *J Allergy Clin Immunol* 1985;76(4):583–590.
82. Mapp C, et al. Protective effect of anti-asthma drugs on late asthmatic reactions and increased airway responsiveness induced by toluene diisocyanate in sensitized subjects. *Am Rev Respir Dis* 1987;136:1403–1407.
83. Hendeles L, Harmen E, Huang D, Cooper R, Delafuente J, Blake K, O'Brien R. Attenuation of allergen induced airway hyperreactivity and late response by theophylline. *Eur Respir J* 1991;14(suppl 4):4815.
83a. Sullivan PJ, Bek S, Jaffar Z, Page CP, Jefferey PK, Costello JF. The effects of low dose theophylline on the bronchial wall infiltrate after antigen challenge. *Am Rev Resp Dir* (in press).
84. Nelson S, Summer WR, Jakab GJ. Aminophylline-induced suppression of pulmonary antibacterial defenses. *Am Rev Respir Dis* 1985;131(6):923–927.
85. Pearce FL, Befus AD, Gauldie J, Bienenstock J. Effects of anti allergic compounds on histamine secretion by isolated mast cells. *J Immunol* 1982;128:2481–2486.
86. Louis RE, Radermecker MF. Substance P induced histamine release from human basophils, skin and lung fragments: effect of nedocromil sodium and theophylline. *Int Arch Allergy Appl Immunol* 1990;92:329–333.
87. Undem BJ, Torphy TJ, Goldman D, Chilton FH. Inhibition by adenosine 3' 5' monophosphate of eicosanoid and platelet activating factor biosynthesis in the mouse PT-18 mast cell. *J Biol Chem* 1990;265(12):6750–6758.
88. Naclerio RM, Bartenfelder D, Proud D, Togias AG, Meyers DA, Kagey-Sobotka A, Norman PS, Lichtenstein LM. Theophylline reduces the response to nasal challenge with antigen. *Am J Med* 1985;79(6A):43–47.
89. Gronneberg R. Inhibition of allergen-induced early reactions in atopic skin by salbutamol and theophylline. *Agents Actions* 1985;16(6):501–503.

90. Kita H, Abu-Ghazaleh RI, Gleich GJ, Abraham RT. Regulation of Ig induced eosinophil degranulation by adenosine 3′ 5′ cyclic monophosphate. *J Immunol* 1991;146 (8):2712–2718.
91. Yukawa T, Kroegel C, Chanez P, Dent G, Ukena D, Chung KF, Barnes PJ. Effect of theophylline and adenosine on eosinophil function. *Am Rev Respir Dis* 1989;140 (2):327–333.
92. Llupia J, Fernandez AG, Berga P, Gristwood RW. Effects of prednisolone, salbutamol and theophylline on bronchial hyperreactivity and leucocyte chemokinesis in guinea pigs. *Drugs Exp Clin Res* 1991;17(8):395–398.
93. Sanjar S, Aoki S, Kristersson A, Smith D, Morley J. Antigen challenge induces pulmonary airway eosinophil accumulation and airway hyperreactivity in sensitized guinea-pigs: the effect of anti-asthma drugs. *Br J Pharmacol* 1990;99(4):679–686.
94. Manzini S, Perretti F, Abelli L, Evanelista S, Seeds EAM, Page CP. Isbufylline, a new xanthine derivative inhibits airways hyperresponsiveness and airways inflammation in guinea pigs. *Eur J Pharmacol* (in press).
95. Zocchi MR, Pardi R, Gromo G, Ferrero E, Ferrero ME, Besana C, Rugarli C. Theophylline induced non specific suppressor activity in human peripheral blood lymphocytes. *J Immunopharmacol* 1985;7(2):217–234.
96. Shore A, Dosch H, Gelfand E. Induction and separation of antigen dependent T helper and T suppressor cells in man. *Nature* 1978;274:586–587.
97. Fink G, Mittelman M, Shohat B, Spitzer SA. Theophylline-induced alterations in cellular immunity in asthmatic patients. *Clin Allergy* 1987;17(4):313–316.
98. Ilfield D, Kitivy S, Fierman M, Topilsky M, Kuperman O. Effect of in vitro theophylline on suppressor cell function of asthmatic patients. *Clin Exp Immunol* 1985; 61:360–367.
99. Lahat N, Nir E, Horenstien L, Colin AA. Effect of theophylline on the proportion and function of T-suppressor cells in asthmatic children. *Allergy* 1985;40(6):453–457.
100. Shohat B, Volovitz B, Varsano I. Induction of suppressor T cells in asthmatic children by theophylline treatment. *Clin Allergy* 1983;13(5):487–493.
101. Guillou PJ, Ramsden C, Kerr M, Davison AM, Giles GR. A prospective controlled clinical trial of aminophylline as an adjunctive immunosuppressive agent. *Transplant Proc* 1984;16(5):1218–1220.
102. Shohat B, Shapira Z, Joshua H, Servadio C. Lack of suppressor T cells in renal transplant recipients and activation by aminophylline. *Thymus* 1983;5(2):67–77.
103. Shapira Z, Shohat B, Yusim A, Servadio C. Suppressor factor in plasma of aminophylline treated renal transplantated patients. *Proc Eur Dial Transplant Assoc* 1983; 19:473–476.
104. Rugarli C, Marni A, Ferrero ME. Prolonged survival of experimental heart transplantation induced by theophylline. *Immunol Lett* 1983;6(5):247–250.
105. Yokoyama A, Yamashita N, Mizushima Y, Yano S. Inhibition of natural killer cell activity by oral administration of theophylline. *Chest* 1990;98(4):924–927.
106. Marshall ME, Phillips B, Riley LK, Rhoades JR, Brown S, Jennings CD. Effects of theophylline on human natural killer cells. *Immunopharmacol Immunotoxicol* 1989; 11(1):1–16.
107. Calhoun WJ, Stevens CA, Lambert SB. Modulation of superoxide production of alveolar macrophages and peripheral blood mononuclear cells by beta-agonists and theophylline. *J Lab Clin Med* 1991;117(6):514–522.
108. O'Neill SJ, Sitar DS, Klass DJ, Taraska VA, Kepron W, Mitenko PA. The pulmonary disposition of theophylline and its influence on human alveolar macrophage bactericidal function. *Am Rev Respir Dis* 1986;134(6):1225–1228.
109. Bessler H, Sirota L, Gilgal R, Dulitzky F, Djaldetti M. In vivo and in vitro effects of theophylline on the peripheral blood mononuclear cells from preterm infants. *Biol Neonate* 1988;54(2):73–78.
110. Brandwein SR. Regulation of interleukin production by mouse peritoneal macrophages. *J Biol Chem* 1986;261(19):8624–8632.
111. Vairo G, Argyriou S, Bordun A, Whittey G, Hamilton JA. Inhibition of signalling pathways for macrophage proliferation by cyclic AMP. *J Biol Chem* 1990;265(5):2692–2701.
112. Condino-Neto A, Vilela MM, Cambiucci EC, Ribeiro JD, Guglielmi AA, Magna LA,

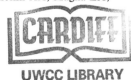

De Nucci G. Theophylline therapy inhibits neutrophil and mononuclear cell chemotaxis from chronic asthmatic children. *Br J Clin Pharmacol* 1991;32(5):557–561.
113. Nielson CP, Crowley JJ, Cusack BJ, Vestal RE. Therapeutic concentrations of theophylline and enprofylline potentiate catecholamine effects and inhibit leukocyte activation. *J Allergy Clin Immunol* 1986;78(4 Pt 1):660–667.
114. Bergstrand H. Phosphodiesterase inhibition and theophylline. *Eur J Respir Dis* 1980; 61:37–44.
115. Ruffin RE, Newhouse MT. Dipyridamole. Is it a bronchodilator? *Eur J Respir Dis* 1981;2:123–126.
116. Kolbeck RC, Speir WA, Carrier GO, Bransome ED. Apparent irrelevance of cyclic nucleotides to the relaxation of tracheal smooth muscle induced by Theophylline. *Lung* 1979;156:173–183.
117. Handslip PDJ, Dart AM, Davies BH. Intravenous salbutamol and aminophylline in asthma: a search for synergy. *Thorax* 1981;36:741–744.
118. Jenne JW. Theophylline as a bronchodilator in COPD and its combination with inhaled beta-adrenergic drugs. *Chest* 1987;92(1 suppl):7S–14S.
119. Murad F. Effects of phosphodiesterase inhibitors and the role of cyclic nucleotides in smooth muscle relaxation. In: Andersson KE, Persson CGA, eds. *Anti-asthma xanthines and adenosine*. Amsterdam: Experta Medica 1985;10–15.
120. Miller WC, Shultz TF. Failure of nitroglycerine as a bronchodilator. *Am Rev Respir Dis* 1979;120:471–478.
121. Mann JS, Holgate ST, Renwick AG, Cushley MJ. Airway effects of purine nucleosides and nucleotides and release with bronchial provocation in asthma. *J Appl Physiol* 1986;61:1667–1676.
122. Finnery MJB, Karlsson J-A, Persson CGA. Effects of bronchoconstrictors and bronchodilators on a novel human small airway preparation. *Br J Pharmacol* 1985;85:29–36.
123. Cushley MJ, Tattersfield AE, Holgate ST. Inhaled adenosine and guanosine on airway resistance in normal and asthmatic subjects. *Br J Clin Pharmacol* 1983;15:161–165.
124. Cushley MJ, Holgate ST. Adenosine-induced bronchoconstriction in asthma: antagonism by inhaled theophylline. *Am Rev Respir Dis* 1984;129:380–384.
125. Persson CGA. Development of safer xanthine drugs for the treatment of obstructive airways disease. *J Allergy Clin Immunol* 1986;78:817–824.
126. Maxwell DL, Fuller RW, Conradson T-B, Dixon CMS, Hughes JMB, Barnes PJ. Opposing effect of theophylline and enprofylline on the cardio-respiratory effects of adenosine infusion in man. *Am Rev Respir Dis* 1987;135:478A.
127. Barnes PJ. Endogenous catecholamines and asthma. *J Allergy Clin Immunol* 1986; 77:791–795.
128. Higbee MD, Kumar M, Galant SP. Stimulation of endogenous catecholamine release by theophylline: a proposed additional mechanism for theophylline effects. *J Allergy Clin Immunol* 1982;70:377–382.
129. Horrobin DF, Manku MS, Franks DJ, Hanet P. Methylxanthine phosphodiesterase inhibitors behave as prostaglandin antagonists in perfused rat mesenteric artery preparations. *Prostaglandins* 1977;13:33–40.
130. Lodfadahl C-G, Barnes PJ. Calcium, calcium channel blockers and airway function. *Acta Pharmacol Toxicol* 1986;58:91–111.
131. Kolbeck RC, Speir WA, Carrier GO, Bransome ED. Apparent irrelevance of cyclic nucleotides to the relaxation of tracheal smooth muscle induced by theophylline. *Lung* 1979;156:173–183.
132. Grandordy BM, Cuss FM, Sampson AS, Palmer JB, Barnes PJ. Phosphatidylinositol response to cholinergic agonists in airway smooth muscle: relationship to contraction and muscarinic receptor occupancy. *J Pharmacol Exp Ther* 1986;238:273–279.
133. Grandordy BM, Barnes PJ. Phosphoinositide turnover in airway smooth muscle. *Am Rev Respir Dis* 1987;(in press).
134. Grandordy B, Cuss FM, Barnes PJ. The effect of anti-asthma drugs on phosphatidylinositol turnover in airway smooth muscle. *Life Sci* 1987;41:1661–1667.
135. Allen SL, Cortijo J, Foster RW, Morgan GP, Small RC, Weston AH. Mechanical and electrical aspects of the relaxant action of aminophylline on guinea-pig isolated trachealis. *Br J Pharmacol* 1986;88:473–483.

136. Woodcock AA, Johnson MA, Geddes DM. Theophylline prescribing, serum concentrations, and toxicity. *Lancet* 1983;2(8350):610–613.
137. Upton RA. Pharmacokinetic interactions between theophylline and other medication (Part II). *Clin Pharmacokinet* 1991;20(2):135–150.
138. Taylor DR, Kinney CD, McDevitt DG. Patient compliance with oral theophylline therapy. *Br J Clin Pharmacol* 1984;17(1):15–20.
139. Shin SG, Juan D, Rammohan M. Theophylline pharmacokinetics in normal elderly subjects. *Clin Pharmacol Ther* 1988;44(5):522–530.
140. Frank WO. Safety: cimetidine and concomitant theophylline or warfarin—drug interactions and their implications. *Clin Ther* 1986;8(suppl A):57–68.
141. LeGatt DF. Theophylline toxicity—a consequence of congestive heart failure. *Drug Intell Clin Pharmacol* 1983;17(1):59–60.
142. Amodio P, Lauro S, Rondana M, Crema G, Merkel C, Gatta A, Ruol A. Theophylline pharmacokinetics and liver function indexes in chronic liver disease. *Respiration* 1991;58(2):106–111.
143. Kishimoto I, Tanigawara Y, Okumura K, Hori R. Blood oxygen tension-related change of theophylline clearance in experimental hypoxemia. *J Pharmacol Exp Ther* 1989; 248(3):1237–1242.
144. Trembath PW, Thorsborne-Palmer DD, Jarrott B, Hammond JJ, Prinsley DM. Theophylline pharmcokinetics in patients from a geriatric hospital: influence of cigarette smoking. *Hum Toxicol* 1986;5(4):265–268.
145. Pokrajac M, Simic D, Varagic VM. Pharmcokinetics of theophylline in hyperthyroid and hypothyroid patients with chronic obstructive pulmonary disease. *Eur J Clin Pharmacol* 1987;33(5):483–486.
146. Gardner MJ, Schatz M, Cousins L, Zeiger R, Middleton E, Jusko WJ. Longitudinal effects of pregnancy on the pharmacokinetics of theophylline. *Eur J Clin Pharmacol* 1987;32(3):289–295.
147. Joad JP, Ahrens RC, Lindgren SD, Weinberger MM. Extrapulmonary effects of maintenance therapy with theophylline and inhaled albuterol in patients with chronic asthma. *J Allergy Clin Immunol* 1986;78(6):1147–1153.
148. Rachelefsky GS, Wo J, Adelson J, Mickey MR, Spector SL, Katz RM, Siegel SC, Rohr AS. Behavior abnormalities and poor school performance due to oral theophylline use. *Pediatrics* 1986;78(6):1133–1138.
149. Furukawa CT, DuHamel TR, Weimer L, Shapiro GG, Pierson WE, Bierman CW. Cognitive and behavioral findings in children taking theophylline. *J Allergy Clin Immunol* 1988;81(1):83–88.
150. Weinberger M, Lindgren S, Bender B, Lerner JA, Szefler S. Effects of theophylline on learning and behavior: reason for concern or concern without reason? *J Pediatr* 1987;111(3):471–474.
151. Lundgren S, Lokshin B, Stromquista A, Weinberger M, Nassif E, McCubbin M, Frasher R. Does asthma or treatment with theophylline limit childrens academic performance. *N Engl J Med* 1992;327(13):296–331.
152. Ekstrom T, Tibbling L. Influence of theophylline on gastro-oesophageal reflux and asthma. *Eur J Clin Pharmacol* 1988;35(4):353–356.
153. Hubert D, Gaudric M, Guerre J, Lockhart A, Marsac J. Effect of theophylline on gastroesophageal reflux in patients with asthma [see comments]. *J Allergy Clin Immunol* 1988;81(6):1168–1174.
154. Levine JH, Michael JR, Guarnieri T. Multifocal atrial tachycardia: a toxic effect of theophylline. *Lancet* 1985;1(8419):12–14.
155. Eiriksson CE Jr, Writer SL, Vestal RE. Theophylline-induced alterations in cardiac electrophysiology in patients with chronic obstructive pulmonary disease. *Am Rev Respir Dis* 1987;135(2):322–326.
156. Gibb WR. Delayed-type hypersensitivity to theophylline/aminophylline [letter]. *Lancet* 1985;1(8419):49.
157. Brook U, Singer L, Fried D. Development of severe Stevens-Johnson syndrome after administration of slow-release theophylline. *Pediatr Dermatol* 1989;6(2):126–129.
158. Hidalgo HA. Severe erythema multiforme (Stevens-Johnson syndrome) after taking sustained release theophylline [letter]. *Pediatr Pulmonol* 1989;6(3):209–210.

159. Niggli F, Fanconi S, Ghelfi D. Hypokalemia in theophylline intoxication [letter]. *J Pediatr* 1987;111(1):157.
160. Greenberg A, Piraino BH, Kroboth PD, Weiss J. Severe theophylline toxicity. Role of conservative measures, antiarrhythmic agents, and charcoal hemoperfusion. *Am J Med* 1984;76(5):854–860.
161. Bertino JS Jr, Walker JW. Reassessment of theophylline toxicity. Serum concentrations, clinical course, and treatment. *Arch Intern Med* 1987;147(4):757–760.
162. Shannon M, Lovejoy FH Jr. The influence of age vs peak serum concentration on life-threatening events after chronic theophylline intoxication. *Arch Intern Med* 1990; 150(10):2045–2048.
163. Greenberg A, Piraino BH, Kroboth PD, Weiss J. Severe theophylline toxicity. Role of conservative measures, antiarrhythmic agents, and charcoal hemoperfusion. *Am J Med* 1984;76(5):854–860.
164. Marchlinski FE, Miller JM. Atrial arrhythmias exacerbated by theophylline. Response to verapamil and evidence for triggered activity in man. *Chest* 1985;88(6):931–934.
165. Bender PR, Brent J, Kulig K. Cardiac arrhythmias during theophylline toxicity [letter]. *Chest* 1991;100(3):884–886.
166. Siemons LJ, Parizel G. Prolonged runs of ventricular tachycardia as a complication of theophylline intoxication. Report of a case. *Acta Cardiol* 1986;41(6):457–464.
167. Friesen RM, Bonet JF. The antiarrhythmic effects of verapamil and propranolol in aminophylline toxic dogs. *Can Anaesth Soc J* 1983;30(2):124–131.
168. Kolander SA, Nydegger CC, Porter RS. T wave inversion associated with severe theophylline toxicity. *Chest* 1989;96(2):429–431.
169. Weinberger M, Hendeles L. Theophylline for chronic asthma: rationale for treatment, product selection, and dosage schedule. *Pediatr Pharmacol New York* 1983;3(3–4):273–285.
170. Singer EP, Kolischenko A. Seizures due to theophylline overdose. *Chest* 1985;87(6):755–757.
171. Bahls FH, Ma KK, Bird TD. Theophylline-associated seizures with "therapeutic" or low toxic serum concentrations: risk factors for serious outcome in adults. *Neurology* 1991;41(8):1309–1312.
172. Hall KW, Dobson KE, Dalton JG, Ghignone MC, Penner SB. Metabolic abnormalities associated with intentional theophylline overdose. *Ann Intern Med* 1984;101(4):457–462.
173. Self-poisoning with theophylline [editorial]. *Lancet* 1985;1(8421):146–147.
174. Ryan T, Coughlan G, McGing P, Phelan D. Ketosis, a complication of theophylline toxicity. *J Intern Med* 1989;226(4):277–278.
175. Whyte KF, Addis GJ. Toxicity of salbutamol and theophylline together [letter]. *Lancet* 1983;2(8350):618–619.
176. Parr MJ, Willatts SM. Fatal theophylline poisoning with rhabdomyolysis. A potential role for dantrolene treatment. *Anaesthesia* 1991;46(7):557–559.
177. Rumpf KW, Wagner H, Criee CP, Schwarck H, Klein H, Kreuzer H, Scheler F. Rhabdomyolysis after theophylline overdose [letter]. *Lancet* 1985;1(8443):1451–1452.
178. Ng RH, Roe C, Funt D, Statland BE. Increased activity of creatine kinase isoenzyme MB in a theophylline-intoxicated patient. *Clin Chem* 1985;31(10):1741–1742.
179. Cusack BJ, Nielson CP, Morgan ME, Vestal RE. Additive effect of theophylline on the cardiac response to isoproterenol. *Clin Pharmacol Ther* 1987;41(3):289–296.
180. Barzu T, Huerta F, Pourrias B. The chronotropic effect of adenosine and ATP in dogs. The antagonism by theophylline. *J Pharmacol* 1985;16(2):197–211.
181. Esquivel M, Burns RJ, Ogilvie RI. Cardiovascular effects of enprofylline and theophylline. *Clin Pharmacol Ther* 1986;39(4):395–402.
182. Lin CI, Chuang IN, Cheng KK, Chiang BN. Arrhythmogenic effects of theophylline in human atrial tissue. *Int J Cardiol* 1987;17(3):289–297.
183. Benditt DG, Benson DW Jr, Kreitt J, Dunnigan A, Pritzker MR, Crouse L, Scheinman MM. Electrophysiologic effects of theophylline in young patients with recurrent symptomatic bradyarrhythmias. *Am J Cardiol* 1983;52(10):1223–1229.
184. Roca DJ, Schiller GD, Farb DH. Chronic caffeine or theophylline exposure reduces gamma-aminobutyric acid/benzodiazepine receptor site interactions. *Mol Pharmacol* 1988;33(5):481–485.

185. Laursen LC, Borga O, Krohn L, Weeke B. Distribution of enprofylline and theophylline between plasma and cerebrospinal fluid. *Ther Drug Monit* 1989;11(2):162–164.
186. Auritt WA, McGeady SJ, Mansmann HC Jr. The relationship of cerebrospinal fluid and plasma theophylline concentrations in children and adolescents taking theophylline. *J Allergy Clin Immunol* 1985;75(6):731–735.
187. Bartel P, Lotz B, Delport R, Ubbink J, Becker P. Electrophysiological indices of central and peripheral nervous system function during theophylline therapy. *Neuropsychobiology* 1989;21(2):104–108.
188. Albertson TE, Joy RM. Modification of excitation and inhibition evoked in dentate gyrus by perforant path stimulation: effects of aminophylline and kindling. *Pharmacol Biochem Behav* 1986;24(1):85–91.
189. Ault B, Olney MA, Joyner JL, Boyer CE, Notrica MA, Soroko FE, Wang CM. Proconvulsant actions of theophylline and caffeine in the hippocampus: implications for the management of temporal lobe epilepsy. *Brain Res* 1987;426(1):93–102.
190. Szot P, Sanders RC, Murray TF. Theophylline-induced upregulation of Al-adenosine receptors associated with reduced sensitivity to convulsants. *Neuropharmacology* 1987;26(8):1173–1180.
191. Czuczwar SJ, Turski WA, Ikonomidou C, Turski L. Aminophylline and CGS 8216 reverse the protective action of diazepam against electroconvulsions in mice. *Epilepsia* 1985;26(6):693–696.
192. Foster PN, Moles EJ, Sheard C, Herbert M, Atkinson M. Low dose aminophylline accelerates recovery from diazepam premedication for digestive endoscopy. *Gastrointest Endosc* 1987;33(6):421–424.
193. Niemand D, Martinell S, Arvidsson S, Ekstrom-Jodal B, Svedmyr N. Adenosine in the inhibition of diazepam sedation by aminophylline. *Acta Anaesthesiol Scand* 1986;30(7):493–495.
194. Marrosu F, Marchi A, De Martino MR, Saba G, Gessa GL. Aminophylline antagonizes diazepam-induced anesthesia and EEG changes in humans. *Psychopharmacology Berlin* 1985;85(1):69–70.
195. Aitken ML, Martin TR. Life-threatening theophylline toxicity is not predictable by serum levels. *Chest* 1987;91(1):10–14.
196. Kossoy AF, Weir MR, Bryant MV. Theophylline toxicity [letter]. *Pediatrics* 1983;72(5):746–747.
197. Mahutte CK, True RJ, Michiels TM, Berman JM, Light RW. Increased serum theophylline clearance with orally administered activated charcoal. *Am Rev Respir Dis* 1983;128(5):820–822.
198. Amitai Y, Lovejoy FH Jr. Characteristics of vomiting associated with acute sustained release theophylline poisoning: implications for management with oral activated charcoal. *J Toxicol Clin Toxicol* 1987;25(7):539–554.
199. Anderson JR, Poklis A, McQueen RC, Purtell JN, Slavin RG. Effects of hemodialysis on theophylline kinetics. *J Clin Pharmacol* 1983;23(10):428–432.
200. Hootkins R Sr, Lerman MJ, Thompson JR. Sequential and simultaneous "in series" hemodialysis and hemoperfusion in the management of theophylline intoxication. *J Am Soc Nephrol* 1990;1(6):923–926.
201. British National Formulary, March 1992. British Medical Association and Royal Pharmaceutical Society of Great Britain.
202. Farrar KT, Dunn AM. Beta-blockers in treatment of theophylline overdose [letter]. *Lancet* 1985;1(8435):983.
203. Amin DN, Henry JA. Propranolol administration in theophylline overdose [letter]. *Lancet* 1985;1(8427):520–521.

Drugs and the Lung,
edited by C.P. Page and W.J. Metzger.
Raven Press, Ltd., New York © 1994

4

Current Drugs for Respiratory Diseases

Glucocorticosteroids

*Ralph Brattsand and *†Olof Selroos

*†*Research and Development, AB ASTRA DRACO, S-221 00 Lund, Sweden;* *†and Mjölbolsta Hospital, SF-10350, Finland*

Glucocorticosteroids (GCSs) have been successfully used for over 40 years in the treatment of airway and lung diseases. As for most types of drugs, the therapeutic development has mainly been governed by empirical findings in the clinic, and mechanistic explanations of their effects have lagged several years or even decades behind. The introduction of GCSs into asthma treatment in the early 1950s was logical, and based on combining two pieces of knowledge: (a) the old knowledge (based on pathology and sputum studies) that severe asthma and asthma deaths are related to eosinophilic inflammation and mucus plugging of the airways, and (b) the new knowledge at that time that GCSs are potent endogenous anti-inflammatory compounds. For a fuller discussion on historical background, the successful clinical introduction, the subsequent misuse with high doses, and elucidation of severe adverse effects, the reader is referred to earlier overviews (1,2).

Researchers in subsequent decades have elucidated parts of the complicated biochemical and pharmacological mechanisms of GCSs, including the possibilities and limitations in differentiating desired steroid actions from the undesired. The GCS receptor seems to be uniform in the human body, which means that there is no basis currently for the development of more selective GCSs for systemic therapy. Fortunately, this limitation is to some extent bypassed by improved clinical understanding of how to use the current systemic compounds in better and safer ways (see subsequent pages). Based on a combination of empiricism and directed pharmacological research, there has been a fruitful development of topical (inhaled) therapy for asthma and rhinitis, and to some extent also of lung parenchymal diseases, especially sarcoidosis. The main benefit of that development has been to markedly improve tolerance, so that anti-inflammatory therapy based on topical steroids can encompass nearly all forms of asthma and be used even as a first-line therapy (3–7). Furthermore, topical therapy also reduces bronchial hyperresponsiveness to nonspecific stimuli, which seldom can be achieved by oral treatment. This successful use of inhalation treatment has in fact been the area where the greatest medical advances of steroid therapy has been achieved over the last two decades. Summarizing that development with its new possibilities is one of the aims of this overview.

GCSs exert a multiplicity of actions (for overview see refs. 1, 2, 8, 9), and it is currently difficult to pinpoint what actions are most essential for ameliorating the symptoms of airway–lung diseases. One way to focus this question further is to go back to the main physiologic functions of GCSs (10). One effect is the "permissive action" securing functional activity of other hormones, e.g., catecholamines, and this action might, in selected patients, protect against receptor subsensitivity on prolonged beta-agonist therapy (1). Another physiological function, which yielded the name "glucocorticosteroid," is to supply glucose to the brain during starvation by enhancing the adrenocorticotropic hormone (ACTH) and cortisol secretions. Metabolically this action is achieved by a combination of catabolic changes in peripheral tissue and anabolic shifts in the liver, and it is mimicked during high-dose systemic therapy leading to some of the well-known catabolic adverse effects of long-term steroid therapy. The third and therapeutically the most important physiologic action is that GCSs can dampen toxic aspects of our host defense actions (11), meaning that they protect tissues outside a localized inflammation against released cytokines, toxic metabolites, and activated cells. To exert such protection in the circulation GCSs have gained the capability of inducing acute and protracted anti-inflammatory actions, and this is the physiological basis that we exploit in therapy by raising GCS concentrations to supraphysiologic levels. The concept of this view of the stress response as an anti-inflammatory feedback system (Fig. 1) is supported by new findings that even subpyrogenic doses of interleukin (IL)-1β can induce cortisol secretion (12), and that systemically administered IL-1β has some anti-inflammatory efficacy via such a mechanism (13). In sensitive animal models it has been possible to show that even physiological GCS levels attenuate inflammation (14).

In asthmatic patients there is still no support for an altered diurnal variation of plasma cortisol (1,15). However, a couple of recent studies suggest that the high morning cortisol levels can attenuate immunoglobulin E (IgE)-mediated inflammation. Mohiuddin and Martin (16) found that the late reaction after bronchial challenge had a shorter latency time and was more severe when the challenge was performed in the evening than in the morning. Another study concluded—based on the late phase allergic inflammation in skin and where the high morning levels of endogenous cortisol was blocked by metyrapone—that IgE-dependent late phase inflammation is dampened by the high physiological level of plasma cortisol (17). It is proposed that we need further studies to elucidate whether the "stress" response to immunologic stimuli may in some way be altered in asthma and other inflammatory lung disorders.

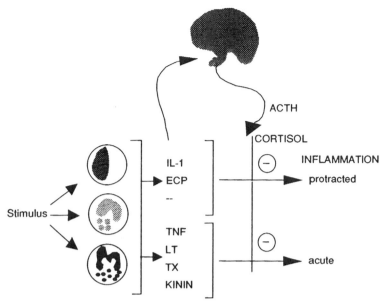

FIG. 1. The stress response: an anti-inflammatory feedback system. The probable physiological purpose of this feedback system is to protect tissues outside a local inflammation site from released toxic mediators. Even subpyrogenic plasma levels of cytokines [e.g., interleukin-1 (IL-1) and tumor necrosis factor (TNF)] can trigger adrenocorticotropic hormone (ACTH) release, and by that enhance cortisol production (see text). (Adapted from ref. 14.)

SUBCELLULAR BASIS OF GCS ACTION

It is generally considered that most GCS actions are mediated through stimulation of the GCS- receptors (GCS-R) (18). This relates also to the anti-inflammatory actions, supported by the demonstrated close correlation between receptor affinity and topical anti-inflammatory potency for a series of GCS-R agonists (19). Furthermore, with GCS-R antagonists (e.g., RU 486) it is possible to block different types of anti-inflammatory actions (20–22). The dogma of actions mediated via steroid receptors is that binding of the steroid to its specific receptor leads to a conformational change of the receptor complex. The complex can then interact with specific binding sites at the promoter-enhancer region of target genes, and by that modulate their transcription (for overviews see refs. 18, 23, 24). The modulation can result in up- or down-regulation of a gene, depending on the organization of its promoter-enhancer region. Also the developmental status of a cell is important, because the ontogeny can shut off some genes and change its setup of steroid receptors and transcriptional factors. There are a few odd examples that GCS can up-regulate a specific gene in one cell type and down-regulate the same gene in other cells (24).

The number of genes strongly modulated by GCS in a given cell does not seem to be large. Based on giant gel electrophoresis Voris and Young (25) found that the synthesis of six to eight proteins was changed in steroid-treated thymocytes. With the "negative hybridization technique" Helmberg et al. (26) showed that GCS up-regulated the synthesis of one and down-regulated the production of two proteins in a mouse macrophage line. However, due to the multitude of cell types (even in the respiratory tract) the total number of GCS-regulated genes is still substantial.

Glucocorticosteroid Receptor (GCS-R)

GCS-R belongs to the family of steroid receptors, which can all be looked upon as a special type of transactivating proteins for genomic modulation (27). These receptors are built up of three domains: the ligand-binding, the DNA-binding and the "modulatory" domains, with the highest structural conservation in the DNA-binding part (24,27,28). The GCS-R is built up of about 780 amino acids, with about 280 in the ligand-binding, 70 in the DNA-binding, and 430 in the "modulatory" domains. In its unliganded state GCS-R exists as a complex together with two molecules of heat shock protein 90-kD (HSP-90) and one molecule of the immunophilin p-59 (Fig. 2). In this complex it is thought that these other proteins cover the DNA-binding domain of the receptor (18,29). There is only one gene for GCS-R (30).

While there are reports on a possible alternative splicing of the receptor formed, there functionally seems to be just one type of GCS-R (18,23,24,28). Most normal cells have a few thousand receptors, but the number varies among cell types as well as with the cell cycle (31). Still, little is known about how many GCS-Rs need to be triggered for inducing a functional response, and whether that number differs for different types of action. In the respiratory tract, *in situ* hybridization shows a higher number of mRNA for GCS-Rs in alveolar and endothelial cells than in airway epithelium and smooth muscle (32). Lavage cells from healthy subjects and patients with sarcoidosis have a similar content of GCS-R mRNA (33). Corticosteroid resistance in asthma does not seem to be caused by a reduced number or affinity of GCS-Rs (34).

Up-Regulation of Genomic Transcription

Up-regulation was the first type of genomic modulation described, and it is still the one best studied, often as the interaction between GCS-R and the promoter-enhancer region of the mouse mammary tumor virus (MMTV) gene. The latter has been used either as the full gene or as just its promoter-enhancer region put before sensitive reporter gene constructs (24,35). Other genes up-regulated by GCSs and of more physiologic-pharmacologic impor-

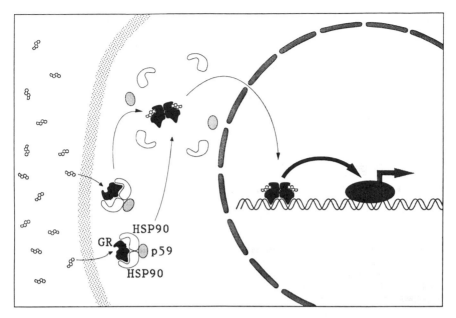

FIG. 2. The different steps for gene modulation by glucocorticosteroids (GCSs) are illustrated schematically. The GCS diffuses by its lipophilicity through the cell membrane and in the cytoplasm it associates to a complex containing the GCS receptor. This complex dissociates and releases its components: two heat shock protein molecules HSP 90, the immunophillin p-59 and the activated, hormone-liganded receptor, which assembles to form a homodimer. This complex is transported to the nucleus, binds to chromatin and interacts with the transcription machinery. Depending on the organization of the individual gene this can lead to up-regulation, when a full transcription complex is formed, or to down-regulation, when the complex blocks other up-regulatory elements to transcription factors (see text). (Adapted from ref. 18.)

tance are tyrosine aminotransferase and phosphoenol pyruvate carboxykinase (enzymes changing the intermediary metabolism of the liver), ribonucleases and endonucleases (decomposing mRNA and DNA—see below), peptidases (inactivating tachykinins), and several receptors including the adrenergic β_2-receptor. A feature of this type of up-regulation is that addition of actinomycin D (inhibitor of mRNA formation) or cycloheximide (inhibitor of protein synthesis) will block the steroid activity (24,36).

When the GCS-R is triggered by a full agonist, the receptor dissociates from the complex with HSP-90 and p-59 and exposes the DNA-binding domain with its two zinc fingers (23,24,28). Via zinc finger II a homodimer forms of two receptors (Fig. 3), and that pair can then couple to specific DNA sequences called glucocorticosteroid responsive elements (GREs), having a partly palindromic sequence (e.g., GGTACAnnnTGTTCT, where n means any nucleotide). The coupling to GRE occurs via zinc finger I, which fits into the major groove of the DNA spiral. The spatial arrangement of that

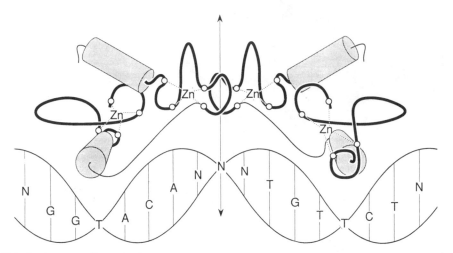

FIG. 3. A model of how the DNA binding domains of the double receptor may associate DNA. A dimer of the GCS receptor DNA-binding domain, consisting each of two "zinc-finger" regions (*thick line*) and two alpha-helices (*shaded cylinders*), is shown on the top of the DNA with the receptor-binding nucleotide sequence indicated. The *double-headed arrow* points out the region of symmetry for both the DNA sequence and the receptor dimer. One of the two alpha-helices within a receptor monomer serves as a recognition helix located in the major groove of the DNA. One region of a zinc-finger is in close contact with the corresponding region of the second receptor monomer (central part of figure). (Adapted from ref. 18.)

complex has been partly elucidated by nuclear magnetic resonance (NMR) (37) and by x-ray crystallography (38). Figure 3 is a model of that interaction (18). Based on co-crystals of the DNA-binding domain and small synthetic GRE (38), it seems likely that the receptor binding fits better to one side than to the other side of the DNA sequence, suggesting that a perfect palindromic structure is not a prerequisite for "docking."

Proper contact between the DNA-binding region of the receptor complex and GRE sites of the promoter is not sufficient for inducing transcription. Thus, there are GCS antagonists that bind efficiently to GRE without inducing any biological activity of their own (22). There are two transactivating regions on the receptor—TAF1 on the modulatory and TAF2 on the ligand binding domain, respectively—which both need to be activated, possibly by phosphorylation (18,23). When properly triggered, a full-transcription complex can be formed and the RNA-polymerase can start to transcribe the gene (39).

Down-Regulation of Genomic Transcription

Reduced transcription of a long series of cytokines, growth factors, and proinflammatory enzymes are of central importance for the anti-inflammatory and immunosuppressive actions of GCSs. The activated GCS-R complex can diminish transcription/translation by at least five partly different mechanisms:

1. A GRE of little importance for the gene can partly overlap other and more important up-regulatory sites. The overlap can occur, e.g., on adenosine 3′,5′-cyclic monophosphate (cAMP) responsive elements (e.g., glucoprotein α-subunit gene) or even on the regions of the TATA box (the nucleotide sequence where the RNA polymerase and its basal transcription factors dock), or on the start site of coding [examples for the two latter types of overlap are the IL-6 gene (40) and the osteocalcin gene (41)]. Closer mutation analyses show that in this latter case the GCS-R binds to flanking nucleotides and not to the TATA-box per se (41).

2. The GCS-R can bind to other types of GRE named nGRE (negative glucocorticosteroid responsive elements), which can directly repress the promoter region. The nGRE seems to have a more variable and less palindromic sequence than GRE (24,28). On the promoter region of the IL-6 gene there are at least two such nGREs, which seem to contribute to the steroid down-regulation of this gene (40).

3. It has recently been demonstrated that GCS-R can, by direct protein–protein contacts, bind to and block the transcription factor activating protein 1 (AP-1) (a heterodimer of the two protooncogenes c-*jun* and c-*fos*—see Fig. 4). This mechanism has been elucidated by the blocking ability of GCS on AP-1–mediated synthesis of the metalloproteases collagenase and stromolysin. However, this type of interaction may refer to down-regulation of many mediators, because AP-1 is a common transcription factor up-regulated during inflammation and proliferation, and at least c-*fos* is known to be up-regulated in asthmatic airways. In cell systems it has been possible to change the balance between AP-1– and GCS-R–mediated actions, and this has resulted in that overexpression of GCS-R–blocked, AP-1–promoted actions, while overexpression of AP-1 reduced steroid actions (35,43–45). Figure 4 illustrates how GCS-R under normal conditions can bind to both GRE and AP-1. However, during severe inflammation there is a possibility that so much GCS-R is bound to the up-regulated AP-1–mediated pathways, that the amount available for GRE binding might be reduced. This type of interaction may possibly explain *in vitro* results demonstrating that a strong cytokine load overcomes GCS actions (46,47).

4. Steroid treatment of lung tissue is reported to diminish the expression and availability of the transcription factor NFkB (48). This may contribute to an attenuation of cytokine-mediated events (cf. NFkB involvement in Fig. 4).

5. For some cytokines (IL-1β, IL-6, GM-CSF, and IFN-α) it has been shown that GCS treatment shortens the turnover time of their mRNA (49,50). The underlying mechanism is that steroids induce ribonucleases,

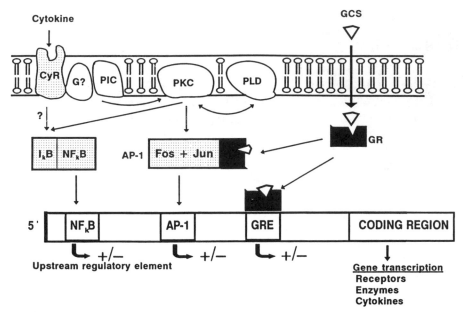

FIG. 4. Effects of cytokines and GCSs on transcription of proinflammatory genes. Cytokines interact with surface receptors leading to changes in gene transcription by activating transcription factors such as activating protein 1 (AP-1) and nuclear factor kappa B (NF$_k$B). AP-1 is a heterodimer of the two protooncogenes c-*fos* and c-*jun* (Fos and Jun, respectively); NF$_k$B is activated by phosphorylation of an inhibitory component. (I$_k$B). Transcription factors bind to particular sequences on the upstream regulatory element of target genes, leading to changes in the rate of transcription and therefore the amount of messenger RNA and target protein. Target genes may include gene coding for surface receptors, for enzymes, and for other cytokines.

GCS may counteract the transcription/translation of cytokines in at least three ways. First, the activated GCS receptor (GR) binds to GCS-responsive elements (GRE) on the same gene, which has the opposite effect on transcription compared to the transcription factor. Second, the activated GR can bind directly to AP-1 via protein–protein interaction, preventing the transcription factor binding to its recognition site on the target gene. Third, GR can up-regulate transcription of ribonucleases, which break down mRNA of the cytokines transcribed. (Adapted from ref. 42.)

which attack adenine-uracil-rich sequences in the 3'-untranslated region of these mRNA. The GM-CSF mRNA seems extrasensitive to this type of attack and in steroid-treated cell cultures its half-life is reduced from several hours to less than half an hour (49).

As for treatment with other hormones, administration of GCS induces some down-regulation of its own receptor (18). Closer analyses of human cell lines showed that steroid treatment reduced the steady-state level of mRNA for GCS-R by about 50% (51), while the turnover time of the mRNA was unaffected ($t_{1/2}$ 2–4 h). With the exception of the small group of GCS-resistant patients, prolonged treatment does not seem to reduce steroid reactivity *in vivo*. Thus, a retained response for "skin blanching" has been demonstrated in asthmatics who have been on long-term oral steroid therapy (52).

Trigger and Latency Times for GCS Actions

There is wide variation in the times required for induction of various actions. A few (e.g., the blocked ACTH secretion) are so rapidly induced that direct and nonreceptor-mediated effects on ion movements have been proposed (1). For initiation of cytotoxic response in rat thymocytes (36), and for reducing vascular exudation in rodents (53,54), the steroid needs to be present in tissue just for the first 5 to 10 min and the surplus can then be washed away. Thus, for some actions GCS can be looked upon as "hit-and-run" drugs that have the ability to trigger a local response, which is then forwarded by the mRNAs and proteins induced. This profile seems ideal for inhalation use, where the drug can trigger a local but protracted message, while the drug itself can be largely absorbed from that site and be subsequently inactivated in the systemic compartment.

However, induction of other actions seem to require continuous GCS exposure for longer periods, as has been shown, e.g., for reduced cytokine production (55) and blocked lymphocyte proliferation. The catabolic actions on connective tissue leading to bruising, skin atrophy, and osteoporosis seem to happen mainly when the GCS peak in plasma or at the local site is markedly protracted. This conclusion can be drawn from the main difference in the diurnal variation of plasma cortisol in normals and patients with morbus Cushing, respectively; while these patients do not have much higher peak level in the morning, they lack the diurnal variation with its low night levels.

ANTI-INFLAMMATORY-IMMUNOSUPPRESSIVE ACTIONS

Due to their multiplicity these actions are listed in Tables 1 through 4, with some details and references included in the tables. Comments are given in the following text on the probable importance of these actions in airway–lung diseases. When available, findings from the airway–lung compartment in humans have been selected but when lacking, data based on human white blood cells or other cells or on animal cells or tissue are given. To simplify Tables 1 and 2, steroid effects are expressed as changes in the synthesis/release of a mediator or as the blockade of its effect. The reader is referred to the references to learn whether alteration in mediator production has been observed as a change in synthesis at the mRNA and/or at the protein level or as a block of release.

TABLE 1. Modulation of interleukins and growth factors (if no species is given the studies refer to human cells or tissue)

Affected mediator	GCS action		Type of study (and mode of GCS administration)	References
IL-1β	Synthesis/release	→	Blood mononuclear cells (in vitro)	63–66
		→	Human lung (in vitro)	67
		→	BAL fluid and cells (in vivo to asthmatics)	68
IL-2	Synthesis/release	→	T cells (in vitro)	69, 70
IL-3	Synthesis/release	→	Murine or blood mononuclear cells (in vitro)	71, 72
	Action	→	Eosinophil survival (in vitro)	73–75
IL-4	Synthesis/release	→	T cells (in vitro)	76, 77
		→	BAL cells (in vivo to asthmatics)	
	Action	→	IL-4 dependent IgE synthesis in mononuclear cells (in vitro)	78
IL-5	Synthesis/release	→	Blood mononuclear cells (in vitro)	79
		→	Serum and BAL cells (in vivo to asthmatics)	77
	Action	→	Eosinophil survival (in vitro)	73–75
		→	Cell recruitment to guinea pig lung (in vivo)	80
IL-6	Synthesis/release	→	Murine and human mononuclear cells, endothelial cells, fibroblasts, alveolar macrophages (in vitro)	49, 64, 81, 82
		→	Bronchial epithelial cells of asthmatic patients (in vitro)	83
IL-8	Synthesis/release	→	Blood mononuclear cells, alveolar macrophages; fibroblasts (in vitro)	49, 84
		→	Bronchial epithelial cells of asthmatic patients (in vitro)	83

IL-10	Synthesis/release	→	Murine splenocytes (*in vivo*)	84a
Neutrophil priming factor	Synthesis/release	→	Mononuclear cells of GCS-sensitive asthmatics (*in vitro*)	61, 63
TNF-α	Synthesis/release	→	Blood mononuclear cells, alveolar macrophages (*in vitro*)	55, 63, 85
		→	Blood mononuclear cells (*in vivo* to asthmatics)	86
		→	Bronchopulmonary secretions of infants with respiratory distress syndrome (*in vivo*)	87
	Action	→	Cytotoxicity on murine fibroblasts or on fibrosarcoma cells (*in vitro*)	88
INF-β	Synthesis/release	→	Fibrosarcoma cells (L929) (*in vitro*)	89
INF-γ	Synthesis/release	→	Blood mononuclear cells (*in vitro*)	90
		←	BAL cells (*in vivo* to asthmatics)	77
	Action	→	Eosinophil survival (*in vitro*)	74
GM-CSF	Synthesis/release	→	Blood mononuclear cells, alveolar macrophages, fibroblasts (*in vitro*)	49, 63, 64, 91
		→	Blood mononuclear cells (*in vivo* to asthmatics)	91
		→	Tracheal cells in culture (*in vitro*)	92
		→	Bronchial epithelial cells of asthmatic patients (*in vitro*)	83
	Action	→	Bronchial epithelium (*in vivo* to asthmatics)	63
		→	Eosinophil survival (*in vitro*)	73–75, 93
		←	Shift in eosinophil buoyant density (*in vitro*)	93, 94
TGF-β	Synthesis/release	←	Lymphocytes (*in vitro*)	95
PDGF		←	Alveolar macrophages or HL60 (*in vitro*)	96

GM-CSF, granulocyte-macrophage colony-stimulating factor; IFN, interferon; IL, interleukin; PDGF, platelet-derived growth factor; TGF, transforming growth factor; TNF, tumor necrosis factor.

Attenuation of Production and Action of Cytokines and Growth Factors
(Table 1)

This key action of attenuation is obvious when one considers that cyto-kines–growth factors and GCSs have opposing profiles of action: the former are proinflammatory and proliferative, whereas steroids have the opposite effect (45). The antagonistic behavior can be seen in the organization of the promoter region of many cytokines–growth factor genes. As shown in Fig. 4, there are up-regulatory sites for cytokine–growth factor–provoked mes-sages, while the GCS-R complex will often down-regulate the gene function by blocking the synthesis/action of transcription factors and by binding to the GRE sites. Table 1 shows that GCS can reduce cytokine synthesis/re-lease along both the Th1 (IL-2) and the Th2 (IL-3, IL-4, IL-5) pathways (see ref. 84a). Blockade of the latter may be of special importance in asthma, because the Th2 pathway has been considered central for IgE production, eosinophil–mast cell proliferation, and the asthmatic type of inflammation (56,57). GCS can intervene with early steps of this pathway (Fig. 5) by reducing the antigen presentation and the cytokine production and action. Steroids in-hibit T-lymphocyte proliferation *in vitro* by blocking the production of IL-1β and IL-2 and by diminishing the expression of the IL-2 receptor (58).

The hypothesis that a key anti-asthmatic action of steroids is to reduce cytokine production/action is supported by a series of human findings. T lymphocytes and monocytes of most subjects are very sensitive *in vitro* to GCS at therapeutic concentrations (57). Based on bronchoalveolar lavage (BAL) or bronchial biopsies steroid treatment *in vivo* has resulted in reduced airway levels of IL-1β, IL-4, IL-5, TNF-α, and GM-CSF (Table 1). There is a small group of GCS-resistant asthmatics (see below) showing a reduced responsiveness to many steroid actions (59), and this group makes it possible to study what steroid actions are the most crucial ones. The inadequate anti-asthmatic response to GCS in these patients correlates with a low sensitivity of their T lymphocytes and monocytes to GCS *in vitro* (60–62). Based on comparison of the block achieved *in vitro* for individual cytokines, Lane et al. (63) concluded that for full anti-asthmatic efficacy a steroid block of the priming factor NPA (neutrophil priming activity, cf. Table 1—not yet chem-ically identified) seems especially important.

The sensitivity for steroid blockade differs not only for various cytokines but also for different cell types. GM-CSF is more sensitive than IL-1β and IL-6, and for all three cytokines there is a much stronger blockade in blood monocytes than in alveolar macrophages (64). It can be speculated that a physiologic function of the weak blockade of IL-1β in alveolar macro-phages is to keep some host defense reactivity within the airway luminal compartment.

In addition to this reduction of cytokine synthesis/release, GCS can also inhibit some actions of already formed cytokines. This effect has been stud-ied by the addition of natural or recombinant cytokines to cell cultures (see

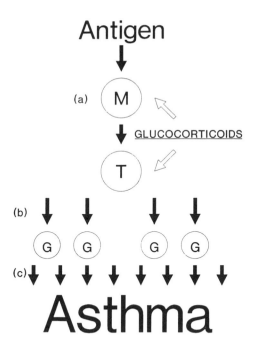

Antigen

(a)

GLUCOCORTICOIDS

(b)

(c)

Asthma

FIG. 5. Postulated cascade of asthmatic inflammation. Local T-lymphocyte activation by antigen presentation in the bronchial mucosa (a) results in the release of several specific lymphokines (b)—probably of the Th2 pathway—which in turn causes the accumulation and activation of a wide range of granulocytes (particularly eosinophils) and their secretion of an even wider range of inflammatory mediators (c). The anti-asthmatic activity of GCS may at least in part be mediated by blockade of the early specific cytokine release. This early intervention may also explain why GCSs have a better efficacy than inhibitors of a single mediator. M, macrophage or related cells; T, T lymphocyte; G, granulocyte. (Adapted from ref. 57.)

Table 1, where the inhibition is listed for the individual cytokine under the subheading "GCS action"). Thus, steroids potently inhibit the priming activity of IL-3, IL-4, IL-5, and GM-CSF on eosinophil survival and density shift and the IL-4–dependent IgE synthesis. The mechanism behind this type of inhibition is not known but may possibly relate to attenuation of synthesis/action of the transactivating factors AP-1 and NFkB (cf. Fig. 4).

The exceptions regarding inhibited production are the two growth factors transforming growth factor (TGF)-β and platelet-derived growth factor (PDGF), for which steroid treatment is reported to enhance transcription (Table 1). For TGF-β the reaction may seem logical, because this factor has some anti-inflammatory activity. However, taking both growth factors together their stimulating rather than blocking activity can explain why GCSs have poor efficacy on later phases of fibrotic processes. There is no information available on whether GCS can inhibit the actions of TGF-β and PDGF.

Modulation of Other Mediators (Table 2)

Proteases and Antiproteases

GCSs can inhibit proteolytic damage by reducing the synthesis/release of several proteases: the metalloproteases collagenase and stromolysine, the

TABLE 2. *Modulation of other proinflammatory factors (if no species is given the studies refer to human cells or tissue)*

Affected mediator	GCS action	Type of study (and mode of GCS administration)		References
Collagenase, elastase, plasminogen activator	Synthesis/release	Macrophages (in vitro)	→	116
Rat mast cell protease II	Synthesis/release	Rat basophilic leukemia cells (in vitro)	→	117
Neutral endopeptidase	Synthesis/release	Airway epithelial cells (in vitro)	⇐	98, 118
Angiotension converting enzyme	Synthesis/release	BAL (in vivo to smokers)	⇐	99
Lipocortin 1	Synthesis/release	Differentiated U-937 cells (in vitro)	⇐	119
		Alveolar macrophages (ex vivo)	⇐	120
Phospholipase A₂ secreted	Synthesis/release	Rat smooth muscle cells (in vitro)	↔	121
Phospholipase A₂ cytosolic	Synthesis/release	WI-38 cells (in vitro)	→	122
Inducible cyclooxygenase	Synthesis/release	Monocytes (in vitro)	→	123
LTB₄	Synthesis/release	Monocytes, alveolar macrophages (in vitro)	→	99, 124, 125
TXA₂	Synthesis/release	Monocytes (in vitro)	→	102
LTB₄, TXB₂, PGF₂, PGE₂	Synthesis/release	BAL cells (in vivo to volunteers or smokers)	→	99, 126
PGI, PAF	Synthesis/release	Rat peritoneal macrophages	→	127
Inducible nitric oxide synthase	Synthesis/release	Murine monocyte/macrophage cell line J 774 (in vitro)	→	104
Endothelin	Synthesis/release	Inflamed rat lung (in vivo)	→	128
		Biopsy or lavage of asthmatic airways (in vivo and in vitro, resp.)	→	129
Surfactant proteins	Synthesis/release	Rat lung tissue (in vitro)	⇐	131
Glycoconjugate secretion	Secretion	Cat tracheal organ in culture (in vitro)	→	132, 1333
		Sputum contents of fucose (in vivo treatment of patients with mucus hypersecretion)	→	110
Fibronectin	Synthesis/release	BAL (in vivo to smokers)	→	99

LT, leukotriene; PAF, platelet-activating factor; PG, prostaglandin; TX, thromboxane.

broadly acting plasminogen activator, and cathepsin B. In addition to this inhibition of proteases, steroid treatment can reinforce the formation of some antiproteases, and Stockley et al. (97) reported that oral prednisolone increased the sputum levels of antileukoprotease, α-1-antichymotrypsin, and tissue inhibitor of metalloproteases. This combination led to a decrease of free proteolytic activity of lung secretions (97).

Another anti-inflammatory action is the induction of the kinin-inactivating enzymes neutral endopeptidase (98) and angiotensin converting enzyme (99). The former enzyme is important for epithelial inactivation of bradykinin and tachykinins, and steroid-induced up-regulation of it has reduced vascular leakiness and local nerve reflexes in experimental systems (100).

Arachidonic Acid Cascade (Table 2)

In mononuclear cells challenged *in vitro,* steroids can decrease the formation of most arachidonic acid metabolites [LTB_4, thromboxanes (TXs), prostaglandins (PGs), prostacyclin, and platelet-activating factor (PAF)]. The blocking potential seems more restricted *in vivo,* but reductions have been reported for LTB_4, TXB_2, and PGE_2 in BAL cells or contents (Table 2). One report describes that high-dose i.v. hydrocortisone given during an acute asthma attack reduces slightly the plasma contents of immunoreactive LTC_4 (101). Based on the urinary excretion of the final metabolite LTE_4, oral or topical steroid treatment does not reduce the excretion of peptidoleukotrienes neither in volunteers (102) nor in asthmatics (103).

When there is a block of the arachidonic acid cascade, the mechanism seems to be down-regulation of key enzymes like phospholipase A_2 (both the secreted and cytosolic types) and the inducible cyclooxygenase (Table 2). The lipocortins may also be involved as competitors for the phospholipid substrate of PLA_2, but the expression of lipocortins seems variable between cell types and even between stages of cellular differentiation.

Other Metabolites (Table 2)

The inducible nitric oxide synthase of macrophages is down-regulated by steroids (104,105). Because macrophages (and possibly also epithelial cells) are using this enzyme for cytotoxic interactions in host defense and inflammation (106), that down-regulation may reduce macrophage-mediated mucosal damage. Also the production of other toxic oxygen metabolites can be attenuated. A high dose of oral prednisolone is reported to reduce the enhanced superoxide ion production in blood neutrophils of emphysematic patients (107).

The smooth muscle contracting peptide endothelin-1 has recently been demonstrated in asthmatic lung (108). Steroids can effectively inhibit endothelin synthesis as demonstrated both in bronchial cells of asthmatics and in animal lung (Table 2).

GCSs can attenuate the cytotoxic action of activated human monocytes or neutrophils on cultured fetal lung fibroblasts (109), with the monocyte as the more steroid-sensitive cell. The protective mechanisms may be a mix of reduced secretion of proteases, cytokines, and oxygen metabolites.

Mucous Secretion (Table 2)

The respiratory secretions originate both from exuded plasma and mucus of submucosal glands and goblet cells. In asthmatic patients steroid treatment can effectively reduce the sputum volume and its albumin contents (110), while these reductions are much less clear in chronic bronchitis. Probable mechanisms in asthma are reduced formation/action of key cytokines and leukotrienes promoting mucus secretion (111), but there may also be some inhibition at the level of glucoconjugate synthesis (Table 2). Furthermore, the steroids can diminish the vascular contribution to sputum by reducing plasma leakage at the endothelial level and its transport into lumen (54,112–115). The importance of reducing plasma leakage is not restricted to lowering mucus production, because this reduction is an important part of the anti-inflammatory efficacy also within mucosal and parenchymal tissue.

Attenuation of IgE-Mediated Events (Table 3)

There is a general agreement that steroid treatment does not reduce the plasma level of IgE (1) but rather tends to raise it slightly. However, with local therapy modulatory effects at the local lymphoid follicle level should not be excluded. In support of this is the finding that GCSs inhibit IL-4–induced IgE synthesis of human tonsil mononuclear cells (78), and also reduce IL-4 expression in BAL cells of steroid-treated asthmatics (77). Furthermore, local steroid treatment counteracts the binding of IgE to local tissue (134). This, and a reduction of mucosal and submucosal mast cell numbers during prolonged inhaled steroid therapy (135–137), as well as some inhibition of IgE-mediated release (138), contribute to an attenuation of the immediate bronchial reaction in allergic patients (139) as well as in IgE-sensitized animals (Table 3). Probably high local steroid levels are required for this attenuation, because conventional oral therapy seems to have a less-dampening effect on the immediate allergic reaction.

The late allergic reaction is more sensitive to steroid action and it is inhibited both by local and systemic therapy. The protective mechanisms are complex but because the steroid can be given even shortly after the immediate reaction, the protection seems to depend on reduced attraction and

TABLE 3. *Attenuation of IgE-mediated actions*

GCS action		Type of study (and mode of GCS administration)	References
IgE production	⇊	IL-4 induced IgE-production in human tonsil mononuclear cells (*in vitro*)	78
Tissue sensitization by IgE	⇊	Tissue binding of intradermally injected IgE in rabbits (local pretreatment)	134
IgE-mediated bronchial challenge			
Immediate reaction	⇊	Sensitized guinea pig lung (*in vitro* or *in vivo*)	144, 147
Late reaction	⇊	Sensitized guinea pig lung and trachea (*in vivo*)	115, 148
	⇊	Sensitized sheep lung (*in vivo*)	149
Hyperresponsiveness	⇊	Sensitized sheep lung hyperresponsiveness to nonspecific stimulus measured 24 h after challenge (*in vivo*)	149

IG, immunoglobulin.
The table is based on animal or tissue culture experiments. For human data, see later sections.

activation of granulocytes, mast cells, and lymphocytes (140–144). Prolonged steroid inhalation attenuates also the nonspecific hyperresponsiveness acquired after allergen challenge (see Table 3 for animal data; see below for human findings) but the underlying mechanisms are not yet defined. As for the blockade of the immediate reaction, attenuation of the hyperresponsiveness is best achieved by high-dose inhalation therapy.

GCSs have much less direct impact on IgG-mediated actions. There is no inhibition of IgG-provoked bronchial constriction (144), and steroids enhance rather than depress IgG synthesis (145). However, due to inhibition of complement expression (146), GCSs can attenuate some consequences of immune complex–provoked reactions. This seems to include also immune complex–mediated activation of blood monocytes of GCS-sensitive asthmatics via the $Fc_{\varsigma}R_2$-receptors (60,63).

Reduced Recruitment of Cells to Inflamed Airway–Lung Tissue and Modulation of their Local Survival

This important anti-inflammatory effect is achieved through a combination of mechanisms:

1. A dampening of inflammation will reduce the proliferation signals (e.g., the growth factor GM-CSF) for progenitor cells in blood and for stem

cells in marrow. It is well known that steroid treatment decreases the numbers of circulating eosinophils and basophils in allergic individuals (150–152). Venge and Dahl (153) demonstrated that a reduced number of blood eosinophils can attenuate the severity of a subsequent late-phase bronchial reaction.

2. While there is some support that GCSs can reduce ICAM-1 expression in a bronchial cell line *in vitro* (130), a lavage and biopsy study in asthmatics does not demonstrate any reduction of ICAM-1 and ELAM-1 (130a). However, GCSs can inhibit a later step in the transmigration process of neutrophils—the passage through the basement membrane (154). This inhibition is probably mediated by a reduced protease secretion (Table 2).

3. Steroids can diminish the production of chemoattractants. This may refer to the total chemotactic activity (functionally determined—ref. 125), as well as to levels of known attractants (LTB$_4$, PAF—Table 2).

4. There is a "priming" action of cytokines on chemokinetic responses of cells already in the circulation (140,155). The specific reduction, e.g., of eosinophilic influx into allergic sites may partially be explained by the high efficacy of steroids to block the formation and priming action of IL-3, IL-5, and GM-CSF on this cell (Table 1).

5. In a couple of very GCS-sensitive types of cell (eosinophils and immature lymphoid cells), steroids can induce apoptosis (programmed cell death) or at least block the life-prolonging action of cytokines on these cells (see Table 1). The direct cytotoxic effect is exerted by induction of endonucleases (75,156), which degrade DNA in a typical pattern (into approximately 200 base pair long segments (157).

Table 4 summarizes published studies in asthmatics, where cellular numbers have been quantified in biopsies or lavage samples before and after steroid treatment. The therapy diminished, more or less uniformly, the numbers of eosinophils and mast cells in the mucosa and submucosa, and at least in some series this reduction was correlated to a decreased hyperresponsiveness (135,158). The reduction in eosinophil and mast cell numbers seems persistent, because Lundgren et al. (159) found a low number of inflammatory cells even after 10 years of steroid treatment. The attenuation of eosinophil function refers also to the airway number of "activated" eosinophils [releasing the cytotoxic protein ECP (160)], to the contents of this protein in BAL fluid (161), as well as to the ability of eosinophils to degranulate [*in vitro* studies (153)].

Steroid therapy has been reported to decrease also the total number of mucosal and submucosal lymphocytes and of submucosal plasma cells (137). Based on activation markers for T-cell subsets lymphocytes expressing IL-2 receptor (CD25$^+$) and memory cells (CD45RO$^+$) were reduced (Table 4). There is some support for an attenuation of antigen presentation due to reduction of HLA-DR expression (162) and of the macrophage subset RFD1$^+$ (Table 4). Lundgren et al. (159) and Laitinen et al. (137) found that

TABLE 4. *Modulation of cell numbers and degranulation products of granulocytes in airway–lung lavage or biopsy specimen of asthmatic patients*

Cell or cell product	Mode of GCS administration	GCS action		References
Eosinophils				
Number	Oral		↓	77a
Number of "activated" (EG2 + positive)	Oral		↓	160a
Number	Inhalation		↓	130a, 135–137, 159, 160a
Eosinophil degranulation product (ECP)				
Number	Inhalation		↓	136, 161
Mast cells				
Number	Oral		↓	160
Number	Inhalation		↓	135–137, 160a
Basophils				
Number	Inhalation to nasal mucosa		↓	163
Lymphocytes				
Number	Oral	T cells (CD3$^+$)	↓	160
		T cells (CD4$^+$)	↓	77a, 162
Number	Inhalation	T cells (CD2,5,8)	↓	162
		T cells (CD45RO$^+$)	↓	164
		T cells (CD25$^+$)	↓	137
		Lymphocytes	↓	137
		Plasma cells	↓	137
Alveolar macrophages				
Number	Inhalation	RFD1$^+$ cells	↓	162
Ratio ciliated/goblet cells	Inhalation		↑	137, 159
Intraepithelial nerves				
Number	Inhalation		↑	137
Fibroblasts				
Number	Inhalation		↑	137
Neutrophils				
Number	Oral	TDI-induced late bronchial reaction	↓	165

ECP, eosinophilic cationic protein; EG, activated eosinophilic granules; RFD, antigen-presenting phenotype; TDI, toluene diisocyanate.

prolonged steroid inhalation improves the ratio between ciliated cells and goblet cells and this important effect helps to explain why steroids decrease the risk of mucus plugging.

Bronchial Smooth Muscle Contraction

GCSs have no bronchorelaxing activity directly at the smooth muscle level in animals (144) or in humans (166). The early reports on direct actions by hydrocortisone are dubious due to vehicle effects and have not been reproduced with the more potent synthetic steroids (1). Even prolonged *in vivo* treatment does not affect the sensitivity of animal tracheal preparations to contractile or relaxant drugs (147,167).

GCSs reinforce transcription of the adrenergic β_2-receptor in animal and human tissue (168) including human lung tissue (169). It has been discussed whether steroid treatment can compensate for the subsensitivity sometimes seen on prolonged β-agonist therapy. With the exception of a subset of asthmatic patients, there is still little support for potentiation of β-receptor action as a major anti-asthmatic mechanism of GCS (for fuller discussion see ref. 1).

PHARMACOLOGICAL PROPERTIES AND DRUG DEVELOPMENT

Due to the apparent uniformity of GCS receptors (GCS-Rs), there is no basis for a differentiation of wanted from unwanted GCS effects at the receptor level. However, by chemical manipulation of the steroid structure it has been possible to develop synthetic derivatives better suited to different types of therapy. These manipulations have shown improvements, as follows: (a) they reduced the cross-affinity for the closely related mineralocorticoid receptor, (b) they enhanced the affinity for GCS-R leading to more potent drugs, and (c) they altered the pharmacokinetic behavior so that uptake, distribution, and biotransformation have been changed. These results have guided development in two main directions—steroids with enhanced biostability for systemic therapy and metabolically more unstable steroids for topical therapy. These developmental lines have been governed more by empiricism than by firm knowledge. In fact, we are still lacking clear answers to the following key questions: (a) What are the main target cells for steroid treatment in airway–lung diseases and do these cells differ in topical and systemic therapy, respectively? (b) What is the GCS concentration required for triggering GCS receptors in these cells? (c) How long do GCSs need to stay in target tissue? (d) How do different airway and lung diseases differ in these regards? The development of GCS drugs in schematically presented in Fig. 6. The development occurred in two phases: an early phase directed to systemic therapy, where little further pharmacological progress

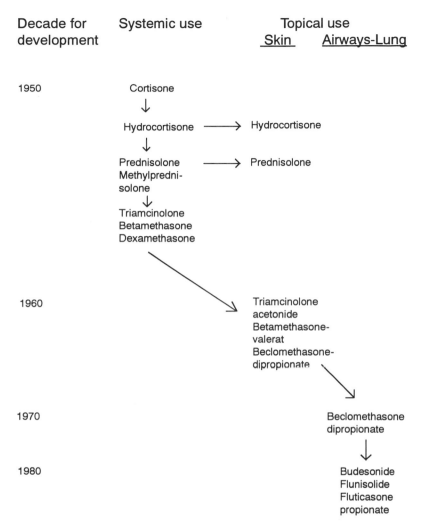

FIG. 6. Schematic overview over development of GCS for systemic and inhalational use. The development can be roughly divided into three phases: an early phase (cortisone to dexamethasone) directed mainly to systemic treatment, and where some compounds can exert also a slight topical efficacy on skin; a later phase based on potent lipophilic acetals and esters primarily developed for topical skin therapy, and where some of these steroids demonstrate topical selectivity also on airway mucosa; and a subsequent phase where the airway selectivity has been further improved by reinforcing the hepatic first-pass metabolism.

has been achieved, and a later and fruitful development in GCS for inhalation therapy.

GCS for Systemic Use (Fig. 7)

Cortisone was the first GCS manufactured for commercial use. Today we know that the 11-keto compounds (position Z in Fig. 7) cortisone and prednisone are prodrugs, which need to be reduced in the liver to the corresponding 11-OH compounds (hydrocortisone and prednisolone) before they acquire affinity for the receptor. Thus, there is no basis for using these 11-keto compounds by the topical route. Hydrocortisone and prednisolone can be used for different types of systemic therapy as well as for the topical treatment of skin (Fig. 6). However, it was shown early that neither of these steroids has significant anti-allergic activity when inhaled (170). Reasons for the poor local activity on airway–lung mucosa was not well understood at that time, but might today be explained, at least partially, by inactivation of these compounds through the enzyme 11β-hydroxy-steroid dehydrogenase. This enzyme has high activity in lung tissue and tracheal epithelial cells (171). Furthermore, on inhalation there is a great surface dilution of administered substance, arguing for the use of steroids more potent than hydrocortisone and prednisolone.

The first synthetic modification of the hydrocortisone skeleton was unsaturation of the 1–2 bond, giving prednisolone (Fig. 7). This modification increases the affinity for GCS-R (but not for the similar mineralocorticoid receptor) and enhances the metabolic stability in liver, explaining the superiority of prednisolone over hydrocortisone for oral therapy. Compared with hydrocortisone, its affinity for GCS receptor is enhanced 12 times (Table 5), while its clearance is halved (Table 6). The mean oral bioavailability of prednisolone is approximately 80%.

A further reduction of the mineralocorticoid activity was obtained by introducing substituents in the 6α and/or 16 positions (X and R_1, respectively, in Fig. 7). While this reduction seems to have been the original rationale for developing 6-α-methylprednisolone, one additional reason for preferring this drug in systemic lung therapy has appeared later (172), and that is its better penetration into the alveolar region. This has been shown in a pharmacokinetic study comparing GCS concentrations in plasma and bronchoalveolar epithelial lining fluid of methylprednisolone and prednisolone (173). For a given concentration of steroid in the plasma of rabbits (after i.v. administration) the concentration of methylprednisolone in the epithelial lining fluid was twice that of prednisolone (174). The reason for the higher lung affinity of methylprednisolone is its higher volume of distribution (Table 6). This is partly due to its lower ability, unlike prednisolone, to bind to transcortin—the specific GCS binding protein in plasma. There are several approaches to optimize systemic therapy with methylprednisolone, prednisolone, and

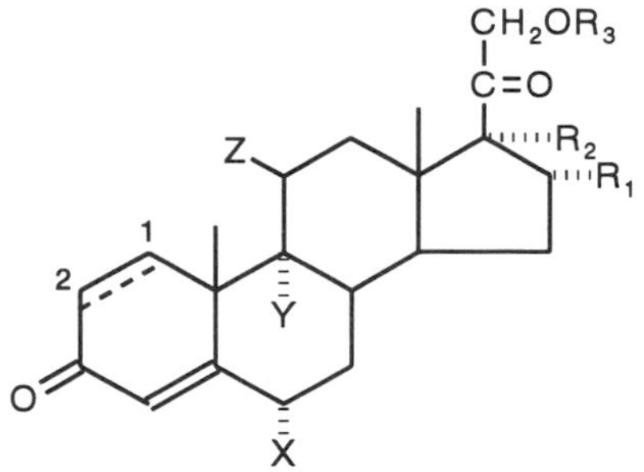

FIG. 7. Structure of GCS used in systemic therapy. Explanation of position numbers in the steroid skeleton: X = 6, Y = 9, Z = 11, R_1 = 16, R_2 = 17, R_3 = 21; Me = methyl.

GCS	1-2	X	Y	Z	R_1	R_2	R_3
Cortisone	sat	H	H	0	H	α–OH	H
Hydrocortisone	"	"	"	β–OH	"	"	"
Prednisolone	unsat	"	"	"	"	"	"
Prednisone	"	"	"	0	"	"	"
6-methylpred-nisolone	"	α-Me	H	β OH	"	"	"
Dexamethasone	"	H	α-F	"	α- Me	"	"
Betamethasone	"	"	α-F	"	β – Me	"	"
Triamcinolone	"	"	α-F	"	α-OH	"	"

prednisone, including splitting the dose over the day or to correct for variations in absorption and clearance in individual patients (175–179).

The next step in substance development was halogenation of the 6α and/or 9α positions of the B-ring (positions X and Y in Fig. 7), leading to triamcinolone, betamethasone, and dexamethasone. In systemic therapy these compounds are several times more potent than prednisolone due to (a) enhanced receptor affinity; (b) reduced binding to trancortin, giving higher free steroid concentration; and (c) a higher biostability leading to prolonged activity. Their pharmacological properties are exemplified with the values for dexamethasone given in Tables 5 and 6. Unfortunately, these compounds do not cause fewer adverse effects in systemic therapy but rather the opposite, which probably depends on their prolonged biological activity. This relates also to inhalation therapy—the enhanced receptor affinity gives dexameth-

TABLE 5. *Relative binding affinity (RBA) for GCS receptor in vitro and relative topical blanching potency in vivo*

GCS	RBA		Topical blanching potency in man
	Rat tissue	Human lung tissue	
Systemic			
Hydrocortisone	0.04		0.13
Prednisolone	0.5		<0.1
Dexamethasone	1	1	1
Topical			
Budesonide	7.8	9.4	980
BDP/BMP	2.3/15.3	0.4/13.5	600/450
Flunisolide	–	1.8	330
Triamcinolone acetonide	3.8	3.6	330
Fluticasone propionate	18	18	1200

BDP, beclomethasone 17α, 21-dipropionate; BMP, beclomethasone 17α-propionate.
RBA adapted from refs. 19, 178, 191–193.
Topical blanching potency adapted from refs. 182, 189, 194.

TABLE 6. *Pharmacokinetic properties after i.v. administration*

GCS	Clearance (L/min)	Volume of distribution (L/kg)	Half-life (h)	Oral bioavailability (%)
Systemic				
Hydrocortisone	0.4	1	1.9	60
Prednisolone	0.2	0.8	3.3	84
Methylprednisolone	0.4	1.3	2.6	90
Dexamethasone	0.2	0.5	4.4	65
Topical				
Budesonide	1.4	4.3	2.8	11
Flunisolide	1.0	1.8	1.6	21
Triamcinolone acetonide	0.8	1.4	1.5	–
Fluticasone propionate	0.9	3.5	3.1	low (see text)

Clearance, volume of distribution, and half-life from refs. 178, 190.
Oral bioavailability from refs. 188, 190, 195–199.

asone anti-asthmatic activity by inhalation—but the high biostability of the absorbed substance leads to as much systemic activity as by the oral route (180).

GCS for Inhalation Use

This development started as a spinoff from topical dermatological therapy. The primary aim was to enhance the poor topical skin activity of triamcinolone and betamethasone (Fig. 6) by introducing lipophilic substituents at the 17α or at the 16α,17α positions (R_1 and R_2 in Fig. 7). Depending on the structure of the 16 position, two types of lipophilic substituents were used— either acetalization of the 16α,17α-OH groups or esterification of the 17α-OH group. This gave the lead compounds triamcinolone 16α,17α-acetonide and betamethasone 17α-valerate, followed rapidly by a series of similar steroids including beclomethasone 17α,21-dipropionate (Fig. 6). During that development little attention was paid to the rates and routes of biotransformation of these compounds, because in topical dermatological therapy systemic absorption is normally strongly restricted by the stratum corneum barrier of skin. However, on mucous membranes—lacking this type of barrier—there is a rapid and profound absorption of topically applied steroids. When betamethasone 17α-valerate and beclomethasone 17α,21-dipropionate were tested by inhalation in asthma and rhinitis (170), it was surprisingly found that they have good systemic tolerance due to a high hepatic first-pass metabolism, compensating for the profound absorption from airway mucosa (181,182). One important metabolic difference between the earlier generation (betamethasone, dexamethasone, and triamcinolone) and selected steroids with lipophilic substituents in the 17α or 16α,17α positions (Fig. 8) is that the latter compounds can be much more effectively inactivated by oxidative biotransformation via the cytochrome P-450 system of liver. This is due to a facilitated binding via hydrophobic interactions to key P-450 enzymes, known to prefer lipophilic substrates, and where bulky substituents do not hinder catalytic activity (183). The metabolic superiority of lipophilic GCS—found serendipitiously for beclomethasone 17α,21-dipropionate and betamethasone 17α-valerate (181,184)—has been further improved in a later steroid generation (Fig. 6), comprising budesonide (185–187), flunisolide (188), and fluticasone propionate (189,190). These compounds have been more specifically designed and selected for high first-pass hepatic metabolism.

Pharmacodynamical and Pharmacokinetical Basis of Inhalation Therapy in Asthma—Exemplified by Budesonide

The introduction of selected lipophilic substituents in the 17α or 16α,17α positions adds at one stroke two key properties to the steroid molecule:

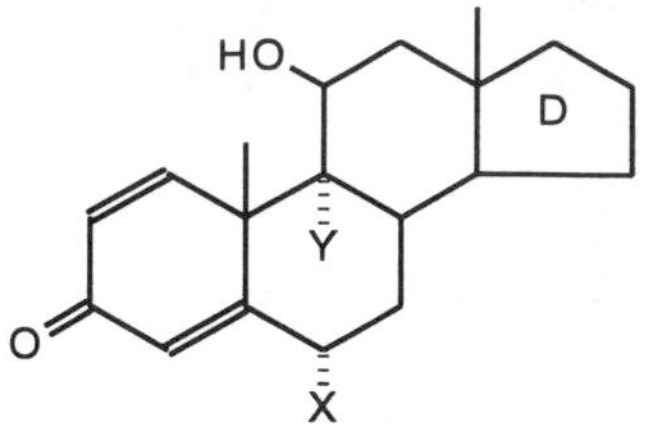

GCS	X	Y	D
Beclomethasone dipropionate	H	Cl	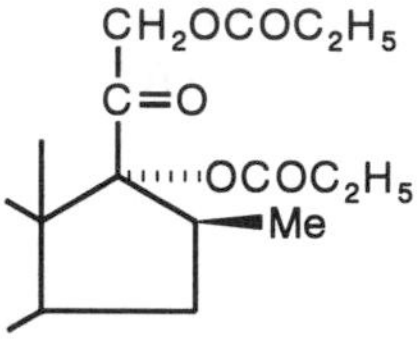 $CH_2OCOC_2H_5$ / $C=O$ / ""$OCOC_2H_5$ / ◀Me
Budesonide	H	H	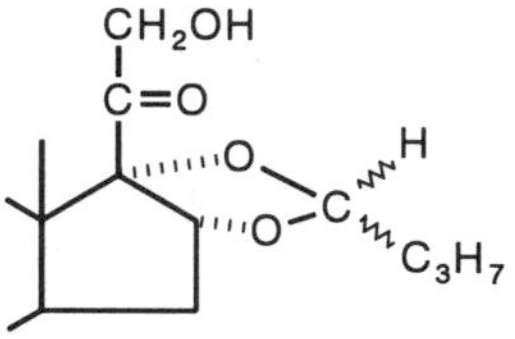 CH_2OH / $C=O$ / O—C—H / O—C_3H_7
Flunisolide	F	H	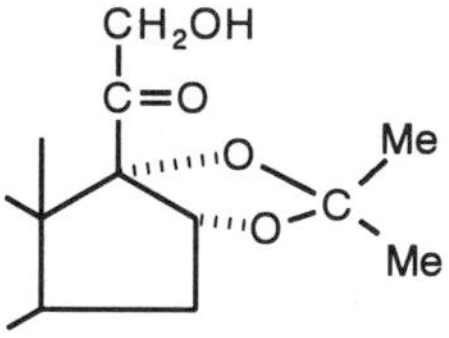 CH_2OH / $C=O$ / O—C—Me / O—Me
Triamcinolone acetonide	H	F	— " —
Fluticasone propionate	F	F	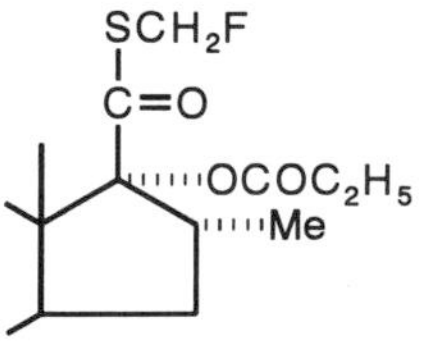 SCH_2F / $C=O$ / ""$OCOC_2H_5$ / ""Me

FIG. 8. Structure of GCS used by inhalation. For explanation of position numbers see Fig. 7.

1. A very high affinity for the receptor, which seems necessary to compensate for the dilution occurring on the vast airway–lung surface and for the potential risk of local metabolic inactivation. As seen in Table 6 the receptor affinity of steroids used by inhalation is at least 100 times higher than that of hydrocortisone. An even greater preference for the lipophilic compounds is seen in the topical blanching test (Table 5), probably depending on their better tissue penetration and binding (see below).
2. An efficient hepatic first-pass metabolism leading to metabolites of negligible steroid activity. The first-pass metabolisms can be measured as clearance and Table 6 illustrates the successful drug development with a three- to five-fold increase from the clearance of the "systemic" steroids (approximately 0.3 L/min) to the "topical" compounds (range 0.8–1.4 L/min). The highest value is close to the maximal hepatic clearance, which is limited by the liver blood flow (approximately 1.5 L/min at rest). The high clearance explains the very low oral bioavailability, which for the best compounds is just a few percentages (Table 6).

The functional importance of this pharmacologic profile is illustrated in Fig. 9. The values of budesonide (Tables 5 and 6) are used to exemplify the figure because this compound has currently the best pharmacokinetic documentation (187). Furthermore, the physicochemical properties of budesonide (notably its relatively high solubility in water—14μg/ml), means that this drug can be delivered by CFC aerosol, by a novel type of multidose dry powder inhaler without additives (Turbuhaler), as well as by nebulization. The systemic contribution of budesonide deposited in the oropharynx and swallowed is rather small due to budesonide's low oral bioavailability (approximately 11%—Table 6). This oral contribution can be further reduced by mouth-rinsing, by adding a big spacer to the metered dose inhaler (200) or by using the dry powder inhaler Turbuhaler, giving an improved airway–lung deposition (201). When such measures are used it has been calculated (192,201) as well as experimentally verified [by blocking the oral uptake with charcoal (201)] that the swallowed fraction constitutes just 15% of total systemic availability. Without these precautions this figure can be 35% to 40% with inhalation from conventional metered dose inhalers (192,201).

Thus, the systemic availability of inhaled steroids is predominantly derived from the airway–lung deposited fraction. Based on experimental studies there seems to be little backwash of steroid substance into the lumen, once absorbed. These studies, as well as studies in man (199), mean that the airway–lung deposited fraction is more or less fully bioavailable through the tracheobronchial and pulmonary circulations (Fig. 9). The uptake rate into systemic circulation may vary somewhat between steroids due to differences in rates of dissolution and absorption and to the extent of local tissue binding. After inhalation of 500 μg budesonide the plasma peak has been determined to be about 2×10^{-9} mol/L, and it was seen at 15 to 30 min, and declined with a half-life of 2 h (199). The peak concentration is restricted

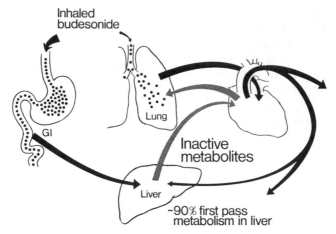

FIG. 9. Schematic overview of *in vivo* pharmacokinetics of inhaled GCS, exemplified with budesonide. (Adapted from ref. 14.)

due to the high volume of distribution (Table 7) and to the efficient hepatic biotransformation of budesonide (199,202,203). This biotransformation occurs along several metabolic routes, among them a splitting of the $16\alpha,17\alpha$-acetal group and a 6β-hydroxylation (204–206). The GCS activity of these metabolites is about 100 times lower than that of the parent drug (19).

    That inhaled budesonide really exerts its major anti-asthmatic activity locally in the airway–lung compartment is supported by a recent study, where the systemic activity of an inhaled dose was matched by a systemic dose of budesonide giving a similar plasma level (area under the curve) as seen after

TABLE 7. *Potential complications of systemic corticosteroid therapy*

Short-term, high dose
    Mental and CNS disturbances including mood swings (euphoria to depression), psychosis (rare)
    Sodium and fluid retention
    Impaired glucose tolerance, hyperosmolar nonketotic coma
    Hypokalemic alkalosis, systemic arterial hypertension, glaucoma, pancreatitis, peptic ulcer and gastrointestinal hemorrhage, proximal myopathy (rare)
Long-term, daily steroids for months or years
    Suppression of the hypothalamic-pituitary-adrenal axis, with adrenal insufficiency
    Cushing's syndrome
    Growth retardation in children
    Osteoporosis with vertebral compression and bone fractures, aseptic necrosis of bone
    Proximal myopathy
    Increased susceptibility to opportunistic infections
    Impaired wound healing, dermal atrophy
    CNS manifestations—depression, lability of mood, anxiety, seizures
    Posterior subcapsular cataract

inhalation (207). The systemic regimen was without significant anti-asthmatic activity. In a comparative dose-response study Toogood et al. (208) estimated that 1 mg inhaled budesonide had a similar anti-asthmatic efficacy as 58 mg oral prednisone, while its plasma cortisol depression was comparable to just 9 mg prednisone. A preferentially local action is supported also by analysis of the budesonide concentration in the airway–lung compartment. After inhalation of 1600 μg budesonide before anesthesia for lung surgery, the lung concentration was found 1 to 4 h later to be 10 times higher than that in plasma, approximately 10^{-8} and 10^{-9} mol/L, respectively (209). Results in rat trachea demonstrated the preference of topical perfusion over mucosal tissue, because the budesonide concentration in the tracheal wall was then more than 100 times higher than when the same dose was administered subcutaneously outside the region (192).

There is experimental evidence that the inhalational 17α or 16α,17α-substituted GCS (Fig. 8) binds better to local airway–lung tissue than do less lipophilic and less airway-selective steroids (e.g., dexamethasone and hydrocortisone). On topical perfusion in a rat tracheal model there was an approximately 15 times better uptake into tracheal tissue of budesonide than of hydrocortisone and dexamethasone. Furthermore, the half-life in the tissue was 2h for budesonide but only 15 to 20 min for the other two steroids (192,210). In the isolated perfused lung Ryrfeldt et al. (211) found that of airway-deposited budesonide a minor fraction bound extensively to lung tissue and needed strong extraction procedure to release it. It can thus be speculated that besides their higher affinity for the GCS receptor (binding depending on specific steroid structure and affinity working in the nanomolar range) the airway-selective GCS may have also a higher nonselective affinity for tissue at the application site (probably via a binding based on general lipophilicity and working more in the micromolar range). It seems logical that when GCSs are slowly released from these still-unidentified binding sites (phospholipid-rich membranes?) they produce prolonged stimulation at local GCS receptors. This type of local depot may explain the possibility of using budesonide even once daily in treatment of stable mild asthma (212,213).

Pharmacological Properties of Other GCSs for Inhalation (Fig. 8 and Tables 5 and 6)

Beclomethasone 17α,21-dipropionate (BDP)

BDP has a much lower water solubility than budesonide (0.1 and 14 μg/ml water, respectively), which means a slower rate of dissolution and absorption (214). BDP itself has just a low affinity for the GCS-R, while its first hydrolysis product beclomethasone 17α-propionate (BMP) has a high affinity (Table 5). This hydrolytic step is rapid in lung homogenate and possibly also in bronchial cells, but slow in bronchial secretions (191,215). Circulating blood contains BMP and just traces of BDP, and in the liver BMP is further biotransformed via at least a couple of metabolic routes (hydrolysis to beclomethasone and/or oxidative biotransformation of BMP). The biotransformation of BMP in human liver cytosolic preparations is slower than that of budesonide (202). This contributes to the observation that BDP in some volunteer and patient studies has demonstrated a greater systemic activity than budesonide (194,216–220). There is no published information on the oral bioavailability and the kinetics of BDP and BMP after i.v. administration or inhalation in man. BDP is administered as a CFC-aerosol or capsule-based dry powder inhaler. The efficacy of the nebulizing formulation is impeded by the very low water solubility of BDP.

Flunisolide

Flunisolide has a lower receptor affinity and blanching potency than budesonide or the BDP/BMP complex (Table 5), but this may be partly compensated for by its much higher water solubility (100 µg/ml). Flunisolide is oxidatively biotransformed in the liver by 6β-hydroxylation (188) into metabolites of low potency, and its clearance and oral bioavailability are 1 L/min and 21%, respectively (Table 6).

Triamcinolone acetonide

This pioneering acetal (Fig. 6) is now delivered also by inhalation. It has a moderate receptor affinity and topical blanching potency similar to flunisolide (Table 5), and also a high water solubility (40 µg/ml). Like flunisolide, triamcinolone acetonide is inactivated by 6β-hydroxylation, but regarding the rate of this deactivation flunisolide may have some preference through the lability of its 6α-F substitution. There is no published figure for its oral bioavailability, while some information is available for the plasma levels reached after inhalation [C_{max} 1.2, 2.3, and 4.5 nmol/L after doses of 400, 800, and 1600 µg, respectively (221)]. Experience from another indication area (slow release formulation for arthritis) suggest that a sustained plasma level greater than 6 nmol/L leads to clinically significant systemic activity.

Fluticasone propionate (FP)

This compound has a new type of 17β side chain and double fluorination of the B ring (Fig. 7). It has a very low water solubility (0.04 µg/ml), suggesting a rather slow absorption rate from airway lumina. Its very high receptor affinity (Table 5) allows the use of a lower dose than that of BDP (222). FP is efficiently inactivated in the liver (but not in lung or blood) by splitting the 17β-thioester and forming a steroid carboxylic acid with negligible receptor affinity (189). The plasma clearance after i.v. infusion has been determined to be 0.9 L/min, and based on that as well as on a proposed low distribution into red cells "a full hepatic extraction and virtually zero oral bioavailability" has been claimed by calculations (190). If the experimentally determined distribution value found by others [20% distribution into red cells (223)] is used in the same type of calculation, the oral bioavailability of FP would be approximately 12%. However, these calculations need to be replaced by values determined through proper pharmacokinetic studies with administration of FP also via the inhalation route.

Pharmacokinetic Interactions

Because all the GCS discussed are inactivated by the cytochrome P-450 system in the liver, there is a risk that liver damage or interactions with other drugs biotransformed along the same route will enhance the circulating steroids levels. The former risk has been investigated in patients with characterized liver damage and with the preliminary conclusion that the presence of portal shunting reduces budesonide clearance, while liver disturbances without shunting only slightly impair its clearance (data in files of Astra Draco). There is still little support that other drugs via hepatic interaction can enhance the systemic effects of inhaled GCS, while there is evidence for positive as well as negative interaction when it relates to the systemic use of steroids (195,224). It is known that cyclosporin can inhibit the metabolism of prednisolone and methylprednisolone (225). Troleandomycin inhibits methylprednisolone elimination and prolongs its duration of effect, and on the whole methylprednisolone seems more susceptible than prednisolone to positive and negative drug interactions (177,224).

TYPES OF ADVERSE EFFECTS

Glucocorticosteroids are frequently associated with fear and unacceptance by patients, and even among some physicians. The side effects of long-term treatment with systemic corticosteroids are well known. It is of outmost importance that the difference in risks of side effects between oral/systemic treatment and inhaled/local treatment is communicated to primary care doctors, patients, relatives, and the general public. Whereas oral corticosteroids cause side effects, the inhaled corticosteroids are mostly free of all types of adverse reactions, or, at least, they cause significantly fewer side effects. The safety of inhaled corticosteroids has been recently reviewed (3).

Oral Corticosteroids

The general side effects of oral corticosteroids have been extensively reviewed (e.g., 2,226). These include serious adverse effects caused by long-term use and those resulting from withdrawal of the drug after prolonged use.

The use of oral corticosteroids for some days or a few weeks does not lead to clinically significant adrenal insufficiency upon cessation of treatment. A course of less than 2 weeks can be discontinued abruptly. If the treatment has continued for some weeks a gradual decrease of the dose is recommended. After long-term treatment with corticosteroids it may take several months until completely normal pituitary and adrenal functions have been achieved. During this recovery period the patient may need substitution therapy with steroids during stressful situations, such as severe infections and surgical procedures. There is no evidence that the administration of ACTH can prevent or reverse the development of glucocorticosteroid-induced adrenal suppression (227).

Short-term, high-dose therapy with corticosteroids may sometimes, although rarely, result in complications of sudden onset (Table 7).

Acute adrenal insufficiency results from a too rapid withdrawal of systemic corticosteroids after prolonged therapy. This is a syndrome characterized by myalgia, arthralgia, stiffness, headache, nausea, anorexia, fatigue, malaise, and fever (228,229). It occurs more commonly if corticosteroids are withdrawn rapidly, but is not related to the dose or duration of treatment. Joint pain seems to occur most frequently in patients with asthma and other lung diseases reducing their doses of glucocorticosteroids, i.e., patients who should not ordinarily have joint symptoms. It is also noteworthy that diseases and symptoms suppressed during treatment with systemic corticosteroids, e.g., eczema, allergic rhinitis, conjunctivitis, etc., may reappear when the dose is reduced. Since many patients with the corticosteroid withdrawal syndrome suffer from concomitant adrenal suppression, appropriate tests to define the adrenal function should be performed.

There are many protocols describing how the gradual reduction of dose should take place in order to avoid the steroid withdrawal syndrome (230,231), but the physician must realize that these are only general guidelines to help design individual reduction protocols. In patients with known or suspected adrenal insufficiency the possibility of reducing the steroids is limited by the status of the underlying disease. Therefore, when the underlying disease is severe or life threatening, the initial reduction must be slow.

In patients receiving a daily dose of 40 mg prednisolone (or equivalent amounts of other corticosteroids) or more, the dose can be rapidly reduced to 40 mg a day. In patients receiving 20 to 40 mg daily the dose can be reduced by 5 mg a week until a dose of 15 mg daily is reached. Thereafter the weekly reduction should be 2.5 mg only. Sometimes the reduction steps can be initially taken every 3 days. When a physiological dose of 5 mg prednisolone has been reached, i.e., a dose not causing disturbances in the function of the pituitary-adrenal axis, the patient can be switched to a single morning dose of 20 mg hydrocortisone daily. Thereafter the hydrocortisone dose can be reduced by 2.5 mg each week until a level of 10 mg daily is reached. Then measurements of early morning plasma cortisol levels and ACTH tests can guide the physician in deciding on subsequent therapy. If the 8 A.M. cortisol level is at least around the lower limit of the reference range, it indicates a sufficiently normal adrenal function and hydrocortisone can be discontinued. However, corticosteroid coverage for major stress situations may be necessary for up to 2 years after complete corticosteroid withdrawal. It is obvious that the pituitary-adrenal function in patients treated with synthetic glucocorticosteroids cannot be reliably estimated from the dose of glucocorticoid, the duration of therapy, or the basal plasma cortisol concentration. This conclusion was reached by Schlaghecke et al. (232), who carried out ACTH tests in 279 patients, and insulin hypoglycemia tests in 61 patients, who had received therapy with 5 to 30 mg prednisolone or its equivalent to treat various chronic diseases for periods up to 15 years.

In addition to adrenal insufficiency, prolonged therapy with systemic corticosteroids may result in fluid and electrolyte disturbances, Cushing's syndrome ("moon face," "buffalo hump," central obesity, supraclavicular fat pads, striae, ecchymoses, acne, and hirsutism), hypertension, hyperglycemia and glycosuria, increased susceptibility to various infections, osteoporosis, aseptic necrosis of bones, peptic ulcers, myopathy, posterior subcapsular cataracts, behavioral disturbances, and growth retardation (Table 7).

To avoid or minimize suppression on the pituitary-adrenal axis glucocorticoids have usually been given as one daily dose in the morning (233). Data obtained in controlled studies, comparing different timings of the dose, is scanty, however. In patients with nocturnal asthma, dosing at 3 P.M. results in improved nighttime sleep and improved lung function, compared with 8 A.M. dosing (234). Dosing of oral corticosteroids every other day instead of daily administration may in some instances reduce the risk of systemic side effects (235). However, a therapeutic regimen with dosing of steroids every other day is not always possible in the treatment of diseases of the lungs, especially not in the treatment of bronchial asthma.

Inhaled Corticosteroids

Inhalation of recommended doses of corticosteroids for treatment of airway diseases is mostly free of adverse effects. However, depending on the inhalation system and technique up to 70% of the delivered dose may impact on surfaces of oropharynx and the upper airways. Inhaled corticosteroids may therefore cause local side effects, such as dysphonia/hoarseness and oropharyngeal candidiasis. These local side effects are mostly transient, and more inconvenient than serious, but sometimes severe enough to warrant temporary or permanent discontinuation of the treatment.

Continued use of high doses of inhaled corticosteroids may result in systemic absorption of drug and consequently in a risk of systemic steroid effects. These systemic effects are, however, almost negligible and always milder than those seen with oral corticosteroids giving the same degree of asthma control.

Local Side Effects

Positive throat cultures for candida in patients using inhaled corticosteroids have been reported in up to 45% in children (236) and in 60% to 70% of adult patients (237,238). The occurrence of clinically significant candidiasis is much lower—about 10% in adults (238,239) and 1% in children (236). The frequency is related to the total daily dose of corticosteroids but not to the duration of treatment (240), and can be reduced by lowering the frequency of administrations and the daily dose, i.e., the number of inhalations per day (238,240). The use of large (750 ml) spacing devices (241) or Aerochamber (242,243) for pressurized metered dose inhalers, and careful mouth rinsing for inspiratory flow-driven powder inhalers (200) also reduce the risk of oropharyngeal side effects. If oral candidiasis develops, it is usually managed with topical antifungal agents. Hoarseness and cough are more frequent side-effects than candidiasis and can be temporarily seen in up to 30% of the patients (238,240). Hoarseness is unrelated to candidiasis and is often seen in patients with voice stress, such as sport coaches, switchboard operators, teachers, singers, etc. A bilateral adductor vocal cord deformity with bowing of the cords on phonation has also been described (244). Hoarseness has been shown to improve with the same measures used for candidiasis, i.e., reduction of dosing frequency and the use of spacing devices (240,241). If hoarseness occurs, voice rest for some time may be appropriate.

More recently attention has been drawn to the local side effects, such as cough and bronchoconstriction, probably caused by the propellants in the metered dose inhalers (245,246). The majority of the patients complaining about cough and local irritation after inhalation from a pressurized metered dose inhaler can use an inspiratory flow-driven drug powder inhaler without carrier powder, such as Turbuhaler, without side effects (200).

Topically applied corticosteroids on the skin will stay there for several hours and may cause adverse effects, e.g., atrophy and bruising. Inhaled corticosteroids are present in low concentrations per surface area of the airway epithelium and they are absorbed within minutes. This difference in pharmacokinetics of corticosteroids applied on the airway mucosa or on the skin probably explains the difference in side effects. Lung fibroblasts also have a lower sensitivity than skin fibroblasts to the catabolic effects of steroids (247). The inhaled steroids have now been available for more than 20 years. Many patients have used them regularly for more than 10 years. No reports on atrophy in the airways have appeared. Biopsy studies have on the contrary demonstrated diminishing inflammation (159), repair of epithelial damage (137), and no signs of atrophy, metaplasia, or malignant transformation (248–251). Inhaled corticosteroids have been found to have no adverse effect on mucociliary clearance (252).

Systemic Side Effects

Inhaled corticosteroids are absorbed from the lung and the orally deposited dose may be swallowed, absorbed from the gastrointestinal tract, and added to the dose that gains access to the systemic circulation. The dose absorbed from the lung is of greater importance because it counts for approximately 90% of the systemically available dose. In adults, low and moderate doses of inhaled budesonide and beclomethasone dipropionate (BDP)—up to 1.0 mg a day—do not have clinically relevant systemic side effects (3). However, depending on the measurements used even doses as low as 0.4 mg BDP have been found to have measurable systemic activity (253). There is also an important intraindividual sensitivity for developing systemic effects with corticosteroids. The systemic effects that will be discussed include effects on the hypothalamic pituitary-adrenal axis, inhibition of growth in children, effects on bone mineralization and turnover in adults, metabolic effects and risk of cataracts, skin bruising, infections, and behaviorial disturbances.

Effects on the Hypothalamic-Pituitary-Adrenal (HPA) Axis

Most of the studies addressing effects on the HPA-axis have measured early morning cortisol in serum, the response to tetracosactrin (ACTH) stimulation, and the excretion of urinary cortisol over 24 h. A short tetracosactrin test and urine free cortisol are equally useful as screening tests and more sensitive than early morning serum cortisol values (254). Insulin stress tests may be slightly more sensitive than urine free cortisol and ACTH tests, as it measures the total hypophysial-pituitary-adrenal function.

Early studies using the low doses of BDP in children, up to 0.1 mg four times daily, did not show signs of adrenal suppression (255). Also in later studies (256) it has been found by using serum cortisol, ACTH stimulation tests, and 24-h urinary free cortisol excretion that doses up to 2.0 mg/1.73 m^2 body surface (daily doses used were 0.8–2.0 mg) can be given with little risk of adrenal suppression. However, Law et al. (257) noted a fall in nocturnal serum cortisol and a delay in its morning rise and peak concentration in children already given 0.3 mg BDP, and Pecora et al. (258), by measuring morning cortisol and ACTH secretion in a controlled study, noted a marked adrenal suppression in children given BDP 0.4 mg daily for 6 months. In a comparative controlled study Pedersen and Fuglsang (218) treated 31 children with doses of BDP and budesonide ranging from 0.8 mg to 1.2 mg daily during two 6-week study periods and measured the 24-h excretion of urinary cortisol. BDP caused a significantly greater suppression on the cortisol excretion than budesonide. The difference was greater on daily doses of 1.0 to 1.2 mg compared with 0.8 mg daily. Furthermore in children, Bisgaard et al. (217,259) found dose-dependent suppression of urinary cortisol with 0.2, 0.4, and 0.8 mg BDP but not with budesonide. Children with asthma have used budesonide, 0.2 to 0.4 mg daily for up to 1 year without changes in their morning serum cortisol values or response to ACTH (260,261).

In adults, no changes in morning plasma cortisol levels were seen in patients taking 1.0 mg BDP daily (262), although some studies indicate suppression occurring with this dose of BDP. However, consistent evidence of significant adrenal suppression is not found until BDP doses of 1.5 mg daily or more have been reached (263–265). And, if the last dose of BDP is taken late, e.g., at midnight, even daily doses of 0.4 mg in adults may result in reduced morning cortisol levels (253).

Budesonide is metabolized more rapidly than BDP. Consequently, in a study in which healthy subjects received increasing doses of budesonide aerosol, given via a spacer, starting from 0.4 mg twice daily, and increasing the dose by 0.8 mg every fortnight up to 12 mg daily, a mean dose of 5.6 mg had to be reached before 50% of the subjects had cortisol suppression below the lower limit of the reference value (266). In addition to serum morning cortisol, Ädelroth (267) performed insulin stress tests in 14 patients with asthma receiving up to 1.6 mg budesonide daily, but no oral corticosteroids. No signs of disturbed HPA function was noted. Of 13 patients treated with a combination of prednisolone and inhaled budesonide (0.8 mg daily in 11 patients and 1.6 mg daily in two patients), seven had an insufficient insulin stress test, and three of the patients had an oral dose of just 2.5 mg prednisolone. Brown et al. (268) studied the HPA axis function in 78 patients using high-dose inhaled corticosteroids (median dose 1.6 mg, range 1.2–2.65 mg daily), 69 on BDP and 9 on budesonide. All patients had 9 A.M. serum cortisol, 24-h urine free cortisol, and a short ACTH test. All tests were done at least 2 weeks after completion of any short course of oral steroids. Twenty-six patients had long-term treatment with oral steroids, which had been discontinued at least 7 months prior to assessment. Suppression of the HPA axis function was defined as abnormal values in at least two of the three tests. Sixteen patients (20.5%) showed signs of suppression on doses of inhaled corticosteroids varying from 1.5 to 2.4 mg daily. No clear relationship was identified between HPA function and daily dose, or between degree of suppression and number of short courses of oral steroids in the preceding 12 months.

Controlled studies comparing the adrenal suppression of budesonide and BDP in healthy adults and in patients with asthma have generally shown budesonide to cause significantly less adrenal suppression (200,216,219,269), although Ebden et al. (271) did not see any difference between 1.5 mg BDP and 1.6 mg budesonide. Johansson et al. (269) performed placebo-controlled dose-response studies by using single doses of 0.2, 0.8, and 3.2 mg inhaled and oral budesonide and BDP. By using administrations at 10 P.M. and measuring cortisol the next day at 8 A.M., 10 A.M., and noon, and calculating the areas under the curves for cortisol, they could detect significant differences between the two drugs by using single doses, with budesonide causing significantly less influence on the adrenals. Similarly, Löfdahl et al. (216) used three dose levels of budesonide and BDP for 3 days in patients known to be sensitive to high doses of BDP. They noted that they could administer budesonide in a 70% higher dose without causing more systemic activity. Selroos and Halme (200) found in a crossover study that patients using BDP 0.5 mg twice daily with a spacing device and mouth rinsing could be changed to budesonide 0.8 mg twice daily delivered via Turbuhaler, and mouth rinsing and spitting out the rinse water, without causing more suppression of serum and urinary cortisol levels. Jennings et al. (219) compared in a randomized, open, crossover study two dose levels, 0.8 and 2.5 mg, of budesonide and BDP for 4 weeks each. The subjects were randomized to one dose level and one treatment sequence, i.e., either budesonide or BDP first. The treatment sequences were balanced for sex and for pre- and postmenopausal women. Nineteen subjects received the 0.8 mg doses and 20 subjects the high-dose regimen. They found that BDP on both dose levels caused significantly more suppression of plasma and urine cortisol as well as of dehydroepiandrosterone.

All studies seem to indicate that in adults, low and moderate doses of inhaled corticosteroids, up to 1.0 mg daily, do not cause systemic activity. The clinical relevance of the statistically significant changes in HPA function in patients using higher doses is not fully clear. On one side the suppression caused by an inhaled dose giving full control of the patients' asthma has to be compared with the dose of oral corticosteroids resulting in the same degree of asthma control. Toogood et al. (208) compared budesonide and oral prednisone and found 1.0 mg budesonide being equipotent with 58 mg prednisone from an efficacy point of view, but equipotent with 9 mg prednisone from a systemic side effect point of view. The relative potencies of inhaled and oral corticosteroids administered separately and for relatively short periods of time as in the above-mentioned study do not necessarily give a complete picture of their long-term performance (272). On the other side, laboratory signs of adrenal suppression during treatment with inhaled corticosteroids may not be a clinical problem in terms of adrenal insufficiency, but may be a sign of an increased risk for other systemic effects such as osteoporosis.

When inhaled corticosteroids have been given to patients on oral steroids (and with suppressed levels of morning cortisol) to allow a reduction of the oral dose, the HPA function has greatly improved (273–277) showing the achieved increase in safety with the inhaled corticosteroids. Therefore, in patients requiring oral steroids, even a slight reduction of the oral dose, with addition of inhaled doses to achieve control, will result in an improved safety. However, it should be kept in mind that full recovery of adrenal function after change from oral to inhaled corticosteroids may be slow, taking up to 3 years or more (278). But there was no evidence of adrenal insufficiency in response to major surgery in 28 steroid-dependent asthmatics using inhaled corticosteroids who previously had abnormal responses to ACTH when using oral corticosteroids (279).

Discontinuation of treatment with inhaled steroids does not result in adrenal insufficiency providing normal clinical doses have been used. Acute adrenal insufficiency has been reported, however, after stopping treatment with 6.4 mg budesonide in an adult patient (280), and 0.2 mg twice daily plus 50 μg nasal spray twice daily in a 7-year-old child (281).

Effects on Growth in Children

There are several factors in addition to hereditary ones influencing the growth rate of children with asthma. Long-term systemic corticosteroid treatment may result in growth retardation (282,283). Poor asthma control as such is a major factor, which undoubtedly causes growth retardation and may also delay puberty (284). The growth pattern may also be different compared with nonasthmatic children with a delayed growth during prepuberty and early puberty, but with normal heights by adulthood (285). It is also well documented that treatment with oral corticosteroids will cause growth retardation, and alternate day dosage regimens may not help to reduce this (286).

Seven long-term studies in children with asthma have failed to show growth retardation when treatment with inhaled corticosteroids in doses up to 0.8 mg daily of BDP or budesonide have been given (287). Growth velocity suppression, however, was noted with BDP (336 μg daily) in a study of 195 children ages 6 to 16 years (288). A recent study in 58 prepubertal children followed for 4.9 years (range 2.6–9.4 years) did not show any evidence for effects of inhaled corticosteroids on growth (289). Knemometry has also been used to measure short-term growth of the lower leg. In this model it has been found that even 2.5 mg prednisolone daily stops short-term growth completely (290). Inhaled budesonide 0.2 and 0.4 mg daily did not influence the short-term growth measured by knemometry, whereas a daily dose of 0.8 mg caused a statistically significant reduction (291). However, this influence was significantly less than that caused by 2.5 mg prednisolone, which will not influence the long-term growth of children. The results of knemometry should therefore be looked upon in relation to the effects of oral steroids. It is obvious that results of short-term knemometry studies cannot be translated into changes in long-term statual growth (292,293). However, it can probably be stated that doses free of any effects in knemometry studies—such as budesonide doses up to 0.4 mg a day—are totally free of effects on the growth of children.

Bone and Mineral Turnover in Adults

Asthma alone can be associated with a decreased bone density (294), probably due to reduction of physical exercise in patients with asthma. Long-term use of oral corticosteroids is associated with decreased bone density (294) and will undoubtedly cause osteoporosis and an increased risk of fractures. Figures as high as 40% have been cited (295,296). Patients on long-term treatment with oral corticosteroids also have significantly reduced levels of serum osteocalcin, suggesting inhibition of bone formation (297). The reduction of serum osteocalcin can be demonstrated with prednisolone 5 mg twice daily given to healthy subjects for 1 week (298).

There are few studies with inhaled corticosteroids assessing their effects on bone and mineral turnover. It was suggested by Reid et al. (294) that inhaled corticosteroids may also affect the bone. They noted a 8% reduction in bone mass of asthmatic patients taking moderate doses of BDP or budesonide. Inhaled budesonide, 0.6 mg daily for 1 week followed by 2.4 mg daily for another week, in normal subjects did not alter the 24-h excretion of urinary calcium or phosphate. Nor were there noted any changes in serum calcium, 25-hydroxy vitamin D, 1-25-dihydroxy vitamin D, or parathyroid hormone levels, indicating that the intestinal absorption of calcium was unaffected (299). These results were obtained when reductions in 24-h urinary cortisol and in blood eosinophils were noted, suggestive of systemic effects. Likewise, Puolijoki et al. (300) did not see any significant changes in urinary calcium/creatinine and hydroxyproline/creatinine ratios, serum parathyroid hormone, calcitonin, D-25-OH- or D-1.25-OH-vitamin, bone-originated alkaline phosphatase, serum carboxyterminal propeptide of human type I procollagen (PICP), or dehydroepiandrosterone values when nine postmenopausal women with newly detected asthma, and not treated with corticosteroids before, received 0.2 mg BDP daily via a spacing device for 3 weeks, followed by 1.0 mg daily for 3 weeks, and then 2.0 mg daily for 3 weeks. However, inhaled BDP in a dose of 2.0 mg daily for 4 weeks to healthy subjects, but not budesonide in the same dose, caused an increase in the urinary hydroxyproline/creatinine ratios and a decrease in serum bone-derived alkaline phosphatase, which is a biochemical marker for bone resorption (220).

The effect of inhaled corticosteroids on osteocalcin, a bone formation marker, has been evaluated in healthy subjects as well as in patients with asthma (Table 8). Pouw et al. (301) measured serum osteocalcin at 9 A.M., 11 A.M., 1 P.M., and 3 P.M. before, during, and after treatment with 2.0 mg BDP for 2 weeks. They studied eight healthy subjects and reported on significantly reduced levels of osteocalcin during treatment. Peretz and Bourdoux (302), however, did not see changes in serum osteocalcin with exactly the same regimen in 10 healthy subjects. The same was true of König et al. (303), who measured serum osteocalcin in 18 children with asthma who used a dose of 20 μg/kg/day (mean daily dose 0.627 mg) for 25 months. Teelucksingh et al. (304) studied 16 healthy subjects in a double-blind, placebo-controlled crossover study administering 0.1, 0.2, 0.35, and 0.5 mg of BDP four times daily for 10 days. Washout periods of 18 days separated the treatment periods. During treatment with BDP there was a significant fall in plasma osteocalcin concentrations relative to placebo even after the lowest dose of 0.4 mg daily on treatment day 5. This effect was dose-dependent up to 1.4 mg daily with a plateau thereafter. With longer treatment the plateau occurred at an even lower dose so that at day 9 of treatment plasma osteocalcin was lowered to the same extent by 0.8, 1.4, and 2.0 mg dosages. Puolijoki et al. (300) also noted a dose-dependent decrease in osteocalcin when nine postmenopausal women with asthma received 0.2 mg, 1.0 mg, and 2.0 mg BDP for 3 weeks each. Meeran et al. (297) also noted a significant reduction in plasma osteocalcin levels when 20 healthy subjects were given 0.5 mg BDP twice daily for 1 week.

Jennings et al. (219) studied the effects of two dose levels of budesonide and BDP, 0.8 mg and 2.5 mg, in 19 and 20 healthy subjects, respectively, in an open, randomized, crossover study. The subjects received either dose for 4 weeks and then changed to the same dose level of the other corticosteroid. There was a 2-week washout period in between. They found a significant dose-related suppression of serum osteocalcin, with BDP causing significantly more suppression than budesonide. Bone-derived alkaline phosphatase, another marker of bone formation, was affected only by the higher dose of BDP. Increased urinary excretion of hydroxyproline, suggesting bone resorption, occurred with BDP but not with budesonide. Serum calcium, as well as the urinary calcium and phosphate/creatinine ratios were normal for both drugs. Serum phosphate levels were increased on both dose levels of BDP and on the high dose level of budesonide. Wolthers et al. (305) studied biochemical markers of bone turnover in 11 children with asthma treated with 2.5 mg and 5 mg prednisolone daily and in 14 other children treated with 0.2 and 0.8 mg budesonide. The two studies were randomized double-blind, crossover trials with five periods of 2 weeks each. The first period was a run-in period and periods 3 and 5 were washout periods. Active treatments were given in periods 2 and 4. A significant decreasing trend of serum osteocalcin and decreased excretion of urinary hydroxyproline were found on prednisolone treatment. Budesonide did not influence the markers of bone turnover.

TABLE 8. *Effects of inhaled corticosteroids on bone mineral metabolism and turnover*

First author (ref. no.)	Year	No. of subjects	Drug	Dose (mg)	Duration of treatment	S-Ca	U-Ca	U-HOP	S-PTH	S-calcitonin	S-osteocalcin	S-alk. phos.
Jennings (219)	1990	6	BUD	0.8	3 weeks	0	0		0	0	0	0
		19	BUD/BDP	1.6–3.2	4 weeks	0	0		0	0	+	0
		20		1.2 2.4/2.5			0				+	BDP +
Pouw (301)	1991	8	BDP	2.0	2 weeks	0	0				+	
Peretz (302)	1991	10	BDP	2.0	2 weeks						0	
König (303)	1991	18[a]	BDP	0.6	25 months						0	
Teelucksingh (304)	1991	16	BDP	0.4–0.8 −1.4–2.0	10 days[c]			0			+	
Puolijoki (300)	1991	9[b]	BDP	0.2–1.0 −2.0	3 weeks[d]		0	0	0	0	+	0
Meeran (297)	1991	20	BDP	1.0	1 week						+	
Wolthers (305)	1992	14[a]	BUD	0.2–0.8	2 weeks						0	
Leech (305a)	1993	21[e]	BUD	0.8 1.6	1 week[f]							
			BDP	1.0 2.0								

BUD; budesonide; BDP, beclomethasone dipropionate.
[a] Children.
[b] Postmenopausal women.
[c] Ten days on each dose level, crossover design.
[d] Three weeks on each does in increasing order.
[e] Premenopausal women.
[f] One week on each dose and on placebo.

A few studies have evaluated the effects of inhaled corticosteroids on bone density. Wolff et al. (306) investigated the long-term effects of inhaled and oral corticosteroids on bone density by using single and dual photon absorptiometry. They studied five asthma patients who inhaled daily an average of 0.326 mg BDP equivalents for 50 months, and a group of five asthma patients who used 12.5 mg prednisolone equivalents daily for an average of 57 months. Unlike patients taking oral steroids, bone density was not reduced in the patients using inhaled corticosteroids. Similarly, Hatton et al. (307) did not find any significant changes in bone mineral density (total body, spine, forearm, and femoral neck) during a 2-year trial period in 11 asthmatic women (three premenopausal, seven postmenopausal, and one had undergone hysterectomy, median age 55, range 36–77) who used >1.0 mg daily of budesonide or BDP (mean dose 1.25 mg daily). Initially the scans of these patients showed significant reductions in lumbar spine bone mineral density when the patients had had oral corticosteroids as well (308). Luengo et al. (309) also treated 21 patients with asthma for 2 years with a mean dose of BDP 0.63 mg daily and were unable to detect any changes in bone density. In children with asthma treated with inhaled BDP for 25 months (mean dose 0.627 mg daily), König et al. (303) did not find differences in bone mineral density and bone mineral content compared with 18 children with asthma not taking corticosteroids. Packe et al. (310) noted a 20% decreased bone density in a group of 20 asthma patients who had taken 1.0 to 2.0 mg BDP daily for at least 1 year and short courses of oral steroids, as well as in 20 patients on a combination of inhaled and oral corticosteroids in comparison with 17 patients who did not use corticosteroids.

Posterior Subcapsular Ocular Cataracts

Cataracts have been diagnosed in a few patients treated with inhaled corticosteroids alone. However, the causal relationship to the treatment with inhaled steroids, and to a particular dose level, is uncertain (3,311–314). Signs of cataracts were neither found in large series of adult patients (315) nor in children with asthma (315a).

Metabolic Effects

Metabolic effects have been studied in healthy adults (219,316,317), elderly patients with diabetes (317), as well as in children with asthma (318–320). Kruszynska et al. (316) studied nine subjects, ages 21 to 44 years, who received BDP 0.5 mg twice daily for 4 weeks, and found marginally increased serum levels of fasting cholesterol, high-density lipoproteins, insulin, lactate, and pyruvate. The blood glycerol levels were slightly decreased. The clinical relevance of the small changes is uncertain. Jennings et al. (219)

measured blood glucose, serum insulin, glucagon, triglycerides, and choles-terol, and carried out a glucose tolerance test in healthy subjects (n = 39) receiving either 0.8 mg (n = 19) or 2.5 mg (n = 20) of BDP and budesonide for 4 weeks in an open, randomized, crossover study. Neither BDP nor bu-desonide affected the carbohydrate metabolism. Small increases in serum triglycerides and cholesterol were noted but the clinical importance of the findings remain unknown. Ebden et al. (317) gave 2.0 mg BDP to young adults and could not detect any changes in cholesterol and insulin levels. The glucose tolerance also remained unchanged in these subjects, as well as in elderly patients with diabetes.

Yernault et al. (318) and Goldstein and König (319) found that doses of 0.4 to 0.5 mg BDP had no effects on blood glucose in children with asthma. Turpeinen et al. (320) treated nine children with asthma, ages 5 to 10 years, with budesonide 0.8 mg/m^2 daily for 1 month, followed by 0.4 mg/m^2 for 4 months. Concomitantly with a clinical improvement they noted a significant increase in high-density lipoprotein cholesterol by 22% during the high-dose treatment. A significant reduction to normal levels was seen when the dose was reduced. No changes were seen in serum total cholesterol, triglycerides, high-density lipoprotein/total cholesterol ratio, body mass index, or glucose tolerance. The high dose increased the ratio of serum insulin to blood glu-cose, calculated from the areas under the incremental 2-h curves in the glu-cose tolerance test. During the lower dose a reduction to the initial ratio level was observed.

Increased Susceptibility for Infections

Increased susceptibility for infections is a common finding in patients treated with oral corticosteroids. These complications have not been re-ported in patients using inhaled corticosteroids. This was first noted in the Brompton Hospital/Medical Research Council study with two dose levels of BDP (321). No increased incidence of respiratory pathogens could be found.

Patients with active pulmonary tuberculosis can be treated with inhaled corticosteroids as soon as there is an effective antituberculosis treatment ongoing. Patients with inactive pulmonary tuberculosis do not need prophy-lactic therapy with isoniazid if treatment with inhaled corticosteroids is started.

Patients with asthma getting an upper respiratory tract infection should not discontinue their treatment with inhaled corticosteroids. On the con-trary, the dose should be increased in order to avoid exacerbations of asthma. In a study in children with asthma Svedmyr et al. (322) showed that increasing the dose of inhaled budesonide when the children started to get a common cold reduced the number of visits to the emergency room and the number of oral steroid courses compared with placebo.

Chicken pox and measles can have a more serious course in patients using corticosteroids in immunosuppressant doses.

Skin Bruising

Skin bruising is a known side effect of long-term oral corticosteroid therapy. There are reports of patients who have developed skin bruising when using high doses of inhaled BDP (323,324). Mak et al. (325) asked 202 patients on inhaled steroids and 204 control patients about skin bruising by using two different types of questionnaires. Forty-seven percent of the patients in the inhaled steroid group, compared with 22% in the control group admitted to easy bruising. The incidence of easy bruising seemed to increase with age, dosage, and duration of treatment.

Behavioral Disturbances

Anxiety/depression and hyperactivity have been reported in patients with asthma. Case reports have been published linking these disturbances to treatment with anti-asthma drugs including corticosteroids. Bender et al. (326) found in a study of 27 severely asthmatic 8- to 16-year-old children and adolescents that a high daily dose of corticosteroids (mean dose 61.5 mg prednisone), but not a low dose (mean dose 3.33 mg daily), resulted in reporting of increased depressive and anxious symptoms. They also performed less proficiently on a test of long-term memory. However, the symptoms remained below clinical levels for depression and anxiety. There were no evidence of steroid-induced psychiatric disturbance. In other studies an association has been reported between treatment with high doses of oral corticosteroids and emotional difficulties and psychological changes (327).

Conclusion

Oral corticosteroids do cause significant systemic side effects, which can be somewhat reduced with alternate day dosing regimens. The nature of side effects with inhaled corticosteroids is predominantly local. Dysphonia and oropharyngeal candidiasis are usually easy to treat, more inconvenient than serious, but sometimes severe enough to warrant temporarily stopping the treatment. Rinsing of the mouth and spitting out the rinse water are important instructions to the patients in order to avoid oropharyngeal candidiasis as well as systemic absorption of the drug. Systemic side effects with inhaled corticosteroids are dose-dependent. Clinically significant side effects are not usually seen with doses up to 0.4 mg in children and with doses below 1.0 mg of budesonide or BDP in adults. With higher doses the frequency of detectable systemic effects increases but their clinical relevance are mostly doubtful. Comparative studies have shown budesonide to be a safer alternative than BDP.

GLUCOCORTICOSTEROIDS IN RESPIRATORY DISEASES

Bronchial Asthma

Acute Severe Asthma

The usefulness of corticosteroids in patients with acute, severe broncho-constriction is still debated (328,329) although most clinicians use them on a more or less routine basis. Recently published guidelines on the management of acute severe asthma also emphasize the importance of systemic corticosteroids (330).

Engel and Heinig (331) recently reviewed the available clinical documentation in this field. They noted that many published papers suffer from methodological problems, that no difference has been seen between oral and intravenous administrations, that dose-response relationships have been difficult to demonstrate, and that a protective effect against relapses has been found only for periods not exceeding 4 weeks. So far, no study has been able to depict the categories of patients who may or may not benefit from the addition of corticosteroids to the symptomatic treatment of acute severe asthma.

Placebo-Controlled Studies in Adults

In 1956 the Medical Research Council published their double-blind, randomized study in 32 patients receiving oral cortisone acetate 350 mg over the first 24 h (332). The final evaluation was done after 2 weeks. Results were evaluated as clinical scores. Compared with placebo, patients treated with cortisone benefited from the treatment. Later studies have shown either some benefits from treatment with corticosteroids or no differences compared with placebo (Table 9). Fanta et al. (333) administered hydrocortisone 2 mg/kg i.v. bolus followed by 0.5 mg/kg/h for 24 h ($n = 11$) or saline ($n = 9$), in a double-blind, randomized study. Both groups had obstruction of the same magnitude before treatment. At the end of 24 h, the subjects given hydrocortisone had significantly greater resolution of airway obstruction; forced expiratory volume in 1 sec (FEV_1) increased $118 \pm 25\%$ (mean $\pm$ SEM) in the steroid-treated group, but only $35 \pm 22\%$ in the saline group. No effect on blood gases was found. Littenberg and Gluck (334) and Schneider et al. (335) administered methylprednisolone i.v. or saline to a large number of patients in their double-blind, randomized studies. They reported on beneficial effects with respect to hospital admissions. In the study by Littenberg and Gluck only nine patients of 48 (19%) treated with methylprednisolone required hospital admission, as compared with 23 of 49 patients (47%) in the control group. In contrast, McFadden et al. (336) and Luksza (337), using hydrocortisone i.v., and Stein and Cole (338) and Morell et al.

TABLE 9. *Placebo-controlled studies in adults on the effects of corticosteroids in acute severe asthma*

First author (ref. no.)	Year	No. of patients	Type of study	Evaluation time point	Corticosteroid	Dose[a]	Effect variable	Effect
MRC (332)	1956	32	db,r,p	14 days	Oral cortisone	350 mg	Clinical score	+
McFadden (336)	1976	38	db,r,p	6 h	I.v. hydrocortisone	0.25 g 0.5 g 1.0 g	FEV_1 sGaw	0 0
Luksza (337)	1982	90	o,p	48 h	I.v. hydrocortisone	0.4 g 1.2 g	PEF	0
Fanta (333)	1983	20	db,r,p	24 h	I.v. hydrocortisone	14 mg/kg	FEV_1 FVC PaO_2	+ + 0
Littenberg (334)	1986	97	db,r,p	4 h	I.v. methylprednisolone	125 mg	FEV_1 FVC Hospital admissions	0 0 +
Schneider (335)	1988	54	db,r,p	6 h	I.v. methylprednisolone	30 mg/kg	Hospital admissions	+
Stein (338)	1990	81	db,r,p	12 h	I.v. methylprednisolone	125 mg	Duration of emergency room treatment Hospital admissions	0 0
Morell (339)	1992	90	db,r,p	48 h	I.v. methylprednisolone	70 mg/kg or 14 mg/kg	FEV_1, FVC, PEF	0

Type of study: db, double-blind; r, randomized; p, placebo; Effect: +, significant effect as compared with placebo; 0, no effect. FEV_1, forced expiratory volume in 1 sec; FVC, forced vital capacity; PEF, peak expiratory flow; sGaw, specific airway conductance; PaO_2, arterial oxygen pressure.
[a]Cumulative dose during first 24 h.

(339), administering methylprednisolone i.v. in double-blind, randomized studies, did not observe any effects compared with saline on lung function tests or on duration of emergency room treatment and hospital admission rate at 12 h.

Placebo-Controlled Studies in Children

Eleven placebo-controlled studies on the effect of corticosteroids in acute asthma in children have been reviewed. They are listed in Table 10. Seven of these 11 studies showed a significant influence on one or more of the pulmonary function tests used.

Six-hourly treatment with oral prednisolone resulted in significant improvement in peak expiratory flow (PEF), which was measured 12 to 48 h after the start of medication (340). After a single oral dose of 30 mg or 60 mg prednisolone, or placebo, in 140 children, PEF was significantly higher in the prednisolone group 6 to 8 h after medication (341). However, the difference disappeared 8 h after medication. A once daily tapering schedule of oral methylprednisolone (starting dose 32 mg) resulted in identical improvements in both the active and the placebo groups 1, 7, and 14 days after start of treatment (342). $FEF_{25-75\%}$ was, however, significantly higher in the steroid group on day 7, as compared with placebo. A faster increase in $FEF_{25-75\%}$, as compared with placebo, was also demonstrated by Younger et al. (343), who treated 45 children who had not responded to standard treatment with beta-agonists, with methylprednisolone i.v. 5 mg/kg or placebo. No differences between the steroid and placebo were seen in FEV_1, forced vital capacity (FVC), or PEF, or in Pao_2. Deshpande et al. (344) gave their patients oral prednisolone, 2 mg/kg on day 1, 1 mg/kg on day 2, and 0.5 mg/kg on day 3 or corresponding placebo. Active treatment resulted in significant improvement in PEF and asthma symptoms. Harris et al. (345) studied the effect of high-dose oral prednisone for 1 week early in the course of an acute exacerbation incompletely responsive to bronchodilators. Twenty-two patients received prednisone and 19 placebo. All prednisone-treated patients improved during the week of treatment (one had a subsequent exacerbation 5 days after discontinuing the study medication). Eight of the placebo-treated patients required rescue intervention with various drugs. Gleeson et al. (346) treated children with nebulized salbutamol and aminophylline i.v. plus either hydrocortisone and oral prednisolone for 5 days, or placebo. The children were observed throughout their hospital stay and for 3 months afterward. On day 2 PEF improved more and the heart rate fell more in the steroid group than in the placebo group. Duration of hospital stay and relapse rate during the succeeding 3 months also favored active treatment.

Four studies failed to show improvement in pulmonary function tests, as compared with placebo. Kattan et al. (347) treated 19 children in an open, randomized study. The children received hydrocortisone i.v. 28 mg/kg or

TABLE 10. *Placebo-controlled studies in children on the effects of corticosteroids in acute asthma*

First author (ref. no.)	Year	No. of patients	Type of study	Evaluation point	Corticosteroid and adm. route	Dose[a]	Effect variable	Effect
Pierson (348)	1974	45	db,r,p	24 h	I.v. hydrocortisone I.v. dexamethasone I.v. betamethasone	14 mg/kg 0.6 mg/kg 0.6 mg/kg	FEV_1 PaO_2	0 +
Kattan (347)	1980	19	r,p	36 h	I.v. hydrocortisone	28 mg/kg	PEF	0
Loren (340)	1980	16	db,r,p	48 h	Oral prednisolone	2 mg/kg	PEF FEV_1 FVC	+ 0 0
Shapiro (342)	1983	28	db,r,p	2 weeks	Oral methylprednisolone	32 mg	FEF_{25-75}	+ (day 7)
Tal (349)	1983	32	db,r,p	4 days	I.v. dexamethasone	0.6 mg/kg	Clinical score	0
Deshpande (344)	1986	50	db,r,p	3 days	Oral prednisolone	2 mg/kg	PEF	+
Harris (345)	1987	40	r,p	2 weeks	Oral prednisolone	40 mg or 80 mg	Rescue intervention PEF	+ +
Storr (341)	1987	140	db,r,p	48 h	Oral prednisolone	30 mg or 60 mg	Clinical score PEF	+ +
Younger (343)	1987	45	db,r,p	3 days	I.v. methylprednisolone	5 mg/kg	FEF_{25-75} PEF,FEV_1,PaO_2 TGV, SGaw V_{maxFRC} Clinical score	+ 0 0 0 0
Springer (350)	1990	50	db,p alternate patient treated	5 days	I.v. hydrocortisone Oral prednisolone	1 mg/kg/h until a defined score, thereafter 2 mg/kg/day		
Gleeson (346)	1990	38	db,r,p	3 months	I.v. hydrocortisone and oral prednisolone	18 mg/kg 1 mg/kg, max 25 mg	PEF SaO_2 Pulse rate Resp. rate Relapse rate	+ (day 2) 0 + 0 (+)

FEF_{25-75}, forced expiratory flow between 25 and 75% of FVC; TGV, total gas volume; SaO_2, arterial oxygen saturation. See table 9 for other abbreviations.

[a] Cumulative dose during first 24 h.

saline every 6 h. Identical improvements in PEF and clinical symptom scores were seen during a 36-h observation period. Pierson et al. (348) treated 45 children with an i.v. bolus followed by a continuous infusion for 24 h of either hydrocortisone, dexamethasone, betamethasone, or placebo saline. No significant differences in improvements in FEV_1 were seen among the four treatments. However, a significant improvement in PaO_2 was found in the steroid-treated children compared with the placebo-treated group. Tal et al. (349) treated 32 wheezy infants, ages 1 to 12 months. The treatments were dexamethasone i.m. or placebo (double-blind), and salbutamol (oral and inhaled), or none (open), in all four possible combinations by using a randomized eight-patient block design with four children in each. No differences were seen between dexamethasone alone, salbutamol alone, or placebo. The combination of dexamethasone plus placebo, however, resulted in more than twice the rate of improvement and was observed within 24 h. Springer et al. (350) treated 50 wheezy infants, ages 1.5 to 11 months, with inhaled salbutamol and either systemic hydrocortisone at a rate of 1 mg/kg/h or placebo, followed by oral prednisolone 2 mg/kg/day or placebo. Treatment with corticosteroids did not change the rate of clinical improvement, nor did it effect lung function 2 to 4 weeks later.

Comparative and Dose-Response Studies

Haskell et al. (351) treated 25 adult patients with acute asthma with methylprednisolone i.v. every 6 h for 3 days at three different dose levels: 15 mg, 40 mg, or 125 mg. FEV_1 was used as an end point. The high-dose group improved significantly by the end of the first day, the medium-dose group improved by the middle of the second day, and the low-dose group did not improve significantly within 3 days. A crossover study in ten patients treated during three consecutive deterioration episodes with three different doses of oral prednisolone, 0.2, 0.4, and 0.6 mg/kg, respectively, also showed a dose-response relationship (352).

There are several other studies evaluating different doses of i.v. as well as of oral corticosteroids but not showing any dose response relationship (336,337,353–360). In some of the studies this may be due to too short an observation period (336,337) or to a small number of patients (353–355,359).

Sue et al. (361) compared hydrocortisone i.v. (100 mg every 6 h), methylprednisolone i.v. (20 mg every 6 h), and dexamethasone i.v. (3.75 mg every 6 h) in a small group of patients with acute severe asthma ($n = 14$). One patient received two treatments. Overall the patients improved on all three i.v. corticosteroid treatments with a degree of improvement becoming significant by 9 h in all three groups.

Brunette et al. (362) investigated the potential for short courses of steroids to prevent or reduce the severity of asthma induced by viral respiratory infections in 32 preschool children. One group received theophylline and orciprenaline during attacks or on a continuous basis. The other group received the same treatment during the first year. During the second year this group got short courses of prednisone 1 mg/kg as soon as the first symptoms of an upper respiratory tract infection appeared and prior to any signs of wheezing. A significant reduction was noted in the number of wheezing days (65%), attacks (65%), visits to emergency room (61%), and hospitalization (90%).

Relapse Rate

Relapse after the treatment of acute asthma in the emergency room is a frequent phenomenon. A short-term benefit from treatment with corticosteroids has been demonstrable. Fiel et al. (363) treated 76 episodes of acute asthma needing emergency therapy with bronchodilators, but not requiring hospitalization. Upon discharge, the patients were treated with a regimen of theophylline, and randomly with placebo or methylprednisolone i.v. 4 mg/kg as a bolus, followed by an 8-day tapering course of oral methylprednisolone. The patients treated with the steroid regimen (34 patient episodes) had fewer respiratory symptoms and a decrease in the need for repeated emergency care. Chapman et al. (364) treated 122 patients in the emergency room. At discharge they were randomly assigned to receive placebo or an 8-day course of prednisone, tapered from 40 mg to 0 mg. The prednisone-treated patients had a significantly reduced risk of relapses during the first 10 days of follow-up, but not thereafter (days 11 through 21 of follow-up).

In the Medical Research Council study (332) patients were followed for 12 weeks but no protection against new exacerbations were seen. Engel et al. (359) could not demonstrate any superiority of high-dose methylprednisolone i.v. pulse therapy compared with an 18-day tapering course of oral prednisolone for the protection against relapses during the 12 weeks following the treatment.

Two placebo-controlled studies in children with acute asthma have shown protection against relapses within a 2-week follow-up period, even though the treatment was stopped after a few days (340,342). The study by Younger et al. (343) showed a protective effect of methylprednisolone i.v. administered during the acute attack against exacerbations during the following 4 weeks.

Maintenance Treatment for Chronic Asthma

The glucocorticosteroids are the single most effective agents for treatment of asthma. When first introduced as cortisone they were looked upon as miracle drugs, but serious systemic side effects limited their long-term use. In an attempt to reduce these side effects, two approaches have been tried:

changing the structure of the steroid skeleton, and the introduction of inhaled corticosteroids. Today oral corticosteroids should be used for maintenance treatment of asthma in only two situations: the few patients who cannot use inhaled drugs properly, and patients who have an adrenal insufficiency because of earlier treatment with systemic corticosteroids. The last-mentioned patients should have the lowest possible substitution dose of oral steroids together with the clinically appropriate dose of an inhaled corticosteroid. If oral corticosteroids have to be used for maintenance treatment of asthma, an alternate-day regimen may be tried. Harter et al. (235) reported their experiences with 58 patients who had various steroid-responsive diseases using a variety of corticosteroid regimens including 10 mg prednisone four times daily and 80 mg every other morning. They concluded that the administration of the total 48-h amount of corticosteroid from a single dose given every other day rather than four times daily reduced the incidence and degree of steroid-induced systemic side effects. Shorter periods between doses, e.g., 12, 24, and 36 h, were accompanied by adrenal suppression similar to that observed in the four times daily regimen, while an interval of 72 h or longer did not appear to be therapeutically effective. Falliers et al. (365) determined an estimate of minimal effective dose of alternate-day prednisone among 6- to 16-year-old children with steroid-dependent asthma. Dosage ranged from 8 to 32 mg of methylprednisolone with a median of 24 mg. It was reported that these children tolerated naturally occurring stress situations such as febrile illness without untoward effects.

Although it has long been recognized that fatal asthma is associated with marked inflammatory changes in the airways (366,367), it is now apparent that inflammation is present even in patients with newly diagnosed mild asthma (368). Biopsies of bronchial tissue from patients with asthma have revealed infiltration by inflammatory cells, particularly eosinophils and lymphocytes, together with epithelial shedding. Bronchoalveolar lavage has also demonstrated an increased proportion of inflammatory cells, especially eosinophils (369), and the number of cells are increased after allergen challenge (370,371). There is a strong association between inflammatory changes in the airway epithelium and the degree of bronchial hyperresponsiveness (372,373). It is also evident that inflammatory changes and hyperresponsiveness precede the development of asthma and the occurrence of smooth muscle contraction (374). Consequently, guidelines for treatment of chronic asthma in adult patients have been developed (375–378); they all stress the importance of early treatment with anti-inflammatory drugs. The inhaled corticosteroids represent today the first-line treatment of patients with asthma (3).

There have been discussions about whether inhaled corticosteroids exhibit their action topically or only systemically as a consequence of absorption from the lungs with secondary redistribution to the airways. Toogood et al. (207), by comparing the relapse rate of patients with steroid-dependent asthma (control maximized by the use of BDP), randomized patients to treatment with inhaled or oral budesonide or placebo. Patients on placebo and oral budesonide had a similar and rapid relapse rate, whereas those on inhaled budesonide remained symptom-free significantly longer and on their earlier PEF levels. These results indicate a local effect of locally applied drug.

Inhaled Corticosteroids as First-Line Therapy of Asthma

Lorentzon et al. (379) studied the effect of two low doses of budesonide, 0.1 mg and 0.2 mg twice daily, in a double-blind, parallel-group study in 103 patients with mild asthma (mean morning PEF before medication approximately 80% of predicted normal, an individual daily mean variation in PEF of 10–30%). The patients had not been treated with anti-inflammatory medication before. Morning PEF values increased by 36 L/min and 47 L/min over placebo with the two doses of budesonide, respectively. Nighttime symptoms and use of bronchodilator aerosol decreased significantly. The authors recommended early introduction of inhaled corticosteroids in patients with mild to moderate asthma.

Juniper et al. (380) studied 32 adult stable nonsteroid-dependent asthmatics who showed hyperresponsiveness to metacholine (PC_{20} <8.0 mg/ml) and whose asthma was well controlled on 0.8 mg or less inhaled salbutamol daily. Control was defined as no limitation of normal daily life, no sputum, not awakened at night by symptoms, and FEV_1 greater than 70% predicted normal before bronchodilator or greater than 80% predicted after bronchodilator. Although it was not stated for how long the patients had suffered from asthma symptoms it is obvious that the patients had a mild disease. Patients were randomized to treatment for 1 year with budesonide 0.4 mg daily or placebo. Patients receiving budesonide showed a fourfold mean improvement in airway responsiveness compared with those receiving placebo, whose responsiveness remained stable. Fifteen of the 16 patients in the budesonide group improved and five returned to the normal range. Largest improvements occurred during the first 3 months of treatment, but some patients showed a gradual improvement throughout the study period. Improvements in responsiveness were accompanied by significant improvements in asthma symptoms, bronchodilator use, and number of asthma exacerbations. Fourteen of these nonsteroid-dependent patients were thereafter randomized to treatment for 3 months with budesonide 0.4 mg daily or placebo (381). The effects seen during the first year of treatment could be maintained in both groups for at least 3 months.

Haahtela et al. (4) investigated in a double-blind, parallel-group study whether treatment of patients with newly detected, mild asthma should be started with an inhaled corticosteroid or with a bronchodilator. They randomized 103 patients to treatment for 2 years with either inhaled terbutaline twice daily, or budesonide, 0.6 mg twice daily. Patients treated with budesonide showed significant improvements in airway function, responsiveness to histamine, use of rescue bronchodilators and in asthma symptom scores. No improvements were seen with the β_2-agonist alone. The authors conclude that treatment of patients with newly diagnosed mild asthma should be started with an anti-inflammatory drug. After completion of the second year of this double-blind study, the patients treated with the inhaled steroid were randomly assigned to further double-blind treatment for a third year with either placebo or a low dose of budesonide, 0.4 mg daily (7). The low-dose budesonide was enough to keep the patients at the improved level, but this was also true of a substantial number of patients in the placebo group. This finding indicated that sufficiently aggressive early treatment with inhaled steroids may result in long-lasting remissions. During the third year patients treated with the β-agonist alone for 2 years received 1.2 mg inhaled budesonide. A gradual improvement was observed but now, 2 years or more after diagnosis, it took a significantly longer time than initially to reach the maximum response. Also, the maximum effect on airway function was significantly lower than that achieved when treatment with budesonide was initiated immediately after diagnosis.

Effects on Bronchial Inflammation

Histopathological studies from patients with asthma who have died during asthma attacks demonstrate marked inflammation in the airways, with infiltration of inflammatory cells, particularly eosinophils, disruption of airway epithelium, and plugging of the airway lumen by viscous secretion (367). Similar, but less severe, pathological changes have been found in bronchial biopsy specimens from patients with even mild asthma (368), mild to moderate asthma (382,383), and after bronchial provocation procedures (370,371,384). The lymphocytes, eosinophils as well as the macrophages are activated (385,386). Bronchoalveolar lavage of patients with asthma has also demonstrated an increase in inflammatory cells, particularly in eosinophils (161,369,387,388). The evidence of asthma as an inflammatory disease has been extensively reviewed (e.g., 56,372,389).

Laitinen et al. (390) compared by using electron microscopy the inflammatory changes in the bronchial mucosa in a patient with newly detected asthma before treatment, during an exacerbation of asthma (when the patient had been treated for 20 weeks with an inhaled β_2-agonist) and after 16 weeks' treatment with budesonide 0.6 mg twice daily. At the time of the clinical exacerbation the patient had signs of epithelial shedding, a decreased number of ciliated cells, and a marked increase in eosinophils. Treatment with budesonide normalized the cellular findings and the ultrastructure of the bronchial mucosa. These findings were confirmed in 14 patients with newly detected mild asthma participating in a double-blind, randomized, parallel-group study (137). Seven patients were randomized to treatment with budesonide 0.6 mg twice daily. Bronchial biopsy specimens were obtained before and after 3 months of therapy, and examined by the use of electron microscopy. Treatment was accompanied by increased numbers of ciliated airway cells and intraepithelial nerves and fewer inflammatory cells, including eosinophils, especially in the epithelium, and lymphocytes. Similar changes of improvement in the epithelium were not seen in seven terbutaline-treated patients. Djukanovic et al. (135) also reported on diminished inflammatory cell findings in ten patients with symptomatic atopic asthma who were biopsied before and after 6 weeks of therapy with BDP 2.0 mg daily for 2 weeks, followed by 1.0 mg daily for 4 weeks. They found a reduction in epithelial and mucosal mast cells and eosinophils and submucosal T lymphocytes, but electron microscopy did not identify any changes in the extent of mast cell and eosinophil degranulation.

Lundgren et al. (159) examined six patients with severe chronic asthma before and after 10 years of treatment with inhaled corticosteroids. Before treatment the patients had an increased number of inflammatory cells compared with the findings in four control subjects. Treatment resulted in a normalization of the number of inflammatory cells as percent of mucosal volume and with a restoration of the ciliated surface epithelium.

Burke et al. (162) studied six patients with stable asthma maintained on inhaled β-agonists alone. Before and after 3 months' treatment with budesonide 0.8 mg daily bronchial biopsies were obtained and examined by the use of a panel of monoclonal antibodies. In parallel with a decrease in bronchial hyperresponsiveness and improvement in airway function they noted marked reductions in the number of T lymphocytes, the number of memory T lymphocytes (CD45RO[+] cells), as well as in the number of antigen-presenting macrophages.

Venge et al. (391) observed that pretreatment with budesonide before allergen challenge both in single dose and after 4 weeks' treatment resulted in significantly reduced levels of eosinophilic cationic protein (ECP) in serum compared with pretreatment values. As ECP is a cytotoxic protein, this is a possible mechanism by which inhaled corticosteroids may prevent epithelial damage and the development of airway hyperresponsiveness. Ädelroth et al. (161) investigated 11 patients with asthma treated only occasionally with inhaled bronchodilators. These patients underwent bronchoalveolar lavage before and after 4 weeks of randomly allocated treatment with either budesonide 0.4 mg daily, or an inhaled β-agonist. The BAL cell findings were not affected by either treatment, probably indicating that the treatment period was too short to result in an effect. However, BAL-ECP levels were significantly decreased by budesonide treatment.

Modulation of Bronchial Hyperresponsiveness

The best practical method of assessing the severity of asthma—in addition to taking a careful medical history and to calculating the variability of daily PEF readings—is to document the position and shape of dose-response curves to histamine or metacholine. It is possible for patients with severe hyperresponsiveness to improve to the point at which their dose-response curves are normal (392). However, shifting of the dose-response curve to the right and achieving a plateau on the curve requires high doses of inhaled corticosteroids for months of treatment (393–395).

Inhaled corticosteroids are the only drugs that have been shown to improve the level of hyperresponsiveness to a clinically important extent in patients with moderate or severe asthma (396). Studies that have used dose-response curves to histamine or metacholine to measure the provoking dose or concentration that causes a 20% fall in FEV_1 ($PD_{20}FEV_1$, $PC_{20}FEV_1$) to assess the response to inhaled corticosteroids have all shown improvements in the severity of hyperresponsiveness (4,368,380,381,394,397–420). Most studies published up to 1989 have been tabulated and discussed by Woolcock and Jenkins (396). The improvements in hyperresponsiveness are dose and time dependent (421,422), but not so in patients with very mild asthma (423). Improvements can be seen after only a few weeks of treatment. In patients with mild, newly detected asthma most improvements occur within the first 3 months (4). There is, however, a further gradual improvement over time (4,380,405,415) and it will take several months until a maximum response is achieved (393).

Dompeling et al. (417) followed patients with asthma for 2 years while treated with bronchodilators alone. Those patients [28 with asthma and 28 with chronic obstructive pulmonary disease (COPD)] who showed an annual decline in FEV_1 of >80 ml/year in combination with at least one exacerbation per year received an inhaled corticosteroid (BDP 0.8 mg daily) for the third year. In the asthmatics the abnormal annual decline in FEV_1 was followed by a significant increase of 562 ml/year during months 1 to 6 of BDP treatment. PC_{20} histamine improved by 3.8 doubling doses and PEF by 16.7%. The diurnal variation in PEF and asthma symptoms also decreased significantly.

Most studies using oral or i.v. corticosteroids have shown little or no effect on hyperresponsiveness (408,424–427), but one study in children receiving up to 2 mg/kg/day prednisone showed that this high dose may influence the hyperresponsiveness (428).

Two studies have compared the effects on hyperresponsiveness of inhaled and oral corticosteroids. Wilmsmeyer et al. (412) compared the use of 1.0 mg BDP with 15 mg prednisone daily for 2 weeks, and showed that the PC_{20} improved with BDP but not with prednisone despite better improvements in airway function with the oral form. Jenkins and Woolcock (408) showed in a crossover study a significant improvement in PD_{20} with 1.2 mg of BDP daily for 3 weeks, but no change in PD_{20} with 12.5 mg prednisone daily for the same period.

Although it is not possible to determine the equipotent doses of oral and inhaled corticosteroids, the available information makes it clear that at conventional therapeutic doses, inhaled forms can ameliorate hyperresponsiveness to a significantly greater extent than can oral forms (396). Comparative studies using inhaled corticosteroids and inhaled chromones [disodium cromoglycate (DSCG), nedocromil] have also shown that the improvements with the latter are small compared with the inhaled steroids (406,407). The effect of the chromones is also present only as long as the drugs are administered immediately before the challenge tests. If challenges are done 12 h or more after stopping treatment with DSCG no protection is seen (409), showing the difference between prophylactic treatment (DSCG, nedocromil) and anti-inflammatory treatment (corticosteroids).

Effects on Early and Late Asthmatic Responses

For long it has been stated that corticosteroids block the late asthmatic reaction (LAR) but do not modify the early asthmatic response (EAR) (429–434). However, some studies have shown that inhaled corticosteroids given for a longer period of time (4 weeks) can ameliorate also the EAR (435). A single dose of budesonide 1.0 mg in the evening and repeated 4h before allergen challenge the next morning did not affect the EAR, although it completely blocked the LAR (139). Treatment for 7 days slightly reduced the EAR, and after 4 weeks' treatment the EAR was almost counteracted. Prednisone does not always reduce the EAR, even after 9 to 16 days of treatment (429). Dose-response studies with inhaled and oral corticosteroids on EAR and LAR have not been done. However, there are some indications that the effects are not only time- but also dose-dependent (435,436). Venge et al. (437) showed that LAR was accompanied by an increase in heat-labile neutrophil chemotactic activity in serum. Inhaled budesonide significantly inhibited the generation of this chemotactic activity, and at the same time it blocked the LAR. This was seen after a single dose as well as after 4 weeks of treatment.

In toluene diisocyanate (TDI)-induced asthma, both inhaled (438) and oral corticosteroids (165,439) have been shown to inhibit the LAR and the associated inflammatory response. Pretreatment with BDP 1.0 mg daily for 1 week also prevents the increase in bronchial hyperresponsiveness following exposure to TDI (438).

Dose Frequency and Maintenance Dose of Inhaled Corticosteroids

When inhaled corticosteroids were introduced in the early 1970s they were used in a fixed dose: BDP 0.1 mg four times daily. If the patient's asthma required more corticosteroids, they were administered as oral corticosteroids in varying doses over time. With increased experience in the use of inhaled corticosteroids the clinical situation is now different. Inhaled corticosteroids are used in individually adjusted doses over a wide dosing range, whereas oral steroids are used only transiently or in the lowest possible fixed dose in order to substitute for a possible adrenal insufficiency, developed during an earlier long-term therapy with oral corticosteroids.

Effects of Dose

One early short-term study (263) failed to find any further benefit from BDP 1.6 mg compared with 0.4 mg daily. Likewise, the first long-term study (321) also partly failed to demonstrate a higher efficacy with a higher dose. This study compared daily doses of 0.4 mg and 0.8 mg BDP in two ways. For the first 28 weeks parallel groups of asthma patients were compared and the higher dose was found to have a greater oral corticosteroid–sparing capacity. For the second 28 weeks, however, those who had failed to halve their oral steroid dose on 0.4 mg daily took twice the dose (0.8 mg). No additional effect was noted. Also Boe et al. (440) in a four-period crossover study in 128 patients did not find differences between BDP and budesonide 0.4 mg daily on the one hand, and a higher dose (BDP 1.0 mg and budesonide 0.8 mg daily) on the other hand. Despite these negative studies, which may have several causes, it is now generally agreed that a dose-response relationship exists also for inhaled corticosteroids (441–444).

Costello and Clark (262) demonstrated a significant improvement in FEV_1 in patients when the dosage of BDP was increased from 0.4 mg to 1.0 mg daily. Ellul-Micallef and Johansson (445) showed a dose-response relationship in improvements in airway function when single doses of budesonide 0.1, 0.4, and 1.6 mg were given to 12 patients with chronic stable asthma. Toogood et al. (443) showed a linear increase in PEF when increasing the dosage of budesonide from 0.4 mg to 1.6 mg daily. Smith and Hodson (239) in a retrospective study in 293 patients showed clinical advantages for the "high-dose" BDP inhaler (0.25 mg per dose) compared with the conventional inhaler (0.05 mg per dose). Laursen et al. (276) in a year-long study, and Tukiainen and Lahdensuo (446) in a 4-week-period crossover study found that 1.6 mg of budesonide compared with 0.4 mg produced greater improvements in PEF. Johansson and Dahl (447) also found dose-dependent increases in PEF when, in a double-blind study, they compared the effects of 0.1, 0.4, and 1.6 mg budesonide daily. Juniper et al. (448) studied steroid-dependent patients and they also found some evidence that the improvements were dose related.

Sears et al (449) clearly demonstrated that increasing the dose of an inhaled steroid in conjunction with use of an inhaled β-agonist only on demand, provided a substantially greater beneficial effect on control of asthma than increasing the dose of the inhaled β-agonist.

Keeping the dose-response relationship with inhaled corticosteroids in mind, the individual maintenance dose should be adjusted to be the lowest possible dose required to keep the patient symptom-free (use of rescue bronchodilators ideally zero, but always less than three doses per week), with a normal exercise tolerance, normal night sleep, and with a normal, or the best possible, airway function. This can usually be achieved when inhaled corticosteroids are used as first-line therapy for patients with newly detected asthma (4). This also means that sometimes quite high doses of inhaled corticosteroids have to be used (444). These doses are clinically more effective and safer still than doses of oral corticosteroids giving the same degree of asthma control.

Dose Frequency

In the beginning, inhaled corticosteroids (BDP, betamethasone) were used four times daily. With the introduction of new corticosteroids for inhalation, studies investigating the importance of different dosing schedules were carried out (450–452). These studies, and subsequent clinical experience, indicate that patients with stable asthma can be successfully maintained on a twice-daily dose regimen for at least several weeks or months (443,453–456). Compared with four times daily administration a twice-daily regimen may improve patient compliance, although this has never been documented in controlled clinical trials.

Toogood et al. (443) and Malo et al. (457) have demonstrated that in terms of clinical efficacy dividing the daily dose into four portions is more effective than twice-daily dosage. This is of clinical importance in patients who gradually start to deteriorate in airway function. Dividing the daily dose into four portions may stabilize the situation without an increase of the total daily dose (139). If the total drug dose per day is increased sufficiently, twice-daily dosing can be just as effective as four-times-daily regimens. This is, however, clinically impractical and hazardous since the drop in anti-asthmatic potency with twice-daily dosing cannot be offset by quadrupling the daily dose (443). It is clinically more effective, and has more favorable cost/benefit and risk/benefit ratios to increase the number of doses per day (443,458,459). This is true of all available inhaled corticosteroids.

Toogood et al. (240) also investigated the importance of timing of the dose. They studied three dose levels of budesonide (0.4, 0.8, and 1.6 mg daily) with two dose frequencies—b.i.d. and q.i.d.—and two dosing schedules, A.M. versus A.M./P.M. dosing. Twice daily A.M. treatment was scheduled at 8:00 and noon, and four times daily A.M. treatments at 7:00, 9:00, 10:30, and noon. Twice daily A.M./P.M. treatments were given at 8 A.M. and 10 P.M., and four times daily A.M./P.M. treatments at 8 A.M., noon, 5:30 P.M., and 10 P.M. In terms of airway function, A.M. dosing slightly reduced the efficacy. The A.M. dosing conserved the HPA function when a high dose of budesonide was used, but there was no parallel sparing of the steroid-induced eosinophilia.

Giving the entire daily dose of inhaled steroids in the forenoon might be expected to reduce the systemic activity as does with oral corticosteroids

(233). Early studies using a once-daily regimen with inhaled corticosteroids failed to show clinical benefits (460–462). More recent studies evaluating the efficacy of once-daily dosing in patients with mild asthma have shown encouraging results (212). With inhaled corticosteroids used as first-line therapy this may further improve the patient compliance, but it needs to be shown.

Prednisolone-Sparing Capacity

As indicated by Toogood et al. (463) results of short-term studies with inhaled corticosteroids are overoptimistic with respect to an oral steroid-sparing capacity. It is not until the treatment with inhaled steroids has continued for several months that the real sparing capacity can be evaluated.

There are 15 studies in adult patients with asthma where the oral steroid-sparing capacity of inhaled corticosteroids has been evaluated over a period of at least 12 months (287). These studies include 1,120 adult patients (239,274,276,321,464–474). The range of a 100% reduction of oral steroids varied in different studies of patients from 25% to 86%; as a mean, a 100% reduction was seen in 45% of the patients. In the first studies with BDP in daily doses of 0.4 to 0.5 mg, an oral steroid withdrawal rate of 70% to 86% was reported. In later studies with this dose the frequency of 100% reduction has been around 30% to 40%. The high-dose inhalers have enabled a complete withdrawal of oral corticosteroids in approximately 50% of the patients. Late failures have been recorded in at least 25% of the cases. These patients, who can only be treated with oral corticosteroids, may be successfully treated with a nebulized steroid suspension. Otulana et al. (475) treated 18 such patients, ages 19 to 62 years with nebulized budesonide over 12 to 18 months. All patients required at least 7.5 mg or more prednisolone to control their symptoms despite treatment with 1.2 to 1.6 mg daily BDP or budesonide. With a daily dose ranging between 4 and 8 mg nebulized budesonide, 14 patients successfully stopped oral corticosteroids, while in three the dose was reduced; only one patient failed to benefit. At the same time there was a significant improvement in airway function and a significant decrease in the number of hospital admissions for acute asthma.

An almost 1-year trial has been reported by Tan et al. (476), who studied patients in Singapore. Twenty-two steroid-dependent patients (mean dose of prednisolone 11.7 ± 4.8 mg) who had required at least three 2-week courses of additional steroids during the preceding 6 months (or demonstrated asthma deterioration when dose reduction was tried) received 1.6 mg budesonide daily. Within 12 ± 10 weeks (range 1–36 weeks) all of them could discontinue their oral steroid treatment. Thereafter the budesonide dose could be reduced to 0.8 mg daily in 21 of the 22 patients. This was achieved within 38 ± 8 weeks (range 28–62 weeks).

Patients on oral corticosteroids have depressed levels of serum and/or urinary cortisol. In studies where the level of serum cortisol and the response to ACTH have been measured before and after institution of inhaled corticosteroids, an increase in serum cortisol and a normalization of the ACTH response have been observed as the oral steroids have been replaced partly or completely with inhaled steroids (274,276,477).

Corticosteroid Resistance

Concerns have been raised regarding corticosteroid resistance appearing in a few patients with asthma, who do not improve symptomatically or with objective changes in lung function when using 30 to 60 mg prednisolone daily (59,478,478a). The steroid-resistant patients were older, had a longer history of asthma, and more nocturnal wheeze and diurnal variability in airway function, but the same level of serum IgE and atopic status as age- and sex-matched control patients. It has long been unclear if this phenomenon exists in reality or if the unresponsiveness is simply undertreatment, poor compliance, abnormal pharmacokinetics, or something else. However, certain abnormalities in cell-mediated immunity have been described (59). These included a reduced susceptibility of peripheral blood monocytes to glucocorticoid-induced complement receptor down-regulation (60). Peripheral blood monocytes of steroid-resistant asthmatics also elaborate a neutrophil activating factor even in the presence of high concentrations of glucocorticosteroids (61). Most important, possibly, is that the corticosteroid-resistant patients have elevated percentages of T lymphocytes expressing the activation molecules IL-2R and HLA-DR, compared with the sensitive patients indicating an ongoing T-lymphocyte activation (62). The phytohemagglutinin-induced proliferation of peripheral blood T lymphocytes from sensitive, but not from steroid-resistant patients, was inhibited by corticosteroids (479,480). The degree of sensitivity of T lymphocytes to corticosteroids correlated with the clinical responsiveness to prednisolone (479). Pharmacokinetic abnormalities have not been found, neither a defect in steroid binding to the receptor, in nuclear transcription of the receptor, nor an evidence for autoantibodies to lipocortin-1. A recent study has suggested an impaired binding of the steroid receptor to glucocorticoid responsive elements (GRE) and also a defect in the inhibitory effect of AP-1 activation on GRE binding (480a). From a clinical point of view, patients who do not respond within 10 days to treatment with high-dose corticosteroids (60 mg prednisolone daily) should be regarded as steroid resistant (481).

Asthma and Pregnancy

Asthma occurs in 0.5% to 1.5% of pregnant women, and thus is a common medical management problem. The influence of pregnancy on the severity of asthma is variable, but in most cases no change is seen. If the patient's disease has improved or deteriorated during one pregnancy it is most likely that it will behave in a similar way during the next pregnancy, too. Early studies indicated that asthma in the mother was associated with increased perinatal morbidity and mortality (482), but this was due, at least partly, to a poor control of the mother's asthma. With current management routines women with asthma are no longer considered high risk-patients by obstetricians (483).

Laboratory studies using high doses of corticosteroids in rodents have shown a correlation between the drugs and fetal and placental malformations and abnormalities. Because of this, and the lack of data in pregnant women, most package inserts for corticosteroids include warnings and restrictions for their use during pregnancy. There are, however, no data indicating a risk for the fetus with commonly used maintenance doses of oral or inhaled corticosteroids. Most steroids do not cross the placenta freely. The fetal/maternal blood concentration of prednisone and prednisolone is only 1:10 (betamethasone 1:3). The inhaled corticosteroids have a significantly lower systemic bioavailability. With the new concentrated forms of inhaled corticosteroids in doses up to 1.6 mg daily, systemic treatment with corticosteroids during pregnancy can be avoided altogether (483).

Pregnant women with asthma should be treated optimally in order to have their best possible lung function. Exacerbations of asthma should be avoided. There is no reason to withhold inhaled or oral corticosteroids in the case where these drugs have been needed before pregnancy. This is the best way to avoid fetal and maternal complications (483,484).

Asthma in Children

An international pediatric asthma consensus group has recently published guidelines on the management of asthma in children (485,486). These guidelines emphasize the inflammatory nature of asthma in children and the early use of anti-inflammatory treatment. Children with asthma are hyperresponsive in the same way as adult patients (487–489), and the degree of responsiveness correlates with the severity of asthma symptoms and medication requirements (487,490), as well as with eosinophil counts and mast cell tryptase levels in the bronchoalveolar lavage fluid (491). Infants considered to be predisposed to asthma on the basis of family history are also more sensitive to histamine than normal infants (492). Lung biopsy specimens from children with stable asthma have shown pathological inflammatory findings similar to findings in children who have died of status asthmaticus (493).

Children with mild asthma can be treated with intermittent use of inhaled bronchodilators. If the use of inhaled β-agonists exceeds three doses per week regular preventive treatment with anti-inflammatory drugs is recommended. In particular those children with persistent cough or wheeze at night, on waking or with exercise, and those with frequent acute episodes of wheezing should have prophylactic treatment. Many pediatricians prefer to start additional treatment with a prophylactic agent, e.g., inhaled DSCG, and to use inhaled corticosteroids only if sufficient control has not been achieved within 6 to 8 weeks of treatment with DSCG. By doing so there is a risk that the child and the parents will be most happy with the result, because the situation is better than before treatment with DSCG. However, it may be that the best possible and optimal control will remain undetected if a trial with inhaled corticosteroids is not instituted (494). In a comparative study BDP was found to be more effective than DSCG and no further advantage was seen of combined therapy over BDP alone (495). Ostergaard and Pedersen (407) compared budesonide 0.1 mg four times daily with DSCG 2 mg four times daily. Although both drugs reduced the bronchial responsiveness to histamine during treatment, budesonide was more efficacious in improving lung function, and in reducing exercise-induced bronchoconstriction and the need of rescue bronchodilator inhalations. Kraemer et al. (496) reported that BDP 0.1 mg (up to a age of 12 years) or 0.2 mg (children older than 12 years) three times daily as powder capsules significantly improved the airway function and reduced the bronchial hyperresponsiveness in children 5 to 15 years of age with mild or moderate asthma in contrast to DSCG and placebo.

Van Essen-Zandvliet et al. (420) included 116 children, ages 7 to 16 years, in a 22-month double-blind, randomized, controlled study. They were hyperresponsive to histamine and showed >15% reversibility to an inhaled bronchodilator. Their FEV_1 had to be 55% to 90% of predicted normal, and/or a FEV_1/FVC ratio of 50% to 75%. They received either inhaled budesonide 0.2 mg plus salbutamol 0.2 mg or placebo plus salbutamol three times daily. After 2 months' treatment there were significant differences in FEV_1, PEF, PD_{20} histamine, and in symptom scores between the two groups, with the corticosteroid treatment revealing better results. The differences were maintained for 22 months, providing evidence that inhaled corticosteroids are important in the long-term treatment of childhood asthma.

Children with perennial asthma not adequately controlled on treatment with DSCG and bronchodilators should have treatment with corticosteroids. Inhaled preparations are preferred since many studies have confirmed that even low doses are effective, give good control, and do not have any significant long-term side effects (e.g., 255,260,261,497–502). Treatment of asthmatic children with corticosteroids results in a decrease of bronchial hyperresponsiveness. This has been shown with oral (428) as well as with inhaled corticosteroids (405,407,411,496,503,504). The study by Bennati et al. (503) was performed during a season of maximal allergen exposure. Kerrebijn et al. (405) noted that the improvement in bronchial hyperresponsiveness was inversely related to the patients baseline status of airway obstruction. In 12 children, ages 7 to 16 years, with mild, stable asthma but with a substantial hyperresponsiveness to inhaled metacholine, treatment with budesonide 0.2 mg three times daily for 6 months reduced the hyperresponsiveness in 11 of the 12 children. Two children became normal. However, in patients with a similar degree of bronchial hyperresponsiveness but with unstable asthma and significant bronchoconstriction, the effect of budesonide 0.6 mg twice daily for two months was minimal (404). Waalkens et al. (504) treated children with mild asthma with either terbutaline alone or with a combination of terbutaline and budesonide 0.2 mg twice daily. Compared with the terbutaline group there was a significant reduction in airway hyperresponsiveness to histamine, improvement in airway function, and a significant reduction of the diurnal variation in peak flow. Inhaled steroids also prevent exercise-induced bronchoconstriction (407,505). In comparative studies with equal doses, budesonide and BDP have been equally effective (450,506,507) or budesonide has been found somewhat more efficacious than the same dose of BDP (508).

Most children can use a metered dose inhaler (MDI) or a powder inhaler and the drug can be given on a twice-daily basis. Young children, ages 4 to 5, can use inspiratory flow-driven powder inhalers or an MDI attached to a spacing device (509). Children younger than 4 requiring treatment with corticosteroids can use an MDI attached to a spacer with a face mask (510–512), nebulizers, or oral preparations. If possible, an oral dose should be given as a single dose every other morning as this results in fewer systemic side effects than daily treatment regimens (365). The control of asthma, however, is not as good as with inhaled corticosteroids, especially on the no-treatment days.

Preparations of both BDP and budesonide to be given by wet nebulization are available. Clinical results with BDP have been disappointing (513,514), whereas results of nebulized budesonide, usually in a dose of 1 mg twice daily, have been very encouraging (515–518). The difference between the drugs appears to be one of dose since the budesonide suspension is about 20 times more concentrated. When a low dose of budesonide, 0.5 mg twice daily, or placebo were given after initial treatment for 2 weeks in a 1-month study, no significant differences were seen between the two drugs (519). In a double-blind, placebo-controlled study the oral steroid-sparing capacity of nebulized budesonide was evaluated in 35 children with severe asthma (ages 10–60 months). Nebulized budesonide significantly reduced the requirements for oral corticosteroids and improved the children's well-being (520).

The steroid-sparing capacity of inhaled BDP in children with steroid-dependent asthma has been evaluated in seven long-term studies (duration of follow-up at least 12 months) including a total of 140 patients (255,498–501,521,522). In 86% of the children the oral steroid could be discontinued, but up to 75% of the children needed short courses of oral steroids during the first year. The frequency of late failures was at least 11%, but probably higher.

It can be concluded that inhaled corticosteroids are beneficial and safe drugs in the treatment of children with moderate to severe asthma. Most patients can be treated with daily doses not exceeding 0.4 mg of budesonide or BDP. The risk of harmful side effects can be neglected when this dose level is used. With higher doses (0.8 mg daily or more) signs of metabolic activity may be detectable. Nevertheless, on these doses children will have a normal growth rate, and possible side effects are milder than those seen when doses of oral steroids are used that give the same degree of asthma control.

Chronic Obstructive Airway Disease

Chronic obstructive airway disease (COAD) or pulmonary disease (COPD) is by definition an inflammatory disease of the airways with irreversible airflow obstruction. It includes chronic bronchitis and pulmonary emphysema in various combinations. Sometimes a component of reversibility may be present. The value of corticosteroids in the treatment of patients with COPD has been repeatedly questioned. Nevertheless, most clinicians have seen clinically significant improvements when corticosteroids have been given to COPD patients with acute exacerbations.

Acute Exacerbations of COPD

There are few controlled clinical trials evaluating the usefulness of steroids in patients with acute exacerbations of COPD. Albert et al. (523) evaluated the role of methylprednisolone in a double-blind, randomized, placebo-controlled study in 44 consecutive patients with chronic bronchitis and severe airflow obstruction. Patients with asthma, atopy, or pneumonia were excluded. Treatment consisted of i.v. aminophylline, inhaled isoprenaline, antibiotics, and either i.v. methylprednisolone 0.5 mg/kg body weight or placebo every 6 h for 72 h. Bedside spirometry was done before and after bronchodilator inhalation three times daily. After 12 h of treatment the methylprednisolone-treated group had a significantly greater improvement in both prebronchodilator and postbronchodilator FEV_1 ($p < .001$). More patients with large improvements in their flow rates (>40% by 72 h) received methylprednisolone ($p < .01$). Emerman et al. (524) performed a randomized, placebo-controlled, double-blind study to determine whether i.v. administration of 100 mg methylprednisolone early in the therapy for acute exacerbations of COPD would improve pulmonary function in the emergency room and reduce the need of hospitalization. They found no greater improvement in FEV_1 in the group receiving the steroid (37%) than in the control group receiving saline (43%). There was also no difference in the rate of hospitalization: 33% in the steroid-treated group, 30% in the control group. It can therefore be concluded that corticosteroids may have a beneficial effect in the treatment of acute exacerbations in patients with COPD, but the effect is not demonstrable until 12 h after the start of therapy.

COPD in a Stable Phase

In patients with COPD, the response to corticosteroids, 30 to 40 mg prednisolone daily or equivalent, has been studied mainly in patients with chronic bronchitis in a stable phase. The results have differed greatly, as many of the studies have involved few patients and different study populations. Nevertheless, the findings suggest that some patients with stable disease may benefit from treatment with corticosteroids. Eosinophilia of blood (525) and of sputum but not of blood (526), variability of FEV_1 (525), and the response to inhaled β-agonists, determined in terms of changes in FEV_1 (526), have been cited as useful criteria for differentiating patients who respond to steroids from nonresponders. Seeing these criteria, it is obvious that it has been difficult to exclude patients with asthma. In fact, when Syed et al. (527) excluded patients with coexistent features of asthma, no significant differences in improvements in airway function were found between prednisone-treated and placebo-treated patients. They studied 18 patients with COPD who received 30 mg prednisone and placebo for 2 weeks each, with a 14 day washout period in between. The authors concluded that careful exclusion of "asthmatic tendencies" may predict nonresponse to corticosteroids in patients with COPD.

Stoller et al. (528) reviewed 14 double-blind, randomized clinical trials with systemic steroids in patients with stable COPD. Overall, eight of the 14 trials showed that the steroids produced some measured benefit, whereas six trials reported no effect. Of the 13 trials that examined FEV_1 as an outcome event, six showed greater improvement with steroids than with placebo, and seven did not. Two of the four trials that measured exercise tolerance (a 12-min walk in three and treadmill exercise performance in one) showed improvement following steroid therapy, whereas two did not.

Although none of the trials satisfied all of the methodological criteria for both validity and clinical pertinence, the trials finding steroids efficacious were generally better designed and more statistically precise than trials failing to show efficacy. The authors also performed a meta-analysis on studies that used a crossover design with a washout period (to assure optimal matching of compared groups and study conditions) and with patients showing stable conditions at baseline (to exclude acute exacerbations). Thereby six studies were identified (526,529–533), of which four showed steroids to work. The two negative trials (529,533) examined small number of patients, 12 and 16 respectively, and did not exclude the possibility of type II error. Thus, the best available randomized clinical trials do suggest that systemic corticosteroids can work, but in none of these six trials was the benefit universal. More recently Callahan et al. (534) performed a meta-analysis by selecting 33 original studies of oral steroid use in patients with COPD since 1951. The quality of the studies was assessed by three investigators by using nine explicit criteria. Ten studies met all nine criteria (526,530–533,535–539). Response to treatment with corticosteroids was defined as a 20% or greater increase in the baseline FEV_1. The selected studies reported effect sizes ranging from 0% to 56%. A calculated weighted mean effect size was 10% (95% CI, 2% to 18%) meaning that patients with COPD receiving corticosteroids approximately 10% more often than patients receiving placebo will improve 20% or more in FEV_1.

Postma et al. (540) performed a long-term study (observation period 14–18 years) on patients with severe chronic obstructive pulmonary disease (COPD) with a FEV_1 <1 L. In the beginning the patients used prednisolone in doses of 10 to 15 mg a day. Later, doses were reduced, if possible. They noted three patterns for the course of FEV_1: no change, initial increase followed by decrease, and a linear progression. At an oral dose of 7.5 mg or less per day, FEV_1 decreased, but often after a considerable time-lag (6–32 months). Their results indicated that, in doses above 7.5 mg daily, prednisolone may slow down the progression of the disease. However, treatment with these doses resulted in a considerable number of severe side effects.

In a later study, Postma et al. (541) reported long-term findings in 139 nonallergic patients with less severe disease (FEV_1 >1.2 L; FEV% 40–55%). They again noted the same three patterns as mentioned above, and a further group of patients with an initial decrease in FEV_1 followed by an increase. The conclusion was similar; in a dose above 7.5 mg a day, prednisolone may slow down the progression of COPD in both patients with irreversible and those with reversible airflow obstruction.

Inhaled Corticosteroids

Little is known about the usefulness of inhaled corticosteroids in the treatment of patients with stable COPD. Harding and Freedman (525) performed two studies on 18 outpatients and 18 inpatients. Both studies involved three consecutive treatment periods, the first with a placebo aerosol, the second with steroid aerosol (betamethasone valerate 0.8 mg daily), and the third with prednisolone 30 mg daily. In both studies, six patients treated with steroids showed significant improvements in airway function. Of the patients who responded, the inpatients did almost as well on inhaled steroids, but the outpatients responded much better to prednisolone. Wardman et al. (542) treated 22 patients with COPD with prednisolone 30 mg daily, BDP 1.5 mg daily, and placebo in a crossover study. The patients received all three treatments for 2 weeks each. Five patients were steroid responsive on both prednisolone and BDP and 17 were not.

Five studies have reported on short-term use of inhaled steroids in patients with COPD (543–547). The overall results of four of the studies (543–546) do not show any attenuation of airway hyperresponsiveness or improvements of FEV_1, even with doses of inhaled steroids and durations of treatment that have a clear effect in patients with asthma. This does not preclude long-term beneficial effects. One placebo-controlled study, however, in 30 patients using inhaled BDP 0.25 mg four times daily for 6 weeks, showed in comparison with placebo-treated patients significant improvements in airway function, bronchitis index, bronchial sample cell count, and in epithelial lining fluid albumin, lactoferrin, and lysozyme concentrations (547).

Results of a double-blind study in 58 nonallergic patients with COPD and moderate airflow obstruction was reported by Renkema et al. (548). The patients were followed prospectively for 2 years when treated with budesonide alone (1.6 mg daily), budesonide plus prednisolone (5 mg daily), or placebo. The results showed that patients with inhaled budesonide added to regular use of bronchodilators had a slower decline in FEV_1 and fewer symptoms after 2-year follow-up than those on bronchodilators alone. Exacerbations also tended to be of shorter duration. Some patients benefited largely from the use of inhaled steroids, but it was not possible to identify characteristics predicting responsiveness. Another study in 274 patients with obstructive airways diseases (asthma and COPD) showed that FEV_1 and airway hyperresponsiveness improved significantly with four-times daily inhaled β_2-agonists (terbutaline 0.5 mg $\times$ 4) and corticosteroids (BDP 0.2 mg $\times$ 4) for 2.5 years compared with β_2-agonists alone, or β_2-agonists and anticholinergics (549). A subgroup analysis showed that patients with COPD improved, although the patients with asthma showed a greater degree of improvement.

Dompeling et al. (417) identified 28 patients with COPD showing an abnormal annual decline in FEV_1 (>80 ml/year during 2 years' follow-up). These patients were included in a prospective study for a third year when they received in addition 0.8 mg BDP. There was an increase in FEV_1 of 232 ml/year during the first 6 months of BDP treatment, which was statistically different from the decline before starting BDP treatment, i.e., -156 ml/year. PEF increased by 4.5%. The diurnal variation in PEF and respiratory symptoms also significantly diminished, but the PC_{20} histamine values remained unchanged.

Selroos (287) performed a long-term study of inhaled budesonide in 52 patients with stable COPD—all smokers or ex-smokers. Patients with atopy, skin tests positive to common allergens, blood or sputum eosinophilia, or with a >15% increase in FEV_1 after an inhaled bronchodilator were excluded. Their mean FEV_1 was 1.7 $\pm$ 0.4 l (mean $\pm$ SD) which was 65 $\pm$ 10% of their predicted normal values and 47 $\pm$ 5% of their measured FVC. No one had taken steroids during the 3 months preceding the study. All patients received prednisolone 30 to 40 mg daily for 10 days. In 12 patients (23%) an increase in FEV_1 of >15% was observed. After the initial course of prednisolone all patients received inhaled budesonide 1.6 mg daily via a spacing device for 6 months. During this period, nine of the 12 responders maintained their improved airway function. In addition, eight of the 40 initial nonresponders to prednisolone responded during treatment with the inhaled preparation. Altogether 17 patients (33%) benefited from the 6-month treatment with inhaled budesonide. During a further mean follow-up time of 2 years, eight of the 17 patients have remained stable on inhaled budesonide only, at doses of 0.8 to 2.0 mg daily. Seven patients have had exacerbations requiring treatment with oral steroids: 11 courses 3 to 8 weeks in duration in five patients, and continuously in two.

Based on the above-cited studies it can be concluded that patients with stable COPD and nonreversible obstruction as measured in reversibility tests with inhaled bronchodilators may respond to long-term treatment with inhaled corticosteroids. However, the responders to inhaled steroids cannot be identified when prednisolone is given, in doses of 30 to 40 mg a day for 10 to 14 days. Inhaled corticosteroids can be used instead of oral steroids at least in some patients with COPD. Because of their more favorable safety profile compared with oral steroids, the inhaled drugs should be tried before long-term maintenance treatment with oral steroids is instituted. It seems reasonable to continue with inhaled steroids for at least 6 months before the results are evaluated.

Elborn et al. (550) described clinically beneficial effects by administering inhaled BDP, 1.5 mg daily, to patients with bronchiectasis. Twenty patients participated in a double-blind, placebo-controlled, crossover study with treatment periods of 6 weeks. Eight patients had a history of whooping cough, one of tuberculosis, and seven patients reported symptoms of hay fever, eczema, or nasal polyposis. An 18% reduction in sputum production, a significant reduction of symptom scores, as well as a small, but statistically significant improvement in airway function were noted.

Interstitial Lung Diseases

Sarcoidosis

Sarcoidosis is a multisystem granulomatous disease of unknown etiology. It mostly effects the lungs, and pulmonary involvement is frequently the indication for starting treatment. Because of the high spontaneous remission rate there was still controversies with respect to when and how to treat patients with pulmonary sarcoidosis. The conservative school starts treatment only when patients are symptomatic with breathlessness or other respiratory symptoms: "Glucocorticoids should be used for the suppression of pulmonary infiltration only in the presence of symptoms troublesome enough to warrant relief by what may be indefinitely prolonged treatment with hormones having potentially dangerous side-effects" (551), whereas other opinion leaders start treatment early and treat patients as long as there are signs of disease activity: "I would compare treatment of pulmonary sarcoidosis to fighting a grass fire. Simply to spray a little water on such a fire for a short time ensures an unfortunate outcome. So long as there is a spark of a whiff of smoke, an adequate suppressant must be applied and withdrawn only when the time is completely quenched" (552). In recent years treatment with inhaled corticosteroids has been evaluated as an alternative to long-term treatment with oral corticosteroids (553).

Early studies showed that short courses of ACTH or cortisone favorably influenced the pulmonary lesions in sarcoidosis, but the side effects were obvious (554,555). Riley et al. (556) found that treatment with corticosteroids improved the vital capacity of three sarcoidosis patients, whereas the reduced diffusion capacity remained unchanged. Repeat biopsies during treatment with cortisone showed remission of granulomas (557). Discontinuation of these short-term courses resulted in relapses of the active manifestations of the disease.

A large number of uncontrolled clinical studies have indicated that more long-term corticosteroid treatment of pulmonary sarcoidosis results in reduction of respiratory symptoms, improvement of radiographic findings, and sometimes in improvement of respiratory functions (558). However, after stopping treatment, reappearance of symptoms and deterioration of radiographic signs have been frequent findings. From these uncontrolled studies the real effect is also difficult to judge because sarcoidosis is characterized by spontaneous recoveries. There is no doubt, however, that patients with widespread pulmonary lesions and respiratory symptoms clinically benefit from treatment with corticosteroids (559–561).

There are a number of controlled clinical studies evaluating the results of treatment of sarcoidosis with corticosteroids (562–572) (Table 11). Young et al. (562) included patients with pulmonary sarcoidosis and with reduced diffusion capacity or arterial oxygen pressure into their study. Alternate patients received prednisone, starting with 60 mg daily, for 6 months. The other patients were observed without treatment. Lung function was somewhat better in the treated group at 6 months. However, a review 1 or 2 years later, and again 10 to 15 years later (568), showed no differences between treated and untreated patients on clinical, radiological, and functional assessments.

Hapke and Meek (563) compared 16 patients treated with prednisolone 15 mg a day for 6 months with 16 patients matched for age, sex, duration of disease, and degree of functional impairment. During the treatment phase the prednisolone-treated group showed more radiographic clearing, but this difference had disappeared at follow-up 4 years later. Israel et al. (564) included 90 patients in a randomized trial with prednisone, 15 mg daily for 3 months. Half of the patients were left untreated. Patients with pulmonary fibrosis or with hypercalcemia or uveitis were excluded. Eighty-three patients were followed for at least 1 year. In 37 patients with stage I disease (bilateral hilar lymphadenopathy without radiographic parenchymal shadows), no differences were seen between treated and untreated patients at any time. In 46 patients with parenchymal infiltrates, improvement was evident at the end of treatment, but after a mean follow-up of 5.4 years no difference was found between treated and untreated patients. Mikami et al. (565) reported on 101 patients randomly allocated to treatment with predni-

TABLE 11. Clinical trials evaluating the effects of oral glucocorticosteroids in patients with sarcoidosis

First author (ref. no.)	Year	No. of patients	Type of disease	Type of study	Active treatment	Follow-up (years)	Results
Young (562)	1970	25	DL_{CO} abnormal or PaO_2 <80 mm Hg	Open Alternate patients treated	Prednisone 60 mg (1 mo) 20 mg (5 mo)	1–2	No difference in DL_{CO}, VC or PaO_2 at rest and exercise
Harkleroad (568)	1982	17	Follow-up of the patients of Young et al.			10–15	As above
Hapke (563)	1971	32	Stage I 2 II 20 III 10	Open Matched controls; alternate patients treated	Prednisolone 15 mg (6 mo)	4	Radiographic improvement during treatment phase; no difference at 4 years
Israel (564)	1973	90	Stage I 37 II–III 46	Open, randomized to treatment or no treatment	Prednisone 15 mg (3 mo)	1	Stage I no difference at any time point; II–III: improvement at 3 mo, but not after 1 year
Mikami (565)	1974	101	Active Stage I 39 II 30 Placebo Stage I 12 II 20	Double-blind randomized placebo-controlled	Prednisolone 30 mg (1 mo) 20 mg (1 mo) 10 mg (1 mo) 5 mg (3 mo)	1	More rapid radiographic improvement in treated patients; no difference at 1-year follow-up
Selroos (566)	1979	39	Stage II not improving spontaneously	Open, randomized to no treatment or to daily or alternate day treatment	Methylprednisolone 32–20 mg (1 mo) 12–16 mg (5 mo) 4–8 mg (1 mo)	2	Treataed patients better at 7 mo (x-ray, VC, DL_{CO}) but no difference at 1 or 2 years; no difference between daily and alternate day therapy

Author	Year	No.	Stage	Study design	Treatment	Duration (y)	Results
Eule (567)	1980	209	Stage I 86 II 123	Open, not randomized (78 patients left untreated)	Prednisolone 40 mg (1 mo) 35–15 mg (5 mo) 10 mg (10 mo or 4 mo)	3	More rapid radiographic improvement in the treated groups; no differences at 18, 24, or 36 months in VC or chest radiographs
Böttger (569)	1980	317	Stage I–II Duration <2 y	Open, not randomized; 100 untreated controls	Prednisolone 20–50 mg (initial dose) 14–28 mo	2	Relapse rate 20–25% irrespective of treatment schedule
Tachibana (570)	1981	118	Stage I 69 II 49	Open, not randomized 38 treated, 80 not treated	Prednisolone alternate days 60–40 mg (6 mo) 30 mg (6 mo) 25–5 mg (6 mo)	0.5–2	Steroid-treated group better at 6 mo and 12 mo but not at 2-year follow-up
Yamamoto (571)	1983	74	Stage I 32 II 42	37 matched pairs of treated and untreated patients	As above	3	No difference in resolution rate between treated and untreated patients
Zaki (572)	1987	183	Stage I 64 II 59 III 19 Other 17	Double-blinnd randomized placebo-controlled	Prednisone 40 mg (3 mo) 20 mg (21 mo)	5	No differences at any time between treated and untreated patients in chest x-ray or lung function tests

solone for 6 months (starting with 30 mg a day) or corresponding placebo. During treatment the prednisolone group showed more rapid clearing of chest radiographic findings. One year later no difference was found between the two groups.

Selroos and Sellergren (566) included 39 patients with pulmonary stage II disease in a randomized trial with methylprednisolone for 7 months. The treated patients received initially methylprednisolone 24 to 32 mg a day and continued with a maintenance dose of 12 to 16 mg a day or every other day. At the end of the treatment period significant improvements in chest radiographs and lung function tests (FVC, DL_{CO}) were recorded compared with the untreated group. No differences were seen between the two treatment modalities. After a follow-up of 24 and 48 months the difference between treated and untreated patients had disappeared.

Zaki et al. (572) included 183 sarcoidosis patients in a double-blind controlled study of 5 years' duration. The treated patients received prednisone, 40 mg daily, for 3 months and then 20 mg daily for at least 2 years. They were unable to document any significant difference between treated and untreated patients with respect to chest radiographic changes and lung function tests.

The results of these controlled clinical trials are negative, in contrast to results seen in clinical practice where patients with pulmonary sarcoidosis respond dramatically to treatment with corticosteroids. The explanation for these contradictory observations could be that normally patients are followed up without treatment in the hope of a spontaneous remission. Treatment is started only when the spontaneous recovery does not take place. These patients are also those usually included in clinical studies. It may be that treatment in these cases is started much too late to be effective. There are no controlled long-term clinical trials evaluating the clinical course and the final outcome of patients with newly detected sarcoidosis treated with corticosteroids immediately after diagnosis.

The indications for starting or not starting treatment with corticosteroids for pulmonary sarcoidosis are the following:

1. Symptom-free patients with bilateral hilar lymphadenopathy (BHL), i.e., stage I disease, and normal lung function, should not be treated with corticosteroids since many patients will have complete spontaneous resolution within 2 years. Development of impaired lung function and/or radiographic parenchymal lesions requires starting therapy.
2. Patients with initial erythema nodosum have good prognosis without treatment irrespective of chest radiographic findings. Treatment with corticosteroids should be avoided.
3. Patients with stage I disease but with dyspnea should have corticosteroids, because they often develop parenchymal lesions and fibrosis. Early treatment of these patients may prevent them from developing respiratory insufficiency.

4. Patients with pulmonary radiographic infiltrates and BHL (stage II) and respiratory symptoms should be treated with doses of corticosteroids high enough to normalize pulmonary function, chest radiographic findings, as well as biochemical signs of disease activity (e.g., serum angiotensin converting enzyme and lysozyme).
5. Asymptomatic patients with stage II disease but with normal lung function can be followed up for 3 to 6 months in the hope of spontaneous recovery. If no improvement occurs treatment should be started.
6. Patients with pulmonary infiltrates without BHL (stage III) may have an active or even inactive disease. Thorough examinations, such as bronchoalveolar lavage, gallium scan, pulmonary function tests, and biochemical activity tests, should be carried out to determine the degree of activity. If there are signs of an active disease, treatment with corticosteroids should be instituted. If activity is not demonstrable, treatment with steroids will not change the clinical picture of the disease and should be withdrawn if already started. The best is not to give treatment in these cases.
7. Patients with irreversible pulmonary fibrosis (stage IV) generally do not respond to treatment but may still require a dose of corticosteroids for symptomatic control of the disease.

Patients with sarcoidosis on treatment with oral corticosteroids should be carefully monitored so that the dose is the smallest required and so that treatment can be stopped if resolution is not apparent. It should also be remembered that extrapulmonary lesions may require treatment with corticosteroids when the pulmonary lesions do not.

Inhaled Corticosteroids

Fear of systemic glucocorticoid side effects during long-term treatment has resulted in the current therapeutic recommendations: observation without steroids in the hope of spontaneous remission. If a clinically effective treatment free of side effects were available, this treatment would probably be instituted early, although with the risk that some patients would be treated unnecessarily.

Early attempts to use inhaled BDP for treatment of pulmonary sarcoidosis were not successful (573), probably because the daily dose of BDP was too low and the disease too advanced to be treatable with inhaled preparations.

Because of favorable lung-specific pharmacokinetic properties the use of the inhaled corticosteroid budesonide in patients with corticosteroid-sensitive pulmonary parenchymal diseases was proposed. Animal experiments with the use of an isolated, perfused, and ventilated rat lung model showed that local instillation of budesonide into the bronchial tree resulted in a higher pulmonary tissue concentration than systemic administration via the circulation (211). Single-dose administration of 1.6 mg budesonide via a spacing device immediately before general anaesthesia to patients undergoing surgery for localized lung lesions also gave interesting results (209). Lung tissue samples were obtained as soon as possible from the periphery of a healthy lobe simultaneously with a plasma sample. The results showed tissue concentrations of budesonide approximately eight times higher than in plasma and high enough to give a good receptor binding and consequently with great likelihood of local anti-inflammatory response.

Clinical studies have shown that patients with active pulmonary sarcoidosis and not spontaneously recovering, can improve when using budesonide 0.8 to 1.6 mg daily as the only anti-inflammatory drug (574,575). Also some 50% of patients treated with oral corticosteroids but relapsing after stopping treatment could be successfully treated with only inhaled budesonide (576,577). The doses in these cases were 1.2 to 2.4 mg daily. An observation in these early studies was that the improvement after initiating therapy was slow compared to the improvement rate usually seen when starting treatment with oral corticosteroids. Therefore, an initial combination of oral and inhaled steroids might result in a more rapid improvement, while the long-term maintenance treatment could be given with only inhaled budesonide (and thereby reducing the risk of systemic side effects). This has also been verified in clinical studies (578–581). A prednisolone sparing capacity of inhaled corticosteroids has also been found in patients who must be treated with oral steroids for longer periods of time (582,583). Published studies evaluating the effects of inhaled corticosteroids in sarcoidosis are summarized in Table 12.

The mechanisms behind the clinical effects of budesonide are not fully understood. It has been shown, however, that budesonide reduces the number and proportion of T lymphocytes in the bronchoalveolar lavage fluid and normalizes an increased ratio of $CD4^+/CD8^+$ (T-helper/T-suppressor) lymphocytes (584,585). Budesonide also reduces the BAL concentrations of hyaluronan, which seems to be a marker of early fibroblast activation (584). Furthermore, a normalization of BAL macrophage subpopulations with budesonide, with a decrease in antigen-presenting macrophages simultaneously with the lymphocytes, indicates that early and pathogenetically important processes can be influenced by local therapy with corticosteroids (585).

Sarcoidosis patients with extrapulmonary lesions requiring treatment cannot be treated with inhaled drugs, because the dose absorbed from the lungs to the circulation is too low to give systemic efficacy. In patients with very severe disease the daily doses of corticosteroids suitable to inhale also seems to be too low to yield a clinically effective treatment (586). Therefore, the place of inhaled steroids in the management of patients with pulmonary sarcoidosis seems to be (a) long-term maintenance therapy after induction of response with high doses of oral steroids, (b) the only therapy for patients with relatively mild disease, and (c) supplement to oral steroids as an oral steroid sparing medication.

Extrinsic Allergic Alveolitis

Extrinsic allergic alveolitis (EAA) (hypersensitivity pneumonitis) is caused by repeated inhalation of organic dust. Farmer's lung is the classical form of EAA and is associated with exposure to moldy hay containing fungal spores, e.g., *Thermoactinomyces vulgaris*. Today, more than 50 different occupational and environmental sources of antigen associated with EAA have been described.

In most cases, and especially in early ones, avoidance of exposure is the treatment of choice and patients will recover spontaneously. However, total avoidance frequently requires a major change in life-style with several types of problems involved. Alternatives to a complete removal of antigen from the environment include avoidance of obvious sources of heavy exposure, the use of face masks, hoods, and air filters, and sometimes prophylactic premedication that may prevent or reduce the reaction. Such prophylactic medication includes disodium cromoglycate or inhaled or oral corticosteroids. To be effective, prophylactic treatment with corticosteroids should be started at least 1 week before exposure. It is not known whether prophylactic treatment influences the long-term prognosis and prevents subsequent development of permanent lung damage.

In the 1950s and 1960s it was found that symptoms associated with EAA could be alleviated by the use of corticosteroids (587,588). Few studies have evaluated the long-term effects of corticosteroid treatment given in the acute stage of EAA. Mönkäre (589) reported that the recovery of pulmonary function during an average 19 months' follow-up was identical whether the patients were treated with corticosteroids for 4 weeks or 12 weeks. This study was not randomized and there was no placebo group included. However, one-third of the patients—those with the mildest symptoms—were left untreated. Recovery of pulmonary function was similar when patients in the corticosteroid groups were compared with untreated patients with a similar degree of initial pulmonary diffusion impairment. These patients with EAA were followed-up for 5 years (590). The initial treatment with corticosteroids had no long-term effect on symptoms or respiratory function parameters.

Kokkarinen et al. (591) performed a double-blind placebo-controlled study in 36 patients with EAA in an acute stage after their first attack of farmer's lung disease. Twenty patients received prednisolone for 8 weeks starting with 40 mg daily. After one month of treatment the diffusion capacity was significantly better in the prednisolone group. After 5 years' follow-up no differences were detected between the groups in diffusion capacity, FVC, or FEV_1. During the follow-up recurrence of EAA was evident in six patients in the corticosteroid group, but in only one in the placebo group.

Although little evidence supports the general use of corticosteroids in patients with EAA there are some results indicating favorable protection against pulmonary fibrosis. Anttinen et al. (592) measured serum markers known to reflect tissue collagen synthesis; the serum procollagen type

TABLE 12. *Clinical trials evaluating the effects of inhaled budesonide in patients with pulmonary sarcoidosis*

First author (ref. no.)	Year	No. of patients	Type of study	Type of disease	Treatment	Results
Selroos (574)	1986	20	Open	Stage II–III without spontaneous regression	1.2–1.6 mg (3–6 mo) 0.8–0.4 mg (ad. 18 mo)	11/20 normalized or markedly improved chest x-rays; sign decrease in S-ACE; FVC increased in 16/20 patients
Selroos (576)	1987	12	Open	Stage II–III relapsing after discontinuation of oral steroids	1.2–2.4 mg (6–27 + mo)	8/12 showed regression of parenchymal lesions, improvement in lung function and decrease of S-ACE
Erkkilä (584)	1988	19	Double-blind, placebo-controlled	Stage I 10 II 9 newly detected	1.6 mg (8 weeks)	Decrease in BAL T cells, T4/T8 ratio, S-ACE, S-β_2-microglobulin, BAL-hyaluronan
Selroos (578)	1988	20	Single-blind, matched controls	Stage II–III	(a) oral steroids (2–3 mo) followed by 1.6 mg (ad. 18 mo) (b) oral steroids (18 mo)	No difference between the groups in radiographic and spirometric improvements, and in biochemical tests in serum
Spiteri (585)	1989	15	Placebo-controlled	Stage III and impaired lung function	1.6 mg (4 mo)	Sign decrease in BAL lymphocytes and antigen-presenting macrophages

	Year	N	Design	Stage	Treatment	Results
Vieira (580)	1990	20	Randomized parallel groups	Stage II	1.2–1.6 mg (12 mo) and prednisone for the first weeks, or oral prednisone 40 mg (12 mo)	Identical improvement rates in the two groups
Zych (579)	1993	40	Double-blind, randomized	Stage II 30 III 10	Prednisolone 40 mg (1 mo) 20 mg (2 w) Thereafter budesonide 1.6 mg or prednisolone 10 mg ad. 12 months	Budesonide as good as prednisolone for maintenance treatment
Alberts (575)	1992	47	Double-blind, placebo-controlled	Stage I 13 II 26 III 8	1.2 mg (6 mo) Follow-up for 6 mo	Significant improvements in symptoms and lung function tests in the treated group, which required significantly fewer courses of oral steroids
Selroos (581)	1992	47	Open	Stage II 31 III 16	Oral methylprednisolone 48–4 mg during 6–8 w Budesonide 1.6 mg from week 5 ad. 18 mo (indiv. adjusted doses)	Chest x-ray normalized in 23, improved in 14; sign increase in FVC and DL_{CO} % predicted; sign decrease in S-ACE and S-β_2-microglobulin.

FVC, forced vital capcity; S-ACE,

III N-terminal peptide and galactosylhydroxylysyl glucosyltransferase (S-GGT). They studied 40 patients with EAA at the time of an acute attack and 6 months later; 20 patients received corticosteroids and 20 patients placebo according to a randomized, double-blind protocol. At 6 months, there were two times more elevated marker values in the nontreated group than in the corticosteroid group. The decrease in S-GGT and increase in diffusion capacity were greater in patients receiving corticosteroids, and all but one patient who developed radiographic pulmonary fibrosis belonged to the placebo group.

Avoidance of antigen exposure remains the key issue in managing patients with EAA. If necessary, acute symptoms can be treated with the use of corticosteroids. When the disease is established and an incomplete recovery, or no recovery, has occurred following removal of all exposure, then corticosteroid therapy is indicated. Prednisolone 40 to 60 mg daily is continued for 10 to 14 days. Thereafter, the dose is tapered gradually. There is no evidence that prolongation of treatment after 4 weeks can influence the prognosis. The treatment has to be reinstituted if recurrences occur.

Idiopathic Pulmonary Fibrosis

Fibrosing alveolitis or idiopathic pulmonary fibrosis (IPF) is a disease characterized by insidious onset of dyspnea, digital clubbing, interstitial and predominantly basal infiltrates on the chest radiograph, restrictive pulmonary ventilation deficiency, impaired diffusion capacity, and arterial hypoxemia, exaggerated or elicited by exercise. The mean survival time after diagnosis is 4 to 6 years, but the clinical course is very variable. The majority of the patients will require therapy (593,594).

The standard approach to treating patients with IPF is to suppress the alveolitis with corticosteroids (595,596). Overall data derived from retrospective studies (594) suggest that about 40% to 50% of patients obtain some subjective improvement of dyspnea and about 15% to 20% obtain objective (partial) improvement in terms of the chest radiograph or lung function tests. Younger and less dyspnoeic patients will respond better to treatment with corticosteroids than do older patients with marked shortness of breath (595). An increased number of lymphocytes and less than 3% eosinophils in the BAL fluid seem to be associated with steroid responsiveness (597–599).

Relatively high doses of oral corticosteroids, 1 to 1.5 mg/kg body weight per day (60–100 mg daily), should be used for at least 2 to 3 months to determine whether corticosteroids are of value or not. High-dose i.v. pulse therapy has been tried with varying effects. Keogh et al. (600) reported on beneficial effects, whereas Gulsvik et al. (601) were unable to find any difference in response between i.v. methylprednisolone 1 g every second day for 10 days followed by prednisolone 60 to 30 mg daily, compared with oral prednisolone 30 mg daily.

It is often difficult to assess any changes in these patients since the disease is of long duration and improvements may be very slow. The responding patient will report on less dyspnea. Objectively reduction in pulmonary radiographic infiltrates and improving diffusion capacity and static lung volumes can be seen together with changes in other parameters of disease activity, e.g., uptake of gallium, and BAL cellular findings. If the patient is responsive—improved or even stabilized—the dose of prednisolone is tapered by 1 to 2 mg a week to obtain a maintenance dose of approximately 0.5 mg/kg/day, while watching for clinical or physiological deterioration. If the disease is still stable or improved, prednisolone is then maintained at 0.25 mg/kg/day for a total of 6 to 18 months. Once the steroid treatment has been stopped the patient should continue to be observed for disease relapse. Patients who do not respond to treatment with corticosteroids should be transferred to treatment with cytotoxic drugs. The results of a recent controlled study of therapy suggest that a combination of cyclophosphamide and prednisolone may in some patients have advantages over prednisolone alone (602).

Eosinophilic Granuloma of the Lung

Eosinophilic granuloma of the lung or pulmonary histiocytosis X is radiographically characterized by diffuse nodular and reticulonodular interstitial infiltrates, and pathologically by infiltration of histiocytes and eosinophils, with special mononuclear phagocytes referred to as histiocytosis X cells. There is no conclusive evidence that any treatment is effective. Prophet (603) summarized the results of eight clinical series. In some patients the disease may arrest without treatment (604), while some show a steady decline despite therapy.

Treatment should be considered for those with symptoms (cough, dyspnea, systemic symptoms such as fever, weight loss, and malaise) or disease progression. Treatment includes oral corticosteroids alone or in combination with cytotoxic drugs. The initial dose of prednisolone should be approximately 1 mg/kg body weight for 4 to 6 weeks. Thereafter the dose should be tapered depending on the response (603).

Bronchiolitis Obliterans and BOOP

Bronchiolitis obliterans includes a variety of bronchiolar diseases caused by toxic fumes, infections, drugs, and may also be associated with connective tissue diseases (605). Davidson et al. (606) described a disease characterized by progressive dyspnoea, patchy chest radiographic shadows, and a histopathological picture of intraalveolar organization and fibrosis. They called it cryptogenic organizing pneumonitis or BOOP (bronchiolitis obliterans with organizing pneumonia). However, later Epler et al. (607) used the term BOOP for an obliterative inflammatory process within the small airways. The terminology has therefore been confusing, which has caused clinical problems as the steroid sensitivity is different for the two entities. Patients with BOOP have a predominantly alveolar and respiratory bronchiolar disease whereas bronchiolitis obliterans is a disease affecting small airways but sparing the alveoli. Lung biopsy is important for the differential diagnosis. Patients with BOOP respond rapidly to treatment with corticosteroids. Corticosteroids are also used in the treatment of bronchiolitis obliterans but the response is often poor.

The management of bronchiolitis obliterans is similar to that described for IPF in that high-dose prednisolone is given for 2 to 3 months. The dose can be tapered to a maintenance dose of 10 to 20 mg, which should be continued for at least 12 months.

Corticosteroid therapy is also used in the management of fume exposure with relatively good results (605). Inhaled corticosteroids (budesonide) have also been recommended to be used after exposure to toxic fumes in an attempt to prevent the development of bronchiolitis and pulmonary edema. As early as possible after exposure five to ten doses (1.0–2.0 mg) are given, followed by 1.0 mg every 5 to 10 min during the first hour until the patient is brought to the hospital (608). It is recommended that firemen at work should have easy access to inhaled corticosteroids.

Connective Tissue Diseases

The group of connective tissue diseases includes distinct disease entities such as systemic lupus erythematosus, rheumatoid arthritis, progressive systemic sclerosis, Sjögren's syndrome, polymyositis, and dermatomyositis as well as mixed connective tissue disease. The pulmonary manifestations may occasionally precede or herald the onset of systemic features. Detailed physiological or histological studies as well as autopsy studies usually show that pulmonary involvement is much more common than it is clinically suspected. Fibrosing alveolitis may be seen in all types of connective tissue diseases. Pneumonia is quite frequent in systemic lupus and rheumatoid arthritis, aspiration pneumonia in polymyositis/dermatomyositis, and systemic sclerosis. Bronchitis may be seen in association with rheumatoid arthritis and Sjögren's syndrome, bronchiolitis in rheumatoid arthritis, and bronchiectasis in systemic sclerosis and rheumatoid arthritis. Pleurisy and effusion may occur in systemic lupus, rheumatoid arthritis, and Sjögren's syndrome (609).

When fibrosing alveolitis occurs in association with these conditions it is otherwise indistinguishable from "lone" idiopathic pulmonary fibrosis. The response to treatment with corticosteroids alone or in combination with immunosuppressive agents is unpredictable.

The following protocol can be used in the treatment of patients with pulmonary manifestations of connective tissue diseases. Initial and maintenance therapy:

1. Oral prednisolone, 1 mg/kg body weight daily (usually not exceeding 100 mg a day) for 4 to 6 weeks.
2. Patient is monitored for signs of improvement, e.g., clinical response, physiological studies, chest radiographs.
3. If stable or improved, taper prednisolone over next 6 weeks to 0.25 mg/kg daily, usually at a rate of 1 to 5 mg per week.
4. Maintain prednisolone at this dose and follow clinical parameters at 3 to 6 months interval. Most patients require 12 to 18 months of therapy before it can be stopped completely. In many cases this is suppressive therapy, which cannot be discontinued until the disease process is completely over. In some cases this means that treatment will continue indefinitely.

Prednisolone failures: if the lung disease does not respond to the initial regimen, or if the disease progresses on a low dose of prednisolone, high-dose prednisolone may be restarted, or cytotoxic, immunosuppressive agents may be added.

Pulmonary Vasculitis

The pulmonary vasculitides are a large and heterogeneous group of seemingly unrelated disorders that are all characterized by blood vessel inflammation. Depending on the particular syndrome, virtually any organ system may be involved in this process, either as the primary site of disease or as a secondary manifestation of a vasculitic disorder elsewhere. There are a number of vasculitic disorders in both groups in which the lung is a major site of clinical involvement. Three examples are given in the following subsections.

Systemic Necrotizing Vasculitis of the Polyarteritis Nodosa (PAN) Type

Within this group of disorders there are three entities whose classification has often caused some difficulties. These syndromes include (a) classic PAN, (b) allergic angiitis and granulomatosis (Churg-Strauss syndrome), and (c) the "overlap" syndrome. Until recently, the therapy of these disorders has been rather disappointing. Without therapy the overall 5-year survival has been less than 15%, which is improved to approximately 50% with the use of corticosteroids. Long-term low-dose combination therapy, cyclophosphamide (1–2 mg/kg/day) in combination with tapering doses of corticosteroids, has induced a dramatic remission and disease regression in most patients.

Wegener's Granulomatosis

Wegener's granulomatosis is a disease characterized by the triad of necrotizing granulomatous vasculitis of the upper and lower respiratory tract, glomerulonephritis, and disseminated small vessel vasculitis. Involvement of the lung is observed in virtually all patients at some time during the course of the disease even though symptoms may be present in only one-third of affected patients (610).

Although trimethoprim/sulfamethoxazole has been shown to be effective in patients with Wegener's granulomatosis (611), the therapy of choice is cyclophosphamide, initially in combination with corticosteroids (612). Prednisolone 1 mg/kg/day is generally begun to decrease the inflammatory lesions until the effects of cyclophosphamide are observed. A few weeks' initial course with corticosteroids is usually enough to reach these objectives.

Lymphomatoid Granulomatosis

Lymphomatoid granulomatosis is a form of vasculitis characterized by granulomatous inflammation associated with angiotrophic and angiodestructive infiltration of various organ systems with a predilection for the lung. The cellular infiltrates are unique as they are pleomorphic and composed of normal and atypical lymphocytoid and plasmacytoid cells. Patients are treated with cyclophosphamide and corticosteroids in the same manner as that used for Wegener's granulomatosis.

Eosinophilic Pneumonias

Eosinophilic pneumonia is a condition in which intra-alveolar spaces are filled with inflammatory cells including eosinophils in abundance. It is mostly accompanied by peripheral blood eosinophilia. The association of blood eosinophilia and pulmonary shadowing has been described under many different terms: Löffler's syndrome, pulmonary eosinophilia, pulmonary infiltrates with eosinophilia (PIE), and eosinophilic pneumonia.

In 1971, McCarthy and Pepys (613) confirmed that 111 of 143 patients with pulmonary eosinophilia had evidence for allergic bronchopulmonary aspergillosis. In addition, eosinophilic pneumonias may be seen in association with parasitic infections, exposure to certain chemicals and drugs, and in patients with asthma. In some cases the etiology remains unknown, e.g.,

Löffler's syndrome (transient pulmonary eosinophilia) and chronic (idio-pathic) eosinophilic pneumonia.

Allergic Bronchopulmonary Aspergillosis

Allergic bronchopulmonary aspergillosis (ABPA) is a clinical syndrome characterized by asthma, systemic symptoms of myalgia, fever, and fatigue, transient or fixed pulmonary infiltrates, and evidence of hypersensitivity to *Aspergillus* species. ABPA is one of five clinical types of aspergillus lung disease. The remaining four are (a) invasive or septicemic aspergillosis, which occurs in individuals with a compromised immune response and is associated with invasion of the bronchial wall; pneumonia, mycotic abscesses, chronic granulomas, and systemic spread are often seen; (b) aspergilloma (fungus ball), which is a superficial invasion of an anatomic abnormality, such as bronchiectatic cavities, bronchogenic cysts, and pulmonary cavities complicating tuberculosis; (c) IgE-mediated bronchial asthma; and (d) extrinsic allergic alveolitis caused by inhalation of spores of *A. clavatus* (malt worker's and cheese worker's lung) or of spores of *A. fumigatus* (papermill worker's lung or farmer's lung).

The use of corticosteroids in asthma and extrinsic allergic alveolitis are discussed above. Corticosteroids are not used in the treatment of invasive aspergillosis or for aspergillomas.

Five stages of ABPA have been described: acute (stage I), remission (stage II), exacerbation (stage III), corticosteroid-dependent asthma (stage IV), and fibrotic end-stage (stage V) (614). The staging of APBA may be made at the time of diagnosis and may change over months and years. The course of the syndrome is variable, so patients may be classified into different stages at different times. The stage should not be considered as phases, with progression to stage V as inevitable.

Oral corticosteroids are the drugs of choice in the treatment of ABPA. The steroids improve clinical symptoms including asthmatic ones, improve lesions seen in chest radiograms, decrease the level of total IgE, and decrease the incidence of positive sputum cultures of *A. fumigatus*. The efficacy of prednisone therapy in maintaining clinical improvement during a 5-year follow-up has been reported to be 80% (615).

The treatment of ABPA including exacerbations is to give prednisolone 0.5 mg/kg/day for 2 weeks. Thereafter the dose can be halved or an alternate-day regimen can be tried. The treatment should be continued for 3 to 6 months. A reduction of the daily dose is possible if a rapid decrease in the level of total IgE is observed, in combination with a normalization or marked improvement of the chest radiographic lesions. Acute exacerbations are usually preceded by sharp elevations in total IgE (616). Therefore, monitoring of serum IgE levels is recommended. Remission may be temporary or permanent. Some patients' asthma appears to become much more severe and they cannot be managed without long-term oral steroids or inhaled steroids. Such patients (stage IV) are usually managed with moderate dosages on prednisolone, 20 to 40 mg on alternate days. When patients are managed and new exacerbations are identified and treated, progressive deterioration does not seem to occur that would otherwise result in emergence of stage V (617,618).

There are several reports discussing the long-term results of oral steroid treatment in patients with ABPA. Wang et al. (619) observed 25 patients for 1 to 10 years (mean 2.6 years) after initial therapy with prednisone, which was then tapered and discontinued unless maintained at minimal doses as required for control of asthma. Thirteen patients had no recurrence, four did not comply with the regimen, and eight patients had 12 recurrent episodes characterized by pulmonary infiltrates. The recurrences were closely correlated with sharp increases in total serum IgE.

There are reports on the use of inhaled corticosteroids instead of oral preparations in the maintenance treatment of patients with ABPA. BDP, (620,621), triamcinolone acetonide (622), and budesonide (623) have been tried. Some patients have been well controlled on inhalation therapy.

Löffler's Syndrome

Löffler's syndrome, pulmonary eosinophilia of unknown etiology occurring in relatively asymptomatic patients, is characterized by transient pulmonary infiltrates and peripheral blood eosinophilia. Therapy with corticosteroids should be avoided because the disease is benign and often self-limited. If absolutely necessary, prednisolone in a dose of 20 to 30 mg daily for 1 to 2 weeks is usually adequate to control symptoms related to the disease and accelerate the clearance of the pulmonary infiltrates. Tapering of the dose is recommended because relapses due to too a rapid withdrawal of the steroids are more easily detected.

Chronic (Idiopathic) Pulmonary Eosinophilia

Chronic pulmonary eosinophilia was described as a condition with persistent blood eosinophilia and eosinophilic pulmonary in filtrates (624). Asthma was not a typical feature of the syndrome and did not predict the clinical course or the response to treatment. Similar cases have later been described by Turner-Warwick et al. (625), who used the term *cryptogenic pulmonary eosinophilia*. The patients often present with a clinical picture of high fever, night sweats, weight loss, and severe dyspnea. The chest radiographic picture shows dense pneumonic infiltrates, mostly along the periphery of the lungs. Treatment with oral corticosteroids, e.g., prednisolone 40 to 60 mg daily, results in clinical, radiographic, and functional improvements within several days. Relapses are common when the corticosteroids are withdrawn or the daily dose reduced. The pulmonary infiltrates reappear in a pattern similar to the original lesions.

Drug-Induced Pulmonary Reactions

A wide range of drugs may cause pulmonary reactions and infiltrates, cytotoxic drugs (626) as well as noncytotoxic drugs (627).

Eosinophilic reactions have been described with cytotoxic drugs, e.g., methotrexate, bleomycin, procarbazine, with antibiotics and chemotherapeutics such as penicillins, nitrofurantoin, sulfonamides and tetracyclines, with antirheumatics such as gold salts and penicillamine, and with drugs such as sulfasalazine, carbamazepine, and phenytoin. A diffuse alveolitis with or without interstitial fibrosis has most frequently been described in association with cytotoxic drugs, nitrofurantoin, amiodarone, and tocainide.

Nitrofurantoin is the most common cause of drug-induced pulmonary reactions (628–630). Chronic reactions may lead to an interstitial lung disease with a restrictive ventilatory defect and abnormalities of gas exchange (631,632). The key to management is removal of the drug. Oral corticosteroids may be useful in the management of acute symptoms but are less effective in the chronic restrictive phase. The doses and regimens to be used follow those described for treatment of allergic alveolitis.

Tuberculosis

All types of *M. tuberculosis* infections should be treated with adequate antituberculosis combination chemotherapy. In most instances chemotherapy alone is sufficient to secure recovery. In some clinical situations corticosteroids are added, such as miliary tuberculosis and tuberculous pleuritis, pericarditis, peritonitis, and meningitis.

Military tuberculosis is a condition in which tubercle bacilli are spread out over the entire body through hematogenous dissemination. The pulmonary fields are filled with small tuberculous foci, giving the chest radiographs its characteristic "miliary" pattern. Due to many extrapulmonary manifestations the patients mostly exhibit great fatigue and fever, and sometimes they are unconscious. Although controversial, the corticosteroids appear to be effective in hastening the reduction in systemic toxicity, the intensity of the inflammatory exudative pulmonary response, and the radiographic changes. After starting adequate chemotherapy a brief course of corticosteroids may be beneficial to some patients. Because of the potentially severe complications these patients need to be followed very carefully (633).

Tuberculous pleuritis is primarily treated with chemotherapy. Drainage of pleural fluid is not necessary and will only result in new formation of inflammatory exudate. In patients with slow resorption of fluid, addition of corticosteroids may be beneficial. A starting dose of 30 to 40 mg prednisolone is appropriate. Tapering the dose during 2 to 3 weeks is recommended. This treatment with steroids seems to inhibit fibroblast proliferation and thereby reduce the risk of chronic fibrotic sequelae. Intrapleural instillation of corticosteroids is not indicated.

Cystic Fibrosis

The use of corticosteroids has been generally avoided in patients with cystic fibrosis because of the infections present in the respiratory tract. As patients on corticosteroids are less suitable for lung transplantation, the reluctance to prescribe steroids has further increased.

The indications for corticosteroids in cystic fibrosis are allergic bronchopulmonary aspergillosis, acute deterioration in lung symptoms that do not respond to antibiotics and physiotherapy, and progressive deterioration in pulmonary function. However, a study by Auerbach et al. (634) has indicated that early treatment with corticosteroids may be useful. They treated 21 patients with alternate-day prednisone for 4 years in a randomized, double-blind, placebo ($n = 24$) controlled study and noted significant advantages over placebo for height, weight, vital capacity, FEV_1, PEF, ESR, and serum IgG. The prednisone-treated group required nine hospital admissions for cystic fibrosis–related pulmonary disease compared with 35 for the placebo group.

Adult Respiratory Distress Syndrome

The adult respiratory distress syndrome (ARDS) is a type of acute respiratory failure, representing a final common pathway of lung response to a variety of clinical states, resulting in direct or indirect insult to the alveolocapillary interface. These states include trauma, burns, shock irrespective of cause, infections (sepsis), aspiration, multiple transfusions, immune and metabolic disorders, intoxications, etc.

Despite a better understanding of the pathophysiological mechanisms involved and new approaches to supported ventilation, the mortality in ARDS is still very high–50% to 90%. Treatment of patients with ARDS remains supportive and aims to maintain sufficient oxygen delivery to all organs. The underlying cause should be treated if possible and any suspected sites of sepsis should be managed aggressively with antibiotics and surgical drainage (635).

Several anti-inflammatory agents have been tried in patients with ARDS. A continuing controversy revolves around the efficacy of high-dose corticosteroid therapy. Sibbald et al. (636) investigated the leakage of serum protein into the bronchial aspirate of patients with established septic ARDS and concluded that steroids, especially when given early, may reverse lung microvascular permeability.

When discussing the possible effects of corticosteroids in the treatment of patients the evaluation should be divided into two separate parts: early intervention and treatment of the fully established ARDS syndrome.

Several clinical studies have attempted to evaluate the efficacy of corticosteroids in conditions predisposing patients to acute lung injury. Some studies are limited to small patient populations or to small number of patients at risk for ARDS (637). In some trials, the study design or inability to standardize therapy has limited the authors' ability to draw firm conclusions about the benefit of corticosteroid therapy (637).

Schumer (638) performed a prospective randomized study of corticosteroid administration to patients with septic shock. Methylprednisolone 30 mg/ kg or dexamethasone 3 mg/kg given once or twice within 24 h reduced the mortality from 38.4% to 10.5%. Different results have been reported by Bone et al. (639) and the Veterans Administration Systemic Sepsis Cooperative Study Group (640). They both showed that corticosteroid therapy did not improve survival in patients with septic syndrome. Bone et al. (641) also performed a randomized, double-blind, placebo-controlled study in 382 patients with a presumptive septic shock syndrome and at risk for developing ARDS. The diagnosis was based on the presence of fever or hypothermia, tachypnea, tachycardia, and the presence of one of the following indices of organ dysfunction: a change in mental status, hypoxemia, elevated lactate levels, and oliguria. The treatment, either methylprednisolone 30 mg/kg or placebo, was given in four 20-min infusions 6 h apart. The development and reversal of ARDS was followed and resulted in data on 304 of the 382 randomized patients. A trend toward increased incidence of ARDS was seen in the methylprednisolone group (50/152, 33%) compared with the placebo group (38/152, 25%). Significantly fewer methylprednisolone patients reversed their ARDS (15/50, 30%) compared with placebo (23/38, 61%); $p = .005$. The 14-day mortality in patients treated with methylprednisolone was 26/50 (52%) compared with placebo 8/22 (36%), $p = .004$. The authors concluded that early treatment of septic syndrome with methylprednisolone does not prevent the development of ARDS. Additionally, methylprednisolone treatment impedes the reversal of ARDS and increases the mortality rate in patients with ARDS.

Bernard et al. (637) performed the first prospective, randomized, double-blind, placebo-controlled study of corticosteroid therapy in patients with established ARDS: refractory hypoxemia, diffuse bilateral infiltrates on chest radiography, and the absence of congestive heart failure documented by pulmonary-artery catheterization. Fifty patients received methylprednisolone 30 mg/kg every 6 h for 24 h, and 49 received placebo. Serial measurements were made of pulmonary shunting, the ratio of partial pressure of arterial oxygen to partial pressure of alveolar oxygen, the chest radiograph severity score, total thoracic compliance, and pulmonary-artery pressure. No statistically significant differences between groups were found in any characteristics upon entry or during the 5 days after entry. Forty-five days after entry there were no differences between the groups either in mortality or in the reversal of ARDS.

The use of corticosteroids in the treatment of patients at risk for developing ARDS, in patients with early septic shock, as well as in patients with established ARDS, is still highly controversial. In many centers the use of high-dose intravenous methylprednisolone is a standard procedure. However, the results of most recent controlled clinical studies seem to indicate that the benefit of corticosteroids for these indications is fairly limited.

Pneumocystis Pneumonia in Patients with AIDS

Pneumocystis cariini pneumonia is the most common life-threatening opportunistic infection defining the acquired immunodeficiency syndrome (AIDS). Despite early diagnosis and rapid initiation of trimethoprim-sulfamethoxazole or parenteral pentamidine therapy, many patients will require hospitalization. Up to 30% of these patients will develop a respiratory distress syndrome (ARDS).

On the basis of uncontrolled data, adjunctive therapy with corticosteroids for AIDS-associated pneumocystis infection has been used as a means to prevent morbidity and mortality, although the steroids have been shown to be without value in the majority of patients with ARDS.

Recently, five randomized trials assessing the efficacy of adjunctive therapy with corticosteroids have been completed, including a total of 406 patients. It was shown that adjunctive corticosteroid therapy reduced the likelihood of death, respiratory failure, or deterioration of oxygenation in patients with moderate-to-severe pneumocystis pneumonia. An expert panel has reviewed these studies and made a consensus statement on how to use corticosteroids in this situation (642). The panel recommended the regimen used by the California Collaborative Treatment Group (643): on days 1 through 5, 40 mg of oral prednisone should be given twice daily; on days 6 through 10, 40 mg daily; and on days 11 through 21, 20 mg daily. If the antipneumocystis therapy is discontinued earlier, the course with steroids can be stopped at the same time.

As AIDS patients frequently have *M. tuberculosis* infections, special attention should be paid to the risk of reactivation of tuberculosis.

Bronchopulmonary Dysplasia

Bronchopulmonary dysplasia (BPD) is a type of chronic inflammatory and emphysematous lung disease that may follow respirator therapy in infants with early respiratory distress. The severity of the respiratory disease seems to correlate with the degree of early-onset airway reactivity (644). Unlike adults with emphysema, with supportive therapy many of these infants seem to recover by growing new lung tissue over the ensuing 1 to 5 years, although their ultimate outcome remains uncertain since the children have not yet reached adulthood.

The rationale for adding corticosteroids to the treatment of ventilator-dependent premature infants with evolving BPD has been to reduce the inflammatory injury caused by neutrophil products (645). A few controlled studies have demonstrated that dexamethasone can acutely improve pulmonary function and decrease the respiratory support required by ventilator-dependent infants with BPD (646,647).

Mammel et al. (646) treated six infants who had BPD in a double-blind, randomized, crossover trial. Each infant received either dexamethasone or placebo for 72 h and then the other treatment for the same period of time. The study was terminated after the respiratory status (ventilation rate, peak airway pressure, oxygen requirement, and alveolar-arterial oxygen gradient) of all six infants improved only during the administration of dexamethasone. The drug was subsequently continued in all six infants for several weeks. Avery et al. (647) used a sequential-analysis design and treated 16 ventilator-dependent infants between 2 and 6 weeks of age with either dexamethasone i.v. 0.5 mg/kg/day or placebo. The initial dose was continued for 72 h, then reduced to 0.3 mg/kg/day for 72 h, and thereafter decreased by 10% of the current dose every 3 days until a dose of 0.1 mg/kg/day was reached. They assessed weaning from ventilator and measured compliance during the first 72 h of treatment. The trial was stopped when 14 infants had been matched to form seven pairs; in each pair, the treated infant was weaned from the ventilator and the control infant was not. Pulmonary compliance increased by 64% in the treated group and only 5% in the control group. No significant difference was found between the groups in mortality and hospital stay.

The studies by Mammel et al. (646) and Avery et al. (647) have not evaluated whether the initially observed clinical improvement after dexamethasone was associated with a decline in pulmonary inflammation.

Yoder et al. (648) performed a placebo-controlled, double-blind study in 17 ventilator-dependent premature infants with BPD (mean age: gestational age 27 weeks; postnatal age approximately 40 days at entry; weight <1500 g). They received intravenous dexamethasone 0.5 mg/kg/day for 3 days or corresponding placebo. Pulmonary inflammation and function as well as respiratory support were assessed. After 3 days of placebo treatment, there was no significant change in any of the measured parameters. In contrast, dexamethasone-treated infants required significantly less respiratory support. Pulmonary inflammation was suppressed in the dexamethasone-treated group. However, all dexamethasone-treated infants stopped experiencing improvement in their respiratory status within several days of drug discontinuation, and most of the infants reverted to pretreatment oxygen and ventilator requirements.

These results show that short-term treatment with intravenous dexamethasone in ventilator-dependent infants with BPD results in acute suppression of pulmonary inflammation, improved pulmonary mechanics, and a decrease in the requirement for supplemental oxygen and assisted ventilation. It is not known whether discontinuation of treatment is accompanied by a return of the inflammatory state and pulmonary mechanics to the level of pretreatment dysfunction.

Cummings et al. (649) evaluated the usefulness of long-term treatment of dexamethasone in infants with BPD in a randomized, double-blind, placebo-controlled trial. Thirty-six preterm infants (birth weight <1250 g; gestational age <30 weeks) dependent on oxygen and mechanical ventilation at 2 weeks of age were included. They received a 42-day course of dexamethasone ($n = 13$), an 18-day course ($n = 12$), or saline placebo ($n = 11$). The starting dose of dexamethasone was 0.5 mg/kg/day and it was gradually lowered during the period of administration as described by Avery et al. (647). Infants in the 42-day dexamethasone group, but not in the 18-day group, were weaned from mechanical ventilation and supplemental oxygen significantly faster than control infants. Follow-up of all 23 survivors at 6 and 15 months of age showed good outcome in seven of nine infants in the 42-day group, but in only two of nine infants in the 18-day dexamethasone group and in two of five in the placebo group. No side effects of the steroid therapy were reported in this study.

Steroid treatment has been associated with a number of side effects in infants treated with dexamethasone. An increased incidence of pneumothorax, sepsis, necrotizing enterocolitis, hyperglycemia, and arterial hypertension has been reported (650). Ng et al. (651) evaluated the risk of adrenal suppression in infants treated with dexamethasone for BPD for 3 weeks. They used tetracosactrin stimulation test in 22 very low birth weight infants. A distinct pattern of cortisol response was found that was quite unlike that found in older children and adults. Using pretreatment data as control they concluded that there was evidence of modest suppression of the adrenal axis during dexamethasone treatment, although there was considerable recovery 1 month after stopping steroids. Basal concentrations, however, remained low in some cases, which may indicate the need for temporary corticosteroid replacement during severe illness.

The high risk of side effects, and at present the limited success of corticosteroids, suggests that this form of treatment should be limited to ventilator-dependent infants in whom no progress with weaning is being made. It is essential to exclude sepsis before starting treatment and throughout treatment blood pressure, serum electrolytes, and blood glucose must be monitored. There is no evidence that repeated courses of steroids are successful and such a policy is likely to increase the risk of side effects. An appropriate dosage regimen is still that proposed by Avery et al. (647). The precise length of time the lowest steroid dosage should be maintained remains uncertain.

While systemic corticosteroids are effective in improving the status of infants with BPD, their use may be associated with many adverse effects. Nebulized therapy with the topically active corticosteroids BDP (25μg/kg/day) (652) and budesonide (1 mg three times daily) (653) have been successfully used in the treatment of a small number of infants with BPD without major side effects. Further studies of aerosolized corticosteroids in BPD is warranted.

Croup (Acute Laryngotracheobronchitis)

The most frequent cause of acute inspiratory stridor in early childhood is acute viral laryngotracheobronchitis (croup). Corticosteroids have been widely used in the treatment of these children, but the scientific evidence for their efficacy has been inconclusive (654). Many of the early studies involved too few patients to detect existing differences, and the doses of steroids used were also too low. However, a meta-analysis of nine randomized studies with 1,126 patients supported the use of corticosteroids in unintubated children in hospital (655).

Recently Tibballs et al. (656) reported their results of a placebo-controlled study in 70 children, using the duration of intubation and the need for reintubation as end points. The children were randomly assigned treatment with prednisolone 1 mg/kg or placebo every 12 h given by nasogastric tube until 24 h after extubation. Treatment with prednisolone was found to be significantly more effective than placebo with respect to duration of intubation (98 vs. 138 hours). Eleven placebo-treated patients but only two steroid-treated patients required reintubation.

Husby et al. (657) used a nebulized suspension of budesonide in a high-pressure ventilator. They treated 32 children with 1 mg budesonide twice with a 30-min interval or with placebo in a randomized, double-blind study. Two hours after the start of treatment there were clinically significant improvements in stridor, cough, and total croup scores in the steroid group compared with the placebo group.

REFERENCES

1. Ellul-Micallef R. Glucocorticosteroids. In: Barnes PJ, Rodger IW, Thomson NC, eds. *Asthma. Basic mechanisms and clinical management*, 2nd ed. London: Academic Press, 1985;613–657.
2. Haynes RC. Adrenocorticotropic hormone; adrenocortical steroids and their synthetic analogs; inhibitors of the synthesis and actions of adrenocortical hormones. In: Goodman Gilman A, Rall TW, Nies AS, Taylor P, eds: *The pharmacological basis of therapeutics,* 8th ed. New York: Pergamon Press, 1990;1431–1462.

3. Barnes PJ, Pedersen S. Efficacy and safety of inhaled corticosteroids in asthma. *Am Rev Respir Dis* 1993;148:S1–S26.
4. Haahtela T, Järvinen M, Kava T, et al. Comparison of a β_2-agonist, terbutaline, with an inhaled corticosteroid, budesonide, in newly detected asthma. *N Engl J Med* 1991;325:388–392.
5. Reed C. Aerosol steroids as primary treatment of asthma. *N Engl J Med* 1991;325:425–426.
6. Geddes DM. Inhaled corticosteroids: benefits and risks. *Thorax* 1992;47:404–407.
7. Haahtela T, Järvinen M, Kava T, et al. First line treatment of newly detected asthma: an inhaled steroid? One year's follow-up after two years treatment. *Eur Respir J* 1992;5(suppl 15):13s.
7a. Pavard I, Knox A. Pharmacokinetic optimization of inhaled steroid therapy in asthma. *Clin Pharmacokin* 1993;25:126–135.
7b. Lipworth BJ. Clinical pharmacology of corticosteroids in bronchial asthma. *Pharmac Ther* 1993;58:173–209.
8. Schleimer RP, Claman HN, Oronsky AL. *Anti-inflammatory steroid action. Basic and clinical aspects.* San Diego: Academic Press, 1989.
9. Sertl K, Clark T, Kaliner M. Supplement: corticosteroids. Their biological mechanisms and application to the treatment of asthma. *Am Rev Respir Dis* 1990;141(2 part 2).
10. Munck A, Guyre PM. Glucocorticoid physiology and homeostasis in relation to anti-inflammatory action. In: Schleimer RP, Claman HN, Oronsky AL, eds: *Anti-inflammatory steroid action. Basic and clinical aspects.* San Diego: Academic Press, 1989;30–47.
11. Munck A, Guyre PM, Holbrook NJ. Physiological functions of glucocorticoids in stress and their relation to pharmacological actions. *Endocr Rev* 1984;5:25–44.
12. Besedovsky J, Del Rey A, Sorkin E, Dinarello C. Immunoregulatory feedback between IL-1 and glucocorticoid hormones. *Science* 1986;233:652–654.
13. Nakamura H, Motoyoshi S, Kadokawa T. Anti-inflammatory action of IL-1 through the pituitary-adrenal axis in rats. *Eur J Pharmacol* 1988;151:67–73.
14. Brattsand R, Pipkorn U. Glucocorticoids: experimental approaches. In: Kaliner MA, Barnes PJ, Persson CGA, eds. *Asthma. Its pathology and treatment.* New York: Marcel Dekker, 1991;667–710.
15. Durham SR, Keenan J, Cookson WOCM, Craddock CF, Benson MK. Diurnal variation in serum cortisol concentrations in asthmatics after allergen inhalation challenge. *Thorax* 1989;44:582–585.
16. Mohiuddin AA, Martin RJ. Circadian basis of the late asthmatic response. *Am Rev Respir Dis* 1990;142:1153–1157.
17. Herrscher RF, Kasper C, Sullivan TJ. Endogenous cortisol regulates immunoglobulin E-dependent late phase reactions. *J Clin Invest* 1992;90:596–603.
18. Muller M, Renkawitz R. The glucocorticoid receptor. *Biochim Biophys Acta* 1991;1088:171–182.
19. Dahlberg E, Thalen A, Brattsand R, et al. Correlation between chemical structure receptor binding and biological activity of some novel, highly active 16α, 17α-acetal-substituted glucocorticoid. *Mol Pharmacol* 1984;25:70–78.
20. Tsurufuji S, Sugia K, Takemasa F, Yoshizawa S. Blockade by antiglucocorticoids, actinomycin D and cycloheximide of anti-inflammatory action of dexamethasone against bradykinin. *J Pharmacol Exp Ther* 1980;212:225–231.
21. Peers SH, Moon D, Flower R. Reversal of the anti-inflammatory effects of dexamethasone by the glucocorticoid antagonist RU 38436. *Biochem Pharmacol* 1988;37:556–557.
22. Lane L, Kawai S, Udelsman R, et al. Glucocorticoid antagonists: pharmacological attributes of a prototype antiglucocorticoid (RU 486). In: Schleimer RP, Claman HN, Oronsky AL, eds. *Anti-inflammatory steroid action. Basic and clinical aspects.* San Diego: Academic Press, 1989;303–329.
23. Munck A, Mendel DB, Smith LI, Orti E, Glucocorticoid receptors and actions. *Am Rev Respir Dis* 1990;141:S2–S10.
24. Miesfeld RL. Molecular genetics of corticosteroid action. *Am Rev Respir Dis* 1990;141:S11–S17.
25. Voris BP, Young DA. Glucocorticoid-induced proteins in rat thymus cells. *J Biol Chem* 1981;256:11319–11329.

26. Helmberg A, Fässler R, Geley S, et al. Glucocorticoid-regulated gene expression in the immune system. Analysis of glucocorticoid-regulated transcripts from the mouse macrophage-like cell line P388DI. *J Immunol* 1990;145:4332–4337.
27. Evans RM. The steroid and thyroid hormone receptor superfamily. *Science* 1988; 240:889–895.
28. Dahlman-Wright K, Wright A, Carlstedt-Duke J, Gustafsson J-Å. DNA-binding by the glucocorticoid receptor: a structural and functional analysis. *J Steroid Biochem Molec Biol* 1992;41:249–272.
29. Albers MW, Chang H, Faber LE, Schreiber SL. Association of a 59-kilodalton immunophilin with the glucocorticoid receptor complex. *Science* 1992;256:1315–1318.
30. Encio PJ, Detgra-Wadleigh SD. The genomic structure of the human glucocorticoid receptor. *J Biol Chem* 1991;266:7182–7188.
31. Hsu S-C, Qi M, DeFranco DB. Cell cycle regulation of glucocorticoid receptor function. *EMBO J* 1992;11:3457–3468.
32. Adcock IM, Brönnegård M, Barnes PJ. Glucocorticoid receptor mRNA localization and expression in human lung. *Am Rev Respir Dis* 1991;43:A628.
33. Andersson O, Brönnegård M, Sonnenfeld T, et al. Glucocorticoid receptor mRNA expression in pulmonary alveolar macrophages in sarcoidosis. *Chest* 1991;99:1336–1341.
34. Lane SJ, Lee TH. Glucocorticoid receptor characteristics in monocytes of patients with corticosteroid resistant bronchial asthma. *Am Rev Respir Dis* 1991;143:1020–1024.
35. Jonat C, Rahmsdorf HJ, Park K-K, et al. Antitumor promotion and antiinflammation: downmodulation of AP-1 (Fos/Jun) activity by glucocorticoids. *Cell* 1990;62:1189–1204.
36. Fahey JV, Guyre PM, Munck A. Mechanisms of antiinflammatory actions of glucocorticoids. *Adv Inflammat Res* 1981;2:21–51.
37. Härd T, Kellenbach E, Boelens R, et al. Crystallographic analysis of the interaction of the glucocorticoid receptor with DNA. *Science* 1990;249:157–159.
38. Luisi BF, Xu WX, Otwinowski Z, Freedman LP, Yamamoto KR, Sigler PB. Crystallographic analysis of the interaction of the glucocorticoid receptor with DNA. *Nature* 1991;352:497–505.
39. Beato M, Brüggemeier U, Chalepakis G, et al. Regulation of transcription by glucocorticoids. In: Cohen P, Foulkes IG, eds. *The hormonal control of gene transcription.* Amsterdam: Elsevier, 1991;117–128.
40. Ray A, Laforge KS, Sehgal PB. On the mechanisms of efficient repression of the interleukin-6 promotor by glucocorticoids: enhancer TATA box and RNA start site occlusion. *Mol Cell Biol* 1990;10:5736–5746.
41. Strömstedt P-E, Poellinger L, Gustafsson J-Å, Carlstedt-Duke J. The glucocorticoid receptor binds to a sequence overlapping the TATA box of the human osteocalcin promotor: a potential mechanism for negative regulation. *Mol Cell Biol* 1991;11:3379–3383.
42. Woolcock AJ, Barnes PJ. Supplement: asthma: the important question—part 2. *Am Rev Respir Dis* 1992;146:1349–1366.
43. Yang-Yen HF, Chambard JC, Sun Y-I, et al. Transcriptional interference between c-jun and the glucocorticoid receptor: mutual inhibition of DNA binding due to direct protein-protein interaction. *Cell* 1990;62:1205–1215.
44. Schule R, Rangarajan P, Kliewers S, et al. Functional antagonism between oncoprotein c-jun and the glucocorticoid receptor. *Cell* 1990;62:1217–1226.
45. Ponta H, Cato ACB, Herrlich P. Interference of pathway specific transcription factors. *Biochim Biophys Acta* 1992;1129:255–261.
46. Szefler SJ, Norton CE, Ball B, Gross JM, Aida Y, Pabst MJ. IFN-γ and LPS overcome glucocorticoid inhibition of priming for superoxide release in human monocytes. *J Immunol* 1989;142:3985–3992.
47. Almawi WY, Lipman MJ, Stevens AC, Zanker B, Hadro ET, Strom TB. Abrogation of glucocorticosteroid-mediated inhibition of T cell proliferation by the synergistic action of IL-1, IL-6 and IFN-γ. *J Immunol* 1991;146:3523–3527.
48. Adcock IM, Gelder CM, Shirasaki H, Yacoub M, Barnes PJ. Effects of steroids on transcription factors in human lung. *Am Rev Respir Dis* 1992;145:A834.
49. Tobler A, Meier R, Seitz M, Dewald B, Baggiolini M, Fey FF. Glucocorticoids down-

regulate gene expression of GM-CSF, NAP-1/IL-8 and IL-6, but not M-CSF in human fibroblasts. *Blood* 1992;79:45–51.

50. Peppel K, Vinci JM, Baglioni C. The AU-rich sequences in the 3'-untranslated region mediate the increased turnover of interferon mRNA induced by glucocorticoids. *J Exp Med* 1991;173:349–355.

51. Rosewicz S, McDonald AR, Maddux BA, Godfine ID, Miesfeld RL, Logsden CD. Mechanism of glucocorticoid receptor down-regulation by glucocorticoids. *J Biol Chem* 1988;263:2581–2584.

52. Brown PH, Teelucksingh S, Matusiewicz SP, Greening AP, Crompton GK, Edwards CRW. Cutaneous vasoconstrictor response to glucocorticoids in asthma. *Lancet* 1991;337:576–580.

53. Svensjö E, Roempke K. Time dependent inhibition of bradykinin and histamine-induced increase in microvascular permeability by local glucocorticosteroid treatment. In: Hogg JC, Ellul-Micallef R, Brattsand R, eds. *Glucocorticosteroids, inflammation and bronchial hyperreactivity.* Amsterdam: Excerpta Medica, 1985;136–144.

54. Miller-Larsson A, Brattsand R. Topical anti-inflammatory activity of the glucocorticoid budesonide on airway mucosa. Evidence for a hit and run type of activity. *Agents Actions* 1990;29(42):127–129.

55. Waage A, Bakke O. Glucocorticoids suppress the production of tumour necrosis factor by lipopolysaccharide-stimulated human monocytes. *Immunology* 1988;63:299–302.

56. Kay AB. Asthma and inflammation. *J Allergy Clin Immunol* 1991;87:893–910.

57. Corrigan C. Mechanism of glucocorticoid action in asthma: too little, too late. *Clin Exp Allergy* 1992;22:315–317.

58. Grabstein K, Dower S, Gillis S, Urdal V, Larsen A. Expression of interleukin-2, interferon and the IL-2 receptor by human peripheral blood lymphocytes. *J Immunol* 1986;136:4503–4508.

59. Carmichael J, Peterson IC, Diaz P, Crompton GK, Kay AB, Grant IWB. Corticosteroid resistance in chronic asthma. *BMJ* 1981;282:1419–1422.

60. Kay AB, Diaz P, Carmichael J, Grant IWB. Corticosteroid-resistant chronic asthma and monocyte complement receptors. *Clin Exp Immunol* 1981;44:576–580.

61. Wilkinson JRW, Crea AEG, Clark TJH, Lee TH. Identification and characterization of a monocyte-derived neutrophil-activating factor in corticosteroid-resistant bronchial asthma. *J Clin Invest* 1989;84:1930–1941.

62. Corrigan CJ, Brown PH, Barnes NC, et al. Glucocorticoid resistance in chronic asthma: glucocorticoid pharmacokinetics, glucocorticoid receptor characteristics and inhibition of peripheral blood T-cell proliferation by glucocorticoids in vitro. *Am Rev Respir Dis* 1991;144:1016–1025.

63. Lane SJ, Wilkinson JRW, Cochrane GM, Lee TH, Arm JP. Differential *in vitro* regulation by glucocorticoids of monocyte-derived cytokine generation in glucocorticoid-resistant asthma. *Am Rev Respir Dis* 1993;147:690–696.

63a. Sousa AR, Poston RN, Lane SJ, Nakhosteen JA, Lee TH. Detection of GM-CSF ini asthmatic bronchial epithelium and decrease by inhaled corticosteroids. *Am Rev Respir Dis* 1993;147:1557–1561.

64. Linden M, Brattsand R. Effects of a corticosteroid, budesonide, on alveolar macrophage and blood monocyte secretion of cytokines: differential sensitivity of GM-CSF, IL-1β and IL-6. (submitted)

65. Knudsen PJ, Dinarello CA, Strom TB. Glucocorticoids inhibit transcriptional and post-transcriptional expression of interleukin 1 in U937 cells. *J Immunol* 1987;139:4129–4134.

66. Lee SW, Tsou AP, Chan H, Thomas J, Petrie K, Eugui E, Allison A. Glucocorticoids selectively inhibit the transcription of the interleukin 1β gene and decrease the stability of interleukin 1β mRNA. *Proc Natl Acad Sci USA* 1988;85:1204–1208.

67. Bochner B, Rutledge BK, Schleimer RP. Interleukin 1 production by human lung tissue. II. Inhibition by anti-inflammatory steroids. *J Immunol* 1987;139:2303–2307.

68. Borish L, Mascali JJ, Dishuck J, Beam WR, Martin RJ, Rosenwasser LJ. Detection of alveolar macrophage derived IL-1β in asthma. Inhibition with corticosteroids. *J Immunol* 1992;149:3078–3082.

69. Gillis S, Crabtree GR, Smith KA. Glucocorticoid-induced inhibition of T-cell-growth factor production. I. The effect of mitogen-induced lymphocyte proliferation. *J Immunol* 1979;123:1624–1631.

70. Vacca A, Felli MP, Forina AR, et al. Glucocorticoid receptor-mediated suppression of the interleukin gene expression through impairment of the cooperativity between nuclear factor of activated T cells and AP-1 enhancer elements. *J Exp Med* 1992;175:637–646.

71. Culpepper P, Lee F. Regulation of IL-3 expression by glucocorticoids in cloned murine cells. *J Immunol* 1985;135:3191–3197.

72. Djaldetti R, Fishman P, Shtatlender V, Sredni B, Djaldetti M. Effect of dexamethasone on IL-1 and IL-3-LA release by unstimulated human mononuclear cells. *Biomed Pharmacother* 1990;44:515–518.

73. Cox G, Ohtoshi T, Vancheri C, et al. Promotion of eosinophil survival by human bronchial epithelial cells and its modulation by steroids. *Am J Respir Cell Mol Biol* 1991;4:525–531.

74. Wallen N, Kita H, Weiler D, Gleich G. Glucocorticoids inhibit cytokine-mediated eosinophil survival. *J Immunol* 1991;147:3490–3495.

75. Her E, Frazer J, Austen KF, Owen WF. Eosinophil hematopoietins antagonize the programmed cell death of eosinophils. *J Clin Invest* 1991;88:1982–1987.

76. Wu CY, Fargeas C, Nakajima T, Delespesse G. Glucocorticoids suppress the production of interleukin 4 by human lymphocytes. *Eur J Immunol* 1991;21:2645–2647.

77. Robinson DS, Hamid Q, Ying S, et al. Prednisolone treatment in asthma is associated with modulation of bronchial lavage cell interleukin-4, interleukin-5 and interferon cytokine gene expression. *Am Rev Respir Dis* 1993;148:401–406.

77a. Corrigan CJ, Hazku A, Gemou-Engesaeth V, et al. CD4 T-lymphocyte activation in asthma is accompanied by increased serum concentrations of interleukin-5: effect of glucocorticoid therapy. *Am Rev Respir Dis* 1993;147:540–547.

78. Renz H, Mazer BD, Gelfand EW. Differential inhibition of T and B cell function in IL-4-dependent IgE production by cyclosporin A and methylprednisolone. *J Immunol* 1990;145:3641–3646.

79. Rolfe FG, Hughes JM, Armour CL, Sewell WA. Inhibition of interleukin-5 gene expression by dexamethasone. *Immunology* 1992;77:494–499.

80. Iwama T, Nagai H, Suda H, Tsuruoka N, Koda A. Effect of murine recombinant interleukin-5 on the cell population in guinea-pig airways. *Br J Pharmacol* 1992;105:19–22.

81. Waage A, Slupphaug G, Shalaby R. Glucocorticoids inhibit the production of IL-6 from monocytes, endothelial cells and fibroblasts. *Eur J Immunol* 1990;20:2439–2443.

82. Hirooka Y, Mitsuma T, Nogimori T, Ishizuki Y. Effect of hydrocortisone on interleukin-6-production in human peripheral blood mononuclear cells. *Mediators of Inflammation* 1992;1:9–13.

83. Marini M, Vittori E, Hollemborg J, Mattoli S. Expression of the potent inflammatory cytokines, granulocyte-macrophage-colony-stimulating factor and interleukin-6 and interleukin-8, in bronchial epithelial cells of patients with asthma. *J Allergy Clin Immunol* 1992;89:1001–1009.

84. Standiford TJ, Kunkel SL, Rolfe MW, Evanoff HL, Allen RM, Strieter RM. Regulation of human alveolar macrophage- and blood monocyte derived interleukin-8 by prostaglandin E_2 and dexamethasone. *Am J Respir Cell Mol Biol* 1992;6:75–81.

84a. Kunicka JE, Tatte MA, Denhardt GH, et al. Immunosupression by glucocorticoids: inhibition of production of multiple lymphokines by *in vivo* administration of dexamethasone. *Cell Immunol* 1993;149:39–49.

85. Strieter RM, Remick DG, Lynch JP, et al. Differential regulation of tumor necrosis factor-α in human alveolar macrophages and peripheral blood monocytes: a cellular and molecular analysis. *Am J Respir Cell Mol Biol* 1989;1:57–63.

86. Vecchiarelli A, Siracusa A, Cenci E, Puliti M, Abbritti G. Effect of corticosteroid treatment on interleukin-1 and tumour necrosis factor secretion by monocytes from subjects with asthma. *Clin Exp Allergy* 1992;22:365–370.

87. Murch SH, MacDonald TT, Wood CBS, Costeloe KL. Tumour necrosis factor in the bronchoalveolar secretions of infants with the respiratory distress syndrome and the effect of dexamethasone treatment. *Thorax* 1992;47:44–47.

88. Tsuijmoto M, Okamura N, Adachi H. Dexamethasone inhibits the cytotoxic activity on tumor necrosis factor. *Biochem Biophys Res Commun* 1988;153:109–115.

89. Gessani S, McCandless S, Baglioni C. The glucocorticoid dexamethasone inhibits synthesis of interferon by decreasing the level of its mRNA. *J Biol Chem* 1988;283:7454–7457.

90. Araya SK, Wong-Staal F, Gallo RG. Dexamethasone-mediated inhibition of human T cell growth factor and interferon messenger RNA. *J Immunol* 1984;133:273–276.
91. Nakamura Y, Ozaki T, Kamei T, et al. Increased granulocyte/macrophage colony-stimulating factor production by mononuclear cells from peripheral blood of patients with bronchial asthma. *Am Rev Respir Dis* 1993;147:87–91.
92. Churchill L, Friedman B, Schleimer RP, Proud D. Production of granulocyte-macrophage colony-stimulating factor by cultured human tracheal epithelial cells. *Immunology* 1992;75:189–195.
93. Lamas AM, Leon OG, Schleimer RP. Glucocorticoids inhibit eosinophil responses to granulocyte-macrophage colony-stimulating factor. *J Immunol* 1991;147:254–259.
94. Evans PM, O'Connor BJ, Fuller RW, Barnes PJ, Chung KF. Effect of inhaled corticosteroids on peripheral blood eosinophil counts and density profiles in asthma. *J Allergy Clin Immunol* 1993;91:643–650.
95. Ayanlar Batuman O, Ferrero AP, Diaz A, Jimenez SA. Regulation of transforming growth factor-β1 gene expression by glucocorticoids in normal human T lymphocytes. *J Clin Invest* 1991;88:1574–1580.
96. Haynes AR, Shaw RJ. Dexamethasone-induced increase in platelet-derived growth factor (B) mRNA in human alveolar macrophages and myelomonocytic HL60 macrophage-like cells. *Am J Respir Cell Mol Biol* 1992;7:198–206.
97. Stockley RA, Lomas D, Burnett D. Inflammatory indices for chronic bronchitis and COAD. Proteases and antiproteases. In: Persson CGA, Brattsand R, Laitinen LA, Venge P, eds. *Inflammatory indices in chronic bronchitis.* Agents and Actions supplements vol 30. Basel: Birkhäuser Verlag, 1990;229–241.
98. Borson DB, Gruenert DC. Glucocorticoids induce neutral endopeptidase in transformed human tracheal epithelial cells. *Am J Physiol* 1991;260(Lung Cell Mol Physiol 4):L83–L89.
99. Bergstrand H, Björnson A, Blaschke E, et al. Effects of an inhaled corticosteroid, budesonide, on alveolar macrophage function in smokers. *Thorax* 1990;45:362–368.
100. Piedimonte G, McDonald DM, Nadel JA. Neutral endopeptidase and kininase II mediate glucocorticoid inhibition of neurogenic inflammation in the rat trachea. *J Clin Invest* 1991;88:40–44.
101. Shiratsuki N, Uyma O, Kitada O, et al. Effects of hydrocortisone and aminophylline on plasma leukotriene C_4 levels in patients during an asthmatic attack. *Prostaglandins Leukot Essent Fatty Acids* 1990;40:285–289.
102. Manso G, Baker AJ, Taylor IK, Fuller RW. In vivo and in vitro effects of glucocorticosteroids on arachidonic acid metabolism and monocyte function in nonasthmatic humans. *Eur Respir J* 1992;5:712–718.
103. Taylor IK, Shaw RJ. The mechanism of action of corticosteroids in asthma. *Respir Med* 1993;87:261–277.
103a. O'Shaughnessy KM, Wellings R, Gillies B, Fuller RW. Differential effects of fluticasone propionate on allergen-evoked bronchoconstriction and increased urinary leukotriene E_4 excretion. *Am Rev Respir Dis* 1993;147:1472–1476.
104. Di Rosa M, Radomski M, Carnuccio R, Moncada S. Glucocorticoids inhibit the induction of nitric oxide synthase in macrophages. *Biochem Biophys Res Commun* 1990;172:1246–1252.
105. Radomski MW, Palmer RMJ, Moncada S. Glucocorticoids inhibit the expression of an inducible, but not the constitutive nitric oxide synthase in vascular endothelial cells. *Proc Natl Acad Sci USA* 1990;87:10043–10049.
106. Barnes PJ. Nitric oxide and airways. *Eur Respir J* 1993;6:163–165.
107. Renkema TEJ, Postma DS, Noordhoek JA, Sluiter HJ, Kaufman HF. Influence of in vivo prednisolone on increased in vitro O_2 generation by neutrophils in emphysema. *Eur Respir J* 1993;6:90–95.
108. Mattoli S, Soloperto M, Marini M, Fasoli A. Levels of endothelin in the bronchoalveolar lavage fluid of patients with symptomatic asthma and reversible airflow obstruction. *J Allergy Clin Immunol* 1991;88:376–384.
109. Brattsand R, Delander EL, Peterson C, Wieslander E. Cytotoxicity of human phagocytes studied in vitro in a novel model based on neutral red absorption. *Agents Actions* 1991;34:35–37.
110. Moretti M, Giannico G, Marchioni CF, Bisetti A. Effects of methyl prednisolone on

sputum biochemical components in asthmatic bronchitis. *Eur J Respir Dis* 1984; 65:365–370.

111. Lundgren JD, Kaliner MA, Shelhamer JH. Mechanisms by which glucocorticosteroid inhibit secretion of mucus in asthmatic airways. *Am Rev Respir Dis* 1990;141:S52–S58.

112. Persson GCS, Erjefält I, Andersson P. Leakage of macromolecules from guinea pig tracheobronchial microcirculation. Effects of allergen, leukotrienes, tachykinins, and anti-asthma drugs. *Acta Physiol Scand* 1986;127:95–105.

113. Boschetto P, Rogers DF, Fabbri LM, Barnes PJ. Corticosteroid inhibition of airway microvascular leakage. *Am Rev Respir Dis* 1991;143:605–609.

114. Van de Graaf EA, Out TA, Loos CM, Jansen HM. Respiratory membrane permeability and bronchial hyperreactivity in patients with stable asthma. *Am Rev Respir Dis* 1991;143:362–368.

115. Erjefält I, Greiff L, Alkner U, Persson CGA. Allergen-induced biphasic plasma exudation responses in guinea-pig large airways. *Am Rev Respir Dis* 1993;148:695–701.

116. Werb Z. Biochemical actions of glucocorticoids on macrophages in culture. Specific inhibition of elastase, collagenase and plasminogen activator secretion and effects on other metabolic functions. *J Exp Med* 1978;147:1695–1712.

117. Saunders PR, Marshall JS. Dexamethasone induces a down regulation of rat mast cell protease II content in rat basophilic leukemia cells. *Agents Actions* 1992;36:4–10.

118. Lang Z, Murlas C. Neutral endopeptidase of a human airway epithelial cell line recovers after hypochlorous acid exposure: dexamethasone accelerates this by stimulating neutral endopeptidase mRNA synthesis. *Am J Respir Cell Mol Biol* 1992;7:300–306.

119. Solite E, Raugei G, Melli M, Parenta L. Dexamethasone induces the expression of the mRNA of lipocortin 1 and 2 and the release of lipocortin 1 and 5 in differentiated, but not undifferentiated U-937 cells. *FEBS Lett* 1991;291:238–244.

120. De Caterina R, Sicari R, Giannessi D, et al. Glucocorticoids, lipocortin 1 and eicosanoid synthesis inhibition in various populations of inflammatory cells: evidence for a cell selectivity in glucocorticoid action. 8th International Conference on Prostaglandins and Related Compounds. Montreal July 26–31, 1992.

121. Nakano T, Ohara O, Teraoka H, Arita H. Glucocorticoids suppress group II phospholipase A_2 production by blocking mRNA synthesis and post-transcriptional expression. *J Biol Chem* 1990;265:12745–12748.

122. Lin L-L, Clark J, Lin A, Sultzman L, Martin D, Knopf J. Hormonal regulation of a cytosolic phospholipase A_2 (cPLA$_2$). 8th International Conference on Prostaglandins and Related Compounds. Montreal July 26–31, 1992.

123. O'Banion MK, Winn W, Young DA. cDNA cloning and functional activity of a glucocorticoid-regulated inflammatory cyclooxygenase. *Proc Natl Acad Sci USA* 1992; 89:4888–4892.

124. Fuller RW, Kelsey CR, Cole PJ, Dollery CT, MacDermot J. Dexamethasone inhibits the production of thromboxane B_2 and leukotriene B_4 by human alveolar and peritoneal macrophages in culture. *Clin Sci* 1984;67:653–656.

125. Wieslander E, Linden M, Håkansson L, et al. Human alveolar macrophages from smokers have an impaired capacity to secrete LTB$_4$ but not other chemotactic factors. *Eur J Respir Dis* 1987;71:263–272.

126. Sebaldt RJ, Sheller JR, Oates JA, Roberts LJ II, Fitzgerald GA. Inhibition of eicosanoid biosynthesis by glucocorticoids in humans. *Proc Natl Acad Sci USA* 1990; 87:6974–6978.

127. Lim WH, Stewart AG. Regulation of eicosanoid generation in activated macrophages. *Int Arch Allergy Appl Immunol* 1991;95:77–85.

128. Andersson SE, Zackrisson C, Hemsen A, Lundberg JM. Regulation of lung endothelin content by the glucocorticosteroid budesonide. *Biochem Biophys Res Commun* 1992;188:1116–1121.

129. Vittori E, Marini M, Fasoli A, De Franchis R, Mattoli S. Increased expression of endothelin in bronchial epithelial cells of asthmatic patients and effect of corticosteroids. *Am Rev Respir Dis* 1992;146:1320–1325.

130. van de Stolpe A, Caldenhoven E, Raaijmakers JAM, van der Saag PT, Konderman L. Glucocorticoid-mediated repression on intercellular adhesion molecule 1 expression in human monocytic and bronchial epithelial cell lines. *Am J Respir Cell Mol Biol* 1993;8:340–347.

130a. Montefort S, Roche WR, Howarth PH, et al. Intercellular adhesion molecule-1 (ICAM-I) and endothelial leucocyte adhesion molecule-1 (ELAM-1) expression in the bronchial mucosa of normal and asthmatic subjects. *Eur Respir J* 1992;5:815–823.

131. Fisher JH, McCormack F, Park SS, Stelzner T, Shannon JM, Hofmann T. In vivo regulation of surfactant proteins by glucocorticoids. *Am J Respir Cell Mol Biol* 1991;5:63–70.

132. Lundgren J, Hirata F, Marom Z, et al. Dexamethasone inhibits respiratory glucoconjugate secretion from feline airways in vitro by the induction of lipocortin synthesis. *Am Rev Respir Dis* 1988;137:353–357.

133. Shimura S, Sasaki T, Ikeda K, Yamauchi K, Sasaki H, Takishima T. Direct inhibitory action of glucocorticoid on glucoconjugate secretion from airway submucosal glands. *Am Rev Respir Dis* 1990;141:1044–1049.

134. Hellewell PG, Williams TJ. An anti-inflammatory steroid inhibits tissue sensitization by IgE in vivo. *Br J Pharmacol* 1989;96:5–7.

135. Djukanovic R, Wilson JW, Britten KM, et al. Effect of an inhaled corticosteroid on airway inflammation and symptoms in asthma. *Am Rev Respir Dis* 1992;145:669–674.

136. Jeffery PK, Godfrey RW, Ädelroth E, Nelson F, Rogers A, Johansson S-Å. Effects of treatment on airway inflammation and thickening of basement membrane reticular collagen in asthma. *Am Rev Respir Dis* 1992;145:890–899.

137. Laitinen LA, Laitinen A, Haahtela T. A comparative study of the effects of an inhaled corticosteroid, budesonide, and a β_2-agonist, terbutaline, on airway inflammation in newly diagnosed asthma: a randomized, double blind, parallel-group controlled trial. *J Allergy Clin Immunol* 1992;90:32–42.

138. Bergstrand H, Lindquist B, Petersson B-Å. The glucocorticosteroid budesonide partially blocks histamine release from human lung tissue in vitro. *Allergy* 1986;41:319–329.

139. Dahl R, Johansson S-Å. Importance of duration of treatment with inhaled budesonide on the immediate and late bronchial reaction. *Eur J Respir Dis* 1982;63(suppl 122):167–175.

140. Schleimer RP. Effects of glucocorticosteroids on inflammatory cells relevant to their therapeutic applications in asthma. *Am Rev Respir Dis* 1990;141:S59–S69.

141. Durham SR. The significance of late responses in asthma. *Clin Exp Allergy* 1991;21:3–7.

142. Turner CR, Spannhake EWM. Acute topical steroid administration blocks mast cells increase and the late asthmatic response of the canine peripheral airways. *Am Rev Respir Dis* 1990;141:421–427.

143. Varney V, Gaga M, Frew AJ, de Vos C, Kay AB. The effect of single oral dose of prednisolone or cetirizine on inflammatory cells infiltrating allergen-induced cutaneous late-phase reactions in atopic subjects. *Clin Exp Allergy* 1992;22:43–49.

144. Andersson PT, Brattsand R. Protective effects of the glucocorticoid budesonide on lung anaphylaxis in actively sensitized guinea-pig: inhibition of IgE but not IgG-mediated anaphylaxis. *Br J Pharmacol* 1982;76:139–147.

145. Fischer A, König W. Influence of cytokines and cellular interactions on the glucocorticoid-induced Ig (E, G, A, M) synthesis of peripheral blood mononuclear cells. *Immunology* 1991;74:228–233.

146. Lappin DF, Whaley K. Modulation of complement gene expression by glucocorticoids. *Biochem J* 1991;280:117–123.

147. Persson CGA, Andersson PT, Gustafsson B. Budesonide reduces sensitivity to antigen but does not alter baseline tone or responsiveness to carbachol, terbutaline and enprofylline in IgE-sensitized guinea-pig trachea. *Int Arch Allergy Appl Immunol* 1989;88:381–385.

148. Andersson PT, Brange C, von Kogerer B, Sonmark B, Stahre G. Effect of glucocorticosteroid treatment on ovalbumin-induced IgE-mediated immediate and late allergic response in guinea-pig. *Int Arch Allergy Appl Immunol* 1988;87:32–39.

149. Abraham WM, Laues S, Stevenson JS, Yerger LD. Effect of an inhaled glucocorticosteroid (budesonide) on post-antigen induced increases in airway responsiveness. *Bull Eur Physiopathol Respir* 1986;22:387–392.

150. Gibson PG, Dolovich J, Girgis-Gabardo A, et al. The inflammatory response in asthma exacerbation: changes in circulating eosinophils, basophils and their progenitors. *Clin Exp Allergy* 1990;20:661–668.

151. Venge P, Dahl R, Karlström R, Pedersen B, Peterson CGB. Eosinophil and neutrophil activity in asthma in a one-year double-blind trial with theophylline and two doses of inhaled budesonide. *J Allergy Clin Immunol* 1992;89:190(A).

152. Wempe JB, Tammeling EP, Koëter GH, Håkansson L, Venge P, Postma DS. Blood eosinophil number and activity during 24 hours: effects of treatment with budesonide and bambuterol. *J Allergy Clin Immunol* 1992;90:757–765.

153. Venge P, Dahl R. Are blood eosinophil number and activity important for the development of the late asthmatic reaction after allergen challenge? *Eur Respir J* 1989;2(suppl 6):430s–434s.

154. Oda T, Katori M. Inhibition site of dexamethasone on extravasation of polymorphonuclear leukocytes in the hamster cheek pouch microcirculation. *J Leuko Biol* 1992;52:337–342.

155. Venge P, Håkansson L. The eosinophil and asthma. In: Kaliner MA, Barnes PJ, Persson CGA, eds. *Asthma, its pathology and treatment*, vol 49. New York: Marcel Dekker, 1991;477–502.

156. Cohen JJ. Lymphocyte death induced by glucocorticoids. In: Schleimer RP, Claman HN, Oronsky AL, eds. *Anti-inflammatory steroid action. Basic and clinical aspects*. San Diego: Academic Press, 1989;110–131.

157. Crompton MM, Cidlowski JA. Identification of a glucocorticoid-induced nuclease in thymocytes. *J Biol Chem* 1987;262:8288–8292.

158. Holgate ST, Wilson JR, Howarth PH. New insights into airway inflammation by endobronchial biopsy. *Am Rev Respir Dis* 1992;145:S2–S6.

159. Lundgren R, Söderberg M, Hörstedt P, Stenling R. Morphological studies of bronchial mucosal biopsies from asthmatics before and after 10 years of treatment with inhaled steroids. *Eur Respir J* 1988;1:883–889.

160. Bentley AM, Robinson DS, Assoufi B, Kay AB, Durham SR. The effect of prednisolone treatment on the local bronchial cellular infiltrate in asthma—reduction in eosinophils, T-lymphocytes and mast cells. *J Allergy Clin Immunol* 1993;91:222.

160a. Duddridge M, Ward C, Hendrick DJ, Walters EH. Changes in bronchoalveolar lavage inflammatory cells in asthmatic patients treated with high dose inhaled beclomethasone dipropionate. *Eur Respir J* 1993;6:489–497.

161. Ädelroth E, Rosenhall L, Johansson SA, Linden M, Venge P. Inflammatory cells and eosinophil activity in asthmatics investigated by bronchoalveolar lavage. *Am Rev Respir Dis* 1990;142:91–99.

162. Burke C, Power CK, Norris A, Condez A, Schmekel B, Poulter LW. Lung function and immunopathological changes after inhaled corticosteroid therapy in asthma. *Eur Respir J* 1992;5:73–79.

163. Bascom R, Wachs M, Naclerio RM, Pipkorn U, Lichtenstein LM, Galli SJ. Basophil influx occurs after nasal antigen challenge: effects of topical corticosteroid pretreatment. *J Allergy Clin Immunol* 1988;81:580–589.

164. Holgate ST, Wilson JR, Howard PH. New insights into airway inflammation by endobronchial biopsy. *Am Rev Respir Dis* 1992;145:S2–S6.

165. Boschetto P, Fabbri LM, Zocca E, et al. Prednisone inhibits late asthmatic reactions and airway inflammation induced by toluene diisocyanate in sensitized subjects. *J Allergy Clin Immunol* 1987;80:261–267.

166. Ramsdell JW, Berry CC, Clausen JL. The immediate effects of cortisol on pulmonary function in normals and asthmatics. *J Allergy Clin Immunol* 1983;71:69–74.

167. Gustafsson B, Persson CGA. Effect of three weeks' treatment with budesonide on in vitro contractile and relaxant airway effects in the rat. *Thorax* 1989;44:24–27.

168. Fraser CM, Venter JC. Beta-adrenergic receptors. Relationship of primary structure, receptor function and regulation. *Am Rev Respir Dis* 1990;141:S22–S30.

169. Mak JCW, Adcock I, Barnes PJ. Dexamethasone increases β_2-adrenoceptor gene expression in human lung. *Am Rev Respir Dis* 1992;145:A834.

170. Morrow-Brown H. The introduction and early development of inhaled steroid therapy. In: Mygind N, Clark TJH, eds. *Topical steroid treatment for asthma and rhinitis*. London: Baillière Tindall, 1980;66–76.

171. Schleimer RP, Kato M. Regulation of lung inflammation by local glucocorticoid metabolism: an hypothesis. *J Asthma* 1992;29:303–317.

172. Vichyanond P, Irvin CG, Larsen GL, Szefler SJ, Hill M. Penetration of corticosteroids

into the lung: evidence for difference between methylprednisolone and prednisolone. *J Allergy Clin Immunol* 1989;84:867–873.

173. Braude AS, Rebuck AS. Prednisolone and methylprednisolone disposition in the lung. *Lancet* 1983;2:995–997.

174. Greos LS, Vichyanond P, Bloedow DC, et al. Methylprednisolone achieves greater concentrations in the lung than prednisolone. A pharmacokinetic analysis. *Am Rev Respir Dis* 1991;144:586–592.

175. Hill MR, Szefler SJ, Ball BD, Bartoszek M, Brenner AM. Monitoring glucocorticoid therapy: a pharmacokinetic approach. *Clin Pharmacol Ther* 1990;48:390–398.

176. Reiss WG, Slaughter RL, Ludwig EA, Middleton E, Jusko WJ. Steroid dose-sparing: pharmacodynamic responses to single versus divided doses of methylprednisolone in man. *J Allergy Clin Immunol* 1990;85:1058–1066.

177. Szefler SJ. Measuring the response to glucocorticoids. *J Allergy Clin Immunol* 1990;85:985–987.

178. Szefler SJ. Glucocorticoid therapy for asthma: clinical pharmacology. *J Allergy Clin Immunol* 1991;88:147–165.

179. Fisher LE, Ludwig EA, Wald JA, Sloan RR, Middleton E, Jusko WJ. Pharmacokinetics and pharmacodynamics of methylprednisolone when administered at 8 am versus 4 pm. *Clin Pharmacol Ther* 1992;51:677–688.

180. Toogood JH, Lefcoe NM. Dexamethasone aerosol for the treatment of steroid dependent chronic bronchial asthmatic patients. *J Allergy* 1965;36:321–332.

181. Martin LE, Tanner RJN, Clark TJH, Cochrane GM. Absorption and metabolism of orally administered beclomethasone dipropionate. *Clin Pharmacol Ther* 1974;15:267–275.

182. Harris DM. Clinical pharmacology of beclomethasone dipropionate. In: Mygind N, Clark TJH, eds. *Topical steroid treatment for asthma and rhinitis*. London: Ballière Tindall, 1980;34–47.

183. Smith DA. Species differences in metabolism and pharmacokinetics: are we close to an understanding? *Drug Metab* 1991;23:355–373.

184. Mygind N, Clark TJH. *Topical steroid treatment for asthma and rhinitis*. London: Ballière Tindall, 1980.

185. Brattsand R, Thalén A, Roempke K, Källström L, Gruvstad E. Influence of 16α,17α-acetal substitution and steroid nuclear fluorination on the topical to systemic activity ratio of glucocorticoids. *J Steroid Biochem* 1982;16:779–786.

186. Clark TJH, Mygind N, Selroos O. Corticosteroid treatment in asthma. *Eur J Respir Dis* 1982;63(suppl 122):9–278.

187. Brogden RN, McTavish D. Budesonide. An updated review of its pharmacological properties and therapeutic efficacy in asthma and rhinitis. *Drugs* 1992;44:375–407.

188. Chaplin MD, Cooper WC, Segre EJ, Oren J, Jones RE, Nerenberg C. Correlation of flunisolide plasma levels to eosinopenic response in humans. *J Allergy Clin Immunol* 1980;65:445–453.

189. Phillips GH. Structure-activity relationship of topically active steroids: the selection of fluticasone propionate. *Respir Med* 1990;84(suppl A):19–23.

190. Harding S. The human pharmacology of fluticasone propionate. *Respir Med* 1990;84(suppl A):25–29.

191. Rohdewald P, von Eift M, Würthwein G. Aktivierung von Beclometason-dipropionat im BronchialSekret sowie Rezeptoraffinität und Löslichkeit inhalativ angewandter Glukokortikoide. *Atemw Lungenkrkh* 1990;16:79–84.

192. Brattsand R, Axelsson B. New inhaled glucocorticosteroids In: Barnes PJ, ed. *New drugs for asthma*. London: IBC Techn Serv, 1992;192–207.

193. Würthwein G, Rehder S, Rohdewald P. Lipophilicity and receptor affinity of glucocorticoids. *Pharm Ztg Wiss* 1992;137:161–167.

194. Johansson S-Å, Andersson K-A, Brattsand R, Gruvstad E, Hedner P. Topical and systemic glucocorticoid potencies of budesonide, beclomethasone dipropionate and prednisolone in man. *Eur J Respir Dis* 1982;63(suppl 122):74–82.

195. Edsbäcker S. *Studies on the metabolic fate and human pharmacokinetics of budesonide*. Thesis, University of Lund, 1986.

196. Toothaker RD, Craig WA, Welling PG. Effect of dose size on the pharmacokinetics of oral hydrocortisone suspension. *J Pharm Sci* 1982;71:1182–1185.

197. Rose J, Yurchak A, Meikle M, Jusko W. Effect of smoking on prednisone, prednisolone and dexamethasone pharmacokinetics. *J Pharmacokin Biopharm* 1981;9:1–14.

198. Derendorf H, Möllman H, Rohdewald P, Rehder J, Schmidt EW. Kinetics of methylprednisolone and its hemisuccinate ester. *Clin Pharmacol Ther* 1985;37:502–507.

199. Ryrfeldt Å, Andersson P, Edsbäcker S, Tönnesson M, Davies D, Pauwels R. Pharmacokinetics and metabolism of budesonide, a selective glucocorticoid. *Eur J Respir Dis* 1982;63(suppl 122):86–95.

200. Selroos O, Halme M. Effect of a volumatic spacer and mouth rinsing on systemic absorption of inhaled corticosteroids from metered dose inhaler and dry powder inhaler. *Thorax* 1991;46:891–894.

201. Thorsson L, Edsbäcker S. Lung deposition of budesonide from Turbuhaler is twice that from a pressurized metered dose inhaler. *Thorax* 1993;48:434.

202. Andersson PH, Ryrfeldt Å. Biotransformation of the topical glucocorticoids budesonide and beclomethasone 17α,21-dipropionate in human liver and lung homogenate. *J Pharm Pharmacol* 1984;36:763–765.

203. Ryrfeldt Å, Edsbäcker S, Pauwels R. Kinetics of the epimeric glucocorticoid budesonide. *Clin Pharmacol Ther* 1984;35:525–530.

204. Edsbäcker S, Jönsson S, Lindberg C, Ryrfeldt Å, Thalén A. Metabolic pathways of the topical glucocorticoid budesonide in man. *Drug Metab Dispos* 1983;11:590–596.

205. Edsbäcker S, Andersson P, Lindberg C, Paulsson J, Ryrfeldt Å, Thalén A. Liver metabolism of budesonide in rat, mouse, and man. Comparative aspects. *Drug Metab Dispos* 1987;15:403–411.

206. Edsbäcker S, Andersson P, Lindberg C, Ryrfeldt Å, Thalén A. Metabolic acetal splitting of budesonide. A novel inactivation pathway for topical glucocorticoids. *Drug Metab Dispos* 1987;15:412–417.

207. Toogood JH, Frankish CW, Jennings BH, et al. A comparison of the antiasthmatic efficacy of inhaled versus oral budesonide. *J Allergy Clin Immunol* 1990;85:872–880.

208. Toogood JH, Baskerville J, Jennings B, Lefcoe NM, Johansson S-Å. Bioequivalent doses of budesonide and prednisone in moderate and severe asthma. *J Allergy Clin Immunol* 1989;84:688–700.

209. Van den Bosch JMM, Westmann CJJ, Aumann J, Edsbäcker S, Tönnesson M, Selroos O. Relationship between lung tissue and blood plasma concentrations of inhaled budesonide. *Biopharm Drug Dispos* 1993;14:455–459.

210. Miller-Larsson A, Lundin P, Brattsand R. Affinity for airway tissue of topical glucocorticosteroid budesonide but not hydrocortisone—study in a rat tracheal model in situ. *Eur Respir J* 1992;5:364s.

211. Ryrfeldt Å, Persson G, Nilsson E. Pulmonary disposition of the potent glucocorticoid budesonide, evaluated in an isolated perfused rat lung model. *Biochem Pharmacol* 1989;38:17–22.

212. Campbell LM, Watson DG, Venables TL, Taylor MD, Richardson PD. Once daily budesonide Turbuhaler compared with placebo as initial prophylactic therapy for asthma. *Br J Clin Res* 1991;2:111–122.

213. Jones AH, Langdon CG, Lee PS, et al. Pulmicort Turbuhaler once daily as initial prophylactic therapy for asthma. *Resp Med* (in press).

214. Chanoine F, Grenot C, Heidmann P, Junien JL. Pharmacokinetics of butixocort 21-propionate, budesonide and beclomethasone dipropionate in the rat after intratracheal, intravenous and oral treatments. *Drug Metab Dispos* 1991;19:546–553.

215. Würthwein G, Rohdewald P. Activation of beclomethasone dipropionate by hydrolysis to beclomethasone-17-monopropionate. *Biopharm Drug Dispos* 1990;11:381–394.

216. Löfdahl C-G, Mellstrand T, Svedmyr N. Glucocorticoids and asthma. Studies of resistance and systemic effects of glucocorticoids. *Eur J Respir Dis* 1984;65(suppl 136):69–77.

217. Bisgaard H, Damkjaer Nilsen M, Andersen B, et al. Adrenal function in children with bronchial asthma treated with beclomethasone dipropionate or budesonide. *J Allergy Clin Immunol* 1988;81:1088–1095.

218. Pedersen S, Fuglsang G. Urine cortisol excretion in children treated with high doses of inhaled corticosteroids: a comparison of budesonide and beclomethasone. *Eur Respir J* 1988;1:433–435.

219. Jennings BH, Larsson B, Andersson K-E, Johansson S-Å. The assessment of systemic

effects of inhaled glucocorticosteroids: a comparison of budesonide and beclomethasone dipropionate in healthy volunteers. In: Jennings BH. *Assessment of systemic effects of inhaled glucocorticosteroids*. Thesis, University of Lund, 1990;VII:1–14.

220. Ali NJ, Capewell S, Ward MJ. Bone turnover during high dose inhaled corticosteroid treatment. *Thorax* 1991;46:160–164.

221. Zaborny BA, Lukacsko P, Barinov-Colligon I, Ziemniak JA. Inhaled corticosteroids in asthma: a dose-proportionality study with triamcinolone acetonide aerosol. *J Clin Pharmacol* 1992;32:463–469.

222. Barnes NC, Marone G, Di Maria GU, Visser S, Utama I, Payne SL. A comparison of fluticasone propionate, 1 mg daily, with beclomethasone dipropionate, 2 mg daily, in the treatment of severe asthma. *Eur Respir Dis* 1993;6:877–884.

223. Andersson PH, Brattsand R, Dahlström K, Edsbäcker S. Oral bioavailability of fluticasone propionate. *Br J Clin Pharmacol* 1993;36:135–136.

224. Nelson HS, Hamilos DL, Corsello PR et al. A double-blind study of troleandomycin and methylprednisolone in asthmatic subjects who require daily corticosteroids. *Am Rev Respir Dis* 1993;147:398–404.

225. Öst L. Effects of cyclosporin on prednisolone metabolism. *Lancet* 1984;1:451.

226. David DS, Grieco MH, Cushman P Jr. Adrenal glucocorticoids after twenty years. A review of their clinically relevant consequences. *J Chron Dis* 1970;22:637–711.

227. Axelrod L. Glucocorticoid therapy. *Medicine (Baltimore)* 1976;55:39–65.

228. Amatruda TT Jr, Hollingsworth DR, D'Esopo ND, Upton GV, Bondy PK. A study of the mechanism of the steroid withdrawal syndrome. Evidence for integrity of the hypothalamic-pituitary-adrenal system. *J Clin Endocrinol Metab* 1960;20:339–354.

229. Dixon RB, Christy NP. On the various forms of corticosteroid withdrawal syndrome. *Am J Med* 1980;68:224–230.

230. Byyny RL. Withdrawal from glucocorticoid therapy. *N Engl J Med* 1976;295:30–32.

231. Christy NP. Corticosteroid withdrawal. In: Bayless TM, Brian MC, Cherniack RM, eds. *Current therapy in internal medicine 1984–1985*. Philadelphia: BC Decker, 1984;535–545.

232. Schlaghecke R, Kornely E, Santen R Th, Ridderskamp P. The effect of long-term glucocorticoid therapy on pituitary-adrenal responses to exogenous corticotropin-releasing hormone. *N Engl J Med* 1992;326:226–230.

233. Myles AB, Bacon PA, Daly JR. Single daily dose corticosteroid treatment. Effect on adrenal function and therapeutic efficacy in various diseases. *Ann Rheum Dis* 1971;30:149–153.

234. Beam WR, Torvik JA, Suh BY, Martin RJ. Timing of prednisone and influence on sleep in nocturnal asthma. *Am Rev Respir Dis* 1992;145(4, part 2):A421.

235. Harter JG, Reddy WJ, Thorn GW. Studies on an intermittent corticosteroid dosage regimen. *N Engl J Med* 1963;269:591–596.

236. Shaw NJ, Edmunds AT. Inhaled beclomethasone and oral candidiasis. *Arch Dis Child* 1986;61:788–790.

237. Cayton RM, Soutar CA, Stanford CS, Turner GC, Nunn AJ. Double-blind trial comparing two dosage schedules of beclomethasone dipropionate aerosol in the treatment of chronic bronchial asthma. *Lancet* 1974;2:303–306.

238. Toogood JH, Jennings B, Greenway RW, Chuang L. Candidiasis and dysphonia complicating beclomethasone treatment of asthma. *J Allergy Clin Immunol* 1980;65:145–153.

239. Smith MJ, Hodson ME. High-dose beclomethasone inhaler in the treatment of asthma. *Lancet* 1983;1:265–269.

240. Toogood JH, Jennings B, Baskerville J, Anderson J, Johansson SA. Dosing regimen of budesonide and occurrence of oropharyngeal complications. *Eur J Respir Dis* 1984;65:35–44.

241. Toogood JH, Baskerville J, Jennings B, Lefcoe NM, Johansson S-A. Use of spacers to facilitate inhaled corticosteroid treatment of asthma. *Am Rev Respir Dis* 1984; 129:723–729.

242. Toogood JH, Jennings B, Baskerville J, Lefcoe N, Newhouse M. Assessment of a device for reducing oropharyngeal complications during beclomethasone treatment of asthma. *Am Rev Respir Dis* 1981;123(4, part 2):113.

243. Salzman GA, Pyszczynski DR. Oropharyngeal candidiasis in patients treated with be-

clomethasone dipropionate delivered by metered-dose inhaler alone and with Aerochamber. *J Allergy Clin Immunol* 1988;81:424–428.
244. Williams AJ, Baghat MS, Stableforth DE, Cayton RM, Shenoi PM, Skinner C. Dysphonia caused by inhaled steroids: recognition of a characteristic laryngeal abnormality. *Thorax* 1983;38:813–821.
245. Engel T. Patient-related side effects of CFC propellants. *J Aerosol Med* 1991;4:163–167.
246. Nicklas RA. Paradoxical bronchospasm associated with the use of inhaled beta agonists. *J Allergy Clin Immunol* 1990;85:959–964.
247. Särnstrand B, Jeppsson Å, Malmström A, Brattsand R. Effect of glucocorticoids on hyaluronic acid synthesis in vitro in human fibroblast-like cells from lung and skin. In: Hogg JC, Ellul-Micallef R, Brattsand R, eds. *Glucocorticosteroids, inflammation and bronchial hyperreactivity.* Amsterdam: Excerpta Medica, 1985;157–166.
248. Andersson E, Smidt CM, Sikjaer B, Ainge G, Poynter D. Bronchial biopsies after beclomethasone dipropionate aerosol. *Br J Dis Chest* 1977;77:35–43.
249. Lundgren R. Scanning electron microscopic studies of bronchial mucosa before and during treatment with beclomethasone dipropionate inhalations. *Scand J Respir Dis* 1977;suppl 101:179–187.
250. Thiringer G, Eriksson N, Malmberg R, Svedmyr N, Zettergren L. Bronchoscopic biopsies of bronchial mucosa before and after beclomethasone dipropionate therapy. *Scand J Respir Dis* 1977;suppl 101:173–177.
251. Laursen LC, Taudorf E, Borgeskov S, Kobayasi T, Jensen H, Weeke B. Fiberoptic bronchoscopy and bronchial mucosal biopsies in asthmatics undergoing long-term high-dose budesonide aerosol treatment. *Allergy* 1988;43:284–288.
252. Holmberg K, Pipkorn U. Influence of topical beclomethasone dipropionate suspension on human nasal mucociliary activity. *Eur J Clin Pharmacol* 1986;30:625–627.
253. Messerli Ch, Studer H, Scherrer M. Systemic side effects of beclomethasone dipropionate aerosols (Becotide, Aldecine, Sanasthmyl) in otherwise non steroid treated asthmatic patients. *Pneumonology* 1975;153:29–42.
254. Brown PH, Blundell G, Greening AP, Crompton GK. Screening for hypothalamo-pituitary-adrenal axis suppression in asthmatics taking high dose inhaled corticosteroids. *Respir Med* 1991;85:511–516.
255. Godfrey S, König P. Treatment of childhood asthma for 13 months and longer with beclomethasone dipropionate aerosol. *Arch Dis Child* 1974;49:591–596.
256. Prahl P, Jensen T, Bjerregard-Andersen H. Adrenocortical function in children on high-dose steroid aerosol therapy. *Allergy* 1987;42:541–544.
257. Law CM, Marchant JL, Honour JW, Preece MA, Warner JO. Nocturnal adrenal suppression in asthmatic children taking inhaled beclomethasone dipropionate. *Lancet* 1986;1:942–944.
258. Pecora R, Cherubini V, Guazzarotti L, et al. Beclomethasone dipropionate in childhood asthma: effect on HPA function and GH secretion. *Allergy* 1992;47(suppl 12):227.
259. Bisgaard H, Pedersen S, Damkjaer Nielsen M, Osterballe O. Adrenal function in asthmatic children treated with inhaled budesonide. *Acta Paediatr Scand* 1991;80:213–217.
260. Ribeiro LB. A 12 months tolerance study with budesonide in asthmatic children. In: Godfrey S, ed. *Glucocorticosteroids in childhood asthma.* Amsterdam: Excerpta Medica, 1987;95–108.
261. Varsano I, Volovitz B, Malik H, Amir Y. Safety of 1 year of treatment with budesonide in young children with asthma. *J Allergy Clin Immunol* 1990;85:914–920.
262. Costello JF, Clark TJH. Response of patients receiving high dose beclomethasone dipropionate. *Thorax* 1974;29:571–573.
263. Gaddie J, Petrie GR, Reid IW, Sinclair DJM, Skinner C, Palmer KNV. Aerosol beclomethasone dipropionate: a dose-response study in chronic bronchial asthma. *Lancet* 1973;2:280–281.
264. Sherman B, Weinberger M, Chen-Walden H, Wendt H. Further studies of the effects of inhaled glucocorticoids on pituitary-adrenal function in healthy adults. *J Allergy Clin Immunol* 1982;69:208–212.
265. Smith MJ, Hodson ME. Effects of long term inhaled high dose beclomethasone dipropionate on adrenal function. *Thorax* 1983;38:676–681.
266. Gordon ACH, McDonald CF, Thomson SA, Frame MH, Pottage A, Crompton GK.

Dose of inhaled budesonide required to produce clinical suppression of plasma cortisol. *Eur J Respir Dis* 1987;71:10–14.
267. Ädelroth E. Prednisolone-sparing effects of budesonide: European experiences and cost savings. In: Hargreave FE, Hogg JC, Malo J-L, Toogood JH, eds. *Glucocorticoids and mechanisms of asthma*. Amsterdam: Excerpta Medica, 1989;125–131.
268. Brown PH, Blundell G, Greening AP, Crompton GK. Hypothalamo-pituitary-adrenal axis suppression in asthmatics inhaling high dose corticosteroids. *Respir Med* 1991;85:501–510.
269. Johansson SA, Andersson KE, Brattsand R, Gruvstad E, Hedner P. Topical and systemic glucocorticoid potencies of budesonide and beclomethasone dipropionate in man. *Eur J Clin Pharmacol* 1982;22:523–529.
270. Selroos O, Backman R, Löfroos A-B, Niemistö M, Pietinalho A, Riska H. Corticosteroid inhalation is more effective with Turbuhaler than with pressurised MDI with spacer. *Allergy* 1993;48(suppl 16):26.
271. Ebden P, Jenkins A, Houston G, Davies BH. Comparison of two high dose corticosteroid aerosol treatments, beclomethasone dipropionate (1500 μg/day) and budesonide (1600 μg/day) for chronic asthma. *Thorax* 1986;41:869–874.
272. Toogood JH, Jennings B, Baskerville JC. Aerosol corticosteroids. In: Weiss EB, Stein MS, Segal M, eds. *Bronchial asthma: mechanisms and therapeutics*. Boston: Little, Brown, 1985;698–713.
273. Lal S, Harris DM, Bhalla KK, Singhal SN, Butler AG. Comparison of beclomethasone dipropionate aerosol and prednisolone in reversible airways obstruction. *BMJ* 1972; 3:314–317.
274. Ädelroth E, Rosenhall L, Glennow C. High dose inhaled budesonide in the treatment of severe steroid-dependent asthmatics. *Allergy* 1985;40:58–64.
275. Petri E. Therapieerfolge mit Budesonide (Pulmicort) beim corticosteroidbedürftigen Intrinsic Asthma. *Schweiz Med Wochenschr* 1985;115:1782–1784.
276. Laursen LC, Taudorf E, Weeke B. High-dose inhaled budesonide in treatment of severe steroid-dependent asthma. *Eur J Respir Dis* 1986;68:19–28.
277. Tarlo SM, Broder I, Davies GM, Leznoff A, Mintz S, Corey PN. Six-months double-blind, controlled trial of high dose, concentrated beclomethasone dipropionate in the treatment of severe chronic asthma. *Chest* 1988;93:998–1002.
278. Harrison BDW, Rees LH, Cayton RM, Nabarro JDN. Recovery of hypothalamo-pituitary-adrenal function in asthmatics whose oral steroids have been stopped or reduced. *Clin Endocrinol* 1992;17:109–118.
279. Toogood JH, Jennings B, Baskerville J, Lefcoe NM. Personal observations on the use of inhaled corticosteroid drugs for chronic asthma. *Eur J Respir Dis* 1984;65:321–338.
280. Wong J, Black P. Acute adrenal insufficiency associated with high dose inhaled steroids. *BMJ* 1992;304:1415.
281. Zwaan CM, Odink RJH, Delemarre-van de Waal HA, Dankert-Roelse JE, Bokma JA. Acute adrenal insufficiency after discontinuation of inhaled corticosteroid therapy. *Lancet* 1992;340:1289–1290.
282. Falliers CJ, Tan LS, Szentivanyi J, Jörgensen JR, Bukantz SC. Childhood asthma and steroid therapy as influences on growth. *Am J Dis Child* 1963;105:127–137.
283. Spock A. Growth pattern in 200 children with bronchial asthma. *Ann Allergy* 1965;23:608–615.
284. Balfour-Lynn L. Growth retardation in asthmatic children treated with inhaled beclomethasone dipropionate. *Lancet* 1988;1:475–476.
285. Balfour-Lynn L. Growth and childhood asthma. *Arch Dis Child* 1986;61:1049–1055.
286. Chang KC, Miklich DR, Barwise G, Chai H, Miles-Lawrence R. Linear growth of chronic asthmatic children: the effects of the disease and various forms of steroid therapy. *Clin Allergy* 1982;12:369–378.
287. Selroos O. The effects of inhaled corticosteroids on the natural history of obstructive lung diseases. *Eur Respir Rev* 1991;1:354–365.
288. Tinkelman DG, Reed CE, Nelson HS, Offord KP. Aerosol beclomethasone dipropionate compared with theophylline as primary treatment of chronic, mild to moderately severe asthma in children. *Pediatrics* 1993;92:64–77.
289. Ninan TK, Russell G. Asthma, inhaled corticosteroid treatment, and growth. *Arch Dis Child* 1992;67:703–705.

290. Wolthers OD, Pedersen S. Short term linear growth in asthmatic children during treatment with prednisolone. *BMJ* 1990;301:145–148.
291. Wolthers OD, Pedersen S. Controlled study of linear growth in asthmatic children during treatment with inhaled glucocorticosteroids. *Pediatrics* 1992;89:839–842.
292. Wales JKH, Milner RDG. Knemometry in assessment of linear growth. *Arch Dis Child* 1987;62:166–171.
293. Hermanussen M, Burmeister J. Standards for the predictive accuracy of short term body height and lower leg length measurements on half annual growth rates. *Arch Dis Child* 1989;64:259–263.
294. Reid DM, Nicholl JJ, Smith MA, Higgins B, Tothill P, Nuki G. Corticosteroids and bone mass in asthma: comparisons with rheumatoid arthritis and polymyalgia rheumatica. *BMJ* 1986;293:1463–1466.
295. Rees HA, Williams DA. Long-term steroid therapy in chronic intractable asthma. *BMJ* 1962;2:1575–1579.
296. Greenberger PA, Hendrix RW, Patterson R, Chmiel JS. Bone studies in patients on prolonged systemic corticosteroid therapy for asthma. *Clin Allergy* 1982;12:363–368.
297. Meeran K, Hattersley A, Burrin J, Shiner R, Ibbertson K. Oral and inhaled corticosteroids suppress bone formation. *Am Rev Respir Dis* 1991;143(4, part 2):A625.
298. Hodsman AB, Toogood JH, Jennings BH, Fraser LJ, Baskerville J. Differential effects of inhaled budesonide and oral prednisolone on serum osteocalcin. *J Clin Endocrinol Metab* 1991;72:530–540.
299. Toogood JH, Crilly RG, Jones G, Nadeau J, Wells GA. Effect of high-dose inhaled budesonide on calcium and phosphate metabolism and the risk of osteoporosis. *Am Rev Respir Dis* 1988;138:57–61.
300. Puolijoki H, Liippo K, Herrala J, Salmi J, Risteli J, Tala E. Does high dose inhaled beclomethasone (BDP) effect the calcium metabolism? *Eur Respir J* 1991;4(suppl 14):483s.
301. Pouw EM, Prummel MF, Oosting H, Roos CM, Endert E. Beclomethasone inhalation decreases serum osteocalcin concentrations. *BMJ* 1991;302:627–628.
302. Peretz A, Bourdoux PP. Inhaled corticosteroids, bone formation, and osteocalcin. *Lancet* 1991;338:1340.
303. König P, Cervantes C, Hillman L, Levine C, Douglas B, Maloney C. Bone mineralization in asthmatic children treated with inhaled beclomethasone. *J Allergy Clin Immunol* 1991;87:312.
304. Teelucksingh S, Padfield PL, Tibi L, Gough KJ, Holt PR. Inhaled corticosteroids, bone formation, and osteocalcin. *Lancet* 1991;338:60.
305. Wolthers OD, Juul Riis B, Pedersen S. Bone turnover in asthmatic children treated with inhaled budesonide. *Eur Respir J* 1992;5(suppl 15):311s.
305a. Leech JA, Hodder RV, Ooi DS, Gay J. Effects of short-term inhaled budesonide and beclomethasone dipropionate on serum osteocalcin in premenopausal women. *Am Rev Respir Dis* 1993;148:113–115.
306. Wolff AH, Adelsberg B, Aloia J, Zitt M. Effect of inhaled corticosteroid on bone density in asthmatic patients: a pilot study. *Ann Allergy* 1991;67:117–121.
307. Hatton MQF, Oldroyd B, Stead R, Belchetz PE, Smith MA, Cooke NJ. Bone mineral density changes in women taking inhaled corticosteroids. *Thorax* 1992;47:228P.
308. Stead RJ, Horsman A, Cooke NJ, Belchetz P. Bone mineral density in women taking inhaled corticosteroids. *Thorax* 1990;45:792.
309. Luengo M, Del Rio L, Guanabens N, Picado C. Long-term effect of oral and inhaled glucocorticoids on bone mass in chronic asthma. A two year follow-up study. *Eur Respir J* 1991;4(suppl 14):342s.
310. Packe GE, Douglas JG, McDonald AF, Robins SP, Reid DM. Bone density in asthmatic patients taking high dose inhaled beclomethasone dipropionate and intermittent systemic corticosteroids. *Thorax* 1992;47:414–417.
311. Rooklin AR, Lampert SI, Jaeger EA, McGeady SJ, Mansmann Jr HC. Posterior subcapsular cataracts in steroid-requiring asthmatic children. *J Allergy Clin Immunol* 1979;63:383–386.
312. Kewley GD. Possible association between beclomethasone dipropionate aerosol and cataracts. *Aust Paediatr J* 1980;16:117–118.

313. Allen MB, Ray SG, Leitch AG, Dhillon B, Cullen B. Steroid aerosols and cataract formation. *BMJ* 1989;299:432–433.
314. Karim AKA, Thompson GM, Jacob TJC. Steroid aerosol and cataract formation. *BMJ* 1989;299:918.
315. Toogood JH, Markov AE, Baskerville J, Dyson C. Association of ocular cataracts with inhaled and oral steroid therapy during long-term treatment of asthma. *J Allergy Clin Immunol* 1993;91:571–579.
315a. Simons FE, Persaud MP, Gillespie CA, Cheang M, Shuckett EP. Absence of posterior subcapsular cataracts in young patients treated with inhaled glucocorticoids. *Lancet* 1993;342:776–778.
316. Kruszynska YT, Greenstone M, Home PD, Cooke NJ. Effect of high dose inhaled beclomethasone dipropionate on carbohydrate and lipid metabolism in normal subjects. *Thorax* 1987;42:881–884.
317. Ebden P, McNally P, Samanta A, Fancourt GJ. The effects of high dose inhaled beclomethasone dipropionate on glucose and lipid profiles in normal and diet controlled diabetic subjects. *Respir Med* 1989;83:289–291.
318. Yernault J-C, Leclercq R, Schandevyl W, Virasoro E, De Coster A, Copinschi G. The endocrinometabolic effects of beclomethasone dipropionate in asthmatic patients. *Chest* 1977;71:698–702.
319. Goldstein DE, König P. Effect of inhaled beclomethasone dipropionate on hypothalamic-pituitary-adrenal axis function in children with asthma. *Pediatrics* 1983;72:60–64.
320. Turpeinen M, Sorva R, Juntunen-Backman K. Changes in carbohydrate and lipid metabolism in children with asthma inhaling budesonide. *J Allergy Clin Immunol* 1991;88:384–389.
321. Brompton Hospital/Medical Research Council. Double-blind trial comparing two dosage schedules of beclomethasone dipropionate aerosol with placebo in chronic bronchial asthma. *Br J Dis Chest* 1979;73:121–132.
322. Svedmyr J, Hedlin G, Nyberg E, Åsbrink Nilsson E. Efficacy of short-term courses of budesonide in children with asthma caused by respiratory infection. *Allergy* 1992;47(suppl 12):172.
323. Maxwell DL, Webb J. Adverse effects of inhaled corticosteroids. *BMJ* 1989;298:827–828.
324. Capewell S, Reynolds S, Shuttleworth D, Edwards C, Finlay AY. Purpura and dermal thinning associated with high dose inhaled corticosteroids. *BMJ* 1990;300:1548–1551.
325. Mak VHF, Melchor R, Spiro SG. Easy bruising as a side effect of inhaled corticosteroids. *Eur Respir J* 1992;5:1068–1074.
326. Bender BG, Lerner JA, Kollasch E. Mood and memory changes in asthmatic children receiving corticosteroids. *J Am Acad Child Adolesc Psychiatry* 1988;27:720–725.
327. Bender BG, Lerner JA, Poland JE. Association between corticosteroids and psychologic change in hospitalized asthmatic children. *Ann Allergy* 1991;66:414–419.
328. Fiel SB. Should corticosteroids be used in the treatment of acute, severe asthma? I. A case for the use of corticosteroids in acute, severe asthma. *Pharmacotherapy* 1985;5:327–331.
329. Mok J, Kattan M, Levison H. Should corticosteroids be used in the treatment of acute severe asthma? II. A case against the use of corticosteroids in acute, severe asthma. *Pharmacotherapy* 1985;5:331–335.
330. British Thoracic Society. Guidelines for management of asthma in adults: II—acute severe asthma. *BMJ* 1990;301:797–800.
331. Engel T, Heinig JH. Glucocorticosteroid therapy in acute severe asthma—a critical review. *Eur Respir J* 1991;4:881–889.
332. Medical Research Council. Controlled trial of effects of cortisone acetate in status asthmaticus. *Lancet* 1956;2:803–806.
333. Fanta CH, Rossing TH, McFadden ER. Glucocorticoids in acute asthma. A critical controlled trial. *Am J Med* 1983;74:845–851.
334. Littenberg B, Gluck EH. A controlled trial of methylprednisolone in the emergency treatment of acute asthma. *N Engl J Med* 1986;314:150–152.
335. Schneider SM, Pipher A, Britton HL, Borok Z, Harcup CH. High-dose methylprednisolone as initial treatment in patients with acute bronchospasm. *J Asthma* 1988;25:189–193.

336. McFadden ER Jr, Kiser R, DeGroot WJ, Holmes B, Kiker R, Viser G. A controlled study of the effects of single doses of hydrocortisone on the resolution of acute attacks of asthma. *Am J Med* 1976;60:52–59.
337. Luksza AR. Acute severe asthma treated without steroids. *Br J Dis Chest* 1982;76:15–19.
338. Stein LM, Cole RP. Early administration of corticosteroids in emergency room treatment of acute asthma. *Ann Intern Med* 1990;112:822–827.
339. Morell F, Orriols R, de Gracia J, Curull V, Pujol A. Controlled trial of intravenous corticosteroids in severe acute asthma. *Thorax* 1992;47:588–591.
340. Loren ML, Chai H, Leung P, Rohr C, Brenner AM. Corticosteroids in the treatment of acute exacerbations of asthma. *Ann Allergy* 1980;45:67–71.
341. Storr J, Barrell E, Barry W, Lenney W, Hatcher G. Effect of a single dose of prednisolone in acute childhood asthma. *Lancet* 1987;1:879–882.
342. Shapiro GG, Furukawa CT, Pierson WE, Gardinier R, Bierman CW. Double-blind evaluation of methylprednisolone versus placebo for acute asthma episodes. *Pediatrics* 1983;71:510–514.
343. Younger RE, Gerber PS, Herrod HG, Cohen RM, Crawford LV. Intravenous methylprednisolone efficacy in status asthmaticus of childhood. *Pediatrics* 1987;80:225–230.
344. Deshpande A, McKenzie SA. Short course of steroids in home treatment of children with acute asthma. *BMJ* 1986;293:169–171.
345. Harris JB, Weinberger MM, Nassif E, Smith G, Milavetz G, Stillerman A. Early intervention with short courses of prednisone to prevent progression of asthma in ambulatory patients incompletely responsive to bronchodilators. *J Pediatr* 1987;110:627–633.
346. Gleeson JGA, Loftus BG, Price JF. Placebo controlled trial of systemic corticosteroids in acute childhood asthma. *Acta Paediatr Scand* 1990;79:1052–1058.
347. Kattan M, Gurwitz D, Levison H. Corticosteroids in status asthmaticus. *J Pediatr* 1980;96:596–599.
348. Pierson WE, Bierman CW, Kelley VC. A double-blind trial of corticosteroid therapy in status asthmaticus. *Pediatrics* 1974;54:282–288.
349. Tal A, Bavilski C, Yohai D, Bearman JE, Gorodischer R, Moses SW. Dexamethasone and salbutamol in the treatment of acute wheezing in infants. *Pediatrics* 1983;71:13–18.
350. Springer C, Bar-Yishay E, Uwayyed K, Avital A, Vilozni D, Godfrey S. Corticosteroids do not affect the clinical or physiological status of infants with bronchiolitis. *Pediatr Pulmonol* 1990;9:181–185.
351. Haskell RJ, Wong BM, Hansen JE. A double-blind, randomized clinical trial of methylprednisolone in status asthmaticus. *Arch Intern Med* 1983;143:1324–1327.
352. Webb JR. Dose response of patients to oral corticosteroid treatment during exacerbations of asthma. *BMJ* 1986;292:1045–1047.
353. Britton MG, Collins JV, Brown D, Fairhurst NPA, Lambert RG. High-dose corticosteroids in severe acute asthma. *BMJ* 1976;2:73–74.
354. Harfi H, Hanissian AS, Crawford LV. Treatment of status asthmaticus in children with high doses and conventional doses of methylprednisolone. *Pediatrics* 1978;61:829–831.
355. Tanaka RM, Santiago SM, Kuhn GJ, Williams RE, Klaustermeyer WB. Intravenous methylprednisolone in adults in status asthmaticus. Comparison of two dosages. *Chest* 1982;82:438–440.
356. Harrison BDW, Stokes TC, Hart GJ, Vaughan DA, Ali NJ, Robinson AA. Need for intravenous hydrocortisone in addition to oral prednisolone in patients admitted to hospital with severe asthma without ventilatory failure. *Lancet* 1986;1:181–184.
357. Raimondi AC, Figueroa-Casas JC, Roncoroni AJ. Comparison between high and moderate doses of hydrocortisone in the treatment of status asthmaticus. *Chest* 1986;89:832–835.
358. Ratto D, Alfaro C, Sipsey J, Glowsky MM, Sharma OP. Are intravenous corticosteroids required in status asthmaticus? *JAMA* 1988;260:527–529.
359. Engel T, Dirksen A, Frölund L, et al. Methylprednisolone pulse therapy in acute severe asthma. A randomized, double-blind study. *Allergy* 1990;45:224–230.
360. Bowler SD, Mitchell CA, Armstrong JG. Corticosteroids in acute severe asthma: effectiveness of low doses. *Thorax* 1992;47:584–587.
361. Sue MA, Kwong FK, Klaustermeyer WB. A comparison of intravenous hydrocorti-

sone, methylprednisolone, and dexamethasone in acute bronchial asthma. *Ann Allergy* 1986;56:406–409.
362. Brunette MG, Lands L, Thibodeau L-P. Childhood asthma: prevention of attacks with short-term corticosteroid treatment of upper respiratory tract infection. *Pediatrics* 1988;81:624–629.
363. Fiel SB, Swartz MA, Glanz K, Francis ME. Efficacy of short-term corticosteroid therapy in outpatient treatment of acute bronchial asthma. *Am J Med* 1983;75:259–262.
364. Chapman KR, Verbeek PR, White JG, Rebuck AS. Effect of a short course of prednisone in the prevention of early relapse after the emergency room treatment of acute asthma. *N Engl J Med* 1991;324:788–794.
365. Falliers CJ, Chai H, Molk L, Bane H, Cardoso A. Pulmonary and adrenal effects of alternate-day corticosteroid therapy. *J Allergy Clin Immunol* 1972;49:156–166.
366. Dunnill MS. The pathology of asthma, with special reference to changes in the bronchial mucosa. *J Clin Pathol* 1960;13:27–33.
367. Dunnill MS, Massarella GR, Anderson JA. A comparison of the quantitative anatomy of the bronchi in normal subjects, in status asthmaticus, in chronic bronchitis, and in emphysema. *Thorax* 1969;24:176–179.
368. Laitinen LA, Heino M, Laitinen A, Kava T, Haahtela T. Damage of the airway epithelium and bronchial reactivity in patients with asthma. *Am Rev Respir Dis* 1985;131:599–606.
369. Godard P, Chantreuil J, Damon M, et al. Functional assessment of alveolar macrophages: comparison of cells from asthmatics and normal subjects. *J Allergy Clin Immunol* 1982;70:88–93.
370. de Monchy JGR, Kauffman HF, Venge P, et al. Bronchoalveolar eosinophilia during allergen-induced late asthmatic reactions. *Am Rev Respir Dis* 1985;131:373–376.
371. Metzger WJ, Zavala D, Richerson HB, et al. Local allergen challenge and bronchoalveolar lavage of allergic asthmatic lungs. Description of the model and local airway inflammation. *Am Rev Respir Dis* 1987;135:433–440.
372. Chung KF. Role of inflammation in the hyperreactivity of the airways in asthma. *Thorax* 1986;41:657–662.
373. Barnes PJ. New concept in the pathogenesis of bronchial hyperresponsiveness and asthma. *J Allergy Clin Immunol* 1989;83:1013–1026.
374. Hopp RJ, Townley RG, Biven RE, Bewtra AK, Nair NM. The presence of airway reactivity before the development of asthma. *Am Rev Respir Dis* 1990;141:2–8.
375. Woolcock A, Rubinfeld AR, Seale P, et al. Asthma management plan, 1989. *Med J Aust* 1989;151:650–653.
376. Hargreave FE, Dolovich J, Newhouse MT. The assessment and treatment of asthma: a conference report. *J Allergy Clin Immunol* 1990;85:1098–1111.
377. British Thoracic Society/Royal College of Physicians. Guidelines for management of asthma in adults: I—chronic persistent asthma. *BMJ* 1990;301:651–653.
378. National Heart, Lung, and Blood Institute/National Asthma Education Program/Expert Panel Report. Guidelines for the diagnosis and management of asthma. *J Allergy Clin Immunol* 1991;88:425–534.
379. Lorentzon S, Boe J, Eriksson G, Persson G. Use of inhaled corticosteroids in patients with mild asthma. *Thorax* 1990;45:733–735.
380. Juniper EF, Kline PA, Vanzieleghem MA, Ramsdale EH, O'Byrne PM, Hargreave FE. Effect of long-term treatment with an inhaled corticosteroid (budesonide) on airway hyperresponsiveness and clinical asthma in nonsteroid-dependent asthmatics. *Am Rev Respir Dis* 1990;142:832–836.
381. Juniper EF, Kline PA, Vanzieleghem MA, Hargreave FE. Reduction of budesonide after a year of increased use. A randomized controlled trial to evaluate whether improvements in airway responsiveness and clinical asthma are maintained. *J Allergy Clin Immunol* 1991;87:483–489.
382. Jeffery PK, Wardlaw AJ, Nelson FC, Collins JV, Kay AB. Bronchial biopsies in asthma. An ultrastructural, quantitative study and correlation with hyperreactivity. *Am Rev Respir Dis* 1989;140:1745–1753.
383. Ollerenshaw SL, Woolcock AJ. Characteristics of the inflammation in biopsies from large airways of subjects with asthma and subjects with chronic airflow limitation. *Am Rev Respir Dis* 1992;145:922–927.

384. Beasley R, Roche WR, Roberts JA, Holgate ST. Cellular events in the bronchi in mild asthma and after bronchial provocation. *Am Rev Respir Dis* 1989;139:806–817.
385. Bradley BL, Azzawi M, Jacobson M, et al. Eosinophils, T-lymphocytes, mast cells, neutrophils, and macrophages in bronchial biopsy specimens from atopic subjects with asthma: comparison with biopsy specimens from atopic subjects without asthma and normal control subjects and relationship to bronchial hyperresponsiveness. *J Allergy Clin Immunol* 1991;88:661–674.
386. Poston RN, Chanez P, Lacoste JY, Litchfield T, Lee TH, Bousquet J. Immunohisto-chemical characterization of the cellular infiltration in asthmatic bronchi. *Am Rev Respir Dis* 1992;145:918–921.
387. Kirby JG, Hargreave FE, Gleich GJ, O'Byrne PM. Bronchoalveolar cell profiles of asthmatics and nonasthmatic subjects. *Am Rev Respir Dis* 1987;136:379–383.
388. Wardlaw AJ, Dunnette S, Gleich GJ, Collins JV, Kay AB. Eosinophils and mast cells in bronchoalveolar lavage in subjects with mild asthma. *Am Rev Respir Dis* 1988;137:62–69.
389. Barnes PJ. The changing face of asthma. *Q J Med* 1987;63:359–365.
390. Laitinen LA, Laitinen A, Heino M, Haahtela T. Eosinophilic airway inflammation during exacerbation of asthma and its treatment with inhaled corticosteroid. *Am Rev Respir Dis* 1991;143:423–427.
391. Venge P, Dahl R, Peterson CGB. Eosinophil granule proteins in serum after allergen challenge of asthmatic patients and the effects of anti-asthmatic medication. *Int Arch Allergy Appl Immunol* 1988;87:306–312.
392. Woolcock AJ. Therapies to control the airway inflammation of asthma. *Eur J Respir Dis* 1986;69(suppl 147):166–174.
393. Woolcock AJ, Yan K, Salome CM. Effect of therapy on bronchial hyperresponsiveness in the long-term management of asthma. *Clin Allergy* 1988;18:165–176.
394. Bel EH, Timmers MC, Zwinderman AH, Dijkman JH, Sterk PJ. The effect of inhaled corticosteroids on the maximal degree of airway narrowing to metacholine in asthmatic subjects. *Am Rev Respir Dis* 1991;143:109–113.
395. Sterk PJ, Bel EH. The shape of the dose-response curve to inhaled bronchoconstrictor agents in asthma and in chronic obstructive pulmonary disease. *Am Rev Respir Dis* 1991;143:1433–1437.
396. Woolcock AJ, Jenkins C. Corticosteroids in the modulation of bronchial hyperresponsiveness. *Immunol Allergy Clin North Am* 1990;10:543–557.
397. Easton JG. Effect of an inhaled corticosteroid on metacholine airway reactivity. *J Allergy Clin Immunol* 1981;67:388–393.
398. Clarke PS. The effect of beclomethasone dipropionate on bronchial hyperreactivity. *J Asthma* 1982;19:91–93.
399. Juniper EF, Frith PA, Hargreave FE. Long-term stability of bronchial responsiveness to histamine. *Thorax* 1982;37:288–291.
400. Hartley JPR. The effect of budesonide on bronchial hyperreactivity. In: Hogg JC, El-lul-Micallef R, Brattsand R, eds. *Glucocorticosteroids, inflammation and bronchial hyperreactivity*. Amsterdam: Excerpta Medica, 1985;110–113.
401. Kraan J, Koeter GH, v d Mark ThW, Sluiter HJ, de Vries K. Changes in bronchial hyperreactivity induced by 4 weeks of treatment with antiasthmatic drugs in patients with allergic asthma: a comparison between budesonide and terbutaline. *J Allergy Clin Immunol* 1985;76:628–636.
402. Ryan G, Latimer KM, Juniper EF, Roberts RS, Hargreave FE. Effect of beclomethasone dipropionate on bronchial responsiveness to histamine in controlled nonsteroid-dependent asthma. *J Allergy Clin Immunol* 1985;75:25–30.
403. Dutoit JI, Salome CM, Woolcock AJ. Inhaled corticosteroids reduce the severity of bronchial hyperresponsiveness in asthma but oral theophylline does not. *Am Rev Respir Dis* 1987;136:1174–1178.
404. Kerrebijn KF, van Essen-Zandvliet EEM, Bosschaart A. The effect of inhaled gluco-corticosteroids on bronchial responsiveness. In: Godfrey S, ed. *Glucocorticosteroids in childhood asthma*. Amsterdam: Excerpta Medica, 1987;37–41.
405. Kerrebijn KF, van Essen-Zandvliet EEM, Neijens HJ. Effect of long-term treatment with inhaled corticosteroids and beta-agonists on the bronchial responsiveness in children with asthma. *J Allergy Clin Immunol* 1987;79:653–659.

406. Svendsen UG, Frolund L, Madsen F, Nielsen NH, Holstein-Rathlou N-H, Weeke B. A comparison of the effects of sodium cromoglycate and beclomethasone dipropionate on pulmonary function and bronchial hyperreactivity in subjects with asthma. *J Allergy Clin Immunol* 1987;80:68–74.
407. Ostergaard PA, Pedersen S. The effect of inhaled disodium cromoglycate and budesonide on bronchial responsiveness to histamine and exercise in asthmatic children: a clinical comparison. In: Godfrey S, ed. *Glucocorticosteroids in childhood asthma*. Amsterdam: Excerpta Medica, 1987;55–65.
408. Jenkins CR, Woolcock AJ. Effect of prednisone and beclomethasone dipropionate on airway responsiveness in asthma: a comparative study. *Thorax* 1988;43:378–384.
409. Molema J, van Herwaarden CLA, Folgering HThM. Effects of long-term treatment with inhaled cromoglycate and budesonide on bronchial hyperresponsiveness in patients with allergic asthma. *Eur Respir J* 1989;2:308–316.
410. Bel EH, Timmers MC, Hermans J, Dijkman JH, Sterk P. The long-term effects of nedocromil sodium and beclomethasone dipropionate on bronchial responsiveness to metacholine in nonatopic asthmatic subjects. *Am Rev Respir Dis* 1990;141:21–28.
411. de Baets FM, Goeteyn M, Kerrebijn KF. The effect of two months of treatment with inhaled budesonide on bronchial responsiveness to histamine and house-dust mite antigen in asthmatic children. *Am Rev Respir Dis* 1990;142:581–586.
412. Wilmsmeyer W, Ukena D, Wagner TOF, Sybrecht GW. First-time treatment with steroids in bronchial asthma: comparison of the effects of inhaled beclomethasone and of oral prednisone on airway function, bronchial reactivity and hypothalamic-pituitary-adrenal axis. *Eur Respir J* 1990;3:786–791.
413. ZuWallack RL, Kass J, Shiue S-T, et al. Effect of inhaled triamcinolone on bronchial hyperreactivity and airways obstruction in asthma. *Ann Allergy* 1990;64:207–212.
414. Fuller RW, Choudry NB, Eriksson G. Action of budesonide on asthmatic bronchial hyperresponsiveness. Effects on directly and indirectly acting bronchoconstrictors. *Chest* 1991;100:670–674.
415. Vathenen AS, Knox AJ, Wisniewski A, Tattersfield AE. Time course of change in bronchial reactivity with an inhaled corticosteroid in asthma. *Am Rev Respir Dis* 1991;143:1317–1321.
416. Orefice U, Struzzo P, Dorigo R, Peratoner A. Long-term treatment with sodium cromoglycate, nedocromil sodium and beclomethasone dipropionate reduces bronchial hyperresponsiveness in asthmatic subjects. *Respiration* 1992;59:97–101.
417. Dompeling E, van Schayck CP, Molema J, Folgering H, van Grunsven PM, van Weel C. Inhaled beclomethasone improves the course of asthma and COPD. *Eur Respir J* 1992;5:945–952.
418. Groot CAR, Lammers J-WJ, Molema J, Festen J, van Herwaarden CLA. Effect of inhaled beclomethasone and nedocromil sodium on bronchial hyperresponsiveness to histamine and destilled water. *Eur Respir J* 1992;5:1075–1082.
419. Wempe JB, Postma DS, Breederveld N, Alting-Hebing D, van der Mark TW, Koeter G. Separate and combined effects of corticosteroids and bronchodilators on airflow obstruction and airway hyperresponsiveness in asthma. *J Allergy Clin Immunol* 1992;89:679–687.
420. van Essen-Zandvliet EE, Hughes MD, Waalkens HJ, Duiverman EJ, Pocock SJ, Kerrebijn KF. Effects of 22 months of treatment with inhaled corticosteroids and/or beta-2-agonists on lung function, airway responsiveness, and symptoms in children with asthma. *Am Rev Respir Dis* 1992;146:547–554.
421. Kraan J, Koeter GH, van der Mark ThW, et al. Dosage and time effects of inhaled budesonide on bronchial hyperreactivity. *Am Rev Respir Dis* 1988;137:44–48.
422. Jenkins C, Goldberg H, Woolcock AJ. The effect of high dose inhaled budesonide on lung function and bronchial responsiveness to histamine in patients with asthma. *Am Rev Respir Dis* 1992;145:A461.
423. Owen S, Pickering CAC, Woodcock A. Effect of increasing doses of beclomethasone dipropionate (BDP) on bronchial hyperreactivity (BHR) in asthma. *Thorax* 1990;45:786.
424. Wolfe JD, Rosenthal RR, Bleecker E, Laube B, Norman PS, Permutt S. The effect of corticosteroids on cholinergic hyperreactivity. *J Allergy Clin Immunol* 1979;63:162.
425. Israel R, Poe RH, Wicks CM, Greenblatt DW. The protective effect of methylprednisolone on carbachol-induced bronchospasm. *Am Rev Respir Dis* 1984;130:1019–1022.

426. Mattoli S, Rosati G, Mormile F, Ciappi G. The immediate and short-term effects of corticosteroids on cholinergic hyperreactivity and pulmonary function in subjects with well-controlled asthma. *J Allergy Clin Immunol* 1985;76:214–222.

427. Sotamayor H, Badier M,Vervloet D, Orehek J. Seasonal increase of carbachol airway responsiveness in patients allergic to grass pollen. Reversal by corticosteroids. *Am Rev Respir Dis* 1984;130:56–58.

428. Bhagat RG, Grunstein MM. Effect of corticosteroids on bronchial responsiveness to metacholine in asthmatic children. *Am Rev Respir Dis* 1985;131:902–906.

429. Booij-Noord H, Orie NGM, de Vries K. Immediate and late bronchial obstructive reactions to inhalation of house dust and protective effects of disodium cromoglycate and prednisolone. *J Allergy Clin Immunol* 1971;48:344–354.

430. Pepys J, Davies RJ, Breslin ABX, Hendrick DJ, Hutchcroft BJ. The effects of inhaled beclomethasone dipropionate (Becotide) and sodium cromoglycate on asthmatic reactions to provocation tests. *Clin Allergy* 1974;4:13–24.

431. Cockcroft DW, Murdock KY. Comparative effects of inhaled salbutamol, sodium cromoglycate, and beclomethasone dipropionate on allergen-induced early asthmatic responses, late asthmatic responses and increased bronchial responsiveness to histamine. *J Allergy Clin Immunol* 1987;79:734–740.

432. Pelikan Z, Pelikan-Filipek M, Schoemaker MC, Berger MPF. Effects of disodium cromoglycate and beclomethasone dipropionate on the asthmatic response to allergen challenge I. Immediate response (IAR). *Ann Allergy* 1988;60:211–216.

433. Pelikan Z, Pelikan-Filipek M, Remeijer L. Effects of disodium cromoglycate and beclomethasone dipropionate on the asthmatic response to allergen challenge II. Late response (LAR). *Ann Allergy* 1988;60:217–225.

434. van der Star JG, Berg WC, Steenhuis EJ, de Vries K. The effect of aerosol administration of beclometasone dipropionate on reactive bronchial obstruction after inhalation of house dust. *Ned T Geneesk* 1976;120:1928–1932.

435. Burge PS. The effects of corticosteroids on the immediate asthmatic reaction. *Eur J Respir Dis* 1982;63(suppl 122):163–166.

436. Burge PS, Efthimiou J, Turner-Warwick M, Nelmes PTJ. Double-blind trials of inhaled beclomethasone dipropionate and fluocortin butyl ester in allergen-induced immediate and late asthmatic reactions. *Clin Allergy* 1982;12:523–531.

437. Venge P, Dahl R, Håkansson L. Heat-labile neutrophil chemotactic activity in subjects with asthma after allergen inhalation: relation to the late asthmatic reaction and effects of asthma medication. *J Allergy Clin Immunol* 1987;80:679–688.

438. Mapp C, Boschetto P, Dal Vecchio L, et al. Protective effect of antiasthma drugs on late asthmatic reactions and increased airway responsiveness induced by toluene diisocyanate in sensitized subjects. *Am Rev Respir Dis* 1987;136:1403–1407.

439. Fabbri LM, Chiesura-Corona P, Dal Vecchio L, et al. Prednisone inhibits late asthmatic reactions and the associated increase in airway responsiveness induced by toluenediisocyanate in sensitized subjects. *Am Rev Respir Dis* 1985;132:1010–1014.

440. Boe J, Rosenhall L, Alton M, et al. Comparison of dose-response effects of inhaled beclomethasone dipropionate and budesonide in the management of asthma. *Allergy* 1989;44:349–355.

441. Toogood JH, Lefcoe NM, Haines DSM, et al. A graded dose assessment of the efficacy of beclomethasone dipropionate aerosol for severe chronic asthma. *J Allergy Clin Immunol* 1977;59:298–308.

442. Toogood JH, Baskerville J, Errington N, Jennings B, Chuang L, Lefcoe N. Determinants of the response to beclomethasone aerosol at various dosage levels: a multiple regression analysis to identify clinically useful predictors. *J Allergy Clin Immunol* 1977;60:367–376.

443. Toogood JH, Baskerville JC, Jennings B, Lefcoe NM, Johansson SA. Influence of dosing frequency and schedule on the response of chronic asthmatics to the aerosol steroid, budesonide. *J Allergy Clin Immunol* 1982;70:288–298.

444. Toogood JH. High-dose inhaled steroid therapy for asthma. *J Allergy Clin Immunol* 1989;83:528–536.

445. Ellul-Micallef R, Johansson SA. Acute dose-response studies in bronchial asthma with a new corticosteroid, budesonide. *Br J Clin Pharmacol* 1983;15:419–422.

446. Tukiainen P, Lahdensuo A. Effect of inhaled budesonide on severe steroid-dependent asthma. *Eur J Respir Dis* 1987;70:239–244.

447. Johansson S-Å, Dahl R. A double-blind dose-response study of budesonide by inhalation in patients with bronchial asthma. *Allergy* 1988;43:173–178.
448. Juniper EF, Kline PA, Vanzieleghem MA, Ramsdale EH, O'Byrne PM, Hargreave FE. Long-term effects of budesonide on airway responsiveness and clinical asthma severity in inhaled steroid-dependent asthmatics. *Eur Respir J* 1990;3:1122–1127.
449. Sears MR, Taylor DR, Print CG, Lake DC, Herbison GP, Flannery EM. Increased inhaled bronchodilator vs increased inhaled corticosteroid in the control of moderate asthma. *Chest* 1992;102:1709–1715.
450. Field HV, Jenkinson PMA, Frame MH, Warner JO. Asthma treatment with a new corticosteroid aerosol, budesonide, administered twice daily by spacer inhaler. *Arch Dis Child* 1982;57:864–866.
451. Willey RF, Godden DJ, Carmichael J, Preston P, Frame M, Crompton GK. Comparison of twice daily administration of a new corticosteroid budesonide with beclomethasone dipropionate four times daily in the treatment of chronic asthma. *Br J Dis Chest* 1982;76:61–68.
452. Munch EP, Taudorf E, Weeke B. Dose frequency in the treatment of asthmatics with inhaled topical steroid. *Eur J Respir Dis* 1982;63(suppl 122):143–153.
453. Slavin RG, Izu AE, Bernstein IL, et al. Multicenter study of flunisolide aerosol in adult patients with steroid-dependent asthma. *J Allergy Clin Immunol* 1980;66:379–385.
454. Orgel HA, Meltzer EO, Kemp JP. Flunisolide aerosol in treatment of steroid-dependent asthma in children. *Ann Allergy* 1983;51:21–25.
455. Meltzer EO, Orgel HA, Kemp JP, Chubb JM, Ward JF. Effect of dosing schedule on efficacy and safety of beclomethasone dipropionate aerosol (BDP) in chronic asthma. *J Allergy Clin Immunol* 1983;71:149.
456. Nyholm E, Frame MH, Cayton RM. Therapeutic advantages of twice-daily over four-times daily inhalation budesonide in the treatment of chronic asthma. *Eur J Respir Dis* 1984;65:339–345.
457. Malo J-P, Cartier A, Merland N, et al. Four-times-a-day dosing frequency is better than a twice-a-day regimen in subjects requiring a high-dose inhaled steroid, budesonide, to control moderate to severe asthma. *Am Rev Respir Dis* 1989;140:624–628.
458. Toogood JH. Concentrated aerosol formulations in asthma. *Lancet* 1983;2:790–791.
459. Toogood JH. An appraisal of the influence of dose frequency on the antiasthmatic activity of inhaled corticosteroids. *Ann Allergy* 1985;55:2–4.
460. McGivern DV, Ward M, Macfarlane JT, Roderick Smith WH. Failure of once daily inhaled corticosteroid treatment to control chronic asthma. *Thorax* 1984;39:933–934.
461. Stiksa G, Glennow C. Once daily inhalation of budesonide in the treatment of chronic asthma: a clinical comparison. *Ann Allergy* 1985;55:49–51.
462. Munch EP, Laursen LC, Dirksen A, Weeke ER, Weeke B. Dose frequency in the treatment of asthmatics with inhaled topical steroids. Comparison between a twice daily and a once daily dosing regimen. *Eur J Respir Dis* 1985;67:254–260.
463. Toogood JH, Jennings B, Baskerville J. Tactics for clinical trials of therapy in patients with chronic asthma. *J Asthma* 1983;20(suppl 1):51–60.
464. Morrow Brown H, Storey G, Jackson FA. Beclomethasone dipropionate aerosol in long-term treatment of perennial and seasonal asthma in children and adults: a report of five-and-half years' experience in 600 asthmatic patients. *Br J Clin Pharmacol* 1977;4:259s–267s.
465. Kass I, Nair SV, Patil KD. Beclomethasone dipropionate aerosol in the treatment of steroid-dependent asthmatic patients. An assessment of 18 months of therapy. *Chest* 1977;71:703–707.
466. Cooper EJ, Grant IWB. Beclomethasone dipropionate aerosol in treatment of chronic asthma. *Q J Med* 1977;183:295–308.
467. Kerigan AT, Pugsley SO, Cockcroft DW, Hargreave FE. Substitution of inhaled beclomethasone dipropionate for ingested prednisone in steroid-dependent asthmatics. *Can Med Assoc J* 1977;116:867–871.
468. Davies G, Thomas P, Broder I, et al. Steroid-dependent asthma treated with inhaled beclomethasone dipropionate. A long-term study. *Ann Intern Med* 1977;86:549–553.
469. Toogood JH, Lefcoe NM, Haines DSM, et al. Minimum dose requirements of steroid-dependent asthmatic patients for aerosol beclomethasone and oral prednisone. *J Allergy Clin Immunol* 1978;61:355–364.

470. Golub JR. Long-term triamcinolone acetonide aerosol treatment in adult patients with chronic bronchial asthma. *Ann Allergy* 1980;44:131–137.
471. Kennedy MCS, Haslock MR, Thursby-Pelham DC. Aerosol therapy for asthma: a 10-year follow-up of treatment with beclomethasone dipropionate in 100 asthmatic patients. *Pharmatherapeutica* 1981;2:648–657.
472. Broder I, Tarlo SM, Davies GM, et al. Safety and efficacy of long-term treatment with inhaled beclomethasone dipropionate in steroid-dependent asthma. *Can Med Assoc J* 1987;136:129–135.
473. Dietemann-Molard A, Tenabene A, Kapps M, Pauli G. Efficacité au long cours d'une corticothérapie en aérosol fortement dosé dans le traitement de l'asthme sévère. *Rev Pneumol Clin* 1988;44:269–272.
474. Book A, Dahl R, Eriksson N, et al. Long-term (12–24 months) safety and efficacy of budesonide aerosol in bronchial asthma: a multicentre study. In: Ellul-Micallef R, Lam WK, Toogood JH, eds. *Advances in the use of inhaled corticosteroids.* Hong Kong: Excerpta Medica, 1987;176–187.
475. Otulana BA, Varma N, Bullock A, Higenbottam T. High dose nebulized steroid in the treatment of chronic steroid-dependent asthma. *Respir Med* 1992;86:105–108.
476. Tan WC, Chan TB, Lim TK, Wong ECK. The efficacy of high dose inhaled budesonide in replacing oral corticosteroid in Asian patients with chronic asthma. *Singapore Med J* 1990;31:142–146.
477. Crowe M, Gay AL, Keelan P. Prednisolone sparing effect of high dose budesonide aerosol in the management of chronic systemic steroid dependent asthmatics. *Ir Med J* 1986;79:39–41.
478. Schwartz HJ, Lowell FC, Melby JC. Steroid resistance in bronchial asthma. *Ann Intern Med* 1968;69:493–499.
478a. Woolcock AJ. Steroid resistant asthma: what is the clinical definition? *Eur Respir J* 1993;6:743–747.
479. Corrigan CJ, Brown PH, Barnes NC, Tsai J-J, Frew AJ, Kay AB. Glucocorticoid resistance in chronic asthma. Peripheral blood T lymphocyte activation and comparison of the T lymphocyte inhibitory effects of glucocorticoids and cyclosporin A. *Am Rev Respir Dis* 1991;144:1026–1032.
480. Poznansky MC, Gordon ACH, Grant IWB, Wyllie AH. A cellular abnormality in glucocorticoid resistant asthma. *Clin Exp Immunol* 1985;61:135–142.
480a. Adcock IM, Brown CR, Virdee H et al. DNA binding of glucocorticoid receptor from peripheral blood monocytes of steroid sensitive and resistant patients. *Am Rev Respir Dis* 1993;147:A244.
481. Kamada AK, Leung DYM, Gleason MC, Hill MR, Szefler SJ. High-dose systemic glucocorticoid therapy in the treatment of severe asthma: a case of resistance and patterns of response. *J Allergy Clin Immunol* 1992;90:685–687.
482. Bahna SL, Bjerkedal T. The course and outcome of pregnancy in women with bronchial asthma. *Acta Allergol* 1972;27:397–406.
483. Stenius-Aarniala B, Piirilä P, Teramo K. Asthma and pregnancy: a prospective study of 198 pregnancies. *Thorax* 1988;43:12–18.
484. Greenberger PA. Asthma in pregnancy. *Clin Chest Med* 1992;13:597–605.
485. Warner JO, Götz M, Landau LI, et al. Management of asthma: a consensus statement. *Arch Dis Child* 1989;64:1065–1079.
486. Special Report. Asthma: a follow up statement from an international paediatric asthma consensus group. *Arch Dis Child* 1992;67:240–248.
487. Murray AB, Ferguson AC, Morrison B. Airway responsiveness to histamine as a test of overall severity of asthma in children. *J Allergy Clin Immunol* 1981;68:119–124.
488. Avital A, Bar-Yishay E, Springer C, Godfrey S. Bronchial provocation tests in young children using tracheal auscultation. *J Pediatr* 1988;112:591–594.
489. Ferguson AC, Wong FWM. Bronchial hyperresponsiveness in asthmatic children. Correlation with macrophages and eosinophils in broncholavage fluid. *Chest* 1989;96:988–991.
490. Avital A, Noviski N, Bar-Yishay E, Springer C, Levy M, Godfrey S. Nonspecific bronchial reactivity in asthmatic children depends on severity but not on age. *Am Rev Respir Dis* 1991;144:36–38.
491. Ferguson AC, Whitelaw M, Brown H. Correlation of bronchial eosinophil and mast

cell activation with bronchial hyperresponsiveness in children with asthma. *J Allergy Clin Immunol* 1992;90:609–613.

492. Young S, Le Souëf PN, Geelhoed GC, et al. The influence of a family history of asthma and parental smoking on airway responsiveness in early infancy. *N Engl J Med* 1991;324:1168–1173.

493. Cutz E, Levison H, Cooper DM. Ultrastructure of airways in children with asthma. *Histopathology* 1978;2:407–421.

494. Pedersen S. Asthma in children. In: Barnes PJ, Rodger IW, Thomson NC, eds. *Asthma. Basic mechanisms and clinical management,* 2nd ed. London: Academic Press, 1992;701–722.

495. Francis RS, McEnery G. Disodium cromoglycate compared with beclomethasone dipropionate in juvenile asthma. *Clin Allergy* 1984;14:537–540.

496. Kraemer R, Sennhauser F, Reinhardt M. Effects of regular inhalation of beclomethasone dipropionate and sodium cromoglycate on bronchial hyperreactivity in asthmatic children. *Acta Paediatr Scand* 1987;76:119–123.

497. Gwynn CM, Morrison Smith J. A 1 year follow-up of children and adolescents receiving regular beclomethasone dipropionate. *Clin Allergy* 1974;4:325–330.

498. Lee-Hong E, Collins-Williams C. The long-term use of beclomethasone dipropionate for the control of severe asthma in children. *Ann Allergy* 1977;38:242–244.

499. Godfrey S, Balfour-Lynn L, Tooley M. A three- to five-year follow-up of the use of the aerosol steroid, beclomethasone dipropionate, in childhood asthma. *J Allergy Clin Immunol* 1978;62:335–339.

500. Graff-Lonnevig V, Kraepelien S. Long-term treatment with beclomethasone dipropionate aerosol in asthmatic children, with special reference to growth. *Allergy* 1979;34:57–61.

501. Brown HM, Bhowmik M, Jackson FA, Thantrey N. Beclomethasone dipropionate aerosols in the treatment of asthma in childhood. *Practitioner* 1980;224:847–851.

502. Bisgaard H, Munck SL, Nielsen JP, Petersen W, Ohlsson SV. Inhaled budesonide for treatment of recurrent wheezing in early childhood. *Lancet* 1990;336:649–651.

503. Bennati D, Piacentini GL, Peroni DG, Sette L, Testi R, Boner AL. Changes in bronchial reactivity in asthmatic children after treatment with beclomethasone alone or in association with salbutamol. *J Asthma* 1989;26:359–364.

504. Waalkens HJ, Gerritsen J, Koeter GH, Krouwels FH, van Aalderen WMC, Knol K. Budesonide and terbutaline or terbutaline alone in children with mild asthma: effects on bronchial hyperresponsiveness and diurnal variation in peak flow. *Thorax* 1991;46:499–503.

505. Henriksen JM, Dahl R. Effects of inhaled budesonide alone and in combination with low-dose terbutaline in children with exercise-induced asthma. *Am Rev Respir Dis* 1983;128:993–997.

506. Kjellman M, Möller C, Glennow C, Konar A. A comparison of Becotide and budesonide in children. *Eur J Respir Dis* 1982;63(suppl 124):127.

507. Springer C, Avital A, Maayan CH, Rosler A, Godfrey S. Comparison of budesonide and beclomethasone dipropionate for treatment of asthma. *Arch Dis Child* 1987;62:815–819.

508. Baran D. A comparison of inhaled budesonide and beclomethasone dipropionate in childhood asthma. *Br J Dis Chest* 1987;81:170–175.

509. Gleeson JGA, Price JF. Controlled trial of budesonide given by the Nebuhaler in preschool children with asthma. *BMJ* 1988;297:163–166.

510. Bisgaard H, Ohlsson S. PEP-spacer: an adaptation for administration of MDI to infants. *Allergy* 1989;44:363–364.

511. McCarthy TP. Nebulised budesonide in severe childhood asthma. *Lancet* 1989;1:379–380.

512. Noble V, Ruggins NR, Everard ML, Milner AD. Inhaled budesonide for chronic wheezing under 18 months of age. *Arch Dis Child* 1992;67:285–288.

513. Storr J, Lenney CA, Lenney W. Nebulised beclomethasone dipropionate in preschool asthma. *Arch Dis Child* 1986;61:270–273.

514. Webb MSC, Milner AD, Hiller EJ, Henry RL. Nebulised beclomethasone dipropionate suspension. *Arch Dis Child* 1986;61:1108–1110.

515. Godfrey A, Avital A, Rosler A, Mandelberg A, Uwyyed K. Nebulised budesonide in severe infantile asthma. *Lancet* 1987;2:851–852.

516. de Jongste JC, Duiverman EJ. Nebulised budesonide in severe childhood asthma. *Lancet* 1989;1:1388.
517. Hultquist C. Nebulised budesonide in severe childhood asthma. *Lancet* 1989;1:380.
518. Pedersen S. Studies with nebulised budesonide. In: Godfrey S, ed. *Budesonide. Nebulising suspension.* Oxford: Henry Ling, Dorset Press, 1989;25–29.
519. van Bever HP, Schuddinck L, Wojciechowski M, Stevens WJ. Aerosolized budesonide in asthmatic infants: a double blind study. *Pediatr Pulmonol* 1990;9:177–180.
520. Ilangovan P, Pedersen S, Godfrey S, Nikander K, Noviski N, Warner JO. Treatment of severe steroid dependent preschool asthma with nebulised budesonide suspension. *Arch Dis Child* 1993;68:356–359.
521. Francis RS. Long-term beclomethasone dipropionate aerosol therapy in juvenile asthma. *Thorax* 1976;31:309–314.
522. Kerrebijn KF. Beclomethasone dipropionate in long-term treatment of asthma in children. *Pediatrics* 1976;89:821–826.
523. Albert RK, Martin TR, Lewis SW. Controlled clinical trial of methylprednisolone in patients with chronic bronchitis and acute respiratory insufficiency. *Ann Intern Med* 1980;92:753–758.
524. Emerman CL, Connors AF, Lukens TW, May ME, Effron D. A randomized controlled trial of methylprednisolone in the emergency treatment of acute exacerbations of COPD. *Chest* 1989;95:563–567.
525. Harding SM, Freedman S. A comparison of oral and inhaled steroids in patients with chronic airways obstruction: features determining response. *Thorax* 1978;33:214–218.
526. Shim C, Stover DE, Williams MH Jr. Response to corticosteroids in chronic bronchitis. *J Allergy Clin Immunol* 1978;62:363–367.
527. Syed A, Hoeppner VH, Cockcroft DW. Prediction of nonresponse to corticosteroids in stable chronic airflow limitation. *Clin Invest Med* 1991;14:28–34.
528. Stoller JK, Gerbarg ZB, Feinstein AR. Corticosteroids in stable chronic obstructive pulmonary disease. Reappraisal of efficacy. *J Gen Intern Med* 1987;2:29–35.
529. Morgan W, Rusche E. A controlled trial of the effect of steroids in obstructive airway disease. *Ann Intern Med* 1964;61:248–254.
530. Mendella LA, Manfreda J, Warren CPW, Anthonisen NR. Steroid response in stable chronic obstructive pulmonary disease. *Ann Intern Med* 1982;96:17–21.
531. O'Reilly JF, Shaylor JM, Fromings KM, Harrison BDW. The use of the 12 minute walking test in assessing the effect of oral steroid therapy in patients with chronic airways obstruction. *Br J Dis Chest* 1982;76:374–382.
532. Lam WK, So SY, Yu DYC. Response to oral corticosteroids in chronic airflow obstruction. *Br J Dis Chest* 1983;77:189–198.
533. Eliasson O, Hoffman J, Trueb D, Frederick D, McCormick JR. Corticosteroids in COPD. A clinical trial and reassessment of the literature. *Chest* 1986;89:484–490.
534. Callahan CM, Dittus RS, Katz BP. Oral corticosteroid therapy for patients with stable chronic obstructive pulmonary disease. A meta-analysis. *Ann Intern Med* 1991;114:216–223.
535. Beerel FR, Vance JW. Prednisone treatment for stable pulmonary emphysema. *Am Rev Respir Dis* 1971;104:264–266.
536. Blair GP, Light RW. Treatment of chronic obstructive pulmonary disease with corticosteroids. Comparison of daily vs alternate-day therapy. *Chest* 1984;86:524–528.
537. Mitchell DM, Gildeh P, Dimond AH, Collins JV. Value of serial peak expiratory flow measurements in assessing treatment response in chronic airflow limitation. *Thorax* 1986;41:606–610.
538. Robertson AS, Gove RI, Wieland GA, Burge PS. A double-blind comparison of oral prednisolone 40 mg/day with inhaled beclomethasone dipropionate 1500 μg/day in patients with adult onset chronic obstructive airways disease. *Eur J Respir Dis* 1986;69(suppl 146):565–569.
539. Strain DS, Kinasewitz GT, Franco DP, George RB. Effect of steroid therapy on exercise performance in patients with irreversible chronic obstructive pulmonary disease. *Chest* 1985;88:718–721.
540. Postma DS, Steenhuis EJ, van der Weele LTh, Sluiter HJ. Severe chronic airflow obstruction: can corticosteroids slow down progression? *Eur J Respir Dis* 1985;67:56–64.

541. Postma DS, Peters I, Steenhuis EJ, Sluiter HJ. Moderately severe chronic airflow obstruction. Can corticosteroids slow down obstruction? *Eur Respir J* 1988;1:22–26.
542. Wardman AG, Simpson FG, Know AJ, Page RL, Cooke NJ. The use of high dose inhaled beclomethasone dipropionate as a means of assessing steroid responsiveness in obstructive airways disease. *Br J Dis Chest* 1988;82:168–171.
543. Engel T, Heinig JH, Madsen O, Hansen M, Weeke ER. A trial of inhaled budesonide on airway responsiveness in smokers with chronic bronchitis. *Eur Respir J* 1989;2:935–939.
544. Weir DC, Gove RI, Robertson AS, Burge PS. Corticosteroid trials in non-asthmatic chronic airflow obstruction: a comparison of oral prednisolone and inhaled beclomethasone dipropionate. *Thorax* 1990;45:112–117.
545. Auffarth B, Postma DS, de Monchy JGR, van der Mark ThW, Boorsma M, Koeter GH. Effects of inhaled budesonide on spirometric values, reversibility, airway responsiveness, and cough threshold in smokers with chronic obstructive lung disease. *Thorax* 1991;46:372–377.
546. Watson A, Lim TK, Joyce H, Pride NB. Failure of inhaled corticosteroids to modify bronchoconstrictor or bronchodilator responsiveness in middle-aged smokers with mild airflow obstruction. *Chest* 1992;101:350–355.
547. Thompson AB, Mueller MB, Heires AJ, et al. Aerosolized beclomethasone in chronic bronchitis. Improved pulmonary function and diminished airway inflammation. *Am Rev Respir Dis* 1992;146:389–395.
548. Renkema TEJ, Sluiter HJ, Koeter GH, Postma DS. A two-year prospective study on the effect of inhaled and inhaled plus oral corticosteroids in chronic airflow obstruction. *Am Rev Respir Dis* 1990;141(4, part 2):A504.
549. Kerstjens HAM, Brand PLP, Hughes MD, et al. A comparison of bronchodilator therapy with or without inhaled corticosteroid therapy for obstructive airways disease. *N Engl J Med* 1992;327:1413–1419.
550. Elborn JS, Johnston B, Allen F, Clarke J, McGarry J, Varghese G. Inhaled steroids in patients with bronchiectasis. *Respir Med* 1992;86:121–124.
551. Mitchell DN, Scadding JG. Sarcoidosis: state of the art. *Am Rev Respir Dis* 1974;110:774–802.
552. deRemee RA. The present status of pulmonary sarcoidosis: a house divided. *Chest* 1977;71:388–392.
553. Selroos O. Inhaled corticosteroids and pulmonary sarcoidosis. *Sarcoidosis* 1988;5:104–105.
554. Siltzbach LE, Posner A, Medine MM. Cortisone therapy in sarcoidosis. *JAMA* 1951;147:927–929.
555. Sones M, Israel HL, Dratman MB, Frank JH. Effect of cortisone in sarcoidosis. *N Engl J Med* 1951;244:200–213.
556. Riley RL, Riley MC, Hill HM. Diffuse pulmonary sarcoidosis: diffusing capacity during exercise and other lung function studies in relation to ACTH therapy. *Bull Johns Hopkins Hosp* 1952;91:345–370.
557. Siltzbach LE. Effects of cortisone on sarcoidosis: a study of 13 patients. *Am J Med* 1952;12:139–160.
558. Scadding JG, Mitchell DN. *Sarcoidosis,* 2nd ed. London: Chapman and Hall, 1985.
559. Johnson Johns C, Macgregor MI, Zachary JB, Ball WC. Extended experience in the long-term corticosteroid treatment of pulmonary sarcoidosis. *Ann N Y Acad Sci* 1976;278:722–731.
560. Middleton WG, Douglas AC. Prolonged corticosteroid therapy in pulmonary sarcoidosis. In: Jones Williams W, Davies BH, eds. *Sarcoidosis and other granulomatous diseases.* Cardiff: Alpha Omega, 1980;632–647.
561. Refvem O, Refvem OK. Long-term corticosteroid treatment of pulmonary sarcoidosis. In: Jones Williams W, Davies BH, eds. *Sarcoidosis and other granulomatous diseases.* Cardiff: Alpha Omega, 1980;648–651.
562. Young RL, Harkleroad LE, London RE, Weg JG. Pulmonary sarcoidosis: a prospective evaluation of glucocorticoid therapy. *Ann Intern Med* 1970;73:207–212.
563. Hapke EJ, Meek JC. Steroid treatment in pulmonary sarcoidosis. In: Levinsky L, Macholda F, eds. *Fifth international conference on sarcoidosis.* Praha: Universita Karlova, 1971;621–625.

564. Israel HL, Fronts DW, Beggs RA. A controlled trial of prednisone treatment of sarcoidosis. *Am Rev Respir Dis* 1973;107:609–614.
565. Mikami R, Hiraga Y, Iwai K, et al. A double-blind controlled trial on the effect of corticosteroid therapy in sarcoidosis. In: Iwai K, Hosoda Y, eds. *Proceedings of the VI international conference on sarcoidosis*. Tokyo: University of Tokyo Press, 1974;533–538.
566. Selroos O, Sellergren T-L. Cortocosteroid therapy of pulmonary sarcoidosis. A prospective evaluation of alternate day and daily dosage in stage II disease. *Scand J Respir Dis* 1979;60:215–221.
567. Eule H, Roth I, Weide W. Clinical and functional results of a controlled clinical trial of the value of prednisolone therapy in sarcoidosis, stage I and II. In: Jones Williams W, Davies BH, eds. *Sarcoidosis and other granulomatous diseases*. Cardiff: Alpha Omega, 1980;624–628.
568. Harkleroad LE, Young RL, Savage PJ, Jenkins DW, London RE. Pulmonary sarcoidosis. Long-term follow-up of the effects of steroid therapy. *Chest* 1982;82:84–87.
569. Böttger D. Results of a controlled therapeutic trial of prednisolone in chronic non-fibrotic pulmonary sarcoidosis. In: Jones Williams W, Davies BH, eds. *Sarcoidosis and other granulomatous diseases*. Cardiff: Alpha Omega, 1980;629–631.
570. Tachibana T, Yamamoto M, Saito N, Hiraga Y, Mikami R. Control trial of corticosteroid therapy in Japan. In: Mikami R, Hosoda Y, eds. *Sarcoidosis*. Tokyo: University of Tokyo Press, 1981;285–290.
571. Yamamoto M, Saito N, Tachibana T, et al. Effects of 18-months corticosteroid therapy on stage I and stage II sarcoidosis patients (a control trial). In: Chrétien J, Marsac J, Saltiel JC, eds. *Sarcoidosis and other granulomatous disorders*. Paris: Pergamon Press, 1983;470–474.
572. Zaki MH, Lyons HA, Leilop L, Huang CT. Corticosteroid therapy in sarcoidosis. A five-year, controlled follow-up study. *N Y State J Med* 1987;87:496–499.
573. Williams MH. Beclomethasone dipropionate. *Ann Intern Med* 1981;95:464–467.
574. Selroos O. Use of budesonide in the treatment of pulmonary sarcoidosis. *Ann N Y Acad Sci* 1986;465:713–721.
575. Alberts C, van der Mark ThW, Jansen HM. Budesonide, inhaled therapy for pulmonary sarcoidosis. *Eur Respir J* 1992;5(suppl 15):268s–269s.
576. Selroos O. Use of budesonide in the treatment of pulmonary sarcoidosis. In: Ellul-Micallef R, Lam WK, Toogood JH, eds. *Advances in the use of inhaled corticosteroids*. Hong Kong: Excerpta Medica, 1987;188–197.
577. Selroos O. Relapsing pulmonary stage II-III sarcoidosis can be treated with inhaled budesonide. *Am Rev Respir Dis* 1987;135:A349.
578. Selroos O. Further experiences with inhaled budesonide in the treatment of pulmonary sarcoidosis. In: Grassi C, Rizzato G, Pozzi E, eds. *Sarcoidosis and other granulomatous disorders*. Amsterdam: Elsevier Science, 1988;637–640.
579. Zych D, Pawlicka L, Zielinski J. Inhaled budesonide in the treatment of pulmonary sarcoidosis. *Sarcoidosis* 1993;10:56–61.
580. Vieira L, Mendes B, Barbara C, Longo C, Amaral-Marques R, Avila R. Oral and inhaled corticosteroids in treatment of pulmonary sarcoidosis. *Eur Respir J* 1990;3(suppl 10):423s.
581. Selroos O, Löfroos A-B. How can inhaled budesonide be used in the treatment of pulmonary sarcoidosis? *Sarcoidosis* 1992;9:151.
582. Morgan AD, Johnson MA, Kerr I, Turner-Warwick M. The action of an inhaled corticosteroid as a steroid sparing agent in chronic pulmonary sarcoidosis. *Am Rev Respir Dis* 1987;135(4, part 2):A349.
583. Gupta SK. Treatment of sarcoidosis patients by steroid aerosol: a ten year prospective study from Eastern India. *Sarcoidosis* 1989;6:51–54.
584. Erkkilä S, Fröseth B, Hellström P-E, et al. Inhaled budesonide influences cellular and biochemical abnormalities in pulmonary sarcoidosis. *Sarcoidosis* 1988;5:106–110.
585. Spiteri MA, Newman SP, Clarke SW, Poulter LW. Inhaled corticosteroids can modulate the immunopathogenesis of pulmonary sarcoidosis. *Eur Respir J* 1989;2:218–224.
586. Bjermer L, Nilsson K, Karlström R. Maintenance therapy with inhaled budesonide 1600 μg once daily vs oral prednisone 20 mg every other day in patients with progressive sarcoidosis. *Sarcoidosis* 1992:9:153.

587. Dickie HA, Rankin J. Farmer's lung: an acute granulomatous interstitial pneumonitis occurring in agricultural workers. *JAMA* 1958;167:1069–1076.

588. Emanuel DA, Wenzel FJ, Bowerman CI, Lawton BR. Farmer's lung. Clinical, pathologic and immunologic study of twenty-four patients. *Am J Med* 1964;37:392–401.

589. Mönkäre S. Influence of corticosteroid treatment on the course of farmer's lung. *Eur J Respir Dis* 1983;64:283–293.

590. Mönkäre S, Haahtela T. Farmer's lung—a 5-year follow-up of eighty-six patients. *Clin Allergy* 1987;17:143–151.

591. Kokkarinen JI, Tukiainen HO, Terho EO. Effect of corticosteroid treatment on the recovery of pulmonary function in farmer's lung. *Am Rev Respir Dis* 1992;145:3–5.

592. Anttinen H, Terho EO, Myllylä R, Savolainen E-R. Two serum markers of collagen biosynthesis as possible indicators of irreversible impairment in farmer's lung. *Am Rev Respir Dis* 1986;133:88–93.

593. Crystal RG, Bitterman PB, Rennard SI, et al. Interstitial lung disease of unknown origin. *N Engl J Med* 1984;310:154–166, 235–244.

594. Turner-Warwick M. Approaches to therapy. *Semin Respir Med* 1984;6:92–102.

595. Turner-Warwick M, Burrows B, Johnson A. Cryptogenic fibrosing alveolitis: response to corticosteroid treatment and its effect on survival. *Thorax* 1980;35:593–599.

596. Tukiainen P, Taskinen E, Holsti P, Korhola O, Valle M. Prognosis of cryptogenic fibrosing alveolitis. *Thorax* 1983;38:349–355.

597. Haslam PL, Turton CWG, Lukoszek A, et al. Bronchoalveolar lavage fluid cell counts in cryptogenic fibrosing alveolitis and their relation to therapy. *Thorax* 1980;35:328–339.

598. Rudd RM, Haslam PL, Turner-Warwick M. Cryptogenic fibrosing alveolitis. Relationship of pulmonary physiology and bronchoalveolar lavage to response to treatment and prognosis. *Am Rev Respir Dis* 1981;124:1–8.

599. Watters LC, Schwarz MI, Cherniack RM, et al. Idiopathic pulmonary fibrosis. Pretreatment bronchoalveolar lavage cellular constituents and their relationships with lung histopathology and clinical response to therapy. *Am Rev Respir Dis* 1987;135:696–704.

600. Keogh BA, Bernardo J, Hunninghake GW, Line BR, Price DL, Crystal RG. Effect of intermittent high dose parenteral corticosteroids on the alveolitis of idiopathic pulmonary fibrosis. *Am Rev Respir Dis* 1983;127:18–22.

601. Gulsvik A, Kjelsberg F, Bergmann A, Froland SS, Rootwelt K, Vale JR. High-dose intravenous methylprednisolone pulse therapy as initial treatment in cryptogenic fibrosing alveolitis. A pilot study. *Respiration* 1986;50:252–257.

602. Johnson MA, Kwan S, Snell NJC, Nunn AJ, Darbyshire JH, Turner-Warwick M, Randomised controlled trial comparing prednisolone alone with cyclophosphamide and low dose prednisolone in combination in cryptogenic fibrosing alveolitis. *Thorax* 1989;44:280–288.

603. Prophet D. Primary pulmonary histiocytosis-X. *Clin Chest Med* 1982;3:643–653.

604. Friedman PJ, Liebow AA, Sokoloff J. Eosinophilic granuloma of lung: clinical aspects of primary pulmonary histiocytosis in the adult. *Medicine* 1981;60:385–396.

605. Epler GR, Colby TV. The spectrum of bronchiolitis obliterans. *Chest* 1983;83:161–162.

606. Davidson AG, Heard BE, McAllister WAC, Turner-Warwick MEH. Cryptogenic organizing pneumonitis. *Q J Med* 1983;52:382–394.

607. Epler GR, Colby TV, McLoud TC, Carrington CB, Gaensler EA. Bronchiolitis obliterans organizing pneumonia. *N Engl J Med* 1985;312:152–158.

608. Möllmann HW, Barth J, Schött D, Ulmer WT, Derendorf H, Hochhaus G. Differentialtherapeutische Aspekte zum Einsatz von Glukokortikoiden nach Reizgasvergiftungen. *Intensivmed* 1989;26:2–15.

609. Chang S-W, King TE. Corticosteroids. In: Cherniack RM, ed. *Drugs for the respiratory system*. Orlando: Grune & Stratton, 1986;77–138.

610. Fauci AS, Wolff SM, Wegener's granulomatosis: studies in eighteen patients and a review of the literature. *Medicine* 1973;52:535–561.

611. deRemee RA, McDonald TJ, Weiland LH. Wegener's granulomatosis: observations on treatment with antimicrobial agents. *Mayo Clin Proc* 1985;60:27–32.

612. Leavitt RY, Fauci AS. Pulmonary vasculitis. State of the art. *Am Rev Respir Dis* 1986;134:149–166.

613. McCarthy DS, Pepys J. Allergic bronchopulmonary aspergillosis—clinical immunology. I. Clinical features. *Clin Allergy* 1971;1:261–286.

614. Greenberger PA. Allergic bronchopulmonary aspergillosis and fungoses. *Clin Chest Med* 1988;9:599–608.
615. Safirstein BH, D'Souza MF, Simon G, Tai EH-C, Pepys J. Five-year follow-up of allergic bronchopulmonary aspergillosis. *Am Rev Respir Dis* 1973;108:450–459.
616. Imbeau SA, Nichols D, Flaherty D, Dickie H, Reed C. Relationships between prednisone therapy, disease activity, and the total serum IgE level in allergic bronchopulmonary aspergillosis. *J Allergy Clin Immunol* 1978;62:91–95.
617. Patterson R, Greenberger PA, Halwig JM, Liotta JL, Roberts M. Allergic bronchopulmonary aspergillosis. Natural history and classification of early disease by serologic and roentgenographic studies. *Arch Intern Med* 1986;146:916–918.
618. Patterson R, Greenberger PA, Lee TM, et al. Prolonged evaluation of patients with corticosteroid-dependent asthma of allergic bronchopulmonary aspergillosis. *J Allergy Clin Immunol* 1987;80:663–668.
619. Wang JLF, Patterson R, Roberts M, Ghory AC. The management of allergic bronchopulmonary aspergillosis. *Am Rev Respir Dis* 1979;120:87–92.
620. Imbeault B, Cormier Y. Usefulness of high-dose corticosteroids in allergic bronchopulmonary aspergillosis. *Chest* 1993;103:1614–1617.
621. Crompton GK. Inhaled beclomethasone dipropionate in allergic bronchopulmonary aspergillosis. Report to the research committee of the British Thoracic Association. *Br J Dis Chest* 1979;73:349–356.
622. Pingleton WW, Hiller FC, Bone RC, Kerby GR, Ruth WE. Treatment of allergic aspergillosis with triamcinolone acetonide aerosol. *Chest* 1977;71:782–784.
623. Heinig JH, Weeke ER, Groth S, Schwartz B. High-dose local steroid treatment in bronchopulmonary aspergillosis. *Allergy* 1988;43:24–31.
624. Carrington CB, Addington WW, Goff AM, et al. Chronic eosinophilic pneumonia. *N Engl J Med* 1969;280:787–798.
625. Turner-Warwick M, Assem ESK, Lockwood M. Cryptogenic pulmonary eosinophilia. *Clin Allergy* 1976;6:135–145.
626. Cooper JAD Jr, White DA, Matthay RA. Drug-induced pulmonary disease. Part 1: cytotoxic drugs. *Am Rev Respir Dis* 1986;133:321–340.
627. Cooper JAD Jr, White DA, Matthay RA. Drug-induced pulmonary disease. Part 2: noncytotoxic drugs. *Am Rev Respir Dis* 1986;133:488–505.
628. Hailey FJ, Glascock HW Jr, Hewitt WF. Pleuropneumonic reactions to nitrofurantoin. *N Engl J Med* 1969;281:1087–1090.
629. Larsson S, Cronberg S, Denneberg T, Ohlsson N-M. Pulmonary reaction to nitrofurantoin. *Scand J Respir Dis* 1973;54:103–110.
630. Sovijärvi ARA, Lemola M, Stenius B, Idänpään-Heikkilä J. Nitrofurantoin-induced acute, subacute, and chronic pulmonary reaction. *Scand J Respir Dis* 1977;58:41–50.
631. Rosenow EC III, deRemee RA, Dines DE. Chronic nitrofurantoin pulmonary reaction. Report of five cases. *N Engl J Med* 1968;279:1258–1262.
632. Selroos O, Edgren J. Lupus-like syndrome associated with pulmonary reaction to nitrofurantoin. Report of three cases. *Acta Med Scand* 1975;197:125–129.
633. Lester TW. Extrapulmonary tuberculosis. *Clin Chest Med* 1980;1:219–225.
634. Auerbach HS, Williams M, Kirkpatrick JA, Colten HR. Alternate-day prednisone reduces morbidity and improves pulmonary function in cystic fibrosis. *Lancet* 1985;2:686–688.
635. MacNaughton PD, Evans TW. Management of adult respiratory distress syndrome. *Lancet* 1992;339:469–472.
636. Sibbald WJ, Anderson RR, Reid B, Holliday RL, Driedger AA. Alveolo-capillary permeability in human septic ARDS. Effect of high-dose corticosteroid therapy. *Chest* 1981;79:133–142.
637. Bernard GR, Luce JM, Sprung CL, et al. High-dose corticosteroids in patients with adult respiratory distress syndrome. *N Engl J Med* 1987;317:1565–1570.
638. Schumer W. Steroids in the treatment of clinical septic shock. *Ann Surg* 1976;184:333–339.
639. Bone RC, Fisher CJ Jr, Clemmer TP, et al. A controlled clinical trial of high-dose methylprednisolone in the treatment of severe sepsis and septic shock. *N Engl J Med* 1987;317:653–658.
640. The Veteran's Administration Systemic Sepsis Cooperative Study Group. Effect of

high-dose glucocorticoid therapy on mortality in patients with clinical signs of systemic sepsis. *N Engl J Med* 1987;317:659–665.
641. Bone RC, Fisher CJ Jr, Clemmer TP, et al. Early methylprednisolone treatment for septic syndrome and the adult respiratory distress syndrome. *Chest* 1987;92:1032–1036.
642. The National Institutes of Health-University of California Expert Panel for Corticosteroids as Adjunctive Therapy for Pneumocystis Pneumonia. Special report: consensus statement on the use of corticosteroids as adjunctive therapy for pneumocystis pneumonia in the acquired immunodeficiency syndrome. *N Engl J Med* 1990;323:1500–1504.
643. Bozzette SA, Sattler FR, Chiu J, et al. A controlled trial of early adjunctive treatment with corticosteroids for Pneumocystis carinii pneumonia in the acquired immunodeficiency syndrome. *N Engl J Med* 1990;323:1451–1457.
644. Motoyama EK, Fort MD, Klesh KW, Mutich RL, Guthrie RD. Early onset of airway reactivity in premature infants with bronchopulmonary dysplasia. *Am Rev Respir Dis* 1987;136:50–57.
645. Gerdes JS, Harris MC, Polin RA. Effects of dexamethasone and indomethacin on elastase, α-1 proteinase inhibitor, and fibronectin in bronchoalveolar lavage fluid from neonates. *J Pediatr* 1988;113:727–731.
646. Mammel MC, Green TP, Johnson DE, Thompson TR. Controlled trial of dexamethasone therapy in infants with bronchopulmonary dysplasia. *Lancet* 1983;1:1356–1358.
647. Avery GB, Fletcher AB, Kaplan M, Brudno DS. Controlled trial of dexamethasone in respirator-dependent infants with bronchopulmonary dysplasia. *Pediatrics* 1985;75:106–111.
648. Yoder MC Jr, Chua R, Tepper R. Effect of dexamethasone on pulmonary inflammation and pulmonary function of ventilator-dependent infants with bronchopulmonary dysplasia. *Am Rev Respir Dis* 1991;143:1044–1048.
649. Cummings JJ, D'Eugenio DB, Gross SJ. A controlled trial of dexamethasone in preterm infants at high risk for bronchopulmonary dysplasia. *N Engl J Med* 1989;320:1505–1510.
650. Greenough A. Bronchopulmonary dysplasia: early diagnosis, prophylaxis, and treatment. *Arch Dis Child* 1990;65:1082–1088.
651. Ng PC, Blackburn ME, Brownlee KG, Buckler JMH, Dear PRF. Adrenal response in very low birthweight babies after dexamethasone treatment for bronchopulmonary dysplasia. *Arch Dis Child* 1989;64:1721–1726.
652. Cloutier MM, McLellan N. Nebulized steroid therapy in bronchopulmonary dysplasia. *Pediatr Pulm* 1993;15:111–116.
653. Dunn M, Magnani L, Anaka R, Kirpilani H. Nebulized steroids for bronchopulmonary dysplasia (BPD)—a randomised, double-blind cross-over study. *Pediatr Res* 1992;31:201A.
654. Smith DS. Corticosteroids in croup: a chink in the ivory tower? *J Pediatr* 1989;115:256–257.
655. Kairys SW, Olmstead EM, O'Connor GT. Steroid treatment in laryngotracheitis: a meta-analysis of the evidence from randomised trials. *Pediatrics* 1989;83:683–693.
656. Tibballs J, Shann FA, Landau LI. Placebo-controlled trial of prednisolone in children intubated for croup. *Lancet* 1992;340:745–748.
657. Husby S, Agertoft L, Mortensen S, Pedersen S. Treatment of croup with nebulised steroid (budesonide): a double blind, placebo controlled study. *Arch Dis Child* 1993;68:352–355.

Drugs and the Lung,
edited by C.P. Page and W.J. Metzger.
Raven Press, Ltd., New York © 1994

5

Prophylactic Anti-Asthma Drugs

*+Jonathan W. Becker and *C. Warren Bierman

*Departments of *+Pediatrics and +Medicine
University of Washington, Seattle, Washington 98195*

A generation ago asthma was viewed as a disease of bronchospasm with mucus plugging. Therapy was directed primarily at the relief of symptoms in order to "break the attack." Although more effective drugs were developed to control asthma symptoms, many patients continued to experience a progressive loss of pulmonary function. Asthma morbidity and mortality continued, with an epidemic of asthma deaths in the late 1960s. This epidemic led to a reassessment of the pathophysiology of asthma and to a new concept of the disease.

Asthma is currently considered to be an inflammatory disease of the airways. The pathologic changes of smooth muscle hypertrophy, inflammatory cell infiltration, deposition of collagen on basement membrane, sloughing of respiratory tract mucosa, and hypersecretion of mucus are all attributed to this inflammatory process. Physiological characteristics of asthma include airway inflammation, reversible airflow obstruction, and bronchial hyperresponsiveness. The precise mechanisms by which inflammation leads to these findings is still not clear.

There are multiple pathways by which inflammation may occur. Clearly the inflammation induced by an infectious disease such as a lobar pneumonia is different from that induced by asthma. Multiple components of inflammatory responses have been identified such as the immunoglobulin supergene family, which includes integrins (three groups), selectins (three groups), ICAMs 1–3, VCAM 1, major histocompatibility complex (MHC) classes I and II, activated CD4 and CD8 lymphocytes, and such markers as CD44. These will all need to be put in perspective in terms of relative contribution to the inflammation of asthma. When this is done, more specific and potent drugs for asthma therapy can be developed.

In this chapter, we first briefly review what is now known about the biochemical basis of airway inflammation, bronchial hyperresponsiveness, and reversible airflow obstruction, and then describe current drugs with prophylactic effects in asthma therapy.

TABLE 1. *Features of early and late asthmatic responses after inhaled antigen*

	Early asthmatic response	Late asthmatic response
Onset	<10 min	3–4 h
Peak	10–30 min	8–12 h
Duration	1.5–3 h	>12 h
Prolonged increase in nonallergic responsiveness	—	+

From ref. 13.

AIRWAY INFLAMMATION

The hallmark pathologic feature of asthma is inflammation. Even the most mild, clinically asymptomatic asthmatics possess abnormal histologic features of chronic inflammation on endobronchial biopsy studies (1). Experimental induction of airway inflammation can be generated by bronchial challenge with specific antigen in sensitized asthmatics. This challenge may result in early bronchospasm, which occurs within minutes after challenge, and/or late phase responses, which occur 4 to 24 h later (Table 1). These responses are biochemically quite distinct, and not necessarily co-associated. The inflammation of chronic asthma resembles the late-phase responses to a great extent (2).

A variety of immunologic and nonimmunologic stimuli can initiate the early phase response (Table 2). A provocatant such as antigen initiates an acute response, with a peak in severity by 30 min. Early phase manifestations include bronchoconstriction, release of preformed mediators into both bronchial lumina and pulmonary circulation, generation of eicosanoids, and elaboration of cytokines (3–5).

The primary source of the early phase mediators are mast cells (Fig. 1), a heterogeneous cell type with two phenotypes in human airways (6,7). In humans these populations are distinguished on the basis of their biochemical profile into tryptase (T-MC)–containing mast cells (mucosal type) or

TABLE 2. *Immunologic and nonimmunologic agents of bronchoprovocation*

Agent	Early phase	Late phase
Histamine	+	−
Methacholine	+	−
Adenosine	+	−
Antigen	+	+ or −
Exercise	+	+/−
Cold air	+	−
SO$_2$	+	−
Fog	+	−

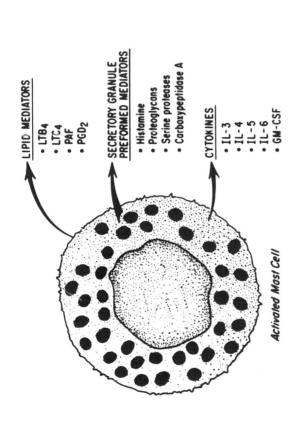

LIPID MEDIATORS
- LTB_4
- LTC_4
- PAF
- PGD_2

SECRETORY GRANULE PREFORMED MEDIATORS
- Histamine
- Proteoglycans
- Serine proteases
- Carboxypeptidase A

CYTOKINES
- IL-3
- IL-4
- IL-5
- IL-6
- GM-CSF

Activated Mast Cell

LEUKOCYTE RESPONSES
- Adherence
- Chemotaxis
- IgE production
- Mast cell proliferation
- Eosinophil activation

FIBROBLAST RESPONSES
- Proliferation
- Vacuolation
- Globopentaosylceramide production
- Collagen production

SUBSTRATE RESPONSES
- Degradation of proteins (e.g. fibronectin, Type IV collagen, and lipoproteins)
- Activation of coagulation cascade

MICROVASCULAR RESPONSES
- Augmented venular permeability
- Leukocyte adherence
- Constriction
- Dilatation

FIG. 1. Biological responses of activated mast cells. When the mast cell immunoglobulin E (IgE) receptor is cross-linked with antigen, the mast cell becomes activated and releases preformed secretory granule mediators and newly synthesized cytokines and plasma-membrane–derived lipid mediators. Some of the biological responses of the activated mast cell are illustrated to demonstrate the diverse functions of this novel cell. (From ref. 7.)

tryptase-chymase (TC-MC)–containing cells, also known as connective tissue mast cells (8). In the airway lumina, T-MCs are present in increased numbers relative to TC-MCs, which are submucosal in location. Preformed mast cell mediators are derived from storage pools, most commonly in the form of mast cell granules. These granules contain histamine, heparin, and a variety of neutral proteases. When activated, preformed mediator release continues until all stored pools are depleted. Alveolar macrophages, which may bear CD23 (FcεRII), may also contribute to this phase, though their role is less clear (9).

Concurrent with degranulation, cellular activation results in mast cell cytokine release and generation of a broad range of eicosanoids (10). Arachidonic acid metabolites generated from the lipoxygenase pathways include leukotrienes (LT) C_4, D_4, and E_4, which were previously known as the "slow reacting substance of anaphylaxis." These metabolites are among the most potent bronchoconstrictors and vasoconstrictors yet identified. Cyclooxygenase products include the prostanoids and thromboxanes, which are capable of inducing bronchoconstriction and increased bronchial hyperresponsiveness, and are vasoactive (11). Prostaglandin D_2 (PGD_2) has been isolated from the airways of human asthmatics both when asymptomatic (5) and following inhaled antigen challenge (3).

Late phase responses of the lower airway are due to the inflammatory infiltrate that develops 4 to 6 h following inhalation challenge (Fig. 2). The infiltrate is composed initially of neutrophils and then of eosinophils (12,13). The bronchoconstriction during an asthmatic late phase response is usually of greater severity and longer duration than that experienced in early phase responses. An animal model with *Ascaris*-sensitized *Macaca arctoides* has been utilized for study of these early and late phase responses (14), while in initial human studies ragweed pollen was utilized (15).

BRONCHIAL HYPERRESPONSIVENESS

Following resolution of the late phase, a period of increased reactivity of asthmatic airways to a variety of immunologic and nonimmunologic stimuli persists. This propensity to asthmatic symptoms at a lowered threshold is termed bronchial hyperresponsiveness (BHR), and has been hypothesized to result in part from late phase response damage to the respiratory tract (2). Findings consistent with this hypothesis have been obtained by bronchoalveolar lavage (BAL) of symptomatic asthmatics with BHR (12). In the absence of overt clinical symptoms, this increased responsiveness can persist for weeks following antigen bronchoprovocation. As a consequence of BHR, increased asthma symptoms, increased inflammation, and increased variability in airflow obstruction may occur, and bronchodilator medications may be needed (16). This effect is less pronounced in adults, and in pediatric patients a wide discrepancy between BHR and clinical severity of symptoms

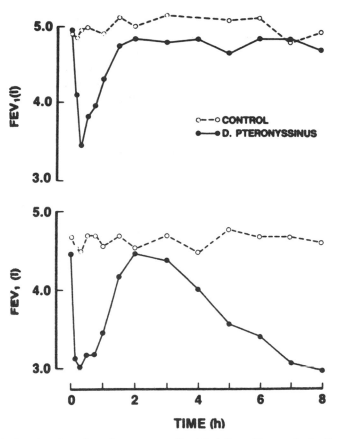

FIG. 2. An isolated early asthmatic response after inhalation of house dust mite extract (*D. pteronyssinus*) (*upper panel*). An early followed by a late asthmatic response after inhalation of house dust mites (*lower panel*). The control measurements (*open circles*) are made after inhalation of the diluent alone. The measurements made after allergen inhalation (*closed circles*) are made at the same time points as the control measurements. (From ref. 13.)

can exist. The degree of BHR has also been used as a prognostic predictor of childhood asthma (17), but all associations between degree of hyperresponsiveness and clinical asthma remain a subject of debate (18).

REVERSIBLE AIRFLOW OBSTRUCTION

The third characteristic of asthma as defined by the National Asthma Education Panel of the United States (19) is reversible obstruction of airway outflow. Obstruction is associated with both early and late phase responses, caused by mucous secretion, airway wall edema, and smooth muscle hypertrophy and spasm. A variety of pulmonary functions are assessed to estimate the degree of obstruction, and these estimates correlate well with clinical severity of asthma flares. A minimum of 15% to 20% reversibility is usually demonstrable in acute asthma or in provocation-induced bronchoconstriction. Relief of obstruction attenuates such clinical symptoms of asthma as wheezing and coughing, but does not reflect the potential for persistent inflammation of the lower airways.

PROPHYLACTIC TREATMENT OF ASTHMA

Development of drugs with prophylactic effects against the characteristic features of asthma has proven to be arduous. Over 5 years of intense testing were required to demonstrate the effectiveness of cromolyn sodium alone (20,21). Screening of potential prophylactic compounds has historically focused on mast cell stabilizing properties, but this has not correlated well with utility in clinical asthma management (22). In addition, classical assessments of efficacy that utilized acute improvement in pulmonary function did not show improvement, as this group of drugs is generally nonbronchodilating. Some 55 prophylactic anti-asthma drugs screened after cromolyn failed to prove efficacious, which underscores the difficulty of developing effective prophylactic agents (23).

Two prophylactic drugs for asthma, cromolyn sodium and nedocromil sodium, have demonstrated efficacy in asthma management. Both drugs possess disease-modifying effects. They reduce inflammation and BHR, which results in a decreased frequency of airflow obstruction (2). This ability to inhibit both early and late phase asthmatic responses is unique to these compounds (22,24), and would be expected to ameliorate the chronic inflammatory changes associated with symptomatic asthma. In this review the basic and clinical pharmacology of these agents, for acute prophylaxis of exercise-induced asthma (EIA) and for chronic asthma management, are addressed. In addition, the prophylactic effects of newer or experimental antihistaminic drugs in asthma are discussed.

CROMOLYN SODIUM–DISODIUM CROMOGLYCATE

This prototypic prophylactic anti-inflammatory drug resulted from research on khellin, a chromone 2-carboxylic acid derived from a Middle Eastern herb Ammi visnaga (21). Derivatives of khellin were synthesized as early as 1956, and found to possess prophylactic, nonbronchodilating properties in asthma. Cromolyn sodium or disodium cromoglycate, which evolved from this research, was synthesized in 1965. Its initial clinical effectiveness was demonstrated by its developer, Dr. Roger Altounyan, whose personal asthma was improved by cromolyn (25).

Basic Pharmacology

Chemistry

Cromolyn is a disodium salt of a bischromone, with pKa of 1.9 (26). At physiologic pH it exists almost entirely in ionized form (21). Its structure is illustrated in Fig. 3.

Mechanisms of Action

Though it was initially thought to be merely a mast cell stabilizer, subsequent studies showed that cromolyn has multiple effects (Table 3) (24).

The timing of cromolyn administration determines the relative effect on the ensuing inflammatory responses. When administered before broncho-provocation, cromolyn inhibits both early and late phase asthmatic responses. If administered after onset of allergen-induced early phase responses, but at least 1 h before the late phase, the late phase can be both delayed in onset and shortened (27).

Effects on the Early Phase

Cromolyn inhibits the early asthmatic responses (28) by inhibiting the release of preformed mast cell mediators and the generation of newly formed substances such as eicosanoids. The inhibitory effect is dose dependent, mast cell subtype specific, and varies within and between species (29). For example, it inhibits the release of mediators from antigen challenge of sensitized rat peritoneal (30,31) and skin (32) mast cells (resemble TC-MC), but not of intestinal mucosal cells (resemble T-MC) (28). Other examples of stimuli inhibited by cromolyn pretreatment in rat TC-phenotype mast cell systems include immunoglobulin E (IgE), compound 48/80, and calcium ionophore A23187 (30,33,34).

In *in vitro* studies of human mast cells, cromolyn has different effects than on animal MCs. Lung strips, mechanically separated (chopped), and enzymatically dispersed human lung contain primarily TC-MC. Antigen-induced

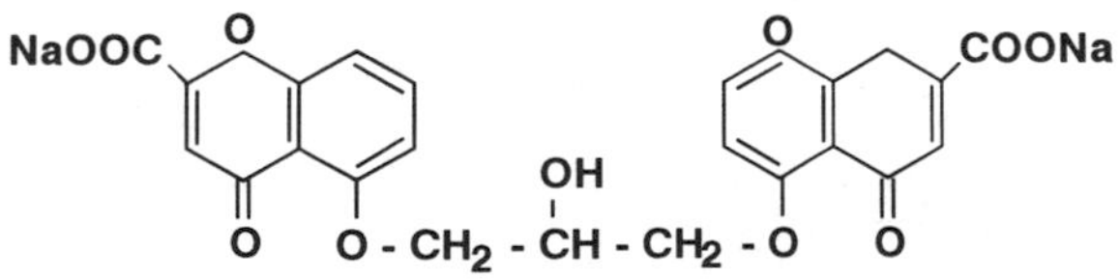

FIG. 3. Chemical structure of cromolyn sodium. (From ref. 36.)

TABLE 3. *Proposed mechanisms of action of cromolyn sodium*

Stabilizes mast cells
Blocks neutrophil chemotactic factor-A (NCF-A) release
Decreases number of lung inflammatory cells
Inhibits protein kinase C
Inhibits activation of inflammatory cells
Decreases bronchial hyperreactivity
Blocks early and late asthmatic reactions
Decreases airway permeability
Inhibits neuronal reflexes within the lung
Prevents down-regulation of β_2-receptors
Inhibits bronchoconstrictor effect of tachykinins

From ref. 24.

histamine and leukotriene release from passively sensitized strips and chopped lung is inhibited 30% to 40% by preincubation in cromolyn containing media (34,35). In dispersed lung, cromolyn inhibits anti-human IgE-induced histamine release by less than 25%, but PGD_2 generation is decreased by 85% (34). The concentrations of cromolyn required (to 1000 μM) to demonstrate even this modest inhibition are unlikely to be attained in clinical use (36). In contrast, T-MCs, which are present on lung mucosal surfaces, are much more sensitive to cromolyn inhibition. Histamine release from anti-human IgE-stimulated BAL-derived T-MC is inhibited 50% at cromolyn concentrations 100-fold less than has been cited for TC-MC (37). Furthermore, this inhibition occurred at a concentration attainable in the lung in clinical practice (36).

Since cromolyn is not fat soluble, the inhibitory effects of cromolyn are postulated to occur through a plasma membrane receptor, which initiates intracellular events. Initial reports of receptor binding studies in mast cells and the RBL-2H3 line reported linkage to a calcium channel (38,39), but the significance of these findings remain uncertain.

Additional controversy continues over cromolyn's intracellular effects. Since calcium is required for mast cell degranulation and cromolyn has mast cell stabilizing properties, some research has focused on cromolyn effects in the inhibition of transmembrane calcium transport and/or intracellular calcium sequestration (38,40). Work with lymphocytes has demonstrated adenosine 3', 5'-cyclic monophosphate (cAMP) accumulation with exposure to cromolyn (41), but no effect on calmodulin, an enzyme modified by other antiallergic drugs (42). Subsequent data have conflicted with these findings and these actions are thought to be less important than other cromolyn effects (43).

Intracellular mechanisms, one involving a phosphorylation reaction, appear to be more important cromolyn effects on mast cells. When anti-IgE and compound 48/80 are utilized to induce rat mast cell histamine secretion, four intracellular membrane proteins of molecular weight 42 kDa, 59 kDa,

68 kDa, and 78 kDa are phosphorylated (44). Phosphorylation of the smaller proteins precedes secretion, which is then followed by phosphorylation of a 78-kDa protein at termination of secretion. Cromolyn sodium induces phosphorylation of this 78-kDa protein, which prevents secretion (45). A second intracellular effect is inhibition of protein kinase C (PKC) (46). This kinase is a calcium- and phosphatidylserine-dependent enzyme, initially thought to be the 78-kDa phosphorylated protein associated with termination of secretion (29,46). Modulation of a phosphatidylinositol pathway guanosine triphosphate (GTP)-binding protein has also recently been suggested (47). Inflammatory cell activation correlates with increased activity of this enzyme, but the interrelationships between the 78-kDa membrane protein phosphorylation, PKC inhibition, and any GTP-binding protein effect caused by cromolyn are unclear at present (28,43).

Cromolyn inhibition of other acute phase responses such as bronchoconstriction have also been studied. Initial work examined the role of neurologically mediated processes and their inhibition by cromolyn, utilizing an anesthetized beagle model (Fig. 4). Findings included inhibition of a vagal-induced increase in total lung resistance and a dose-dependent inhibition of histamine-induced vagal-mediated bronchoconstriction. There was no effect on basal total lung resistance or on inhibition of bronchoconstriction induced by direct electrical stimulation of the vagus. In subsequent work with this model using capsaicin, bronchospasm associated with C-fiber excitation was inhibited by cromolyn (48). A cromolyn dose of 100 μg/kg administered intravenously inhibited C-fiber impulses stimulated by an intravenous dose of 10 μg/kg of capsaicin. These fibers also respond to prostaglandins (49).

Effects on the Late Phase

Cromolyn also attenuates late phase asthmatic responses. Inhibitory effects on multiple inflammatory cells in late responses have been demonstrated, including eosinophils, neutrophils, and monocytes in a variety of *in vitro* systems (Table 4). Cromolyn appears to decrease cellular activation and cytotoxic functions in late phase cells, which correlates most closely with inflammation of chronic asthma (28). The inhibitory effects on activation demonstrated may reflect the clinical effectiveness of cromolyn in suppressing chronic asthma.

Decreased antigen-induced pulmonary infiltrates were detected post-challenge in sensitized guinea pigs, if pretreated with cromolyn (51). This effect has been postulated to be due to decreased responsiveness of inflammatory cells (52,53). In sensitized sheep, cromolyn administered after the early phase response to *Ascaris suum,* inhibited the late phase response (54).

Both early and late phase response inhibition are noted in humans over a single dose range of 10 mg to 40 mg (55,56). In one study of atopic asthmat-

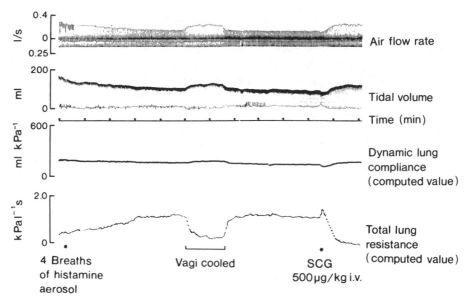

FIG. 4. The effects of sodium cromoglycate (SCG) 500 mg/kg intravenously on a sustained reflex bronchoconstriction induced in a dog anesthetized with chloralose. (From ref. 47.)

ics, after 28 days of cromolyn administration, the clinical responders (14 of 19 in the active treatment group) had decreased numbers of eosinophils in BAL fluid and mucus compared with pretreatment values, consistent with late phase inhibition (57).

Altered late phase responses have also been observed in human inflammatory cells studied following exercise challenge. Cromolyn pretreatment inhibits neutrophil and monocyte activation that may follow exercise (58).

TABLE 4. *Effects of cromolyn on inflammatory cells of the late phase response*

Cell type	System	References
Eosinophil	1, 2, 3	50–53
Neutrophil	1, 2, 3	50–53
Monocyte	1	52

System:

1. Activation of *N*-formyl-methionyl-leucyl-phenylalanine(fMLP)-induced percent complement and IgG Fc receptor positive rosettes. Cellular cytotoxicity by killing of *Schistosoma mansoni.*

2. Ovalbumin sensitized guinea pig lung anaphylaxis model.

3. Granulocyte-macrophage colony stimulating factor and tumor necrosis factor stimulated antibody-dependent, cell-mediated cytotoxicity.

Effects on BHR

Persistent increases in BHR following late phase responses to antigen challenge have been well described. Attenuation of late phase responses by cromolyn would be expected to have significant effects on BHR. This effect has been demonstrated with a variety of immunologic and nonimmunologic challenges (Table 5). While short-term cromolyn use has variably protected against bronchoprovocation, more consistent effects are observed when the drug is administered for more than 8 weeks (36).

When administered prior to bronchoprovocation in animals such as cats or rabbits, cromolyn may be protective for up to 1 h. Similar findings are noted in humans. Protection against early and late phase responses to antigen inhalation have been demonstrated in several studies of atopic asthmatics (24,27,56). Common aeroallergens utilized in challenges include ragweed and birch. In studies with cromolyn administered after early phase response to allergen, variable effectiveness against late phase responses is noted, but

TABLE 5. *Effect of long-term cromolyn sodium administration or treatment upon bronchial responsiveness*

Reference (year)	No. of patients	Duration	Challenge	Decrease in responsiveness
Ryo (1971)	17	2 weeks	Allergen	Yes
Bleeker (1982)	11	4 weeks	Allergen	Yes
Griffin (1983)	11	4 weeks	Cold air	Yes
Numeroso (1983)	6	4 weeks	Nebulized water	Yes
Dickson (1970)	24	1 year	Exercise	Yes
Cockcroft (1977)	21	1 week	Histamine	No
Ryo (1971)	17	2 weeks	Histamine	No
Lowhagen (1985)	14	4 weeks	Histamine	No
Laitenen (1986)	14	4 weeks	Histamine	No
Reques (1985)	56	8 weeks	Histamine	No
Svendsen (1987)	38	8 weeks	Histamine	No
Szmidt (1979)	17	3 weeks	Histamine	Yes
Altounyan (1970)	10	2–7 weeks	Histamine	Yes
Rocchiccioli (1984)	12	6 weeks	Histamine	Yes
Lowhagen (1985)	22	6 weeks	Histamine	Yes
Lowhagen (1984)	40	6–8 weeks	Histamine	Yes
Stafford (1984)	16	12 weeks	Histamine	Yes
Dickson (1970)	24	1 year	Histamine	Yes
Dickson (1979)	50	10 years	Histamine	Yes
Ryo (1971)	17	2 weeks	Methacholine	No
Griffin (1983)	11	4 weeks	Methacholine	No
Bleeker (1982)	11	4 weeks	Methacholine	No
Shapiro (1988)	27	8 weeks	Methacholine	Yes
Furukawa (1984)	46	12 weeks	Methacholine	Yes
Petty (1989)	68	12 weeks	Methacholine	Yes
Kraemer (1984)	32	8 weeks	Carbachol	Yes
Orefice (1984)	51	12 weeks	Acetylcholine	Yes

From ref. 36.

BHR by histamine or methacholine challenge is ablated (27,55). In a 6-week double-blind placebo-controlled (DBPC) trial, atopic asthmatics were protected against the seasonal increase in BHR they usually experienced by natural exposure. Protection was assessed by the histamine dosage needed in provocative challenge to produce a 20% fall in forced expiratory flow in one second (PC_{20}) in subjects (59). Fourteen atopic asthmatics treated for 4 weeks out of season, however, had no significant change in PC_{20} to histamine noted (60).

In longer term trials, more consistent effects are observed (Table 5). A 3-month study with atopic adult asthmatics in season found cromolyn treatment significantly increased the histamine required to reach the PC_{20}. The placebo-treated group had a decrease in histamine necessary to reach the PC_{20} (61). Several 12-week studies have demonstrated decreased BHR by histamine or methacholine PC_{20} (62,63). A 12-week, multicenter study in atopic and nonatopic asthmatics found significantly increased histamine PC_{20} compared with baseline (64). However, in a 1-year DBPC crossover design study that included 16 weeks of cromolyn 20 mg q.i.d., no significant improvement in BHR by PC_{20} to histamine was found (65). In a 3-year study, cromolyn monotherapy demonstrated persistent protection against histamine challenge (66).

Bronchoprovocation with nonimmunologic stimuli include exercise (see acute usage), nebulized water followed by methacholine, hyperosmolar saline, cold air, SO_2, and adenosine (17,67,68). Cromolyn has a protective effect against each of these challenges, but is least protective against histamine or methacholine after a single dose of drug (17,69). No protection against toluene diisocyanate challenge in sensitized subjects was found with a single dose of cromolyn (70).

Pharmacokinetics

Cromolyn sodium is used for asthma by the inhaled route. Distribution of cromolyn follows a single compartment model due to the extent of ionization at physiologic pH. This property makes cromolyn poorly lipid soluble, which results in an inability to diffuse across cellular membranes. It therefore does not cross the placenta or blood-brain barrier, and has no teratogenic effects or sedating properties.

As a polar compound, gastrointestinal tract absorption of cromolyn is poor, estimated at <1%. In contrast, absorption of the small fraction of drug that deposits in distal airways is rapid (26). In animal species, 80% to 90% of the drug is absorbed rapidly in the lung, with a small second fraction absorbed over hours (21). Based on excretion kinetics, human absorption is believed to follow this model and is the rate-limiting step in disposition kinetics. The drug is rapidly cleared from plasma by the kidney and liver, from which it is excreted in urine and bile unmetabolized (21,26).

Clinical Pharmacology: Human Studies

Cromolyn sodium has been evaluated exhaustively in numerous clinical studies, with over 5,700 related publications in 1988 (24). Despite this wealth of information and experience there are no consistent clinical predictors to identify potential cromolyn responders (71). Current use of cromolyn for asthma falls into two categories: acute prophylaxis against a known or potential exposure and prophylaxis against symptoms of chronic asthma.

Acute Usage

The primary acute use of cromolyn is for prophylaxis against exercise-induced asthma (EIA), though other studies have shown it to be effective in bronchoprovocation (see Effects on BHR).

Two to four puffs of cromolyn by metered dose inhaler (MDI) can attenuate EIA if given 10 to 15 min before exercise (19). As EIA is very common in asthmatics, control of these symptoms is important to enhance opportunities for recreation and performance at high levels of competition (72). The first report of a role for cromolyn in EIA prevention was in 1968 (73); subsequent studies supported the initial finding (74,75). By 1 h, much of cromolyn's protective effect against bronchospasm disappears, but inhibition of the late phase response (76), release of neutrophil chemotactic factor-A (77), and cellular activation that may follow EIA (58) persist. The effectiveness of cromolyn is more variable and less potent than the response to β-agonists, and must be considered on an individual basis (75,78). Spinhaler and nebulized preparations are equally efficacious in attenuating EIA (71).

There is no role for the drug in relief of acute asthmatic symptoms. At the same time, cromolyn need not be discontinued during asthma exacerbations. The initial recommendation of discontinuation of cromolyn in acute asthma was made when it was largely administered in powdered form, which tended to increase cough and bronchial hyperreactivity. In liquid aerosols it need not be stopped for acute asthma, unless it exacerbates coughing.

Chronic Usage

Studies of chronic use are divided into short-term and long-term groups due to the distinctive pattern of efficacy that has emerged with years of trials.

Adult Patients

Cromolyn was approved for use in adults in the United Kingdom and United States in 1968 and 1973, respectively (24). A widely held impression that cromolyn is less efficacious in adults persists, resulting in its more prevalent use in children. The U.S. National Asthma Education Panel has recommended the use of cromolyn as first-line therapy for adult chronic moderate asthma, and as an adjunct in chronic severe asthma (19).

Short-term efficacy studies, of less than 8 weeks' duration, demonstrate inconsistent benefits in control of symptoms of chronic asthma (35). Two early studies appeared to demonstrate subjective asthma control (79,80). In a 6-week trial examining the effects of cromolyn on BHR in atopic asthmatics, a coincident reduction was noted in bronchodilator use among active drug-treated subjects (59). Another 6-week DBPC study of 132 seasonal atopic asthmatics and 48 intrinsic asthmatics found beneficial effects of cromolyn treatment. In the atopic group, moderate to severe exacerbations occurred in 21% of subjects in active treatment versus 83% in the placebo group. Further, 58% of the cromolyn treated group were wheeze-free through the pollen season versus 5% who received placebo. Among the intrinsic asthmatics, 70% on active drug improved versus 27% on placebo. A steroid-sparing effect was also noted in a majority of the 12 patients on oral corticosteroids during treatment with cromolyn (81).

In long-term studies, of greater than 8 weeks, efficacy has been more consistently demonstrated. A multicenter study of 12 weeks in atopic and nonatopic asthmatics noted reduced clinical symptom scores, concomitant bronchodilator use, and BHR in those treated with cromolyn and a modest improvement in pulmonary function (64). In a review of two additional 12-week DBPC studies, significant improvements in asthma symptom scores and evening peak expiratory flow rate (PEFR) were found (24). Several 1-year trials have demonstrated significant, persistent benefits of cromolyn therapy. An international multicenter DBPC trial included 397 patients whose asthma was not adequately controlled on bronchodilators; they were enrolled for a 1-year period. Significant improvements were noted by 8 weeks, in that symptom scores improved as did evening PEFR (82). Significant improvement in clinical and objective assessments on cromolyn was noted in a 1-year Brompton Hospital study. The trial was initiated with 103 patients who received placebo, isoproterenol, cromolyn, or cromolyn plus isoproterenol. Study completion rates on medication as prescribed by protocol were 16%, 25%, 67%, and 80%, respectively (83). The study was repeated in Edinburgh with 41 additional patients, with a similar demonstration of efficacy (84,85). Forty-one patients from both centers entered a second year of treatment during which cromolyn continued to provide a protective effect at a reduced dosage. In contrast, a 1-year DBPC crossover study found no significant improvements in asthma symptoms, pulmonary function, or BHR at 1 year. A subgroup of 13 of the 44 patients studied demonstrated significant improvement in morning and evening PEFR while on cromolyn, but without change in BHR (65).

Pediatric Patients

Cromolyn was first approved in the United Kingdom for the pediatric age group in 1968 and in the United States in 1973. Studies have evaluated the efficacy of cromolyn for both short-term and chronic management of asthma. As a result, cromolyn has been recommended by the U.S. National Asthma Education Panel for all pediatric asthmatics who require regular use of anti-asthma therapy (19).

Studies of short-term efficacy have generally examined the effects of less than 8 weeks of treatment. In one of the earliest assessments of efficacy, a 4-week DBPC crossover design in severe asthmatics was utilized. Improvement occurred in 65% of subjects, while an additional 20% became asymptomatic (24). In an 8-week double-blind trial with or without terbutaline, cromolyn provided significant reduction of symptom scores, cough, increased evening peak flows, and decreased reactivity to methacholine (86). A large-scale study of the American Academy of Allergy reported on 252 patients in a placebo-controlled crossover design with 4 weeks of cromolyn sodium. Subjective assessments and reduction of concomitant medication favored cromolyn over placebo, but there were no statistically significant objective assessments (87).

Numerous long-term trials of cromolyn have been published, ranging from 8 weeks to 10 years. Longitudinal studies over years are difficult to perform, but have the potential to assess disease modifying effects of agents. In most long-term studies with cromolyn 60% to 87% of patients report subjective improvement in their asthma control (88,89).

Among the 8-week trials reviewed, a randomized DBPC crossover design study of 38 patients found a significant reduction in pulmonary symptoms in the active drug group (24). A total of 33 out of 38 continued on in an open-label trial for 12 months, again with a reduction in asthma morbidity. Similar findings were noted in a study with 17 children under 5 years of age who used nebulized cromolyn (90). In a study of 46 children with moderate to severe asthma randomized to a DBPC 12-week crossover design, those on cromolyn showed improvement in both asthma symptom control and pulmonary function at 3 and 6 weeks versus placebo (91). In a 6-month trial with 30 corticosteroid-dependent adults using beclomethasone (mean dose 1040 μg/d), subjects received either cromolyn 20 mg q.i.d. or placebo and underwent a 50% reduction of inhaled corticosteroid use. In this study no beclomethasone-sparing effect and a worsening of asthma symptoms were noted; however, 10 of 20 patients had not previously improved with cromolyn use (92). In a 1-year trial with cromolyn added to a stable bronchodilator regimen, subjects had a decrease in BHR to histamine challenge, improved exercise tolerance, and improved clinical symptoms, as noted by decreased concomitant medication use and fewer hospitalizations (93). In a DBPC study of severe perennial asthmatics 71% were "well controlled" after 1 year, compared with 24% in the placebo group (94). In a study of 36 patients with severe asthma, 23 dependent on oral corticosteroids, subjects were treated with cromolyn 20 mg q.i.d. or placebo. After treatment for 4 weeks only subjective improvement was noted. These subjects continued in an open-end 1-year trial and seven patients discontinued corticosteroids, ten experienced a dose reduction, while one increased corticosteroid use (95). In a 3- to 5-year study of 46 children with perennial asthma, 65% of patients at 5 years of treatment were maintained on cromolyn, without need for corticosteroids (96).

Comparative Trials in Chronic Asthma

Initial comparative trials tested cromolyn versus oral and inhaled bronchodilators, while more recent interest has been on trials of cromolyn versus inhaled corticosteroids.

In a 3-month DBPC parallel trial of cromolyn versus sustained release theophylline in 46 children, the initial cromolyn dose of 20 mg q.i.d. was reduced to b.i.d. There was a decrease in number of office visits, BHR, and side effects in the cromolyn-treated group. There were no significant differences between cromolyn and theophylline for symptom control, pulmonary function, or requirement for supplemental medication (97). Other investigators have also demonstrated efficacy of cromolyn comparable to theophylline (98,99). In an 8-week DB crossover study versus terbutaline, cromolyn treated subjects had less cough, BHR, and improved evening PEFR (86).

Many studies have compared cromolyn with inhaled corticosteroids. In most, inhaled corticosteroids have been more effective than cromolyn (100,101) and no significant steroid-sparing effect was found with combination therapy (91,102,103). Several studies, however, have found cromolyn equipotent with inhaled corticosteroids in chronic use (101,104). A DBPC study of 38 atopic adults assessed out of season for their respective pollen sensitivities were divided into treatment groups who received 200 µg of beclomethasone dipropionate (BDP) b.i.d. or cromolyn 2 mg q.i.d. in 8-week blocks. Significant increases in pulmonary function and decreased BHR were found in subjects treated with BDP. Of those patients treated with cromolyn, 37% noted similar improvements (100). Twenty-four children were treated over 6 months in 2-month segments with 20 mg cromolyn and/or 100 µg BDP q.i.d. BDP was found significantly superior for wheeze-free days and morning PEFR, but not for evening PEFR or supplemental bronchodilator use. No steroid-sparing effect or advantage in dual therapy was noted (102).

Clinical Administration

Clinically, cromolyn is most often administered by MDI or nebulizer. Selection of a particular formulation is commonly a result of patient preference, as all routes appear to be equally efficacious in acute and chronic management (74,82).

The MDI formulation is currently marketed with a chlorinated fluorocarbon-driven propellant system that releases a fine aerosol mist. Each actuation releases 5 mg of drug in the European packaging and 800 µg of drug in the United States packaging, with an estimated delivery of less than 10% to the lower airway. Use of a spacing device significantly enhances delivery of medication to the distal airways (105). Two puffs four times daily of the United States formulation are clinically equivalent to one Spinhaler cap four times daily (24).

The nebulizer formulation is available as a 20-mg-unit dose in a 2-ml ampule as a 1% solution in distilled water. Delivery by a motor-driven nebulizer is the preferred route for children under 6 and those unable to properly utilize a MDI. Cromolyn is stable for at least 1 h after mixing with solutions of albuterol, terbutaline sulfate, metaproterenol, isoproterenol, isoetharine hydrochloride, epinephrine hydrochloride, atropine, and acetylcysteine (106,107). Twenty-one asthmatics who utilized an ampule of cromolyn to which 0.2 ml of 10% saline was added had a greater reduction in EIA symptoms and a significant increase of PC_{20} to methacholine (108). This mixture forms an isotonic solution compared to the hypotonic 1% solution.

A Spinhaler formulation is also available, with a capsule unit dose of 20 mg drug plus 20 mg lactose carrier. The capsule is placed in a handheld device that punctures the capsule, held in a rotator receptacle, which releases drug on inspiration. Since substantial amounts of medication are deposited in the device and oropharynx, only 3.2% of each 20-mg dose are delivered to the lung, and 0.8% is swallowed and absorbed from the gastrointestinal tract (21,26). The delivery of medication is strongly dependent on inspiratory flow rate, and reduced flow rates during symptomatic asthma may markedly decrease drug delivery to distal airways by this formulation, in contrast to nebulization.

The usual single dosages for these preparations in the United States are 1.6 mg by MDI or 20 mg by nebulizer or Spinhaler, with the maximal daily dosage four times these amounts.

Adverse Effects

Cromolyn is widely considered to be nontoxic. In animal toxicity studies (21), the monkey LD_{50} was 2000 to 4000 mg/kg i.v. and no deaths occurred in rats and mice fed 8000 mg/kg. Renal tubular degeneration was present in 25% of rats treated with 80 mg/kg in subcutaneous (SQ) doses, administered for 90 consecutive days. No teratogenetic effects were found in doses up to 540 mg/kg, administered SQ to mice. No effects on rat fertility were detected at 100 mg/kg/day.

In humans the most common adverse experiences with cromolyn are cough and pharyngeal irritation by the Spinhaler formulation, particularly in symptomatic asthmatics. There are a few hypersensitivity reports of urticaria and of anaphylaxis to cromolyn (21,109,110) or of immunologic responses such as lymphocyte proliferation, MIF release, and IgG production (111); however, clinically significant adverse responses are exceedingly rare.

There are no known significant drug interactions with cromolyn. Preclinical studies with asthma medications and *in vitro* minimum inhibitory concentration tests for selected antibiotics and microorganisms were not altered by cromolyn (21).

NEDOCROMIL SODIUM

Nedocromil sodium is a compound chemically unrelated to cromolyn, developed from subsequent research on nonbronchodilating prophylactic drugs for asthma.

Basic Pharmacology

Chemistry

Nedocromil is a sodium salt of pyranoquinoline tricyclic dicarboxylic acid, with a pKa of 2.5 (23). The structure is illustrated in Fig. 5.

Mechanisms of Action

The timing of nedocromil administration in relation to proinflammatory stimuli determines the relative effect on the ensuing early and late phase responses. Nedocromil inhibits activation of multiple inflammatory cell types and reduces bronchial hyperresponsiveness with chronic administration. These effects likely account for the clinical utility of nedocromil and each will be considered separately.

Effects on the Early Phase

The pharmacologic profile of nedocromil is very similar to cromolyn, with up to 100-fold greater potency (112–115). Nedocromil stabilizes both T- and

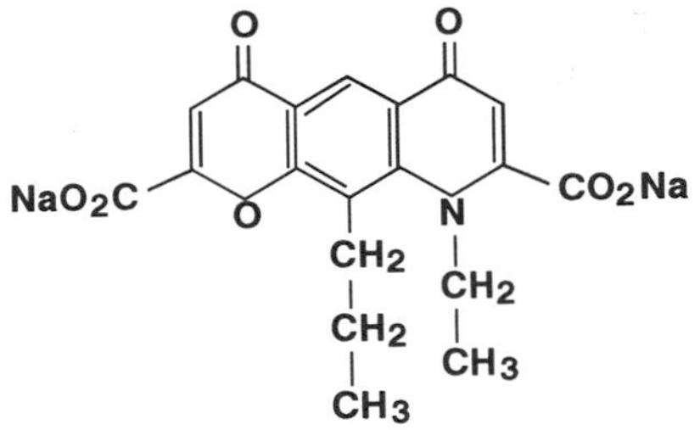

FIG. 5. Chemical structure of nedocromil sodium. (From ref. 36.)

TC-MC, and ranges from equipotent to 100-fold greater inhibitory effect than cromolyn (31,115). This difference is most pronounced in the *Ascaris*-sensitized Macaca monkey model. BAL-derived T-MCs were significantly inhibited by nedocromil against antigen stimulation, as assessed by histamine release and eicosanoid production (LTC_4, PGD_2), while cromolyn demonstrated minimal inhibitory activity. In companion experiments, nedocromil was equipotent with cromolyn in inhibiting anti-IgE stimulated rat peritoneal mast cell (TC-MC phenotype) histamine release (113). Other mast cell studies utilizing a variety of immunologic and nonimmunologic stimuli have demonstrated similar inhibitory effects (31,116,117).

This *in vitro* profile, together with phosphorylation of the same 78-kDa intracellular protein as cromolyn, suggests that nedocromil also acts through a plasma membrane receptor that is similarly distributed (31). Phosphorylation of this protein is not associated with a direct inhibition of the cyclooxygenase or lipoxygenase pathways (113).

Other early phase effects have also been described. Modulation of bronchial nerves, particularly C fibers, have been noted in animal studies (22,118). Cultured human bronchial epithelial cells incubated in nedocromil release decreased amounts of 15-hydroxyeicosatetraenoic (15-HETE) (119) and interleukin (IL)-8 (120) when exposed to total dose infusion (TDI) and IL-1β, respectively. Recently, nedocromil pretreatment was found to modulate human alveolar macrophage cytokine production. A significant decrease in IL-6 release from BAL-derived alveolar macrophages challenged *in vitro* with allergen or anti-human IgE was found (9).

Effects on the Late Phase

Nedocromil has varying inhibitory effects on asthmatic late phase responses (22). When administered before bronchoprovocation, nedocromil inhibits both early and late phase asthmatic responses (121). If administered after onset of allergen-induced early phase responses, but preceding the late phase, results are inconclusive from current studies (22,122). Inflammatory cells associated with late phase responses are modulated by nedocromil, including eosinophils (123), neutrophils (53), and monocytes/macrophages (9). Effects on eosinophils include inhibition of activation and chemotaxis to leukotriene (LT) B_4 and platelet-activating factor (PAF), with decreased eosinophil granule protein release, eicosanoid production, and cytotoxicity (51, 53,123,124). Normodense cells were less sensitive, with no inhibitory effect on PAF and LTC_4 generation in calcium ionophore A23187 stimulated nor unopsonized zymosan-stimulated cells (125). Lymphocyte modulation has been less studied. *Dermatophagoides farinae* allergen reactive human TH-2 clones were not inhibited from proliferation by nedocromil pretreatment (126).

Effects on BHR

When given chronically, nedocromil's potent anti-inflammatory effects would be expected to result in decreased BHR as assessed by bronchoprovocation.

In animal models of BHR with antigen challenge, nedocromil inhibits early and late phase responses of guinea pigs (127) and sheep (128). Nedocromil is protective against inhaled *Ascaris suum* antigen in sensitized *Macaca arctoides* monkeys in a dose-dependent manner. In this challenge, nedocromil is significantly more potent than cromolyn, consistent with effects found in *in vitro* studies of BAL-derived cells (129).

In humans, nedocromil is also protective against a variety of stimuli in bronchoprovocation studies, as shown in Table 6. In immunologic challenge, attenuation of early and late phase responses (114,122) have been demonstrated for both single antigen challenge (121) and antigen provocation during a period of natural exposure (130). In a study of 14 asthmatics and five placebo controls, subjects were challenged with aerosolized *Dermatophagoides pteronyssinus* antigen. Pretreatment with 6 mg nedocromil by MDI resulted in attenuated early and late phase responses and decreased BHR to methacholine 3 and 24 h after antigen challenge (121). Atopic asthmatics challenged in grass pollen season demonstrated decreased BHR by histamine challenge after 2 or 4 weeks of nedocromil (131). In nonimmunologic challenges, nedocromil was protective against challenge with cold air (132), fog (133), SO_2 (134), adenosine monophosphate (135), neurokinin A (136), and in exercise (see also Acute Usage). There was decreased BHR to histamine and methacholine after 6 and 16 weeks of treatment with nedocromil in two studies (137,138) but not in a third (139). Nedocromil is more potent than cromolyn in challenges with cold air, SO_2, and adenosine (36,112).

Pharmacokinetics

Approximately 10% of the dose inhaled by MDI is deposited in the lungs, with the remainder deposited on oropharyngeal tissues. Approximately 2.5%

TABLE 6. *Effect of nedocromil upon bronchial responsiveness*

Reference (year)	No. of patients	Challenge	Result
Dahl (1986)	9	Allergen	N>P
Rak (1986)	12	Allergen	N>P
Robuschi (1986)	6	Allergen	N>P
Svendsen (1986)	11	Allergen	N>P
Younchaiyud (1986)	10	Allergen	N>P
Nair (1989)	12	Allergen	N>P
del Bono (1986)	12	Cold air	N>C>P
Rocchiccioli (1986)	10	Cold air	N>P
Robuschi (1987)	12	Fog	N>P
Bauer (1986)	10	Exercise	N>P
Bleeker (1985)	9	Exercise	N=C
Debelic (1986)	12	Exercise	N>P
Henricksen (1986)	12	Exercise	N>P
Konig (1987)	12	Exercise	N=C
Roberts (1985)	9	Exercise	N>P
Shaw (1986)	8	Exercise	N>P
Altounyan (1986)	10	Adenosine	N>P
Crimi (1986)	18	Adenosine	N>P
Crimi (1986)	15	Adenosine	N>C>P
Altounyan (1986)	6	Sulfur dioxide	N>C>P
Bigby (1986)	10	Sulfur dioxide	N>C>P
Fuller (1986)	6	Sulfur dioxide	N>P
Altounyan (1985)	6	Histamine[a]	↓ responsiveness
Dorward (1986)	12	Histamine[b]	↓ responsiveness

From ref. 36.
[a]Grass pollen season challenge, nedocromil given for 2 weeks.
[b]Grass pollen season challenge, nedocromil given for 4 weeks.
All other studies used nedocromil as a single dose before challenge.
N, nedocromil sodium; C, cromolyn sodium; P, placebo.

of the serum fraction is from gastrointestinal tract absorption of the swallowed medication (112). It is well absorbed from the lung, though slowly, as this is the rate-limiting pharmacokinetic property (23,112). The drug is rapidly eliminated unmetabolized from plasma into urine and bile, and does not accumulate in the bloodstream with multiple doses (22).

Clinical Pharmacology: Human Studies

Nedocromil sodium has undergone extensive clinical investigation in adults since 1984 (36). A recent review cited 52 studies with 554 patients for bronchoprovocation alone (140).

Acute Usage

Acutely, nedocromil attenuates EIA and protects from bronchospasm induced by various bronchoprovocation experiments. A 2 to 4 mg dose inhaled

10 to 15 min before exercise significantly inhibits EIA in both children and adults (140–142), with equal or greater potency to cromolyn (114). In a study dose of 8 mg nedocromil protected 62.5% of patients against a 15% or greater drop in forced expiratory volume in 1 sec (FEV_1) while cromolyn only protected 25%. A dose-response study found nebulized doses of 0.5 mg to 20 mg equally protective to 4 mg inhaled by MDI, with the protective effect persistent for at least 4 h (143). Nedocromil, like cromolyn, inhibits EIA with greater variability than β-agonists (75) and its ultimate role has yet to be determined.

Nedocromil does not relieve acute asthmatic symptoms, but it need not be discontinued during acute asthma unless it exacerbates symptoms, such as cough.

Chronic Usage

Since nedocromil is active in prophylaxis in substantially less time than cromolyn, there is less need for β-agonists and steroids than with cromolyn, and the time to control of asthma symptoms is also shortened.

Adult Patients

Large numbers of studies in adults have been carried out in both short- and long-term nedocromil administration.

In efficacy assessments of less than 8 weeks duration, nedocromil has significant beneficial effects. One early study cites nine placebo-controlled trials, of which eight showed significant improvement versus placebo (114). In a 6-week study of asthmatics treated with theophylline and β-agonists, there was a reduction of these medications to use for symptoms only while nedocromil 4 mg b.i.d., q.i.d., or placebo was added to their regimen. Improvement was noted within 2 weeks on nedocromil, which was significant at 5 to 6 weeks in both groups (143).

In studies longer than 8 weeks, efficacy of nedocromil has been generally maintained. In initial 12-week studies, three of five found significant improvement versus placebo, and two additional trials had a similar trend (114). In a 12-week study of 30 mild to moderate atopic adult asthmatics whose maintenance medication was inhaled bronchodilators, the active treatment group received 4 mg nedocromil by MDI b.i.d. (144). They had decreased nocturnal and daytime asthma, cough, daytime β-agonist use, and increased FEV_1 by week 4 as compared with those in the placebo control group. These differences, however, were not significant at week 12 except for the difference in PEFR variability between groups. FEV_1 was improved throughout the study in the active drug group, but by week 12 placebo and active drug–treated subjects had similar PEFR and forced vital capacity

(FVC). Unfortunately 11 of 30 subjects dropped out of the study, two from the nedocromil treated group and nine from the placebo group. Despite the lack of persistent improvement in the nedocromil-treated group, a majority of patients and clinicians rated the drug as "moderately effective." In a 16-week DBPC study of 127 adults (116 completed the study) with mild to moderate asthma, subjects receiving active drug experienced significantly decreased asthma symptom scores, decreased variability in PEFR, and improved FVC, FEV_1, and PEFR. The effects persisted through week 12, except for improvement in nocturnal asthma, despite withdrawal of theophylline and decreased β-agonist use in the nedocromil-treated group (145). In a 12-month open study of 55 asthmatics on oral bronchodilators, a dose of 4 mg q.i.d. was studied (146). Improvements occurred early, reached significance by 4 months, and were maintained through the duration of the study for PEFR and symptom scores. Concomitant medication use remained significantly reduced from the fourth month for the study's duration.

Pediatric Patients

Little information is yet available from controlled studies in pediatric age groups, yet controversy already exists over the appropriate role for nedocromil in this age group (64,81). The majority of published studies to date have focused on protective effects against EIA; however, one short-term trial in atopic asthmatics has been reported (147). This 5-week DBPC study utilized a 4 mg q.i.d. dose by MDI after a 1-week baseline period. Significant differences in morning chest tightness, morning PEFR, bronchodilator usage, clinic visit spirometry (FVC, FEV_1, and PEFR), and parent's opinion favored nedocromil. No significant differences were found for cough, day- or nighttime asthma, and mean evening PEFR. Adverse effects were reported more often than in adult studies, but occurred with equal frequency in nedocromil and placebo groups.

Comparative Trials in Chronic Asthma

The greater potency of nedocromil compared with cromolyn generated substantial interest in potential steroid sparing effects and comparative efficacy versus the inhaled corticosteroids. In 12 early studies (114), some steroid sparing effect and/or improved symptom control was observed in patients on chronic inhaled corticosteroids, provided the corticosteroid was slowly withdrawn while subjects were treated with nedocromil. In a 6-week DBPC study of patients on maintenance inhaled corticosteroids, nedocromil 4 mg q.i.d. resulted in improved lung function and symptom scores not shown by addition of placebo (148). One study demonstrated improved control of asthma symptoms in a group maintained on inhaled corticosteroids who underwent a dose reduction, followed by randomization to nedocromil 4 mg q.i.d. or placebo (149). In a 1-year open assessment trial, 44 of 51 patients completed the study, with no dropouts due to treatment failure. Of these, 38 of 43 on inhaled corticosteroids either discontinued their use or had a significant dose reduction through the year. At year's end decreased corticosteroid use was maintained while inhaled bronchodilator use had returned to baseline (150). In other studies, little to no steroid sparing effect was noted (92,95).

Clinical Administration

Nedocromil is administered by MDI or nebulizer. The MDI formulation is currently marketed with a chlorinated fluorocarbon–driven propellant system that releases an aerosol mist. Each actuation releases 2 mg of drug in the European formulation and 1.75 mg in the United States formulation. As with cromolyn, an estimated less than 10% of drug reaches the lower airway, and use of a spacing device enhances drug delivery to distal airways (105,151).

Nedocromil solutions have been nebulized in concentrations of 0.5 to 20 mg/ml, and have been well tolerated in doses of 0.5 to 20 mg (143).

Adverse Effects

Nedocromil appears to be as safe as cromolyn. The preclinical studies used very high doses in acute and chronic exposures of multiple species without evidence of toxicity (152). Only minor adverse effects were reported in the majority of human trials (112,114,144). The most common adverse experience is an unpleasant taste of the medication, reported by 13% to 25% of subjects (112,146). This has not been a significant cause of subject dropouts in studies. Other reported side effects include headache (4.8%), nausea (4%), vomiting (1.8%), and dizziness (1.2%). To date there are no reported hypersensitivity responses to nedocromil or significant drug interactions.

ANTIHISTAMINES

Anti-allergic drugs, most with antihistaminic properties, have historically played a limited role in the management of asthma. Classical antihistamines are plagued by limitations including a relative lack of anti–H_1-receptor specificity, higher doses required to attain significant clinical effects in the lung, and increased central nervous system side effects at higher doses. Newer compounds have been designed with increased antihistaminic specificity and nonsedating properties. Many of these drugs also have additional anti-inflammatory properties. While initial trials are promising, the roles for these drugs in prophylaxis of asthma awaits further clinical investigation (153–155).

Astemizole

This is an anti-allergic drug with potent antihistaminic effects, notable clinically for its long tissue half-life and nonsedating properties. Its effects in asthma are limited to prophylaxis against bronchoprovocation and EIA. Doses of 10 to 30 mg increase PC_{20} for antigen in adults and histamine in pediatric populations (156,157). A 10-mg dose is protective against an exercise-induced decrease in FEV_1 in adult asthmatics (158).

The most common side effects are appetite stimulation and weight gain in a few subjects. An increasing frequency of reports of serious cardiac arhythmias have occurred, either from overdosage or in association with underlying cardiac disease.

Azelastine

This anti-allergic compound, notable for its antihistaminic properties and modest bronchodilatation, has prolonged tissue binding properties and a long half-life on oral administration (159,160). Its mechanism of action is unknown, but effects include attenuated mast cell degranulation, inhibition of release of products of the 5-lipoxygenase pathway, and altered intracellular calcium metabolism (161–163).

In bronchoprovocation challenges, the PC_{20} for histamine is increased by a single 8.8-mg dose (164). Allergen-induced PC_{35} is increased by chronic administration of azelastine, with a significant effect at a minimum dose of 4.4 mg (165). A single 4.4-mg dose 4 h prior to exercise protects against EIA in young adults (166).

The drug is well tolerated, with the most frequent complaints being of sedation and a chronic bitter taste, present in 26% and 41.2% of subjects, respectively, on 4.4 mg b.i.d. (160,165). This drug is projected to obtain U.S. Food and Drug Administration approval in 1993–1994.

Cetirizine

This drug is a metabolite of hydroxyzine, with anti-allergic properties and highly specific H_1-receptor antagonism. The drug is well absorbed orally and is excreted unmetabolized in the urine. Minimal sedation and no anticholinergic effects are noted. In addition to potent anti–H_1-receptor effects, cetirizine inhibits skin mast cell PGD_2 release and late phase eosinophil and neutrophil migration (155,167,168).

In clinical use, significant bronchodilatation and increased PC_{20} to histamine are noted with single doses of 5 to 20 mg. In prophylaxis for exercise challenge, oral cetirizine was ineffective while 5 to 10 mg of drug administered by nebulizer protected against a fall in FEV_1 (169).

Ketotifin

This anti-allergic agent has antihistaminic H_1- and H_2-receptor binding and mast cell stabilizing (decreased eicosanoid and histamine release) properties. Calcium metabolism is also altered (170,171).

Variable results for prophylactic use in bronchoprovocation have been obtained. In bronchoprovocation a 2-mg oral dose for 4 weeks protected against methacholine-induced rise in respiratory resistance and 0.5 mg by nebulizer increased the PC_{20} to histamine (172). In contrast no prophylactic effects against EIA were noted in single-dose challenges (173). A 1-year DBPC trial of 1 mg b.i.d. in moderate asthmatics found significant improvement in symptom scores, reduced concomitant medication use, and improved pulmonary function (174). A positive responder phenotype was noted consisting of younger, milder, more athletic asthmatics. The drug was well tolerated for the duration of the study.

Loratadine

This anti-allergic drug has highly specific anti–H_1-receptor effects, is long-acting, and nonsedating. In bronchoprovocation studies with dosages of 10 or 20 mg, an increased PC_{20} versus placebo was found for histamine, but no significant protection against inhaled methacholine or antigen (175). In a DBPC crossover study with inhaled corticosteroid-dependent asthmatics, trends toward significant improvement in symptom scores and pulmonary function were found. These effects were achieved on a tapered dose of corticosteroid (176). The drug became available in the United States in 1993 for use at a dose of 10 mg daily (for individuals over 12 years of age with seasonal rhinitis).

Mizolastine

This benzimidazole derivative has anti-allergic properties and highly specific and potent H_1 antagonism. A long half-life and mild sedating effects at higher doses have been noted in limited human trials. Prophylactic effects in preclinical studies include mast cell stabilizing effects for both T and TC-like phenotypes. Preliminary studies in humans with asthma are encouraging (177).

Pemirolast

This long-acting, nonbronchodilatory anti-allergic drug was developed specifically for asthma prophylaxis. A review (178) of its known effects includes mast cell stabilizing properties, as demonstrated by decreased mediator release from sensitized, antigen-stimulated cells. No protection against bronchoprovocation with methacholine was found, but EIA was reduced significantly. Limited clinical experience has found the drug to be well tolerated.

Picumast

This benzylpiperazine residue-substituted coumarin derivative is an antihistaminic anti-allergic drug with prolonged activity (179). Picumast is an antagonist to H_1 and LTC_4 receptors and its metabolites are also biologically active, with increased H_1-receptor antagonism but decreased effects on leukocyte activation versus the parent compound (69). Anti-allergic effects include mast cell stabilization (180) significantly greater than cromolyn (69). Other anti-inflammatory effects include decreased eosinophil and neutrophil activation (179). Its mechanism of action is due partially to inhibition of calmodulin-dependent enzymes phosphodiesterase and a calcium adenosine triphosphatase (ATPase) (41).

Studies in humans have shown the drug to be well tolerated, with protective effects against asthma (181) and decreased BHR (182).

Terfenadine

Terfenadine is a potent, specific H_1-receptor antagonist that also produces modest bronchodilatation (183). It is nonsedating, with no significant anticholinergic or antiserotonergic properties.

In bronchoprovocation studies with allergen, a single dose is protective against early and late phase responses, including a decrease in FEV_1 (184). In nonimmunologic challenges, terfenadine is protective against PC_{20} to histamine, nebulized distilled water, hyperosmolar saline, and cold air hyperventilation, but not against methacholine challenge (153,185,186). Multiple studies have demonstrated inhibition of EIA, with a dose-dependent effect (187,188).

While usually well tolerated, reports of serious cardiac arrhythmias have occurred with terfenadine, including torsades de pointes. The most common cause of this toxic interaction is related to elevated serum concentrations of terfenadine when drugs are administered simultaneously that compete for the same hepatic oxidative enzyme system, such as ketoconazole (or similar antifungals) or macrolide antibiotics (e.g., erythromycin) (189). Underlying hepatic or cardiac disease [especially prolonged QTc (the corrected QT interval on ECG)] may also predispose to toxicity.

CONCLUSIONS

The shift from symptomatic to preventive therapy has slowly gained acceptance in the practice of primary care physicians. Sales of anti-asthma medications have begun a shift from traditional agents targeted at the relief of bronchoconstriction, toward a variety of compounds with immunomodulatory properties, but continue to lag substantially behind.

The current management of children with asthma includes use of cromolyn sodium for all children who require regular medication. Unlike inhaled steroids, cromolyn and nedocromil do not result in decreased linear growth rates of prepubertal or pubertal males (2,19). Not all pediatric asthmatics are controlled on this regimen. Those with severe disease or who fail to respond to cromolyn after an 8-week trial are likely to benefit from the addition of an inhaled corticosteroid. This combined anti-inflammatory therapy is based on their underlying differences in mechanisms of action and the varied potential steroid-sparing effect of cromolyn.

In adults, cromolyn should also be given an initial trial because of its safety. If control of symptoms after 8 weeks is incomplete, and a further increase in dosage is not effective, a change to inhaled corticosteroid is indicated.

Available in the United States only since 1993, nedocromil sodium will likely play a more significant role in asthma management after further clinical investigation. The drug may replace cromolyn sodium or, in selected patients, replace inhaled corticosteroid. To date other agents such as anti-histaminic/anti-allergic drugs play only a minor role in asthma therapy. As more potent agents are evaluated they may have much more important roles in asthma management.

Future prophylactic strategies will initially target a variety of inflammatory mediators—eicosanoids, cytokines, neuropeptides, etc.—prioritized as their respective roles are clarified. Also under development are soluble cytokine receptors, a potentially effective method of preventing these short-lived molecules from reaching their target cells. Further in the future antisense drugs, active on a transcriptional level, may be developed to prevent mediator generation and release by activated immune cells.

ACKNOWLEDGMENT

The authors would like to express sincere thanks for technical assistance in preparation of this manuscript provided by Lisa Hales.

REFERENCES

1. Beasley R, Roche WR, Roberts JA, Holgate ST. Cellular events in the bronchi in mild asthma and after bronchial provocation. *Am Rev Respir Dis* 1989;139:806–817.
2. Barnes PJ. A new approach to the treatment of asthma. *N Engl J Med* 1989; 321(22):1517–1527.
3. Murray JJ, Tonnel AB, Brash AR, et al. Release of prostaglandin D_2 into human airways during acute antigen challenge. *N Engl J Med* 1986;315:800–804.
4. Piacentini GL, Kaliner MA. The potential roles of leukotrienes in bronchial asthma. *Am Rev Respir Dis* 1991;143:S96–99.
5. Liu MC, Bleecker ER, Lichtenstein LM, et al. Evidence for elevated levels of histamine, prostaglandin D_2, and other bronchoconstricting prostaglandins in the airways of subjects with mild asthma. *Am Rev Respir Dis* 1990;142:126–132.
6. Barrett KE, Metcalfe DD. Heterogeneity of mast cells in the tissues of the respiratory tract and other organ systems. *Am Rev Respir Dis* 1987;135:1190–1195.
7. Stevens RL, Austen KF. Recent advances in the cellular and molecular biology of mast cells. *Immunol Today* 1989;10(11):381–386.
8. Schwartz LB. Heterogeneity of mast cells in humans. In: Galli SJ, Austen KF, eds. *Mast cell and basophil differentiation and function in health and disease*. New York: Raven Press, 1989;93–105.
9. Borish L, Williams J, Johnson S, Mascali JJ, Miller R, Rosenwasser LJ. Anti-inflammatory effects of nedocromil sodium: inhibition of alveolar macrophage function. *Clin Exp Allergy* 1992;22:984–990.
10. Henderson WR Jr. Eicosanoids and platelet-activating factor in allergic respiratory diseases. *Am Rev Respir Dis* 1991;143:S86–90.
11. Fuller RW, Dixon CMS, Dollery CT, Barnes PJ. Prostaglandin D_2 potentiates airway responsiveness to histamine and methacholine. *Am Rev Respir Dis* 1986;133:252–254.
12. Metzger WJ, Richerson HB, Worden K, Monick M, Hunnighake GW. Bronchoalveolar lavage of allergic asthmatic patients following allergen bronchoprovocation. *Chest* 1986;89:477–483.
13. O'Byrne PM, Dolovich J, Hargreave FE. Late asthmatic responses. *Am Rev Respir Dis* 1987;136:740–751.
14. Pritchard DI, Eady RP, Harper ST, et al. Laboratory infection of primates with *Ascaris suum* to provide a model of allergic bronchoconstriction. *Clin Exp Immunol* 1983; 54:469–476.
15. Robertson DG, Kerigan AT, Hargreave FE, Chalmers R, Dolovich J. Late asthmatic responses induced by ragweed pollen allergen. *J Allergy Clin Immunol* 1974;54:244–254.
16. Holgate ST, Beasley R, Twentyman OP. The pathogenesis and significance of bronchial hyper-responsiveness in airways disease. *Clin Sci* 1987;73:561–572.
17. Magnussen H, Rabe KF, Nowak D. Therapy of bronchial hyper-responsiveness. *Clin Exp Allergy* 1991;21:379–389.
18. Josephs LK, Gregg I, Mullee MA, Holgate ST. Nonspecific bronchial reactivity and its relationship to the clinical expression of asthma. *Am Rev Respir Dis* 1989;140:350–357.
19. Sheffer AL, chairman. Guidelines for the diagnosis and management of asthma. National Heart, Lung and Blood Institute. National Asthma Education Program. Expert Panel Report. *J Allergy Clin Immunol* 1991;88:425–534.
20. Orr TSC. Development of preclinical models for testing antiasthma drugs. *Drugs* 1989;37(suppl 1):113–116.
21. Cox JS, Beach JE, Blair AM, et al. Disodium cromoglycate. *Adv Drug Res* 1970;5:115–196.
22. Ford DM, Filcek SAL. An introduction to nedocromil sodium. In: Barnes PJ, ed. *New drugs for asthma*. London: IBC Press, 1989;131–148.
23. Auty RM. The clinical development of a new agent for the treatment of airway inflammation, nedocromil sodium (Tilade). *Eur J Respir Dis* 1986;69(suppl 147):120–131.
24. Murphy S. Cromolyn sodium: basic mechanisms and clinical usage. *Pediatr Asthma Allergy* 1988;2:237–254.

25. Holgate ST. Reflections on the mechanism(s) of action of sodium cromglycate (Intal) and the role of mast cells in asthma. *Respir Med* 1989;83:25–31.
26. Walker SR, Evans ME, Richards AJ, Paterson. The fate of [^{14}C]disodium cromglycate in man. *J Pharm Phamacol* 1972;24:525–531.
27. Mattoli S, Foresi A, Corbo GM, Valente S, Ciappi G. Effects of two doses of cromolyn on allergen-induced late asthmatic response and increased responsiveness. *J Allergy Clin Immunol* 1987;79:747–754.
28. Church MK. Inflammatory cell stabilizers and antihistamines. *Agents Actions* 1989; 28(suppl):349–363.
29. Kay AB. The mode of action of anti-allergic drugs. *Clin Allergy* 1987;17:153–164.
30. Garland LG. Effect of cromoglycate on anaphylactic histamine release from rat peritoneal mast cells. *Br J Pharmacol* 1973;49(1):128–130.
31. Pearce FL, Al-laith M, Bosman L, et al. Effects of sodium cromoglycate and nedocromil sodium on histamine secretion from mast cells from various locations. *Drugs* 1989;37(suppl 1):37–43.
32. Goose J, Blair JN. Passive cutaneous anaphylaxis in the rat, induced with two homologous reagin-like antibodies and its specific inhibition with disodium cromglycate. *Immunology* 1969;16:749–760.
33. Marshall R. Protective effect of disodium cromglycate on rat peritoneal mast cells. *Thorax* 1972;27:38–43.
34. Church MK. Reassessment of mast cell stabilizers in the treatment of respiratory disease. *Ann Allergy* 1989;62:215–221.
35. Church MK, Young KD. The characteristics of inhibition of histamine release from human lung fragments by sodium cromglycate, salbutamol and chlorpromazine. *Br J Pharmacol* 1983;78:671–679.
36. Furukawa CT. Antiasthma agents. Cromolyn sodium and nedocromil sodium. *Immunol Allergy Clin North Am* 1990;10(3):503–514.
37. Mazurek N, Berger G, Pecht I. A binding site on mast cells and basophils for the antiallergic drug cromolyn. *Nature* 1980;286:722–723.
38. Mazurek N, Bashkin P, Petrank A, Pecht I. Basophil variants with impaired cromoglycate binding do not respond to an immunological degranulation stimulus. *Nature* 1983;303:528–530.
39. Mazurek N, Bashkin P, Loyter A, Pecht I. Restoration of Ca^{2+} influx and degranulation capacity of variant RBL-2H3 cells upon implantation of isolated cromolyn binding protein. *Proc Natl Acad Sci USA* 1983;80:6014–6018.
40. Lavin N, Rachelefsky GS, Kaplan SA. An action of disodium cromoglycate: inhibition of cyclic 3′,5′-AMP pholphodiesterase. *J Allergy Clin Immunol* 1976;57:80–88.
41. Gigl G, Hartweg G, Sanchez-Delgado E, Metz G, Gietzen K. Calmodulin antagonism: a pharmacological approach for the inhibition of mediator release from mast cells. *Cell Calcium* 1987;8:327–344.
42. Holian A, Hamilton R, Scheule RK. Mechanistic aspects of cromolyn sodium action on the alveolar macrophage: inhibition of stimulation by soluble agonists. *Agents Actions* 1991;33:318–325.
43. Wells E, Mann J. Phosphorylation of a mast cell protein in response to treatment with anti-allergic compounds. Implications for the mode of action of sodium cromglycate. *Biochem Pharmacol* 1983;32:837–842.
44. Theoharides TC, Sieghart W, Greengard P, Douglas WW. Antiallergic drug cromolyn may inhibit histamine secretion by regulating phosphorylation of a mast cell protein. *Science* 1980;207:80–82.
45. Lucas AM, Shuster S. Cromolyn inhibition of protein kinase C activity. *Biochem Pharmacol* 1987;36:562–565.
46. Schatz-Munding M, Ullrich V. Priming of human polymorphonuclear leukocytes with granulocyte-macrophage colony-stimulating factor involves protein kinase C rather than enhanced calcium mobilisation. *Eur J Biochem* 1992;204:705–712.
47. Jackson DM, Richards IM. The effects of sodium cromoglycate on histamine aerosol-induced reflex bronchoconstriction in the anaesthetized dog. *Br J Pharmacol* 1977; 61:257–262.
48. Dixon M, Jackson DM, Richards IM. The action of sodium cromoglycate on "C" fibre endings in the dog lung. *Br J Pharmacol* 1980;70:11–13.

49. Coleridge HM, Coleridge JCG, Ginzel KH, Baker DG, Banzett RB, Morrison MA. Stimulation of "irritant" receptors and afferent C-fibres in the lungs by prostaglandins. *Nature* 1976;264:451–453.
50. Rand TH, Lopez AF, Gamble JR, Vadas MA. Nedocromil sodium and cromolyn (sodium cromoglycate) selectively inhibit antibody-dependent granulocyte-mediated cytotox. *Int Arch Allergy Appl Immunol* 1988;87:151–158.
51. Hutson PA, Holgate ST, Church MK. The effect of cromolyn sodium and albuterol on early and late phase bronchoconstriction and airway leukocyte infiltration after allergen challenge of nonanesthetized guinea pigs. *Am Rev Respir Dis* 1988;138:1157–1163.
52. Kay AB, Walsh GM, Moqbel R, et al. Disodium cromoglycate inhibits activation of human inflammatory cells in vitro. *J Allergy Clin Immunol* 1987;80:1–8.
53. Moqbel R, Walsh GM, Macdonald AJ, Kay B. Effect of disodium cromoglycate on activation of human eosinophils and neutrophils following reversed (anti-IgE) anaphylaxis. *Clin Allergy* 1986;16:73–83.
54. Patalano F, Ruggieri F. Sodium cromoglycate: a review. *Eur Respir J* 1989;2(suppl 6):556s–560s.
55. Cockcroft DW, Murdock KY. Comparative effects of inhaled salbutamol, sodium cromoglycate, and beclomethasone dipropionate on allergen-induced early asthmatic responses, late asthmatic responses, and increased bronchial responsiveness to histamine. *J Allergy Clin Immunol* 1987;79:734–740.
56. Booji-Noord H, Orie NGM, de Vries K. Immediate and late bronchial obstructive reactions to inhalation of house dust and protective effects of disodium cromoglycate and prednisolone. *J Allergy Clin Immunol* 1971;48:344–354.
57. Diaz P, Galleguillos FR, Gonzalez MC, Pantin CFA, Kay AB. Bronchoalveolar lavage in asthma: the effect of disodium cromoglycate (cromolyn) on leukocyte counts, immunoglobulins, and complement. *J Allergy Clin Immunol* 1984;74:41–48.
58. Moqbel R, Durham SR, Carroll M, et al. Enhanced neutrophil and monocyte cytotoxicity after exercise induced asthma. *Thorax* 1985;40:218–219.
59. Lowhagen O, Rak S. Modification of bronchial hyperreactivity after treatment with sodium cromoglycate during pollen season. *J Allergy Clin Immunol* 1985;75:460–467.
60. Lowhagen O, Rak S. Bronchial hyperreactivity after treatment with sodium cromoglycate in atopic asthmatic patients not exposed to relevant allergens. *J Allergy Clin Immunol* 1985;75:343–347.
61. Stafford WP, Mansfield LE, Yarbrough J. Cromolyn modifies histamine bronchial reactivity in symptomatic seasonal asthma. *Ann Allergy* 1984;52:401–405.
62. Orefice U, Struzzo PL, Pitzalis G. Non specific bronchial hyperresponsiveness study in asthmatic subjects before and after medium-term treatment with nedocromil sodium and sodium cromoglycate. *Am Rev Respir Dis* 1989;139(2):A509.
63. Chhabra SK, Gaur SN. Effect of long-term treatment with sodium cromoglycate on nonspecific bronchial hyperresponsiveness in asthma. *Chest* 1989;95:1235–1238.
64. Petty TL, Rollins Dr, Christopher K, Good JT, Oakley R. Cromolyn sodium is effective in adult chronic asthmatics. *Am Rev Respir Dis* 1989;139:694–701.
65. Jenkins CJ, Breslin AB. Long term study of the effect of sodium cromoglycate on nonspecific bronchial hyperresponsiveness. *Thorax* 1987;42:664–669.
66. Watanabe H. The effect of DSCG against bronchial hyperreactivity in asthmatic children. *N Engl Reg Allergy Proc* 1988;9:354.
67. Koenig JQ, Marshall SG, van Belle G, et al. Therapeutic range cromolyn dose-response inhibition and complete obliteration of SO_2-induced bronchoconstriction in atopic adolescents. *J Allergy Clin Immunol* 1988;81:897–901.
68. Cushley MJ, Holgate ST. Adenosine-induced bronchoconstriction in asthma: role of mast cell-mediator release. *J Allergy Clin Immunol* 1985;75:272–278.
69. Phillips MJ, Ollier S, Gould CAL, Davies RJ. Effect of antihistamines and antiallergic drugs on responses to allergen and histamine provocation tests in asthma. *Thorax* 1984;39:345–351.
70. Mapp C, Bochetto P, Dal Vecchio L, et al. Protective effect of antiasthma drugs on late asthmatic reactions and increased airway responsiveness induced by toluene diisocyanate in sensitized subjects. *Am Rev Respir Dis* 1987;136:1403–1407.
71. Shapiro GG, Konig P. Cromolyn sodium: a review. *Pharmacotherapy* 1985;5:156–170.
72. Shapiro GG, Bierman CW. Exercise-induced asthma. *J Asthma* 1983;20(5):383–389.

73. Davies SE. Effect of disodium cromoglycate on exercise-induced asthma. *Br Med J* 1968;3:593–594.
74. Corkey C, Mindorff C, Levison H, Newth C. Comparison of three different preparations of disodium cromoglycate in the prevention of exercise-induced bronchospasm. *Am Rev Respir Dis* 1982;125:623–626.
75. Morton AR, Ogle SL, Fitch KD. Effects of nedocromil sodium, cromolyn sodium, and a placebo in exercise-induced asthma. *Ann Allergy* 1992;68:143–148.
76. Bierman CW. A comparison of late reactions to antigen and exercise. *J Allergy Clin Immunol* 1984;73:654–659.
77. Bierman CW, Spiro SG, Petheram I. Characterization of the late response in exercise-induced asthma. *J Allergy Clin Immunol* 1984;74:701–706.
78. Bierman CW. Management of exercise-induced asthma. *Ann Allergy* 1992;68:119–122.
79. Chen JL, Moore N, Norman PS, Van Metre TE. Disodium cromoglycate, a new compound for the prevention of exacerbations of asthma. *J Allergy* 1969;43:89–100.
80. Toogood JH, Lefcoe NM, Rose DK, McCourtie DR. A double-blind study of disodium cromoglycate for prophylaxis of bronchial asthma. *Am Rev Respir Dis* 1971;104:323–330.
81. Ford RM. Disodium cromoglycate in the treatment of seasonal and perennial asthma. *Med J Aust* 1969;2:537–540.
82. Eigen H, Reid JJ, Dahl R, et al. Evaluation of the addition of cromolyn sodium to bronchodilator maintenance therapy in the long-term management of asthma. *J Allergy Clin Immunol* 1987;80:612–621.
83. Brompton Hospital/Medical Research Council Collaborative Trial. Long-term study of disodium cromoglycate in treatment of severe extrinsic or intrinsic bronchial asthma in adults. *Br Med J* 1972;4:383–388.
84. Northern General Hospital, Brompton Hospital, and Medical Research Council Collaborative Trial. Sodium cromoglycate in chronic asthma. *Br Med J* 1976;1:361–364.
85. Turner-Warwick M. Are the results of early long-term trials of sodium cromoglycate valid? *Respir Med* 1989;83:7–10.
86. Shapiro GG, Furukawa CT, Peirson WE, Sharpe MJ, Menendez R, Bierman CW. Double-blind evaluation of nebulized cromolyn, terbutaline, and the combination for childhood asthma. *J Allergy Clin Immunol* 1988;81:449–454.
87. Bernstein IL, Siegel SC, Brandon ML, et al. A controlled study of cromolyn sodium by the drug committee of the American Academy of Allergy and Immunology. *J Allergy Clin Immunol* 1972;50:235–245.
88. Berman BA, Fenton MM, Girsh LS, et al. Cromolyn sodium in the treatment of children with severe, perennial asthma. *Pediatrics* 1975;55:621–629.
89. Crisp J, Ostrander C, Giannine A, Stroup G, Deamer WC. Cromolyn sodium therapy for chronic perennial asthma. *JAMA* 1974;229:787–789.
90. Hiller JE, Milner AD, Lenney W. Nebulized sodium cromoglycate in young asthmatic children. *Arch Dis Child* 1977;52:875–876.
91. Geller-Bernstein C, Levin S. Sodium cromoglycate pressurised aerosol in childhood asthma. *Curr Ther Res* 1983;34:345–349.
92. Toogood JH, Jennings B, Lefcoe NM. A clinical trial of combined cromolyn/beclomethasone treatment for chronic asthma. *J Allergy Clin Immunol* 1981;67:317–324.
93. Dickson W. A one year's trial of Intal compound in 24 children with severe asthma. In: Pepys J, Frankland AW, eds. *Disodium cromoglycate in allergic airways disease.* London: Butterworths, 1970;105–114.
94. Silverman M, Connolly NM, Balfour-Lynn L, Godfrey S. Long-term trial of disodium cromoglycate and isoprenaline in children with asthma. *Br Med J* 1979;3:378–381.
95. Friday GA, Facktor MA, Bernstein TA, Fireman P. Cromolyn therapy for severe asthma in children. *J Pediatr* 1973;83:299–304.
96. Godfrey S, Balfour-Lynn L, Konig P. The place of cromolyn sodium in the long-term management of childhood asthma based on a 3- to 5-year follow-up. *J Pediatr* 1975;87:465–473.
97. Furukawa CT, Shapiro GG, Bierman CW, Kraemer MJ, Ward DJ, Pierson WE. A double-blind study comparing the effectiveness of cromolyn sodium and sustained-release theophylline in childhood asthma. *Pediatrics* 1984;74:453–459.

98. Hambleton G, Weinberger M, Taylor J, et al. Comparison of cromoglycate (cromolyn) and theophylline in controlling symptoms of chronic asthma, a collaborative study. *Lancet* 1977;1:381–385.
99. Edmunds AT, Carswell F, Robinson P, Hughes AO. Controlled trial cromoglycate and slow-release aminophylline in perennial childhood asthma. *Br Med J* 1980;281:842.
100. Svendsen UG, Frolund L, Madsen F, Neilson N, Holstein-Rathlou NH, Weeke B. A comparison of the effects of sodium cromoglycate and beclomethasone dipropionate on pulmonary function and bronchial hyperreactivity in subjects with asthma. *J Allergy Clin Immunol* 1987;80:68–74.
101. Mitchell I, Paterson IC, Cameron SJ, Grant IWB. Treatment of childhood asthma with sodium cromoglycate and beclomethasone dipropionate aerosol singly and in combination. *Br Med J* 1976;2:457–458.
102. Francis RS, Mcenery G. Disodium cromoglycate compared with beclomethasone dipropionate in juvenile asthma. *Clin Allergy* 1984;14:537–540.
103. Hiller EJ, Milner AD. Betamethasone 17 valerate aerosol and disodium cromoglycate in severe childhood asthma. *B J Dis Chest* 1975;69:103–106.
104. Shapiro GG, Sharpe M, DeRouen TA, et al. Cromolyn versus triamcinolone acetonide for youngsters with moderate asthma. *J Allergy Clin Immunol* 1991;88:742–748.
105. Newman SP, Moren F, Pavia D, Little F, Clarke SW. Deposition of pressurized suspension aerosols inhaled through extension devices. *Am Rev Respir Dis* 1981;124:317–320.
106. Lesko LL, Miller AK. Physical-chemical compatibility of cromolyn sodium nebulizer solution-bronchodilator inhalant solution admixtures. *Ann Allergy* 1984;53:236–238.
107. Emm T, Metcalf JE, Lesko LJ, Chai MF. Update on the physical-chemical compatibility of cromolyn sodium nebulizer solution: bronchodilator inhalant solution admixtures. *Ann Allergy* 1991;66:185–189.
108. Weiner P, Saaid M, Reshef A. Isotonic nebulized disodium cromoglycate provides better protection against methacholine- and exercise-induced bronchoconstriction. *Am Rev Respir Dis* 1988;137:1309–1311.
109. Menon MPS, Das AK. Asthma and urticaria during disodium cromoglycate treatment, a case report. *Scand J Respir Dis* 1977;58:145–150.
110. Brown LA, Kaplan RA, Benjamin PA, Hoffman LS, Shearer WT. Immunoglobulin E-mediated anaphylaxis with inhaled cromolyn sodium. *J Allergy Clin Immunol* 1981;68:416–420.
111. Sheffer AL, Rocklin RE, Goetzl EJ. Immunologic components of hypersensitivity reactions to cromolyn sodium. *N Engl J Med* 1975;293:1220–1224.
112. Gonzalez JP, Brogden RN. Nedocromil sodium. A preliminary review of its pharmacodynamic and pharmacokinetic properties, and therapeutic efficacy on the treatment of reversible obstructive airways disease. *Drugs* 1987;34:560–577.
113. Wells E, Jackson CG, Harper ST, Mann J, Eady RP. Inhibition of histamine, LTC$_4$, PGD$_2$ release from primate bronchoalveolar mast cells and a comparison with rat peritoneal mast cells. *J Immunol* 1986;137:3941–3945.
114. Holgate ST. Clinical evaluation of nedocromil sodium in asthma. *Eur J Respir Dis* 1986;69(suppl 147):149–159.
115. Leung KBP, Flint KC, Brostoff J, Hudspith BN, Johnson NMcI, Pearce FL. A comparison of nedocromil sodium and sodium cromoglycate on human lung mast cells obtained by bronchoalveolar lavage and by dispersion of lung fragments. *Eur J Respir Dis* 1986;69(suppl 147):223–226.
116. Riley PA, Mather ME, Keogh RW, Eady RP. Activity of nedocromil sodium in mast-cell-dependent reactions in the rat. *Int Arch Allergy Appl Immunol* 1987;82:108–110.
117. Enerback L, Bergstrom S. Effect of nedocromil sodium on the compound exocytosis of mast cells. *Drugs* 1989;37(suppl 1):44–50.
118. Eady RP. The pharmacology of nedocromil sodium. *Eur J Respir Dis* 1986;69(suppl 147):112–119.
119. Mattoli S, Mezzetti M, Fasoli A, Patalano F, Allegra L. Nedocromil sodium prevents the release of 15-hydroxyeicosatetraenoic acid from human bronchial epithelial cells exposed to toluene diisocyanate in vitro. *Int Arch Allergy Appl Immunol* 1990;92:16–22.

120. Vittori E, Sciacca F, Colotta F, Mantovani A, Mattoli S. Protective effect of nedo-cromil sodium on the interleukin-1-induced production of interleukin-8 in human bronchial epithelial cells. *J Allergy Clin Immunol* 1992;90:76–84.
121. Aalbers R, Kauffman HF, Groen H, Koeter GH, de Monchy JGR. The effect of ne-docromil sodium on the early and late phase reaction and allergen-induced bronchial hyperresponsiveness. *J Allergy Clin Immunol* 1990;87:993–1001.
122. Crimi E, Brusasco V, Crimi P. Effect of nedocromil sodium on the late asthmatic re-action to bronchial antigen challenge. *J Allergy Clin Immunol* 1989;83:985–990.
123. Sedgwick JB, Bjornsdottir U, Geiger KM, Busse WW. Inhibition of eosinophil density change and leukotriene C4 generation by nedocromil sodium. *J Allergy Clin Immunol* 1992;90:202–209.
124. Spry CJF, Kumaraswami V, Tai PC. The effect of nedocromil sodium on secretion from human eosinophils. *Eur J Respir Dis* 1986;69(suppl 147):241–243.
125. Burke LA, Crea AEG, Wilkinson JRW, Arm JP, Spur BW, Lee TJ. Comparison of the generation of platelet-activating factor and leukotriene C_4 in human eosinophils stim-ulated by unopsonized zymosan and by the calcium ionophore A23187: the effects of nedocromil sodium. *J Allergy Clin Immunol* 1990;85:26–35.
126. O'Hehir RE, Moqbel R. Action of nedocromil sodium and sodium cromoglycate on cloned human allergin-specific CD4+ lymphocytes. *Drugs* 1989;37(suppl 1):23–25.
127. Church MK, Hutson PA, Holgate ST. Effect of nedocromil sodium on early and late phase responses to allergen challenge in the guinea pig. *Drugs* 1989;37:101–108.
128. Abraham WM. Effect of nedocromil sodium in antigen-induced airway responses in allergic sheep. *Drugs* 1989;37(suppl 1):78–86.
129. Richards IM, Eady RP, Jackson DM, et al. Ascaris-induced bronchoconstriction in primates experimentally infected with *Ascaris suum* ova. *Clin Exp Immunol* 1983; 54:461–468.
130. Altounyan REC, Cole M, Lee TB. Effect of nedocromil sodium on changes in bronchial hyperreactivity in non-asthmatic, atopic rhinitic subjects during the grass pollen sea-son. *Eur J Respir Dis* 1986;69:271–273.
131. Altounyan REC, Cole M, Lee TB. Effects of nedocromil sodium on changes in bron-chial hyperreactivity in non-asthmatic atopic rhinitic subjects during the grass pollen season. *Prog Respir Res* 1985;19:397.
132. Juniper EF, Kline PA, Morris MM, Hargreave FE. Airway constriction by isocapnic hyperventilation of cold, dry air: comparison of magnitude and duration of protection by nedocromil sodium and sodium cromoglycate. *Clin Allergy* 1987;17:523–528.
133. Robuschi M, Vaghi A, Simone P, Bianco S. Prevention of fog-induced bronchospasm by nedocromil sodium. *Clin Allergy* 1987;17:69–74.
134. Altounyan REC, Cole M, Lee TB. Inhibition of sulphur dioxide-induced bronchocon-striction by nedocromil sodium and sodium cromoglycate in non-asthmatic, atopic sub-jects. *Eur J Respir Dis* 1986;69(suppl 147):274–276.
135. Crimi N, Palermo F, Oliveri R, et al. Comparative study of the effects of nedocromil sodium (4 mg) and sodium cromoglycate (10 mg) on adenosine-induced bronchocon-striction in asthmatic subjects. *Clin Allergy* 1988;18:367–374.
136. Joos GF, Pauwels RA, Van Der Straeten ME. Effect of nedocromil sodium on the bron-choconstrictor effect of neurokinin A in asthmatics. *Drugs* 1989;37:109–112.
137. Svendsen UG, Frolund L, Madsen F, Nielsen NH. A comparison of the effects of nedocromil sodium and beclomethasone dipropionate on pulmonary function, symp-toms and bronchial responsiveness in patients with asthma. *J Allergy Clin Immunol* 1989;84:224–231.
138. Bel EH, Timmers MC, Hermans JO, Dijkman JH, Sterk PJ. The long-term effects of nedocromil sodium and beclomethasone dipropionate on bronchial responsiveness to methacholine in nonatopic asthmatic subjects. *Am Rev Respir Dis* 1990;141:21–28.
139. Crimi E, Brusasco V, Brancatisano M, Losurdo E, Crimi P. Effect of nedocromil so-dium on adenosine- and methacholine-induced bronchospasm in asthma. *Clin Allergy* 1987;17:135–141.
140. Rocchiccioli KMS, Riley PA. Clinical pharmacology of nedocromil sodium. *Drugs* 1989;37(suppl 1):123–126.
141. Bauer CP. The protective effect of nedocromil sodium in exercise-induced asthma. *Eur J Respir Dis* 1986;69:252–254.

142. Albazzaz MK, Neale MG, Patel KR. Dose-response study of nebulised nedocromil sodium in exercise induced asthma. *Thorax* 1989;44:816–819.
143. van As A, Chick TW, Bodman SF, et al. A group comparative study of the safety and efficacy of nedocromil sodium (Tiladel') in reversible airways disease: a preliminary report. *Eur J Respir Dis* 1986;69(suppl 147):143–148.
144. Fairfax AJ, Allbeson M. A double blind group comparative trial of nedocromil sodium and placebo in the management of bronchial asthma. *J Int Med Res* 1988;16:216–224.
145. North American Tilade Study Group. A double-blind multicenter group comparative study of the efficacy and safety of nedocromil sodium in the management of asthma. *Chest* 1990;97:1299–1306.
146. Carrasco E, Sepulveda R. The acceptability, tolerability and safety of nedocromil sodium in long-term clinical use. *Eur J Respir Dis* 1986;69:311–313.
147. Businco L, Cantani A, Di Fazio A, Bernardini L. A double-blind, placebo controlled study to assess the efficacy of nedocromil sodium in the management of childhood grass pollen asthma. *Clin Exp Allergy* 1990;20:683–688.
148. Greif J, Fink G, Smorzik Y, et al. Nedocromil sodium and placebo in the treatment of bronchial asthma. *Chest* 1989;96:583–588.
149. Dorow P. A double-blind group comparative trial of nedocromil sodium and placebo in the management of bronchial asthma in steroid-dependent patients. *Eur J Respir Dis* 1986;69:317–319.
150. Lal S, Malhotra S, Gribben D, Hodder D. An open assessment study of the acceptability, tolerability and safety of nedocromil sodium in long-term clinical use in patients with perennial asthma. *Eur J Respir Dis* 1986;69(suppl 147):136–142.
151. Dolovich MB, Newhouse MT. Aerosols: Generation, methods of administration, and therapeutic applications in asthma. In: Middleton E, Reed CE, Ellis EF, et al., eds. *Allergy: principles and practice.* St. Louis: CV Mosby, 1988;559–578.
152. Clark B, Clarke AJ, Bamford DG, Greenwood B. Nedocromil sodium preclinical safety evaluation studies: a preliminary report. *Eur J Respir Dis* 1986;69:248–251.
153. Townley RG. Antiallergic properties of the second-generation H_1 antihistamines during the early and late reactions to antigen. *J Allergy Clin Immunol* 1992;90:720–725.
154. Holgate SI, Finnerty JP. Antihistamines in asthma. *J Allergy Clin Immunol* 1989; 83:537–547.
155. Rafferty P. Antihistamines in the treatment of clinical asthma. *J Allergy Clin Immunol* 1990;88:647–650.
156. Cistero A, Abadias M, Lleonart R, et al. Effect of astemizole on allergic asthma. *Ann Allergy* 1992;69:123–127.
157. Backer V, Bach-Mortensen N, Becker U, et al. The effect of astemizole on bronchial hyperresponsiveness and exercise-induced asthma in children. *Allergy* 1989;44:209–213.
158. Clee MD, Ingram CG, Reid PC, Robertson AS. The effect of astemizole on exercise-induced asthma. *Br J Dis Chest* 1984;78:180–183.
159. McTavish D, Sorkin EM. Azelastine, a review of its pharmacodynamic and pharmacokinetic properties, and therapeutic potential. *Drugs* 1989;38(5):778–800.
160. Kemp JP, Meltzer EO, Orgel HA, et al. A dose-response study of the bronchodilator action of azelastine in asthma. *J Allergy Clin Immunol* 1987;79:893–899.
161. Fields DAS, Pillar J, Diamantis W, Perhach JL, Sofia RD, Chand N. Inhibition by azelastine of nonallergic histamine release from rat peritoneal mast cells. *J Allergy Clin Immunol* 1984;73:400–403.
162. Achterrath-Tuckermann U, Simmet T, Luck W, Szelenyi I, Peskar BA. Inhibition of cysteinyl-leukotrine production by azelastine and its biological significance. *Agents Actions* 1988;24:217–223.
163. Nakamura T, Nishizawa Y, Sato T, Yamato C. Effect of azelastine on the intracellular Ca^{2+} mobilization in guinea pig peritoneal macrophages. *Eur J Pharmacol* 1988; 148:35–41.
164. Albazzaz MK, Patel KR. Effect of azelastine on bronchoconstriction induced by histamine and leukotriene C4 in patients with extrinsic asthma. *Thorax* 1988;43:306–311.
165. Ollier S, Gould CAL, Davies RJ. The effect of single and multiple dose therapy with azelastine on the immediate asthmatic response to allergen provocation testing. *J Allergy Clin Immunol* 1986;78:358–364.

166. Magnussen H, Reuss G, Jorres R, Aurich R. The effect of azelastine on exercise-induced asthma. *Chest* 1988;93(5):937–940.
167. Bernheim J, Arendt C, De Vos C. Cetirizine: more than an antihistamine? *Agents Actions* 1991;34:269–293.
168. Sheffer AL, Samuels LL. Cetirizine: antiallergic therapy beyond traditional H1 antihistamines. *J Allergy Clin Immunol* 1990;86:1040–1046.
169. Ghosh SK, De Vos C, McIlroy I, Patel KR. Effect of cetirizine on exercise induced asthma. *Thorax* 1991;46:242–244.
170. Nagata M, Kamino T, Kimura I, et al. The effect of ketotifen on bronchial hyperresponsiveness in patients with bronchial asthma. *Immunol Allergy Pract* 1991;13 (11):445–449.
171. Wilhelms OH. Inhibition profiles of picumast and ketotifen on the in vitro release of prostanoids, slow-reacting substance of anaphylaxis, histamine and enzyme from human leukocytes and rat alveolar macrophages. *Int Arch Allergy Appl Immunol* 1987;82:547–549.
172. Lai CKW, Ollier S, Lau CK, Holgate ST. Effect of azelastine and ketotifen on the bronchial and skin responses to platelet-activating factor in humans. *Clin Exp Allergy* 1991;21:489–496.
173. Petheram IS, Moxham J, Bierman CW, McAllen M, Spiro SG. Ketotifen in atopic asthma and exercise-induced asthma. *Thorax* 1981;36:308–312.
174. Podleski WK, Zelenak TM, Schmidt JL. Long term trial of ketotifen in bronchial asthma. *Ann Allergy* 1984;52:406–410.
175. Town GI, Holgate ST. Comparison of the effect of loratadine on the airway and skin responses to histamine, methacholine, and allergen in subjects with asthma. *J Allergy Clin Immunol* 1990;86:886–893.
176. Dirksen A, Engel T, Frolund L, Heinig JH, Svendsen UG, Weeke B. Effect of a nonsedative antihistaminic (loratidine) in moderate asthma. *Allergy* 1989;44:566–571.
177. Rosenzweig P, Thebault JJ, Caplain H, et al. Pharmacodynamics and pharmacokinetics of mizolastine (SL 85.0324), a new nonsedative H_1 antihistamine. *Ann Allergy* 1992; 69:135–139.
178. Kemp JP, Bernstein IL, Bierman CW, Li JT, Siegel SC, Spangenberg RD, Tinkelman DG. Pemirolast, a new oral nonbronchodilator drug for chronic asthma. *Ann Allergy* 1992;68:488–492.
179. Moqbel R, Hartnell A, Kay AB. The effects of picumast on human eosinophil and neutrophil activation. *Clin Exp Allergy* 1991;21(suppl 3):39–44.
180. Rosch A, Schaumann W, Wilhelms OH. Picumast and mast cell function. *Clin Exp Allergy* 1991;21(suppl 3):17–22.
181. Boerner D, Metz K, Eberhardt R. Efficacy and tolerability of picumast dihydrochloride in comparison with placebo in asthmatic patients. *Drug Res* 1989;39:1363–1367.
182. Slapke J, Muller S, Boerner D. A one-year double blind clinical study of the efficacy and tolerability of picumast dihydrochloride versus ketotifen in patients with bronchial asthma. *Drug Res* 1989;39:1368–1372.
183. Rafferty P, Holgate ST. Terfenadine (Seldane) is a potent and selective histamine H1 receptor antagonist in asthmatic airways. *Am Rev Respir Dis* 1987;135:181–184.
184. Hamid M, Rafferty P, Holgate ST. The inhibitory effect of terfenadine and flurbiprofen on early and late-phase bronchoconstriction following allergen challenge in atopic asthma. *Clin Exp Allergy* 1990;20:261–267.
185. Finney MJB, Anderson SD, Black JL. Terfenadine modifies airway narrowing induced by the inhalation of nonisotonic aerosols in subjects with asthma. *Am Rev Respir Dis* 1990;141:1151–1157.
186. Patel KR. Effect of terfenadine on methacholine-induced bronchoconstriction in asthma. *J Allergy Clin Immunol* 1987;79:355–358.
187. Pierson WE, Furukawa CT, Shapiro GS, Altman LC, Bierman CW. Terfenadine blockade of exercise-induced bronchospasm. *Ann Allergy* 1989;63:461–464.
188. O'Hickey SP, Belcher N, Rees PJ, Lee TH. Effect of terfenadine on the bronchoconstrictor response to hypertonic saline and exercise in asthmatic subjects. *Thorax* 1988;43:865.
189. Monahan BP, Ferguson CL, Killeavy ES, Lloyd BK, Troy J, Cantilena LR Jr. Torsades de pointes occurring in association with terfenadine use. *JAMA* 1990;264:2788–2790.

Drugs and the Lung,
edited by C.P. Page and W.J. Metzger.
Raven Press, Ltd., New York © 1994

6

Antihistamines

Philip G. Bardin and Stephen T. Holgate

*Immunopharmacology Group, Southampton General Hospital,
Southampton S09 4XY, United Kingdom*

Histamine, a potent effector agent in allergic diseases, was first synthesized in 1907 by Vogt (1). Dale and Laidlaw (2) discovered that the substance had a smooth muscle relaxing action, decreased blood pressure, and that its pharmacological activity resembled that of many tissue extracts. The observation that the immediate response of an animal to an inert protein to which it had been sensitized was similar to histamine toxicity prompted them to speculate that histamine may play a pivotal role in anaphylactic reactions. However, many scientists held the view that histamine was the result of tissue degeneration and putrefaction and it was only in 1927 that Best and coworkers (3) were able to show convincingly that it was present in impeccably fresh samples of liver and lung. This was followed by demonstration of its presence in a variety of other tissues, hence the name *histamine* after the Greek word for tissue, *histos.*

The association of histamine with asthma was made by Weiss and coworkers (4), who demonstrated wheezing in asthmatics after intravenous injection of the amine. Later work by Schild et al. (5) extended this observation, showing that histamine was released from lung tissue after allergen challenge, and that this coincided with the induction of bronchoconstriction.

The first recorded evidence of a histamine antagonist was by Bovet and Staub (6) from the Pasteur Institute, who noticed that a compound designated F929 (2-iso-propyl-5-methyl-phenoxyethyl-diethylamine) attenuated some of the actions of histamine. It had dramatic effects on guinea pigs, protecting them against lethal doses of histamine and reducing or ablating many of the features of anaphylaxis. Contractile effects of histamine on tracheal and intestinal smooth muscle was also attenuated. The discovery led to synthesis of the first two antihistamines, phenbenzamine and pyrilamine maleate; the latter is still in use today.

ENDOGENOUS HISTAMINE

Biosynthesis

Most mammalian tissues are able to synthesize histamine from histidine by way of L-histidine decarboxylase, an enzyme specific for histidine. In most tissues the chief site of synthesis and storage of histamine is the mast cell or, in the blood, its circulating counterpart, the basophil. It is stored in secretory granules in association with heparin proteoglycan and a variety of other preformed mediators (7).

Concentrations of histamine are very low in plasma and other body fluids, but has been found to be high in skin, lung, and intestinal mucosa. Turn-over rate of histamine from mast cells is slow and after depletion it may take weeks for concentrations of the amine to return to normal. This contrasts with non–mast cell sites of synthesis and storage such as human epidermis, gastric mucosal cells, neurons within the CNS, and in rapidly growing or regenerating tissues where production is high and turnover is rapid, mediated by induction of L-histidine decarboxylase. The functional importance of this difference in histamine synthesizing capacity is not clear.

During mast cell activation, histamine and the remaining granule constituents are released when antigen interacts with specific immunoglobulin E (IgE) $F_c R_1$ receptors on the surface of the mast cell (8). Ligand-receptor binding stimulates membrane phospholipid metabolism followed by influx of extracellular calcium and mobilization of intracellular calcium stores, an intracellular signal that produces secretion of granule contents as well as mobilization of arachidonic acid from membrane phospholipid stores. Histamine is expelled along with other constituents of the secretory granules that comprise heparin, proteins and peptides, including eosinophil chemotactic factor (ECF-A) and neutrophil chemotactic factor (NCF-A). Enzymes such as β-glucuronidase, neutral proteases, peroxidase, and superoxide dismutase are also released into the extracellular environment, as are a host of metabolites derived from arachidonic acid, platelet-activating factor (PAF), and kinins. Many of these substances have potent biological activities related to allergic disease and their effects may in some situations dominate the clinical picture (9).

Pharmacological Effects

Histamine has varied effects in different organ systems, some of which are of great relevance to the pathogenesis of asthma (Table 1).

TABLE 1. *Physiological effects of histamine on different tissues*

Vascular system
  Resistance vessels: vasodilation (H_1 and H_2 receptors)
  Capillaries: increased permeability, extravascular plasma leakage, edema (H_1 receptors)
  Large blood vessels: vasoconstriction
  Veins: constriction
Extravascular smooth muscle
  H_1 receptors: contraction, bronchoconstriction
  H_2 receptors: relaxation
Peripheral nerve endings
  Afferent nerves: ? neuropeptide release via axon reflex
  Efferent nerves: bronchoconstriction via cholinergic mechanisms
Inflammatory cells
  T-cell H_1 and H_2 receptors: release of inhibitory or stimulatory cytokines

Vascular System

Vasodilation is the characteristic action of histamine on resistance vessels and involves both H_1 and H_2 receptor subtypes. H_1 responses are relatively rapid in onset and short lived whereas H_2 responses produce dilation that develops more slowly but is more sustained in nature. A combination of H_1 and H_2 antagonists are required to abolish this response and to prevent decreases in blood pressure. In contrast to its effects in small blood vessels, histamine tends to constrict larger blood vessels, in some species more than in others.

Histamine increases vascular permeability in capillary vessels, resulting in outward passage of plasma protein and fluid into the extracellular spaces, a response mediated principally by H_1 receptors. The response is mediated by effects on postcapillary venules where contraction and separation of endothelial cells expose the basement membrane, which is freely permeable to plasma protein and fluid. Edema forms and this produces the typical wheal visible when histamine is injected intradermally; an identical mechanism also operates in other situations (anaphylaxis, early asthmatic reaction) where histamine release causes clinical symptoms attributable to increased small blood vessel permeability.

Extravascular Smooth Muscle

Histamine has a dual action on various smooth muscles, contraction being due to H_1 receptor activation and relaxation being mediated by H_2 receptors. In human bronchial smooth muscle the spasmogenic influence of H_1 receptors is dominant and H_2 antagonists have no clinically discernible bronchodilator effects. However, *in vitro* studies have demonstrated slight potentiation of histamine-induced bronchospasm by H_2 blockade (10). In asthmatic patients in particular, bronchoconstriction induced by histamine may be a reflex component that arises from irritation of afferent vagal nerve endings.

Nerve Endings

Histamine can elicit responses via stimulation of various nerve endings including autonomic afferents and efferents. The neuronal receptors for histamine are generally of the H_1 subtype (11).

Cells Mediating Inflammation

Histamine may have immunoregulatory functions mediated by receptors on mast cells, lymphocytes, neutrophils, and eosinophils. An inhibitory cytokine secreted by T lymphocytes in response to histamine stimulation (histamine-induced suppressor factor) suppresses T and B cell proliferative responses as well as suppressing production of migration inhibitory factor (MIF), an effect abolished by H_2-receptor blockade but not by H_1-receptor antagonism (12). When stimulated with histamine, T lymphocytes bearing H_1 receptors have also been found to suppress IgG production by B cells *in vitro* (13).

Differential stimulation of H_1 and H_2 receptors on T lymphocytes produces either MIFs or a lymphocyte chemoattractant factor (LCF) and such findings have suggested a model for the immunoregulatory role of histamine (14). This model proposes that allergen challenge releases histamine from mast cells and basophils and at the same time stimulates lymphocytes to produce colony stimulating factors to increase production of mast cells and basophils. Histamine releasing factors may also be liberated to augment histamine release; the released amine then acts on T lymphocytes via H_2 receptors to stimulate the release of a suppressor or inhibitory factor that reduces lymphocyte proliferation and other effector functions (Fig. 1).

Mast Cells and Basophils

Great morphological and functional similarity exists between mast cells and basophils. Basophils are derived from precursors in the bone marrow, whereas tissue mast cells are thought to derive from connective tissue cells. Basophils stay in the blood for a short period only (approximately 5–6 h) before migrating into tissues. There is no evidence that they transform into tissue mast cells. However, some evidence suggests that blood monocytes may serve as a precursor pool for tissue mast cells (15).

Basophils are smaller and usually less granular than mast cells and have a bilobed or trilobed nucleus in contrast to the mononuclear character of

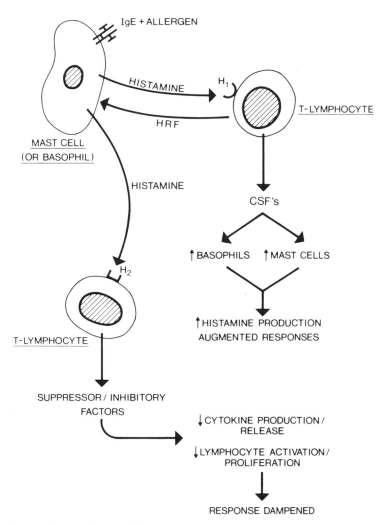

FIG. 1. Proposed model for the differential regulation of immune responses and modulation of T-cell function by histamine acting on H_1 and H_2 receptors. HRF, Histamine releasing factors; CSF, Colony stimulating factors.

mast cells. Both basophils and eosinophils exhibit a diurnal rhythm, the highest blood concentration occurring during the night and the lowest in the morning (16). Steroid hormones and corticosteroid therapy cause a parallel decrease in basophil and eosinophil concentration in the blood and a common influence of the hypothalamus-pituitary-adrenal system on both cell lines has been postulated (17).

Basophils and tissue mast cells have a major secretory function releasing their granule contents outside the cell (degranulation) in response to a wide variety of stimuli. IgE is bound to basophils and mast cells of both normal and atopic individuals via the F_C portion of IgE and allergen binding to the F_{AB} position initiates the classic sequence of events leading to mediator release from such cells.

The release of histamine, leukotrienes, prostaglandins, and other substances during degranulation is pivotal in the development of early (EAR) and probably also late asthmatic responses (LAR). Recent studies have indicated that a wide variety of stimuli besides allergens are able to initiate release of preformed mediators from basophils. A 30-kDa histamine releasing factor has been described, produced by mononuclear cells from ragweed-sensitive subjects (18) and a similar "factor" secreted into the supernatant of neutrophils incubated with PAF and leukotriene (LT) B_4 may stimulate histamine release from human lung sections (19). The cytokines interleukin (IL) -3, -4, and -5 have recently been implicated in important aspects of allergic cellular and immune responses and Piona et al. (20) have demonstrated that IL-3, -5, and -6 significantly enhanced anti-IgE–induced histamine release from human basophils. It is not yet known whether release of other intracellular constituents of mast cells such as sulfidopeptide leukotrienes are similarly affected; it is also possible that IL-4 and other cytokines present in human nasal mast cells (21) may be released or functionally modulated by interactions with extracellular cytokines. Other modulatory peptides (including the platelet-derived growth factors: connective tissue-activating peptide-III and neutrophil-activating peptide-2) also possess histamine releasing activity in human basophils and may conceivably play some role in allergic inflammation if this involves platelet participation.

An important aspect of the role of mast cells in allergic diseases may involve cytokine production and release, and recent studies by Plaut et al. (22) have demonstrated that mast cell lines in culture are able to secrete several cytokines including IL-3, -4, -5, and -6, an observation that has been extended by Moller et al. (23) to include IL-8. Using double-staining techniques our group has recently demonstrated that tryptase-positive mast cells from human nasal biopsies also give positive staining for IL-4. This implies that mast cells may play a controlling role in allergic responses and it is possible that antihistamines may exhibit inhibiting or other effects not only on mediator release itself, but through cytokine actions may modulate regulating mechanisms in the development and perpetuation of inflammation. Basophils and mast cells are responsive to pharmacological manipulation and release of histamine and other mediators can be inhibited *in vitro* by antihistamines and corticosteroids as well as by other glucocorticoids such as dihydrotestosterone (24). Further exploration of the effects of such compounds on cytokine release may explain changes in cutaneous reactions and inhibition of eosinophil migration seen recently with cetirizine (25), a specific H_1-receptor antagonist.

Recent morphological and functional evidence supports a biologically significant interaction between mast cells and peripheral nerves. It appears that neural impulses can promote mast cell degranulation through axon reflexes or other mechanisms (26). Further evidence suggest that allergen-induced mast cell degranulation may release mediators that communicate with local nerves, producing axon reflexes and further transmission of signals to the spinal cord and central nervous system. It is not known how this function of mast cells is influenced by antihistamine compounds and it seems possible that such drugs may have an important role to play in the prevention of neurogenic inflammation.

HISTAMINE RECEPTORS

Three distinctive receptors of histamine have been described to date. Stimulation by histamine leads to distinctive changes in various tissue types and organ systems, reflecting the divergent actions of histamine acting as a ligand at such receptors.

Mepyramine, a typical antihistamine drug, was used in 1965 by Ash and coworkers (27) to show that prior administration blocked classic contractile responses in smooth muscle to histamine. The pharmacological receptors involved in these mepyramine-sensitive responses were defined as H_1 receptors. However, histamine-induced secretion of acid by the stomach, increases in heart rate, and uterine contraction cannot be antagonized by mepyramine and related drugs. Black and coworkers (28) demonstrated that such effects are mediated via burinamide-sensitive receptors, defined as H_2 receptors. Subsequent work has led to the development of more potent H_2-receptor antagonists that found clinical application as inhibitors of gastric acid secretion in the management of peptic ulcer disease.

Recently it was observed that histamine inhibits its own synthesis and release in brain slices by a negative feedback mechanism operating at the level of histaminergic nerve endings (29). Using an agonist (α-methylhistamine) and antagonist (thioperamide), Arrang and coworkers (29) have demonstrated the presence of a third (H_3) subclass of histamine receptor in brain tissues. The function of H_3 receptors seems to be analogous to that of other classes of presynaptic receptors mediating feedback regulation of several neurotransmitters. Since stimulation of H_3 receptors modulates cholinergic neurotransmission in human airways *in vitro* (30) and nonadrenergic noncholinergic bronchoconstriction in guinea pigs *in vivo* (31), and neurogenic mechanisms probably contribute to asthmatic bronchoconstriction, stimulation of H_3 receptors may be beneficial in asthma.

ANTIHISTAMINE COMPOUNDS

Development of antihistamine drugs binding to the H_1 receptor has widened the scope of pharmacological manipulation and intervention in human diseases such as rhinitis and asthma. Targeting and blocking of H_1 receptors has been used to counter and decrease classic effects associated with histamine release and relieve symptoms such as itching, excessive nasal secretions, as well as chest wheezing following bronchial smooth muscle contraction. This was initially accomplished by use of the earlier "classic" compounds with good clinical effect, but often accompanied by unacceptable CNS and anticholinergic side effects. Recent developments have produced a new generation of nonsedating H_1 antagonists that may be distinguished from the classic compounds by (a) relative lack of sedatory and other CNS side effects, and (b) kinetics of receptor binding and dissociation leading to variable prolongation of clinical effects. A brief description of the different groups of antihistamines will be given to explain the differential effects of some compounds and place their clinical use in context.

Classic H_1-Receptor Antagonists

Histamine is a hydrophilic molecule comprised of an imidazole ring and an amino group connected by two methylene groups. In contrast, the majority of the H_1 antagonists are composed of one or often two heterocyclic or aromatic rings connected via a nitrogen, carbon, or oxygen linkage to the amine group. The nitrogen of this group is tertiary, having two substituents (Fig. 2).

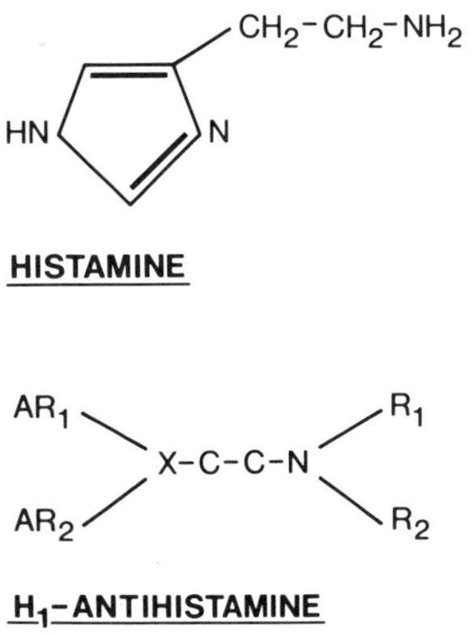

HISTAMINE

H₁-ANTIHISTAMINE

FIG. 2. Chemical structure of histamine and the general formula for six major groups of antihistamine compounds (see text).

The classic H_1 antagonists can be divided into six major groups based on their chemical structure (Table 2). Most classic antagonists are lipophilic as a result of alkyl substituents present in the chemical structure. In general they are well and rapidly absorbed after oral or parenteral administration and clinical benefits can be detected within 15 to 45 min. Duration of action is 3 to 6 h although some compounds have a longer period of activity. Tissue distribution is wide and includes the central nervous system and cross-placental transfer. Metabolism occurs in the liver via hydroxylation and excretion is in the urine. Because the affinity of histamine is approximately ten times higher for H_1 compared with H_2 receptors (32), the H_1 effects often predominate physiological responses and can be effectively blocked by the classic compounds on the basis of direct competition with histamine for the H_1 receptor. This binding of antihistamines is readily reversible and the number of receptors occupied will be determined primarily by the concentrations of drug in the vicinity of the receptor site. This accounts for the relatively short duration of action of such compounds and may explain their relative lack of efficacy in the bronchial tree where up to 10^{-4} to 10^{-3} mol/L histamine may be released in response to allergen challenge (33). Increased doses of drug are associated with significant side effects and limit the extent to which more drug can be delivered at the H_1 receptor to compete with histamine for binding.

The most common side effects of the classic H_1 antihistamines are sedation, anticholinergic effects via a dose-dependent blocking of cholinergic muscarinic receptors, CNS disturbances of mood, and gastrointestinal side effects. Although some tolerance may develop after repeated use, such side effects restrict clinical use of these compounds and has led to the search for nonsedating H_1-receptor antagonists with a longer duration of action.

TABLE 2. *The six major groups of class H_1-receptor antagonists*

General group	Linkage atom	Compounds	Characteristics
Alkylamines	Carbon	Chlorpheniramine Brompheniramine Triprolidine	Less drowsiness Rarely: CNS stimulation
Ethanolamines	Oxygen	Clemastine Diphenhydramine Carbinoxamine	Anticholinergic side effects Drowsiness
Ethylenediamines	Nitrogen	Pyrilamine Methapyrilene Antazoline	Drowsiness and sedation Gastrointestinal side effects
Piperazines	Nitrogen	Cyclizine Buclizine Hydroxyzine	Mild side effects Useful for motion sickness
Piperidines	Nitrogen	Cyproheptadine Azatadine	Drowsiness
Phenothiazines	Nitrogen	Promethazine Trimeprazine	Sedative side effects Anticholinergic side effects

Nonsedating H_1-Receptor Antagonists

The development of compounds that compete specifically for binding to the H_1 receptor, but lack the classical side effects, has enabled renewed evaluation of their efficacy in the treatment of diseases requiring almost total blockade of histamine receptors for clinical efficacy. This has rekindled interest in the treatment of asthma, rhinitis, and allergic eczema and also enabled studies of other therapeutic and possible immunomodulatory actions of some compounds such as cetirizine (34). The best known antihistamines making up this group are terfenadine, astemizole, azelastine, cetirizine, mequitazine, loratidine, temelastine, and acrivastine.

Modification of the original chemical structure has enabled synthesis of novel chemical substances and account for the development of some of the above new compounds. Loratidine is a derivative of the piperidine group, mequitzine is a phenothiazine-like compound, and acrivastine is derived from the alkylamines. Although both astemizole and terfenadine contain a piperidine ring, they are not considered to be part of that group because of marked structural and pharmacological differences. All are characterized by a lack of CNS penetration compared to the classic compounds (35), explaining their relative lack of side effects at higher doses. The kinetics of their interaction with the H_1 receptor may also be different and are regarded as slower in onset, more specific, and more avidly binding to H_1 receptors coupled to a prolonged duration of action ascribed to competitive as well as possibly non competitive mechanisms (36). The latter observation may be related to prolonged functional antagonism at the H_1 receptor. Some of the newer and more interesting compounds will be discussed briefly.

Terfenadine

Oral terfenadine is well absorbed and peak plasma levels can be measured 60 to 90 min later. The drug is distributed widely through body tissues and organs as measured by radiolabeled ^{14}C-terfenadine (37). As with astemizole, low levels were present in the CNS and high levels in lung and liver. Almost all of the absorbed drug is metabolized to two major metabolites that exhibit weak H_1 antagonism in guinea pig ileum (38). After hydroxylation and glucuronidation, terfenadine is excreted in urine and bile in roughly equal proportions (39).

In contrast to astemizole, terfenadine has a relatively short duration of action of about 8 h when measured as inhibition of histamine-induced skin reactions (40). Cumulative doses (five consecutive doses of 60 mg given every 12 h) only prolonged H_1 antagonism by 90 to 180 min as assessed by the above methods.

Sedative side effects are very mild or absent, contributing to better patient compliance. Prolonged H_1-receptor blockade produced by terfenadine, astemizole, and other drugs in this group can reduce or eliminate histamine-associated "breakthrough" effects, and have enabled critical assessment of their potential in diseases such as asthma, where large amounts of histamine are released in the bronchial tree and clinical efficacy of this type of compound depends on potent and effective pharmacological receptor antagonism.

Astemizole

Chemically this compound is similar to the piperidine group of H_1 antagonists but with marked pharmacological differences. Good absorption occurs from the gastrointestinal tract and peak plasma concentration are present 60 to 90 min later. Food in the stomach may retard absorption and the drug should therefore be taken before meals. Distribution studies have demonstrated drug presence in the lung, intestine, liver, kidney, and thyroid with no measurable levels in the CNS, indicating poor blood-brain barrier penetration (41).

Metabolism via hydroxylation, glucuronidation, and dealkylation occurs with formation of metabolites that appear to have comparable pharmacological activity. Elimination is very slow; approximately 60% is excreted in the feces via biliary excretion and 10% in the urine by 14 days postdosing with a 10-mg tablet (42).

The slow onset of action of astemizole and its prolonged effects are well documented. In a study using 10 mg daily the maximal effect on inhibition of the flare response to intradermal histamine was seen after 6 days and this was still present (83% inhibition) 18 days after the last dose was administered (43). Astemizole appears devoid of antagonist activity at beta-adrenergic and cholinergic receptors, and although it has weak affinity for alpha-adrenergic and serotonin receptors, this is not clinically significant.

No side effects related to the classic compounds occur with astemizole and it is devoid of any interactions with alcohol or diazepam (44).

Cetirizine

Although cetirizine is the major human metabolite of the classic antihistamine hydroxyzine, its high molecular polarity and protein-binding capacity results in poor penetration of the blood-brain barrier (45). Potency and duration of receptor binding are greater than for either hydroxyzine or terfenadine when compared using cutaneous wheal and flare responses to histamine (46). A single 20-mg dose of cetirizine produced 70% suppression of the wheal and flare reaction at 24 h (47).

The mean half-life of cetirizine is approximately 9 h in adults and 6 h in children. Up to 60% of the drug is excreted in unchanged form in the urine

(45), and pharmacokinetic studies with ^{14}C-cetirizine have demonstrated that there is little metabolism of the compound in humans and that only one minor metabolite is formed (48).

Recent evidence suggests that the anti-allergic actions of cetirizine may implicate mechanisms other than H_1-receptor antagonism, since the drug also inhibits release of PAF and prostaglandin D_2 (PGD_2) as well as decreasing inflammatory cell migration in late phase cutaneous reactions (49). Inflammatory events may thus be modulated, an action particularly beneficial in various forms of allergic rhinitis and asthma, conditions in which allergic inflammation may be pivotal in the pathogenesis of hyperresponsiveness and development of symptoms. Combination of H_1-receptor antagonism and anti-inflammatory actions in one compound is an attractive concept because, in addition to control of symptoms, the underlying pathology may be treated as well.

Azelastine

Azelastine hydrochloride is a novel phthalazinone derivative that exhibits potent histamine H_1-receptor, serotonin, and LTD_4-receptor antagonism (50,51). Peak blood levels occur approximately 4 to 5 h after oral ingestion and there is a linear relationship between increasing dosage and peak plasma concentrations. Bronchodilating effects occur on doses of 4 mg and higher, but this was only marginally increased by 8- and 16-mg doses; consequently the 4-mg dose has been considered optimal (52). Side effects include a bitter taste and sleepiness. Such effects are usually mild and are not sufficient to cause interruption of medication or problems with normal daily activities.

After single oral doses, azelastine produced bronchodilatation lasting 4 to 6 h (53) and a dose-related displacement of histamine-induced bronchoconstriction (54). It also afforded at least a fivefold protection again the EAR provoked by allergen (55), and in a clinical study lasting 2 weeks, both the symptoms and frequency of exacerbations of wheezing were reduced (56). Our group has also shown that a dose of 8.8 mg significantly inhibited the EAR and LAR in atopic asthmatics (57), and this prompted speculation that the effect on the late phase may be mediated by inhibition of LTD_4 or as a result of changes in nonspecific bronchial responsiveness. Other possible mechanisms for this observation include inhibition of superoxide release by neutrophils and eosinophils (58) or inhibition of macrophage activation (59). Although both IgE-mediated and nonallergic histamine release is inhibited by azelastine *in vitro* (60,61), a recent study has suggested that *in vivo* the compound does not inhibit mast cell activation but rather opposes the consequences of released histamine, namely sneezing, edema, and kinin generation (62).

Early clinical studies have been promising and azelastine may prove to have a useful therapeutic role in selected asthmatic subjects.

Mequitazine

Although a phenothiazine derivative, mequitazine causes only very mild sedation and impairment of performance at its recommended therapeutic dose of 5 mg twice daily (63). This may be attributable to decreased affinity for cerebral H_1 receptors coupled to impaired movement across the blood-brain barrier. As a phenothiazine, mesquitazine inhibits calmodulin and interferes with mobilization of membrane phospholipids via inhibition of phospholipase A_2, an action that may partly explain its effective bronchodilating action against leukotrienes and prostaglandins (64).

Acrivastine

Acrivastine is an alkylamine derivative that attains high plasma levels after oral ingestion with a short serum half-life of approximately 2 h (65). Although it has only mild sedative and cholinergic side effects, clinical utility remains to be established.

ANTIHISTAMINES WITH ADDITIONAL BENEFICIAL ACTIONS

Possible anti-inflammatory actions via reduced mediator release and impaired cellular responses have already been discussed for cetirizine. Other antihistamines such as azelastine and ketotifen may possess additional characteristics particularly beneficial in allergic disease, primarily by inhibition of mediator release from mast cells.

Cromolyn sodium was the first compound used clinically to prevent mediator release, but because of poor intestinal absorption it has not been useful as an oral drug. New compounds synthesized subsequently have been demonstrated to possess varying efficacy when taken orally to suppress mast cell mediator release via inhibition of degranulation. Their mode of action is controversial but may involve at least three possible mechanisms that may lead to a decrease in intracellular free Ca^{2+}. First, it has been postulated that an action on mast cell and basophil plasma membranes may directly inhibit Ca^{2+} influx or, second, stabilize the cell membrane to prevent Na^{2+} entry, an event that promotes intracellular Ca^{2+} release. A third mechanism proposed is that the drugs may directly decrease intracellular Ca^{2+} release from the sarcoplasmic reticulum (66).

Azelastine, ketotifen, and oxatomide are three antihistamines considered to possess some mast cell stabilizing activity in addition to classical H_1-receptor antagonism. They exhibit varying effects on histamine, cholinergic, serotonin, and leukotriene receptors. At histamine receptors a dual action may be detected with characteristics of both competitive and noncompetitive binding, making quantitative comparison with other antihistamine drugs difficult. These three compounds show little or no anticholinergic activity at therapeutic concentrations.

Azelastine decreased leukotriene C_4 (LTC_4), LTD_4, and LTE_4 from rat peritoneal mast cells (67), and demonstrated inhibition of allergen-induced bronchoconstriction in guinea pigs (68). It remains unclear whether the latter responses are mediated by inhibition of leukotriene release, events at the leukotriene receptor, or directly via Ca^{2+} antagonism in airway smooth muscle.

ANTIHISTAMINES IN EXPERIMENTAL ASTHMA

The discovery that drugs could compete with and antagonize the target tissue effects of histamine has provided new insights into the role of histamine in asthma and opened new possibilities for pharmacological intervention. Although early preparations appeared effective in the treatment of allergic rhinitis, their efficacy in the treatment of clinical asthma was low (69,70). Their lack of specificity for H_1 receptors with additional actions at muscarinic, cholinergic, and serotonin receptors suggested that other pharmacological effects contributed significantly to bronchodilator actions. Critical assessment of the influence of effective H_1-receptor antagonism in asthma was also confounded by sedation at high doses. The situation 15 years ago could be summarized as antihistamines having little use in the treatment of asthma. The advent of the new highly potent and selective H_1-receptor antagonists has permitted a reappraisal of histamine's role in asthma.

Inhalation of histamine in the laboratory has been shown to be a powerful and reproducible bronchoconstrictor agonist to which asthmatic airways are hyperresponsive, the basis for widely used laboratory and field testing of nonspecific bronchial hyperresponsiveness (BHR) (71). Using this convenient test system it has been possible to examine the efficacy and selectivity of antihistamines on the airways; the former an be determined by measuring the degree of displacement of the histamine dose-response curve with the relevant antagonist(s). Our group has shown in atopic asthmatic subjects that oral doses of terfenadine (180 mg), astemizole (10 mg), and azelastine (8.8 mg) provided 35-fold, 17-fold, and 50-fold protection, respectively, against histamine-induced bronchoconstriction (72–74). The specificity of the protection provided by these drugs is indicated by an absence of significant effect on the bronchoconstriction provoked by methacholine, a specific agonist for smooth muscle muscarinic (M_3) receptors.

The component of bronchoconstriction produced by histamine in response to natural stimuli such as allergen and exercise has also been investigated. A single oral dose of 180 mg of terfenadine inhibits the allergen-induced early asthmatic reaction by 50% (75), at a time (15 min) when most mast cell–derived histamine is released from airway mast cells. Increasing the dose of terfenadine to 600 mg has no additional protective effect against allergen, suggesting that approximately 50% of the airways bronchoconstrictor response is contributed by histamine, the rest coming from other constrictor mediators.

The nonsedating H_1 antihistamines are also effective in attenuating acute bronchoconstriction provoked by stimuli other than allergen. An important role for mast cell mediators including histamine has been suggested in exercise-induced asthma (EIA) following reports of increases in measured plasma histamine during EIA (76,77). However, other groups have failed to show histaminemia accompanying EIA (78), and in those that did, its origin from circulating basophils increased during exercise could not be excluded (79). Hypertonicity may be the relevant stimulus for EIA (80), and Gravelyn et al. (81) have shown that after local bronchial challenge with hypertonic saline solution, histamine levels rise in lavage fluid, a finding compatible with mast cell degranulation.

Several investigators have now shown that prior treatment of patients with adequate doses of potent and selective nonsedative antihistamines inhibits the subsequent bronchoconstrictor response to exercise (82,83). Our own work has indicated that terfenadine in an oral dose of 180 mg reduced EIA by about 35% with the peak effect observed within the first 10 to 15 min after exercise. The protective effect was not consistent between patients— some were more responsive than others and the protective effect of terfenadine could not be accounted for by the observed bronchodilation caused by the compound.

Other bronchoconstrictor stimuli that exhibit at least some antihistamine-sensitive components include hypertonic saline solution (84), adenosine 5'-monophosphate (85), and benzalkinium chloride (86). Antihistamines do not inhibit the bronchial response to bradykinin and SO_2, suggesting that smooth muscle contraction induced by such agents is mediated via nonhistaminergic pathways (87).

Recently the protective efficacy of aerosolized thiazinamium chloride against histamine-induced and exercise-induced bronchoconstriction was evaluated by Gong et al. (88), after other studies had suggested significant prolonged bronchodilator effects for this mode of administration (89). Gong et al. observed a modest bronchodilator effect and attenuation of the airway obstruction induced by histamine, but no effect on exercise-induced bronchoconstriction. Another study has shown attenuation of the EAR to allergen and of methacholine-induced bronchoconstriction after premedication with the same inhaled compound, and the authors proposed that results were sufficiently encouraging to warrant therapeutic trials in chronic asthma (90).

Further studies on cetirizine by Gong et al. (91) examined the effect of single oral doses (5, 10, and 20 mg) on the allergen-induced EAR and also on EIA. Cetirizine was not uniformly effective in preventing bronchoconstriction elicited by such stimuli, although individual cases did benefit. The authors commented that histamine is only one of many mediators participating in immediate asthmatic responses and that selective H_1 antagonists may not completely block these airway events. Clinical benefit can be expected in selected patients, especially those with allergic rhinitis or urticaria. Unfortunately, subjects were not evaluated for late phase responses and the influence of cetirizine on the LAR was not assessed.

Late Phase Responses

Approximately 60% to 70% of atopic patients with asthma will develop "late" bronchoconstriction, usually 3 to 10 h after inhalation of allergen, and this response is accompanied by an increase in BHR.

Little is known about the effect of histamine in the late phase asthmatic reaction, a surprising omission in view of the data that have accumulated on the role of histamine in immediate reactions. In both animals and humans this late phase of bronchoconstriction involves the selective recruitment of eosinophils and other circulating leukocytes, and this has been useful as a model for the more chronic inflammatory events of clinical asthma (92,93).

Only a small number of studies have investigated the role of histamine as an effector mediator in late phase asthma. De Monchy et al. (94) were unable to demonstrate increased levels of the major metabolite N-methylhistamine in association with late phase bronchoconstriction, whereas elevated plasma concentrations were present after the early response provoked by allergen. Other studies have suggested that elevated circulating serum levels of histamine may occur during late phase allergen responses (95) and that the amine may also be elevated in nasal late phase responses after allergen instillation (96). The latter study found some inhibition of the late phase by chlorpheniramine, although this may have been caused by nonspecific anticholinergic or antiserotonin actions. Recently we have found that azelastine administered in an oral dose of 8.8 mg produced complete inhibition of the late phase response to inhaled allergen (97), an observation that may relate to histamine antagonism or some other as yet unknown effect of the compound. The effects of azelastine on eosinophil function *in vitro* suggests that its inhibition of the late phase reaction may be related to possible anti-inflammatory actions of this group of drugs.

ANTIHISTAMINES IN CLINICAL ASTHMA

Clinical trials with some of the earlier generation of antihistamines administered orally to patients over a period of several weeks failed to demonstrate efficacy in asthma (97). Recent development of the potent and specific nonsedative antihistamines has permitted a reappraisal of their therapeutic potential in a clinical setting.

Single-dose studies with terfenadine, azelastine, and cetirizine have demonstrated dose-related bronchodilatation similar to that achieved with inhalation of β_2-agonist drugs (98–100). Because this bronchodilation is likely to be the result of specific H_1-receptor antagonism, it has been suggested that some basal histamine tone exists in the airways of asthmatics attributed to ongoing mast cell and basophil degranulation (101). This phenomenon may be of more importance in asthmatics with significantly reduced baseline airway caliber and suggests that H_1-receptor-specific antihistamine compounds may benefit this particular group to a greater extent.

A number of studies have evaluated response to the nonsedative antihistamines in a clinical setting measuring symptoms, peak expiratory flow (PEF), and forced expiratory volume in 1 sec (FEV_1), changes in BHR, and skin reactivity (Table 3). Although most studies have shown some benefit to patients, this has often been of marginal clinical significance. This is exemplified by the study of Taytard et al. (102) who found a (statistically) significant reduction in overall symptoms scores (2.4 to 1.8 on scale of 0 to 12) and increased PEF from 420 to 427 L/min. Clearly such slight improvements make no difference to the clinical expression of the disease in asthmatic patients, and the drugs cannot be judged to be effective in a clinical setting. Some studies have indicated that antihistamines may be beneficial in certain subgroups of asthmatics, notably young patients or those with seasonal pollen-induced asthma. Rafferty et al. (103) found that treatment with terfenadine in this group during the summer pollen season decreased cough by 77% and wheeze by 47%, coupled to modest increases in PEF of 5.5% (morning) and 6.2% (evening). The subjects also reported a 40% reduction in bronchodilator use. It appears likely that seasonal exposure to aeroallergens leads to increased mast cell degranulation in the airways of susceptible individuals, and that at least some clinically useful effect of a potent antihistamine administered across the pollen season might be anticipated.

A Canadian multicenter study with ketotifen in 138 children with chronic asthma measured symptom scores, spirometry (including morning and evening PEF), and the need for additional medication over a 6-month period (104). Although 60% of children on ketotifen could stop the use of theophylline (versus 34% of patients taking placebo), changes in FEV_1 and PEF were small and clearly of marginal clinical significance. Since patient symptoms at baseline were controlled in this study, it was difficult to show a clinically significant reduction in symptoms on treatment with ketotifen.

Other studies (Table 3) have shown the same trend and have provided some measure of encouragement for the clinician to try the use of antihistamines in selected asthmatics. Patients who may benefit include (a) young asthmatics, (b) seasonal pollen-induced asthma patients, and (c) severe asthma patients with reduced baseline airway caliber and presumed high basal histamine tone in the airways. Variations in design and execution make evaluation and comparison of many clinical trials with antihistamines diffi-

TABLE 3. Clinical studies of H_1 receptor antagonists in asthma

Investigator (reference)	Drug(s)	Study design	Patient characteristics	Duration	Symptom scores	PFs	BHR	Skin/allergen challenge	Additional medication
Finnerty et al. (105)	Cetirizine 10 mg bid	PC,C,DB	14 Asthmatics (8 atopic)	2 weeks	–	NC in FEV_1	NC	–	–
Rafferty et al. (106)	Cetirizine Oral 15 mg bid	PC,C,DB	10 Asthmatics (10 atopic)	Oral × 3 days	–	NC in FEV_1	–	NC in EAR/LAR	–
Gould et al. (107)	Azelastine 4.4 mg bid	PC,DB	24 Asthmatics (all atopic)	7 weeks	↓ (wheeze only)	PEF ↑ NC in FEV_1	↓ (H) NC(M)	↓ Skin wheal diameter	→
Spector et al. (108)	Terfenadine 60/120 mg bid	PC,DB,C	12 Asthmatics	1 week	–	FEV_1 ↑	–	–	–
Rackham et al. (104)	Ketotifen 1 mg bid	PC,DB	138 Asthmatics (children)	7 months	→	PEF ↑ FEV_1 NC	–	–	→
Boerner et al. (109)	Picumast dihydrochloride 1 mg bid	PC,DB	107 Asthmatics ("mixed" group)	6 weeks	→	PEF ↑	–	–	→
Rafferty et al. (103)	Terfenadine 180 mg tds	PC,DB,C	18 Asthmatics (grass pollen sensitive)	9 weeks	→	PEF ↑	↑ (but NS)	–	→
Kopferschmitt-Kubler et al. (110)	Cetirizine 10 mg bid	PC,DB,C	5 Asthmatics (all atopic)	4 days	–	–	–	↓ EAR (NS)	–
Brutman et al. (111)	Cetirizine 5 mg AM 10 mg PM	DB,PC	57 Asthmatics	2 weeks	–	PEF↑ FEV_1	–	–	→
Bousquet et al. (112)	Cetirizine 10 mg bid 15 mg bid Terfenadine 60 mg bid	Open	26 Asthmatics	4 weeks	→	PEV ↑ (Cetirizine 15 mg)	–	–	→
Dijkman et al. (113)	Cetirizine 10 mg bid Terfenadine 60 mg bid	Open	39 Asthmatics (grass pollen sensitive)	6 weeks	→	PEF ↑ (C>T)	–	–	→
Taytard et al. (102)	Terfenadine 120 mg bd	PC,DB,C	52 Asthmatics (pollen sensitive)	2 weeks	→	PEF ↑	–	–	→
Cookson et al. (114)	Terfenadine 120 mg bd	PC,DB,C	22 Asthmatics (17 atopic)	4 weeks	NC	NC (↑ PEF in young subjects)	–	–	NC

PC, placebo controlled; DB, double-blind; C, crossover; PEF, peak expiratory flow rate; FEV, forced expiratory flow in 1 sec; NC, no change; BHR, bronchial hyperresponsiveness; H, histamine; M, methacholine; NS, not statistically significant; EAR, early asthmatic reaction; LAR, late asthmatic reaction; ↓, decreased; ↑, increased.

cult, but the lack of a clear and significant beneficial effect in many studies suggests that their clinical application is currently not clearly established.

Novel effects of specific H_1 antagonists on other cellular and immune functions are exciting and may provide new insights into the functions of histamine as well as provide useful therapeutic options in the management of clinical asthma. Such non–H_1-receptor characteristics exhibited by azelastine, cetirizine, and other similar compounds have to be evaluated in outpatient studies to assess their clinical impact and benefit in asthmatic subjects.

CONCLUSIONS

Histamine has a pivotal role in many physiological processes in the body, as well as in the development of allergic skin reactions, anaphylaxis, and in early asthmatic responses. Its importance in late asthmatic responses remain to be defined. Antagonism of specific receptors for histamine has useful clinical applications in allergic disease, while some newer compounds may also have immunological and other characteristics applicable to their use in allergic inflammation.

Although definitive conclusions cannot be drawn from available data, current evidence indicates that antihistamines, particularly the new nonsedating H_1-receptor antagonists, may have a role to play in improving lung function and clinical symptoms in adults and children with asthma. Such compounds may exert a protective effect by enhancing the threshold for stimuli to induce bronchoconstriction, as shown by short-term studies in both groups of patients.

Several important questions have yet to be addressed: What degree of protection might be expected?; Can the effect be sustained for prolonged periods?; and, importantly, Which patients could derive the most benefit from antihistamine therapy? At present, the role of this group of compounds may be predicted to be that of adjuvant therapy in patients stabilized on maintenance asthma treatment, but who require additional medication under conditions that exacerbate their disease. Answers to the questions posed above are required before their place in asthma therapy can be defined with certainty.

ACKNOWLEDGMENT

This research was supported by the Medical Research Council of South Africa.

REFERENCES

1. Windaus A, Vogt W. Syntheses des imidazolylathyamines. *Ber Dtsh Chem Ges* 1907;3:3691–3695.

2. Dale HH, Laidlaw PP. The physiological action of betaimidazolylethylamine. *J Physiol* 1910;41:318.
3. Best CH, Dale HH, Dudley HW, Thorpe WV. The nature of vasodilator constituents of certain tissue extracts. *J Physiol* 1927;62:397–417.
4. Weiss S, Robb GP, Ellis LB. The systemic effects of histamine in man with special reference to the response of the cardiovascular system. *Arch Intern Med* 1932;49:360–396.
5. Schild HO, Hawkins DF, Mongar JL, Herxheimer H. Reactions of isolated human asthmatic lung and bronchial tissue to a specific antigen. *Lancet* 1951;2:376–382.
6. Bovet D, Staub A. Action protectrice des ethers phenoliques au cours de l'intoxication histaminique. *CR Soc Biol (Paris)* 1937;124:547–549.
7. Uvnas B, Aborg CH, Bergendorff A. Storage of histamine in mast cells: evidence for ionic binding of histamine to protein carboxyls in the granule heparin protein complex. *Acta Physiol Scand* 1970;336(suppl):1–26.
8. Ishizaka T. Analysis of triggering events in mast cells for immunoglobulin E-mediated histamine release. *J Allergy Clin Immunol* 1981;67:90–96.
9. Dahlen SE, Hansson G, Hedquist P, Bjorck T, Granstrom E, Dahlen B. Allergen challenge of lung tissue from asthmatics elicits bronchial contraction that correlates with the release of leukotrienes C_4, D_4, and E_4. *Proc Natl Acad Sci USA* 1983;80:1712–1716.
10. Dunlop LS, Smith AP, Piper PJ. The effect of histamine antagonists on antigen-induced contractions of sensitised human bronchus in vitro. *Br J Pharmacol* 1977;59:475.
11. Ganellin CR, Parsons ME, eds. *Pharmacology of histamine receptors*. Bristol: Wright/PSG, 1982.
12. Rocklin RE. Histamine suppressor factor (HSF): effect on migration inhibitory factor (MIF) production and proliferation. *J Immunol* 1977;118:1734–1740.
13. Garovoy MR, Reddish MA, Rocklin RE. Histamine induced suppressor factor (HSF): inhibition of helper T-cell generation and function. *J Immunol* 1983;130:357–362.
14. Beer DJ, Rocklin RE. Histamine induced suppressor-cell activity. *J Allergy Clin Immunol* 1984;73:439–452.
15. Thiede A. Preliminary report on the origin of rat mast cells. *Klin Wochenschr* 1971;49:435.
16. Boseila A. The normal count of basophilic leukocytes in human blood. *Acta Med Scand* 1959;163:526.
17. Wintrobe MM. Leucocyte kinetics and function. In: Wintrobe MM, Lee GRR, eds. *Clinical haematology*, Philadelphia: Lee and Febiger 1981;8:228–230.
18. Jobin M, Brunet C, Hebert J. Isolation and biological activities of a molecular weight specie of histamine-releasing factor. *J Allergy Clin Immunol* 1991;87:252(abstract).
19. Nagakura T, Ohno K, Masaki T, Iikura Y, Maekawa K. Neutrophil-derived NCA and histamine-releasing activity from human lung tissue. *J Allergy Clin Immunol* 1991;87:252(abstract).
20. Piona A, Tedeschi A, Lorini M, Tech M, Parma M, Arquati M, Miadonna A. Different effects of interleukins on in vitro histamine release from human basophils. *J Allergy Clin Immunol* 1991;87:157(abstract).
21. Bradding P, Feather I, Wilson S, Holgate ST, Howarth PH. Interleukin-4 immunoreactivity is localised to mast cells in the upper respiratory tract. *Thorax* 1992;47:231P.
22. Plaut M, Pierce JH, Watson CJ, Hanley-Hyde J, Nordan RP, Paul WE. Mast cell lines produce lymphokines in response to cross-linkage of Fc RI or to calcium ionophores. *Nature* 1989;339:64–67.
23. Moller A, Schadendorf D, Lippert U, Forster E, Luger TA, Czarnetski BM. Human mast cell and basophil cell lines produce interleukin 8 and 6. *J Allergy Clin Immunol* 1991;87:209(abstract).
24. Soler M, Morel A, Ferrt V, Vervloet D. Immediate inhibition on basophil histamine release by steroids. *J Allergy Clin Immunol* 1991;87:171(abstract).
25. Fadel R, David B, Herperin-Richard N, Borgnon A, Rassemont R, Rihoux JP. *In vivo* effects of cetirizine on cutaneous reactivity and eosinophil migration induced by platelet activating factor (PAF-acether) in man. *J Allergy Clin Immunol* 1990;86:314–320.
26. Bienenstock J, Macqueen G, Sestini P, Marshall JS, Stead RH, Perdue MH. Mast cell/nerve interactions *in vitro* and *in vivo*. *Am Rev Respir Dis* 1991;143:555–558.
27. Ash ASF, Schild HO. Receptors mediating some actions of histamine. *Br J Pharmacol Chemother* 1966;27:429–439.

28. Black JW, Duncan WAM, Durant CJ, Ganellin CR, Parsons EM. Definition and antagonism of histamine H_2 receptors. *Nature* 1977;236:385–390.
29. Arrang JM, Garbarg M, Lancelot JC, Leconte JC, Pollard H, Robba M, Schunach W, Schwartz JC. Highly potent and selective ligands for histamine H_3 receptors. *Nature* 1987;327:117–123.
30. Itchinose M, Stretton CD, Schwartz JD, Barnes PJ. Histamine H_3 receptors inhibit cholinergic bronchoconstriction in guinea-pig airways. *Br J Pharmacol* 1989;97:13–15.
31. Itchinose M, Barnes PJ. Inhibitory histamine H_3 receptors on cholinergic nerves in human airways. *Eur J Pharmacol* 1989;163:383–386.
32. Black JW. Histamine receptors. In: Klinge E, ed. *Proceedings of the Sixth International Congress of Pharmacology,* vol 1. Helsinki: Finnish Pharmacological Society, 1975.
33. Adams GK, Lichtenstein LM. *In vitro* studies of antigen-induced bronchospasm: effect of antihistamine and SRS-A antagonist on response of sensitised guinea-pig and human airways to antigen. *J Immunol* 1979;122:555–562.
34. Michel L, de Vos C, Rihoux J-P, Burtin C, Benveniste J, Dubertret L. Inhibitory effect of oral cetirizine on *in vivo* antigen-induced histamine and PAF-acether release and eosinophil recruitment in human skin. *J Allergy Clin Immunol* 1988;82:101–109.
35. Nicholson AN. Antihistamines and sedation. *Lancet* 1983;2:211.
36. Cheng HC, Woodward JK. Antihistaminic effect of terfenadine: a new piperidine type antihistamine. *Drug Dev Res* 1982;2:181–187.
37. Castaner J, Thorpe P. Terfenadine. *Drugs Future* 1978;3:220.
38. Garteiz DA, Hook RH, Walker BJ, Okerholm RA. Pharmacokinetics and biotransformation studies of terfenadine in man. *Arzneimittelforschung* 1982;32:1185.
39. Okerholm RA, Weiner DL, Hook RH. Bio-availability of terfenadine in man. *Biopharm Drug Dispos* 1981;2:185–188.
40. Huther KJ, Renftle G, Barraud N. Inhibitory activity of terfenadine on histamine-induced skin wheals in man. *Eur J Clin Pharmacol* 1977;12:195.
41. Landrow PM, Jannsen PFM, Gommeren W, Heysen JE. *In vitro* and *in vivo* binding characteristics of a new long-acting histamine H_1 antagonist, astemizole. *Mol Pharmacol* 1984;21:294–298.
42. Richards DM, Brogden RM, Heel RC. Astemizole. A review of its pharmacodynamic properties and therapeutic efficacy. *Drugs* 1985;29:34–42.
43. Brugmans J, Van den Bussche S, Scheijgrond H. Inhibitory activity of astemizole on histamine-induced skin reactions in man. Twelfth International Congress Chemotherapy, Florence, July 19–24, 1981.
44. Moser L, Huther KJ, Kock-Weser J, Lundt PV. Effect of terfenadine and diphenhydramine alone or in combination with diazepam and alcohol on psychomotor performance and subjective feelings. *Eur J Clin Pharmacol* 1978;14:417–421.
45. Simons FE, Simons KJ, Chung M, Yeh J. The comparative pharmacokinetics of H_1-receptor antagonists. *Ann Allergy* 1987;59:20–24.
46. Ghys L, Rihoux JP. Pharmacological modulation of cutaneous reactivity to histamine: a double-blind acute comparative study between ceterizine, terfenadine and astemizole. *J Int Med Res* 1989;17:24–27.
47. Gengo FM, Dabronzo J, Yarchak A, Love S, Miller JK. The relative antihistaminic and psychomotor effects of hydroxyzine and cetirizine. *Clin Pharmacol Ther* 1987;42:265–272.
48. Wood SG, John BA, Chasseaud LF, Yeh J, Chung M. The metabolism and pharmacokinetics of ^{14}C-cetirizine in humans. *Ann Allergy* 1987;59:31–34.
49. Charlesworth EN, Kagey-Sobotka A, Norman PS, Lichtenstein M. Effect of cetirizine on mast cell-mediator release and cellular traffic during the cutaneous late-phase reaction. *J Allergy Clin Immunol* 1989;83:905–912.
50. Zechtel HJ, Brock N, Leuk D, Acterrath-Tuckerman A. Pharmacological and toxicological properties of azelastine: a novel antiallergic agent. *Arzneimittelforschung* 1981;31:1184–1191.
51. Chand N, Nolan K, Diamantis W, Perhach JL, Sofia RD. Inhibition of leukotriene mediated lung anaphylaxis by azelastine: a novel orally effective anti-asthmatic drug. *Allergy* 1986;41:473–478.
52. Spector SL, Perhach JL, Rohr AS, Rachelefsky GS, Katz RM, Siegel SC. Pharmaco-

dynamic evaluation of azelastine in subjects with asthma. *J Allergy Clin Immunol* 1987;80:75–80.

53. Kemp JP, Meltzer EO, Orgel HA, Welch MJ, Lockey RF, Middleton E, Spector SL, Perhach JL, Newton JJ. A dose response study of the bronchodilator action of azelastine in asthma. *J Allergy Clin Immunol* 1986;77:249(abstract).

54. Rafferty P, Harrison PJ, Holgate ST. Effect of azelastine on the airway response to histamine and methacholine in asthmatic subjects. *Allergol Immunol Clin* 1987;2:188.

55. Rafferty P, Harrison PJ, Holgate ST. Effect of azelastine on histamine and allergen-induced bronchoconstriction in asthmatic subjects. *Thorax* 1988;43:220(abstract).

56. Storms W, Middleton E, Dvorin D. Azelastine in the treatment of asthma. *J Allergy Clin Immunol* 1985;75:167.

57. Rafferty P, Ng WH, Philips G, Clough J, Church MK, Aurich R, Ollier S, Holgate ST. The inhibitory actions of azelastine hydrochloride on the early and late bronchoconstrictor responses to inhaled allergen in atopic asthma. *J Allergy Clin Immunol* 1989;84:649–657.

58. Busse W, Randlev B, Sedgwick J, Sofia RD. The effect of azelastine on neutrophil and eosinophil generation of superoxide. *J Allergy Clin Immunol* 1989;83:400–405.

59. Honda M, Miura K, Tanigawa T. Effect of azelastine hydroxichloride on macrophage chemotaxis and phagocytosis *in vitro*. *Allergy* 1982;37:417.

60. Little MM, Casale TB. Azelastine inhibits IgE-mediated human basophil release. *J Allergy Clin Immunol* 1989;83:862–865.

61. Fields AS, Pillar J, Diamantis W, Perhach JL, Sofia RD, Chand N. Inhibition by azelastine of nonallergic histamine release from rat peritoneal mast cells. *J Allergy Clin Immunol* 1984;73:400–403.

62. Shin MH, Baroody F, Proud D, Kagey-Sabotka A, Lichtenstein LM, Naclerio RM. The effect of azelastine on the early allergic response. *Clin Exp Allergy* 1992;22:289–295.

63. Nicholson AN, Stone BM. The H_1-antagonist mequitazine: studies on performance and visual function. *Eur J Clin Pharmacol* 1983;25:563–567.

64. Rossoni G, Omini C, Folco GC. Bronchodilating activity of mequitazine. *Arch Int Pharmacodyn Ther* 1984;268:128–134.

65. Cohen AF, Hamilton MJ, Liao SH, Findlay JWA, Peck AW. Pharmacodynamics and pharmacokinetics of BW825C: a new antihistamine. *Eur J Clin Pharmacol* 1985;28:197–204.

66. Truneh A, White JR, Pearce FL. Effects of ketotifen and oxatomide on histamine secretion of mast cells. *Agents Actions* 1982;12:206–211.

67. Diamantis W, Chand N, Harrison JE. Inhibition of release of SRS-A and its antagonism by azelastine, an H_1 antagonist anti-allergic agent. *Pharmacologist* 1982;24:200–206.

68. Chand N, Diamantis W, Sofia RD. Antagonism of leukotrienes, calcium and histamine by azelastine. *Pharmacologist* 1984;26:152–157.

69. Curry JJ. The effect of antihistamine substances and other drugs on histamine bronchoconstriction in asthmatic subjects. *J Clin Invest* 1946;25:792–799.

70. Karlin JM. The use of antihistamines in asthma. *Ann Allergy* 1972;30:342–347.

71. Cockcroft DW, Killian DN, Mellon JJA, Hargreave FE. Bronchial reactivity to inhaled histamine: a method and clinical survey. *Clin Allergy* 1977;7:235–243.

72. Rafferty P, Holgate ST. Terfenadine is a potent and selective histamine H_1 receptor antagonist in asthmatic airways. *Am Rev Respir Dir* 1987;135:181–184.

73. Howarth PH, Holgate ST. Astemizole, an H_1 antagonist in allergic asthma. *J Allergy Clin Immunol* 1985;75:166.

74. Rafferty P, Harrison PJ, Aurich R, Holgate ST. The *in vivo* potency and selectivity of azelastine as an H_1-receptor antagonist in human airways and skin. *J Allergy Clin Immunol* 1989;84:649–657.

75. Holgate ST, Mann JS, Church MK, Cushley MJ. Mechanisms and significance of adenosine-induced bronchoconstriction in asthma. *Allergy* 1987;42:727.

76. Lee TH, Nagy L, Nagakura T, Walport MJ, Kay AB. Identification and partial characterisation of an exercise-induced neutrophil chemotactic activity in bronchial asthma. *J Clin Invest* 1982;69:889–899.

77. Barnes PJ, Brown MJ. Venous plasma histamine in exercise and hyperventilation-induced asthma in man. *Clin Sci* 1981;61:159–162.

78. Deal EC, Wasserman SE, Soter NA, Ingram RH, McFadden ER. Evaluation of role played by mediators of immediate hypersensitivity in exercise-induced asthma. *J Clin Invest* 1980;65:659–665.
79. Howarth PH, Pao G-K, Church MK, Holgate ST. Exercise and isocapnic hyperventilation-induced bronchoconstriction in asthma: relevance of circulating basophils to measurement of plasma histamine. *J Allergy Clin Immunol* 1984;73:391–399.
80. Smith CM, Anderson SO. Hyperosmolarity as the stimulus to asthma induced by hyperventilation. *J Allergy Clin Immunol* 1986;77:729–736.
81. Gravelyn TR, Pan PM, Eschenbacher WL. Mediator release in an isolated airway segment in subjects with asthma. *Am Rev Respir Dis* 1988;137:641–646.
82. Patel JR. Terfenadine in exercise-induced asthma. *Br Med J* 1984;288:1496–1497.
83. Finnerty JP, Holgate ST. Role of histamine and prostaglandins in EIA. *J Allergy Clin Immunol* 1988;81:240.
84. Wilmot C, Finnerty JP, Holgate ST. Role of histamine and prostaglandins in the bronchial response to inhaled hypertonic saline. *Thorax* 1988;43:865.
85. Philips GD, Holgate ST. Effect of oral Terfenadine alone and in combination with flurbiprofen on adenosine 5-monophosphate-induced bronchoconstriction in non-atopic asthma. *Thorax* 1987;42:939–945.
86. Miszkiel KA, Beasly R, Rafferty P, Holgate ST. The influence of ipratropium bromide and sodium cromoglycate on benzalkonium chloride-induced bronchoconstriction in asthma. *Br J Clin Pharmacol* 1988;26:295–301.
87. Dixon CMS, Barnes PJ. Bradykinin-induced bronchoconstriction: inhibition by nedocromil sodium and sodium cromoglycate in non-asthmatic atopic subjects. *Br J Clin Pharmacol* 1989;27:831–836.
88. Gong H, Brik A, Tashkin DP, Duphinee B. Effects of inhaled thiazinamium chloride on histamine-induced and exercise-induced bronchoconstriction. *Ann Allergy* 1989; 62:230–235.
89. Falliers CJ, Freeland GR, Daniel WC. Single dose, double-blind comparison of thiazinamium chloride, albuterol and placebo in asthma. *Am Rev Respir Dis* 1985; 131:A96(abstract).
90. Reed CE, Welso PW, Freeland GR. Prophylactic effect of aerosolised thiazinamium chloride on methacholine and allergen-induced bronchoconstriction. *Am Rev Respir Dis* 19895;131:A8(abstract).
91. Gong H, Tashkin DP, Dauphinee B, Djahed B, Wu T-C. Effects of oral certirizine, a selective H_1 antagonist, on allergen and exercise-induced bronchoconstriction in subjects with asthma. *J Allergy Clin Immunol* 1990;85:632–641.
92. Larsen GL, Wilson MC, Marsh WR, Haslett C, Murphy KR. Neutrophils and late phase reactions. In: Kay AB, ed. *Allergy and inflammation.* London: Academic Press, 1987;225–244.
93. Abraham WM, Delhunt JC, Herger L, Marchette B. Characterisation of a late phase pulmonary response following allergen challenge in allergic sheep. *Am Rev Respir Dis* 1983;128:839–844.
94. De Monchy JG, Keyser JJ, Kauffman HF, Beaumont F, de Vries K. Histamine in late asthmatic reactions following housedust mite inhalation. *Agents Actions* 1985;16:252–255.
95. Nagy L, Lee TH, Kay AB. Neutrophil chemotactic activity in antigen-induced late asthmatic reactions. *N Engl J Med* 1987;306:497–501.
96. Booij-Noord H, de Vries K, Sluiter HJ, Orie NGM. Late bronchial obstruction reaction to experimental inhalation of house dust extract. *Clin Allergy* 1972;2:43–61.
97. Holgate ST, Finnerty JP. Antihistamines in asthma. *J Allergy Clin Immunol* 1989;83:537–547.
98. Patel KR. Effect of terfenadine on methacholine-induced bronchoconstriction in asthma. *J Allergy Clin Immunol* 1987;79:893–899.
99. Kemp JP, Metzer EO, Orgel HA. A dose response study of the bronchodilator action of azelastine in asthma. *J Allergy Clin Immunol* 1987;79:893–899.
100. Tashkin DP, Brik A, Gong H. Cetirizine inhibition of histamine-induced bronchospasm. *Ann Allergy* 1987;59:49–52.
101. White J, Eiser NM. The role of histamine and its receptors in the pathogenesis of asthma. *Br J Dis Chest* 1983;77:215–226.

102. Taytard A, Beaumonth D, Pujet JC, Sapere M, Lewis PS. Treatment of bronchial asthma with terfenadine: a randomised controlled trial. *Br J Clin Pharmacol* 1987;24:743–746.
103. Rafferty P, Holgate ST. Terfenadine, a potent histamine H_1-receptor antagonist in the treatment of grass pollen sensitive asthma during the hay fever season. *Br J Clin Pharmacol* 1990;30:229–235.
104. Rackham A, Brown CA, Chandra RK, Hoogerwerf PE, Kennedy RJ, Knight A, et al. Canadian multicentre study with ketotifen in the treatment of asthma in children aged 5–17 years. *J Allergy Clin Immunol* 1989;84:286–296.
105. Finnerty JP, Holgate ST, Rihoux J-P. The effect of 2 weeks treatment with cetirizine on bronchial reactivity to methacholine in asthma. *Br J Clin Pharmacol* 1990;29:79–84.
106. Rafferty P, Ghosh SK, de Vos C, Patel KR. The effect of oral and inhaled certifizine on the early bronchoconstrictor response to inhaled allergen in asthmatic subjects. *Am Rev Respir Dis* 1991;143:A756.
107. Gould CAL, Ollier S, Aurich R, Daview RJ. A study of the clinical efficacy of azelastine in patients with extrinsic asthma, and its effect on airway responsiveness. *Br J Clin Pharmacol* 1988;26:515–525.
108. Spector S, Lee N, Huster W, McNutt B, Siegel S, Katz R, et al. Bronchodilator activity of terfenadine, single and steady state bid dosing in allergic asthmatics. *J Allergy Clin Immunol* 1991;86:345.
109. Boerner D, Metz K, Eberhardt R. Efficacy and tolerability of picumast dihydrochloride in comparison with placebo in asthmatic subjects. *Arzneimittelforschung* 1989;39:1363–1367.
110. Kopferschmitt-Kubler MC, Couchot A, Pauli G. Evaluation of the effect of oral cetirizine on antigen-induced immediate asthmatic responses. *Ann Allergy* 1990;65:501–503.
111. Bruttman G, Pedrali P, Adrendt C, Rihoux JP. Protective effect of cetirizine in patients suffering from pollen asthma. *Ann Allergy* 1990;4:224–228.
112. Bousquet J, Emonot A, Germoutly J. Multi-centre double-blind parallel study to investigate the efficacy and toleration of cetirizine in the treatment of hay fever-associated asthma. *Allergology* 1989;10:119(abstract).
113. Dijkman JH, Hekking PRM, Molkenboer JF. Prophylactic treatment of grass-pollen induced asthma with cetirizine. *Clin Exp Allergy* 1990;20:483–490.
114. Cookson WOCM, Higgins RM, Chadwick GA. A clinical trial of the H_1 antihistamine terfenadine in atopic asthma. *Am Rev Respir Dis* 1987;135:387A(abstract).

Drugs and the Lung,
edited by C.P. Page and W.J. Metzger.
Raven Press, Ltd., New York © 1994

7

Immunosuppressive Agents in the Treatment of Asthma

Christine A. Sorkness, *Jutta C. Joseph, and †William W. Busse

*Department of Pharmacy and Medicine (CHS), University of Wisconsin–Madison School of Pharmacy, Madison, Wisconsin 53706 *Department of Pharmacy Practice, College of Pharmacy, Washington State University at Spokane, Spokane, Washington 99204-0399 and †Department of Medicine, Allergy/Clinical Immunology, University of Wisconsin Medical School, Madison, Wisconsin 53792*

Airway inflammation is a significant component of asthma and is considered to play a major role in airway hyperresponsiveness (1). Corticosteroids are the most effective therapy available to reduce the inflammatory response in patients with asthma. However, the long-term administration of systemic corticosteroids carries a risk of significant side effects (Table 1). Most patients with asthma can be treated successfully with combinations of beta-agonists, inhaled corticosteroids, theophylline, and cromolyn, reserving systemic corticosteroids to treat a life-threatening attack or severe exacerbation. There are patients with asthma, the so-called steroid-dependent asthmatic, who experience repeated asthma exacerbations even after careful systemic corticosteroid withdrawal, and require long-term administration of corticosteroids to control symptoms and maintain lung function. This has led to investigations evaluating the use of alternative anti-inflammatory agents in the treatment of corticosteroid-dependent asthma in an attempt to reduce or eliminate the need for chronic administration of systemic corticosteroids to maintain lung function. We will review these alternative therapies, including gold, dapsone, hydroxychloroquine, cyclosporine A, immunoglobulins, and methotrexate, the agent with the greatest clinical experience.

GOLD THERAPY

Gold therapy (chrysotherapy) has proven efficacy in the treatment of inflammatory diseases such as rheumatoid arthritis (2) and pemphigus (3,4).

TABLE 1. *Complications associated with chronic use of systemic corticosteroids*

Adrenal suppression
Osteoporosis
Cataract formation
Glucose intolerance
Obesity
Hypertension
Myopathy
Capillary fragility and bruising

Recent evidence also suggests that gold salts may be effective in the treatment of asthma (Table 2). Consequently, gold therapy may permit reduction in corticosteroids without pulmonary function deterioration in the severe asthmatic patient.

The immunologic mechanisms and pharmacologic actions of the gold salts are not defined. Parenteral gold salts, gold sodium thiomalate, and aurothioglucose inhibit *in vitro* responses of lymphocytes to mitogens (5). Parenteral gold salts have also been shown to inhibit the activity of lysosomal enzymes and prevent prostaglandin synthesis. In animals, the administration of gold salt results in decreased airway responsiveness to inhaled histamine (6) and histamine-induced smooth muscle contraction in guinea pig tracheal rings (7).

The reported incidence of adverse effects associated with parenteral gold salt administration in arthritis patients ranges between 25% and 50%. Common adverse effects include skin rash, stomatitis, leukopenia, thrombocytopenia, and proteinuria (8). The oral gold salt preparation auranofin is associated with less toxicity than that encountered with parenteral forms of gold. This may be due to less accumulation of auranofin in body tissue compared with its parenteral form (9). Auranofin may also have unique immunologic properties compared with the injectable gold preparations. Unlike parenteral formulations, auranofin inhibits the activity of antibody-forming cells and suppresses *in vitro* production of antibodies in animals (10). Other *in vitro* effects of auranofin include inhibition of basophil histamine release and leukotriene- and histamine-induced contraction of isolated guinea pig tracheal smooth muscle (10,11). Recent studies have also demonstrated inhibition of histamine release from rat mast cells, as well as anti-immunoglobulin E (IgE)–induced release of histamine and leukotriene C_4 from human lung mast cells by auranofin (12,13).

Based upon this experimental evidence, gold compounds could potentially modulate several immunologic and inflammatory effects associated with asthma. Muranaka et al. (14) evaluated gold sodium thiomalate in a double-blind placebo-controlled trial of 79 asthma patients. The active treatment group was given a total cumulative dose of 1540 mg over 30 weeks. In physician global evaluations, 71% of the gold-treated patients versus 44% of

TABLE 2. Summary of gold clinical trials in asthma

Authors	Reference	No. of patients	Age (years)	Duration of steroid dependence	Study design	Treatment regimen	Results	Adverse effects
Muranaka et al.	14	79	Gold 40.3 Placebo 40.6	Gold 11.5 years Placebo 11.1 years	Double-blind placebo-controlled	Gold thiomalate IM/week × 30 weeks (10 mg–100 mg)	67.8% of gold-treated patients improved vs. 43.6% of placebo-treated patients	Dermatitis, stomatitis, proteinuria, fever
Klaustermeyer et al.	16	10	45–72	1–20 years	Blind crossover (1st interval double-blind)	Aurothioglucose 50 mg IM vs placebo × 22 weeks	5/10 reduced prednisone requirement with stable or improved lung function	Proteinuria, rash, metallic taste
Bernstein et al.	17	20	47	25.9 months	Open-label	Auranofin 3 mg bid × 24 weeks	1) Cumulative prednisone dose 7 days before and 10 days after methacholine test 293 ± 125 mg (baseline) to 192 ± 115 mg (week 16) 2) 9 patients had decreased methacholine responsiveness 3) FEV$_1$ unchanged—2.07 L (baseline) to 2.09 L (week 24)	Loose stools/diarrhea, rash, stomatitis

placebo-treated subjects reported subjective improvement. Side effects were observed in 14 out of 38 (37%) gold-treated patients, consisting primarily of dermatitis and stomatitis. In a subsequent study, Muranaka et al. (15) reported results of a 5-year open-label study in which three groups of adult patients with asthma of the paroxysmal type were subjected to either intramuscular aurothiomalate, antigen immunotherapy, or symptomatic treatment with bronchodilators and corticosteroids. Efficacy of treatment was measured by patient requirements for both bronchodilators and corticosteroids as well as by changes in airway responsiveness as determined by acetylcholine bronchoprovocation. After 5 years of treatment, there was a significant decrease ($p < .05$) in bronchial responsiveness to acetylcholine only in patients who received chrysotherapy. In the other two treatment groups, no changes in bronchial responsiveness to acetylcholine were observed. Five of the 14 patients who were treated with gold salt became asymptomatic and reported no requirements for bronchodilators or corticosteroids for at least 3 years. None of the patients in the other treatment groups entered a state of long-term remission during the treatment. Fourteen patients (ten gold-treated patients, two patients on antigen immunotherapy, two on symptomatic treatment) discontinued their particular treatment during the course of the trial. Seven of the gold-treated patients stopped treatment due to the development of dermatitis, stomatitis, or proteinuria, all of which resolved after treatment was interrupted. All other patients (three gold-treated patients, two on immunotherapy, two on symptomatic treatment) discontinued treatment because of amelioration of asthmatic attacks or they moved out of the area. The results of this study suggest that chrysotherapy may decrease the necessity for symptomatic medications such as bronchodilators and corticosteroids. It also demonstrates that long-term therapy with gold salt reduces bronchial hyperresponsiveness to acetylcholine in some patients. Side effects of gold therapy, however, were a significant limiting factor in its use for the treatment of asthma.

Klaustermeyer et al. (16) conducted a blind, crossover trial (first interval double-blind) of eight corticosteroid-dependent asthma patients treated with aurothioglucose over 22 weeks. Five patients received aurothioglucose but were not crossed over to placebo because of a suspected long washout time. The three patients who received placebo crossed-over after 22 weeks to receive aurothioglucose therapy. Efficacy of treatment was measured by changes in forced expiratory volume in 1 sec (FEV_1) and corticosteroid dose. All patients were maintained on oral theophylline, oral β-agonists, and inhaled bronchodilator therapy throughout the study. Five of eight patients showed a reduction in corticosteroid requirements while maintaining or improving lung function. Two patients developed significant proteinuria that resolved with cessation of gold. This study suggests the corticosteroid-sparing effect of chrysotherapy. A major limitation of this study was the small number of patients involved.

The first study that investigated the use of oral auranofin in the treatment of asthma was conducted by Bernstein et al. (17). Eighteen corticosteroid-dependent patients with asthma received auranofin 3 mg twice a day for 20 weeks in an open clinical trial. Concomitant treatment with β_2-agonists, xanthine products, and corticosteroids was not altered until after 8 weeks of auranofin therapy, on the assumption that the therapeutic effect of auranofin would not be attained until that period of time. Prospective evaluation of bronchial responsiveness to methacholine was determined before and 16 weeks after initiation of auranofin therapy. Serial spirometry was measured prior to and 10 and 20 weeks after treatment. All patients recorded concomitant medications, symptom scores as well as morning and evening peak expiratory flow rates. *In vitro* immunologic studies performed before and after 8 and 20 weeks of auranofin therapy included leukocyte histamine release (LHR) in response to antihuman IgE, lymphocyte blast transformation (LBT) in response to the mitogens, and leukocyte inhibitory factor (LIF) responses to tetanus toxoid and candida antigens.

There were no significant differences between baseline and posttreatment spirometry lung volumes and single breath carbon monoxide diffusing capacity. After 16 weeks of treatment, the total prednisone dose administered from 7 days before through 10 days after each methacholine test day decreased from a mean 293 ± 125 mg at baseline to 192 ± 115 mg. Fifty percent of patients exhibited decreased methacholine responsiveness, as defined by an increase in the concentration of methacholine causing a 20% decrease in FEV_1 at week 16. A significant correlation ($r = .60$) was observed between the increase in the concentration of methacholine causing a 20% decrease in FEV_1 and the decrease in corticosteroid cumulative dose after 16 weeks of treatment.

No significant changes occurred in daily or nocturnal symptoms during the active auranofin treatment period compared with the pretreatment period. However, there was a 34% and 22% reduction in the mean number of nighttime and daytime asthma attacks, respectively.

There was a significant decrease in antigen-IgE–induced leukocyte histamine release after 20 weeks of auranofin therapy ($p < .005$). *In vitro* mitogen-induced lymphocyte proliferative responses to specific plant mitogens remained unchanged. Serial LIF assays demonstrated a significant increase in cloning inhibitory factor (CIF) activity to tetanus toxoid and *Candida albicans* antigens at varying concentrations.

Gastrointestinal symptoms were the most frequently reported adverse effects. Loose stools and diarrhea were reported by 65% of the patients. Most patients developed these symptoms during the first month of treatment, improving after dose reduction or resolving spontaneously on the full dose. Cutaneous reactions occurred in 15% of patients. One patient was withdrawn from the study due to a cutaneous hypersensitivity reaction. None of the patients exhibited clinically significant hematological changes.

In summary, this study demonstrates that auranofin therapy may have potential benefit in the treatment of corticosteroid-dependent asthma but has significant side effects that require close monitoring. This study also demonstrates that auranofin may exert immunomodulatory activity without compromising cellular immune function as demonstrated by the cell-mediated functional assays. Multicenter, controlled clinical trials are in progress to establish the efficacy and safety of auranofin therapy in corticosteroid dependent asthma.

DAPSONE AND HYDROXYCHLOROQUINE

Dapsone, a sulfone (4,4'-diaminodiphenyl sulfone) has been used in the treatment of leprosy and a variety of cutaneous and rheumatologic disorders. Its primary effect appears to be the inhibition of neutrophil function. It decreases neutrophil production of reactive oxygen species, chemotaxis, and injury to pulmonary epithelial cells.

Berlow et al. (18) conducted an open-label trial of dapsone (100 mg twice a day) in ten patients (ages 23–80 years) with chronic corticosteroid-dependent asthma over a period of 7 to 20 months. Average daily baseline prednisone dose ranged from 5 to 60 mg. FEV_1, symptom scores, and daily peak flow rates remained stable despite a significant reduction in the average cumulative monthly prednisone dose (428 mg to 8 mg). Five of ten patients stopped corticosteroids by month 6 and two additional patients by month 13.

Since its introduction in the 1940s, dapsone has been reported to produce a variety of adverse reactions (19), but it has had a generally acceptable safety profile. Neurologic reactions, including neuropathy and psychosis; gastrointestinal reactions, including hepatitis; cutaneous reactions; and hematologic reactions, including methemoglobinemia, hemolysis, leukopenia, and agranulocytosis have been reported. The most common adverse reaction is dose-dependent hemolytic anemia secondary to methemoglobinemia, with average drops in hemoglobin of 2 g/dl.

In Berlow's study, nine of the ten patients developed significant anemia, averaging hemoglobin drops of 3.6 g/dl (range unreported). The authors stated there was no obvious clinical impact and attributed the high prevalence to the relatively large dose of dapsone administered. One subject developed a digoxin-responsive tachyarrhythmia of questionable relationship to the dapsone. Three additional patients did not complete the study (one patient due to malaise and weakness, another due to rash and thrombocytopenia at month 2, and a third due to acute psychosis at month 7). This third patient had a history of psychological problems, so the relationship of this adverse event to dapsone is unclear.

Hydroxychloroquine is a known membrane stabilizer of inflammatory cells and inhibitor of phospholipase A_2, and has proven efficacy in inflammatory disease. An open-label 28-week trial of hydroxychloroquine (300 mg to 400 mg/day to a maximum of 6.5 mg/kg/day) resulted in the improvement (not statistically significant) of mean forced vital capacity (FVC) and FEV_1 in severe symptomatic noncorticosteroid ($n = 4$) and corticosteroid-dependent ($n = 7$) asthmatic patients (20). Among the corticosteroid-dependent patients, the cumulative monthly prednisone dosage required also decreased 50% from 383 mg to 191 mg at week 28. Comparison of pretreatment IgE levels to levels during treatment in ten patients demonstrated a decrease from a mean of 645 to 339 IU/ml ($p < .05$).

Charous (20) concluded that the study patients demonstrated few side effects during the 28-week trial. One patient exhibited transient gastrointestinal upset, which resolved without alteration in hydroxychloroquine dosage. A second patient developed a facial rash, initially attributed to hydroxychloroquine therapy; a dermatology consult later assessed the rash to be seborrheic flare induced by prednisone taper. This patient continued the study drug, with control of the rash by topical corticosteroids.

In spite of the low prevalence of adverse events in this 28-week trial, it must be cautioned that prolonged therapy (especially with high dosages) may result in serious and sometimes irreversible toxicity including retinopathy. Adverse hematologic effects can occur and the drug must be administered with caution to patients with glucose 6-phosphate dehydrogenase (G-6-PD) deficiency.

Larger, randomized controlled studies are needed to evaluate possible therapeutic roles for dapsone and hydroxychloroquine in the treatment of corticosteroid-dependent asthma, especially in view of their potential adverse reaction profiles in long-term use.

CYCLOSPORINE A

Cyclosporine A (CsA) is a cyclic undecapeptide metabolite extracted from the fungus, *Tolypocladium inflatum;* it has been used to prevent and treat organ allograft rejection and a variety of inflammatory and autoimmune diseases.

The precise mechanism for its anti-inflammatory action is unknown. It is thought to act mainly through inhibition of activation of T lymphocytes by interfering with the synthesis of lymphokines. More specifically, CsA may bind to cytoplasmic and nuclear regulatory proteins, thereby blocking gene activation of T cells and lymphokines (21).

The importance of the T cell in the pathogenesis of corticosteroid-dependent asthma and the potential role of cyclosporine in the treatment of steroid-dependent asthma and the potential role of cyclosporine in the treatment of steroid-dependent asthma was demonstrated by Alexander et al. (22). Thirty-three patients (mean age 27 years) with long-standing asthma

TABLE 3. *Summary of cyclosporine (CsA) clinical trials in asthma*

Author	Reference	No. of patients	Age (mean)	Duration of steroid dependence	Study design	Treatment regimen	Results	Side effects
Alexander et al.	22	33	49	9.3 years	Double-blind, placebo-controlled, crossover trial	Cyclosporine 5 mg/kg/day × 12 weeks orally	12.0% and 17.6% increase in mean PEFR and FEV_1, respectively during CsA therapy compared to placebo	Hypertrichosis, paresthesias, tremor, headache, HTN
Szceklik et al.	23	12	47	16 years	Open label	Cyclosporine 3 mg/kg/day × 9 months	Prednisone reduction 30 mg to 11 mg per day in 6 patients	TIA, septic cholangitis, peripheral neuropathy

HTN, hypertension nephropathy; TIA, transient ischemic attack.

who required continuous oral corticosteroids (mean duration 9.3 years) were treated in a randomized, double-blind, placebo-controlled, crossover trial for 12 weeks. All treatment except inhaled bronchodilator and systemic corticosteroid (prednisolone) usage was kept constant during the trial. Corticosteroid dosage was increased if required for asthma exacerbations.

During cyclosporine therapy, there was a significant increase in the mean morning peak expiratory flow rate (PEFR) and FEV_1 (12.0% and 17.6%, respectively) compared to placebo. Cyclosporine therapy also resulted in a 27.6% decrease in the diurnal variation in PEFR. Side effects from cyclosporine did not differ significantly from placebo. Two patients failed crossover to second treatment period (one to cyclosporine and one to placebo) due to asthma exacerbations that required hospital admission. Another patient withdrew at the end of the first treatment period with cyclosporine due to hypertrichosis.

Szceklik et al. (23) have demonstrated the steroid-sparing effects of cyclosporine in asthma. Twelve patients with severe asthma who required daily systemic corticosteroids (average duration 16 years) were treated in an open-trial with cyclosporine (average whole-blood trough levels of 105 ng/ml) over a 9-month period. The mean daily dose of oral prednisone was reduced from 30 mg to 11 mg in six patients, while symptom scores and peak expiratory flows improved significantly. This was also accompanied by a reduction in the number of asthma exacerbations. Six other patients failed to reduce corticosteroid dosage after 4 to 7 months of cyclosporine therapy. No clinical differences were detected between the group of nonresponders compared with the group of responders to cyclosporine. After 9 months of therapy, three patients had worsening of preexisting hypertension and one patient developed transient peripheral neuropathy of the lower extremities. Therapy was stopped temporarily in one patient due to a transient ischemic attack (second month of therapy) and septic cholangitis (ninth month of therapy). Mild, transient elevations of serum creatinine were also reported.

These studies (Table 3) suggest that cyclosporine might have a beneficial role in the treatment of corticosteroid-dependent asthma in some patients; side effects, however, are substantial. Larger, randomized studies are needed to determine its mechanism and role in treating steroid-dependent asthma.

IMMUNOGLOBULINS

The administration of intravenous immunoglobulins (IVIG) has shown remarkable efficacy in the treatment of humoral immune deficiencies and diseases mediated by immune-effector mechanisms, most notably autoimmune diseases. Intramuscularly administered immunoglobulins can be painful, absorbed slowly, and subject to local proteolysis. Advancements in the manufacturing process have led to the development of intravenous immunoglobulin preparations that are safe with minimal adverse reactions and no known long-term side effects. Intravenous immunoglobulin injections are also less painful than intramuscular injections, larger doses can be administered, and high serum levels of antibody can be achieved immediately. Side effects from immunoglobulin administration occur in approximately 10% of the injections or infusions (24,25). Side effects are usually mild and may consist of fever, chills, headache, dizziness, myalgias, nausea, and dyspnea. Since there is a direct correlation between the i.v. infusion rate and adverse reactions, many side effects can be minimized by slowing the rate of infusion. These reactions are thought to be caused by complement activation arising from infusion or injection of aggregates formed in solutions (26).

IgA-deficient individuals are also more likely to experience severe reactions after injection or infusions of immunoglobulin. This is the result of immunoglobulin preparations containing sufficient IgA to react with circulating anti-IgA antibody in IgA-deficient individuals. These antibodies are found in up to 40% of sera of IgA deficient donors (26,27) and in 20% of patients with common variable immunodeficiency (28). For this reason, an IgA-depleted immunoglobulin preparation is preferred in IgA-deficient individuals who require replacement therapy. All preparations should be administered with caution, with patients monitored closely. Intravenous preparations approved by the Food and Drug Administration and available in the United States are shown in Table 4.

The exact mechanisms of actions of immunoglobulins on the immune response are unclear. Nevertheless, the use of immunoblobulins in the treatment of immune deficiencies and autoimmune diseases have led to the discovery of a number of immunomodulatory activities by this therapeutic modality. *In vitro,* immunoglobulins inhibit proliferation of peripheral blood mononuclear cells stimulated with phytohemagglutinin or allogeneic cells (31) and the differentiation of B cells to antibody-secreting cells after stimulation with the polyclonal B cell activator pokeweed mitogen (32). There is also evidence to suggest that IVIG may down-regulate antibody responses by providing a source of anti-idiotypic antibodies (33). These anti-idiotype antibodies can suppress auto-antibody production (34) and even IgE-specific antibodies (35).

IVIG has been very successful in the treatment in children with Kawasaki disease. Leung (36) has provided evidence of the potential immunomodulatory effects of IVIG therapy on immune activation, and cytokine release and activity in children with the acute form of Kawasaki disease. His results indicate that IVIG repairs the immunoregulatory imbalance in Kawasaki disease by (a) increasing the number of activated T-suppressor cells and (b) decreasing the number of activated T cells and the number of B-lineage cells spontaneously secreting antibodies.

The immodulatory effect of IVIG has also been demonstrated in the treatment of corticosteroid-dependent asthma. Mazer and Gelfand (37) con-

TABLE 4. *Intravenous immunoglobulins marketed in the United States*

Product name	Manufacturer	Product form	Approximate IgA content (mcg/ml)	Characteristics
Gamimune	Cutter Laboratories—No longer available	5% in maltose; 50 ml vial (2.5 g)		Low in IgG3 and IgG4
Gamimune-N	Cutter Biological, Miles Laboratories	5% in maltose; 10-, 50-, or 100-ml vials	270	Delivery pH 4.25; low IgG4
Sandoglobulin	Sandoz Pharmaceuticals	3% or 6% in sucrose; 1-, 3-, or 6-g lyophilized powder; diluent provided for reconstitution	720	Delivery pH 6.6; can be reconstituted in 0.9% NaCl, H$_2$O, D5W
Gammagard	Hyland Division, Baxter Healthcare Corp. (Another preparation, marketed by the American Red Cross, is prepared by Baxter Hyland with plasma from Red Cross volunteer donors)	5% in glucose and glycine; 0.5, 2.5, 5, or 10 g lyophilized powder; d luent provided for reconstitution	0.4–1.9	Delivery pH 6.8; lowest in IgA, low IgG4
Gammar-IV	Armour Pharmaceutical	5% in sucrose in lyophilizec powder	20	Delivery pH 7.0
IVEEGAM	Immuno-US, Inc.	5% in glucose as lyophilizec powder, 0.5, 1, 2.5, or 5 g	5	Delivery pH 6.8
Venoglobulin-I	Alpha Therapeutics	5% in mannitol as lyophilized powder, 2.5 or 5 g	24	Delivery pH 6.8

Adapted from refs. 24, 29, 30.

ducted an open-label study in eight children who had been receiving oral corticosteroids continuously for at least 1 year before their enrollment in the study. These patients had also been maintained with oral and inhaled bronchodilators and inhaled corticosteroids and had required bursts of oral steroids for exacerbations of asthma. None of these patients had a documented immunoglobulin deficiency, antibody-deficiency, or a history of susceptibility to infection. The patients were treated with 2 g/kg IVIG (Sandoglobulin), administered during 2 days every 4 weeks for a period of 6 months. There was a significant reduction in the maintenance oral corticosteroid dose (32.6 mg every other day to 11.5 mg every other day) and in the extra oral corticosteroids needed for control of asthma exacerbations (158 mg/month to 49.2 mg/month). This was accompanied by significant reduction ($p < .001$) in clinical symptoms scores. Interestingly, methacholine responsiveness and exercise-induced bronchospasm remained unchanged, suggesting that IVIG had no effect on bronchial hyperresponsiveness. Seven of the eight treated patients also showed a progressive decrease in immediate skin test reactions to a panel of allergens as well as reduction in total IgE (324 ± 110 IU to 133 ± 57 IU) after 6 months of IVIG therapy.

We have also observed a 60-year-old woman on 14 g/month (200 mg/kg) IVIG for the past 2 years. Prior to starting immunoglobulin therapy, she experienced approximately 3 sinus infections per year and required an average of four corticosteroid bursts per year to control her asthma over a 6-year period. Laboratory evaluation revealed a general IgG and IgA deficiency. Further evaluation showed the patient was deficient in all four IgG subclasses. Since starting immunoglobulin therapy 2 years ago, she has experienced fewer sinus infections per year and required only two steroid bursts to control her asthma. More recently within the past year, she has not experienced any bacterial sinus infections and had one viral upper respiratory infection requiring her only steroid burst. Her FEV_1 has also remained relatively stable throughout the year. After 2 years of therapy, IgG immunoglobulin levels are back to normal. The patient has tolerated IVIG well. The only major side effect was a serum sickness–like reaction that she experienced after two doses, which did not recur after switching to a different brand of immunoglobulin.

The exact mechanism of action of IVIG in asthma is unknown, but preliminary findings are encouraging. Larger, randomized, placebo-controlled trials are essential to evaluate the use of IVIG in the treatment of corticosteroid-dependent asthma.

METHOTREXATE

Methotrexate (MTX) is an antimetabolite that inhibits the enzyme dihydrofolate reductase, which converts dihydrofolate to the coenzyme tetrahydrofolate. This enzyme participates in the single carbon transfer necessary for methionine, purine, and thymidylate synthesis.

Methotrexate's anti-inflammatory effect has been demonstrated *in vivo* and *in vitro* and appears to be due, primarily, to a decrease in neutrophil chemotaxis to LTB_4 and C5a (38–41). Phagocytosis or killing by neutrophils (42) is unaffected by low-dose methotrexate therapy. It is unclear whether any of these observations are related to methotrexate inhibition of dihyrofolate reductase.

Methotrexate has been widely used as an anti-inflammatory agent to treat a variety of chronic inflammatory diseases, including rheumatoid arthritis and psoriasis, and causes few side effects and minimal toxicity (43) if appropriately dosed and monitored. Five clinical trials on the use of methotrexate in corticosteroid-dependent asthma have been published and are summarized in Table 5.

Mullarkey et al. (44) were the first to publish a randomized, double-blind crossover study on the use of methotrexate in corticosteroid-dependent asthma. Patients received a 15-mg oral dose per week or identical placebo. Randomized patients had used inhaled beta-agonists and inhaled corticosteroids at least three times a day, as well as theophylline to the limits of tolerance, for a year before study entry. Each patient had required prednisone or its equivalent for control of asthma during the preceding year, at a minimum average dose of 10 mg per day.

Twenty-two patients were initially enrolled, and 14 patients completed the study (mean age of 49 years; average months of steroid therapy 82.6 ± 52.2; average prednisone dose at entry 173.5 ± 107 mg/week). Thirteen of the 14 patients decreased their use of prednisone while receiving one of the treatments; one of the 14 patients who completed the study was excluded by the authors from subsequent analyses because he underwent elective sinus surgery just before crossover.

All but one of the 13 analyzed patients decreased the prednisone dosage while receiving methotrexate. This prednisone reduction ranged from 16.2% to 73.5% (average 36.5%) and was independent of the treatment of initial randomization ($p = .01$). One patient discontinued prednisone, four reduced the dosage by over 50%, and three reduced by $\geq 40\%$. There was no significant deterioration in mean FVC and FEV_1; patients' subjective asthma symptom ratings also showed statistically significant improvement. Nine patients continued to take MTX after completion of the double-blind study. All nine patients had further reductions in corticosteroid requirements; four discontinued prednisone. Adverse reactions reported due to MTX included mild nausea (three), pruritic rash (one), and elevated serum aspartate aminotransferase level (AST) (one).

In a prospective, open-label study, Mullarkey et al. (45) treated 25 patients with corticosteroid-dependent asthma (with MTX) for 18 months or more (average duration MTX = 22.8 months, range 18–28). The average age of

TABLE 5. Summary of methotrexate (MTX) clinical trials in asthma

Author (Reference)	No. of patients	Age (mean)	Duration of steroid dependence (mean)	Study design	Treatment regimen	Results	Significance	MTX adverse effects	Comments
Mullarkey et al. (44)	14	49	82.6 ± 52.2 mos.	Randomized, double-blind, crossover trial of 24 weeks duration	Placebo—12 weeks MTX 15 mg per week po—12 weeks	Prednisone (mg/week): MTX—116.20 mg Placebo—183.10 mg FEV_1 (L/sec): MTX—1.84 Placebo—1.74	.01 .17	Nausea (3), rash (1), elevated AST (1)	16 patients continued in open label
Mullarkey et al. (45)	25	49.4 (19–69)	4.7 yrs (1–11)	Prospective, open trial	(a) 22.8 months (18–28) (b) MTX-po/IM 15–50 mg/week	Prednisone: 26.8–6.3 mg/d FEV_1: 1.7–1.9 L/sec	.0001 .0513	Nausea (5), rash (2), stomatitis (1), thinning of hair (3), elevated AST (12)	
Erzurum et al. (46)	18	MTX 53.8±11.3 Placebo 42.4±16.7	MTX 5.6 ± 5.3 yrs Placebo 9.8 ± 9.1 years	Randomized, double-blind, parallel, placebo controlled, 13-week trial	13 weeks—MTX 10 mg IM q week vs. placebo	Prednisone: MTX 39.6% reduction Placebo 40.2% reduction FEV_1: No significant difference	NS NS	Nausea (3), diarrhea, (6), elevated transaminases (2)	
Shiner et al. (47)	60 MTX = 32 Placebo = 28	MTX 49 (22–73) Placebo 48 (22–75)	Minimum of 1 year	Randomized, double-blind, placebo-controlled of 24 weeks duration	MTX 15 mg po q week vs. placebo	Prednisone: MTX 50% reduction Placebo 14% reduction	p <.005.	Significantly elevated transaminases (3), GI symptoms (2)	No PFT changes during study
Dyer et al. (48)	10	54 (38–64)	Minimum of 2 years	Randomized, double-blind, placebo-controlled, crossover of 3 months duration each	MTX 15 mg po q week vs. placebo	Prednisone: MTX 30% reduction FEV_1: No significant difference	p <.01 NS	GI symptoms (2), hair thinning (2), stomatitis (1)	Initial 3-week steroid taper period; 4-week washout period

these patients was 49.4 years, with an average duration of asthma of 10.6 years (range 3–33). Patients received either oral or intramuscular doses of MTX of 15 to 50 mg per week.

The average daily prednisone dose was reduced from 26.8 mg to 6.3 mg with MTX therapy ($p = .0001$). There was no deterioration in pulmonary function tests during the same time interval. Reported adverse events included nausea (five), rash (two), stomatitis (two), thinning of hair (three), and elevated AST (12).

Erzurum et al. (46) conducted a double-blind, parallel, placebo-controlled, 13-week clinical trial with follow-up of patients in an open trial of methotrexate at the conclusion of the double-blind study. Nineteen patients were enrolled in the study; two of these patients were excluded from the analysis. These enrolled patients were selected from 46 patients referred by local physicians as being severe, corticosteroid-dependent asthma patients. To be eligible, patients must have been treated with corticosteroids daily, or every other day, for more than 1 year, required a minimum of 15 mg of prednisone daily (or equivalent) for at least 3 months prior, shown an inability to taper below this dose, and had at least one documented corticosteroid toxicity event.

During the 13-week study, patients received methotrexate 15 mg or color-matched placebo (Folvite 5 mg) IM once weekly. At week 6, steroid taper was initiated with guidelines set for reductions of 5 mg in daily prednisone dosage per week. At the end of the double-blind period, patients were categorized as success (ability to taper prednisone dose by at least 33%) or failure. Patients on placebo who had successfully tapered their corticosteroid dose by 33% returned to their referring physician (four patients). Those on placebo who failed to taper more than 33% (five patients) were openly placed on MTX and their minimum required prednisone dosage; steroid taper was attempted as in the double-blind protocol. Those patients initially randomized to MTX therapy continued on this drug. If patients on MTX had difficulty tapering the prednisone dose during the follow-up, the MTX dose was increased to 30 mg weekly and prednisone taper was again attempted.

Patients on MTX and placebo significantly decreased their prednisone dose by 39.6% and 40.2%, respectively. Tests of pulmonary function did not differ significantly between the MTX and placebo groups; airway responsiveness and symptom scores were unchanged as well. No significant toxicity was reported in the 13-week double-blind study. The authors concluded that no significant benefit of MTX on asthma control could be shown in the patients they studied.

Shiner et al. (47) recruited 69 patients with corticosteroid-dependent asthma from 11 treatment centers, and enrolled them in a randomized, double-blind, placebo-controlled trial of 24 weeks' treatment with an oral weekly dose of 15 mg MTX. A 4-week run-in and 10-week run-out period were included in the study design. The patients were evaluated by the same physician every 4 weeks, with reduction of the daily prednisolone dose by 2.5 mg if symptom scores and spirometry were unchanged or improved.

After 24 weeks of MTX therapy, the prednisolone dose had been reduced by a significantly greater proportion of patients in the MTX than in the placebo group (50% vs. 14%); the reduction was not sustained after the study treatment was stopped. Five of the 38 patients taking methotrexate developed significant elevations in liver function tests.

Dyer et al. (48) reported the results of a double-blind, placebo-controlled crossover study of MTX 15 mg a week or identical placebo for 12 weeks each. Before entry to the initial period, patients began a 3-week steroid-taper period to ensure the minimal steroid dosage. There was a 4-week washout period between the two crossover periods. To be eligible, patients required a minimum of 7.5 mg/day or 20 mg every other day of prednisone, with steroid dependency for at least 2 years. During the crossover segments, prednisone was tapered by 2.5 mg every 2 weeks, if tolerated.

Twelve patients entered the study and 10 completed (mean age = 54 years and mean prednisone dose = 13.12 mg/day). The initial taper resulted in a mean 1.4-mg prednisone reduction before randomization to treatment groups. The average prednisone dose of the placebo trial was 11.97 mg/day and 8.37 mg/day with the MTX trial. The steroid requirement was reduced by 3.6 mg/day or 31% while patients received MTX ($p < .01$). There was no deterioration in clinical status or spirometry during the two trials. No patient discontinued MTX due to toxicity. Seven patients successfully continued on low-dose MTX after completion of the protocol.

To determine the long-term benefit and safety profile of low-dose methotrexate in corticosteroid-dependent asthma, Sorkness et al. (49) initiated a prospective open-label study in highly selected adult patients with asthma. Patients had been enrolled in the clinic practices of the primary investigators and had been unable to withdraw from oral corticosteroids on multiple attempts despite optimal bronchodilator and high-dose aerosolized corticosteroid therapies. These individuals had been on a minimum of 10 mg prednisone per day, or equivalent, for at least 1 year and had evidence of corticosteroid complications. Entry assessments included spirometry, single breath carbon monoxide diffusing capacity (DL_{CO}), chest x-ray, urine pregnancy test, laboratory safety studies (CBC, creatinine, AST), and liver biopsy (if the patient had risk factors such as previous history liver disease, diabetes, or obesity). Patients were requested to abstain from alcohol. Patients were treated with weekly oral doses of 10 to 15 mg MTX and evaluated at monthly intervals. The corticosteroid dose was gradually reduced based on individual asthma patient stability and tolerance; spirometry and home peak expiratory flow readings were the primary efficacy parameters assessed.

The demographic and clinical characteristics of the 25 enrolled patients are outlined in Table 6. The mean age of these patients was 54.4 years (17

TABLE 6. *Demographic and clinical characteristics for patients in prospective, open-label MTX study*

Patient no.	Age/gender	Years of asthma	Years of corticosteroid therapy	Enrollment FEV$_1$ (% predicted)	Prednisone dosage at enrollment (mg/day)
1	50/M	4	4	67.1	30
2	54/M	5	5	69.5	20
3	57/M	30	18	79.2	10
4	37/F	7	2	86.4	20
5	65/M	10	10	48.5	15
6	59/M	8	4	43.4	20
7	65/M	7	7	62.7	10
8	60/F	28	21	66.1	15
9	55/F	25	4	86.7	15
10	66/M	11	8	47.1	25
11	49/M	4	2	60.7	20
12	65/M	4	3	17.0	20
13	51/F	7	6	82.1	30
14	35/M	5	1.5	82.6	20
15	51/F	15	13	72.3	10
16	64/M	21	15	93.6	15
17	63/M	7	7	54.0	15
18	55/M	13	10	65.3	32.5
19	39/M	3.5	3	68.4	25
20	40/F	3.5	3.5	60.0	40
21	62/F	20	15	51.5	40
22	57/M	52	4	48.7	22.5
23	51/F	26	5	80.8	10
24	50/M	15	5	40.5	22.5
25	60/M	5	5	43.2	15
	$\mu = 54.4 \pm 9.2$ yrs	$\mu = 13.4 \pm 11.7$	$\mu = 7.2 \pm 5.3$	$\mu = 63.1 \pm 18.1$	$\mu = 20.7 \pm 8.6$

males and 8 females), with an average duration of asthma of 13.4 years and duration of corticosteroid dependency of 7.2 years. At the time of enrollment, the average percent predicted FEV_1 was 63.1% ± 18.1%; the average prednisone dose at entry was 20.7 ± 8.6 mg/day. All patients had corticosteroid complications, including obesity, glucose intolerance, hypertension, cataracts, and osteoporosis.

Table 7 compares the mean dose of daily prednisone in the 25 patients over 24 months and the mean percent predicted FEV_1 over the same time period. At 12 months, the mean daily prednisone dose had been reduced to 9.4 mg; this represents a 49.6% reduction. At 24 months, the mean daily prednisone dose had been reduced to 6.8 mg, representing a 63.6% reduction. Three of the 25 patients were able to discontinue prednisone. This reduction in corticosteroid dose over the 24-month interval was significant ($p < .01$, analysis of variance). Paired contrasts of baseline versus 6, 12, 18, and 24 months are also significant ($p < .01$). Importantly, these patients' percent predicted FEV_1 remained stable over the 24-month study period.

Adverse reactions observed in this 24-month study are comparable to those previously reported with MTX use. Four patients developed gastrointestinal distress or diarrhea (this did not require discontinuation of MTX) and three reported mouth tenderness, or sores, which were successfully managed with folic acid administration. No hematologic or other laboratory test abnormalities required MTX discontinuation. One patient developed pneumonitis; this was manifested by an infiltrate on chest and reduced DL_{CO}; this patient has successfully restarted MTX, and did not experience pneumonitis during an additional 2 years of treatment. Two deaths occurred during the study. One death was associated with acute bronchospasm and occurred within 3 months of MTX initiation; prednisone was not being reduced at the time of death. An autopsy documented hyperinflated lungs but failed to document airway inflammation, mucous plugs, or methotrexate pneumonitis. The other death was unrelated to asthma.

We also observed a case of allergic bronchopulmonary aspergillosis (ABPA), which developed during corticosteroid dose reduction while on

TABLE 7. *Twenty-four month analysis of patients in prospective, open-label MTX study*

Study period	No. of patients	FEV_1 (% predicted)	Prednisone	
			Mean dose (± S.D.)	% Reduction
Enrollment	25	63.1 ± 18.1	20.7 ± 8.6	
6 months	23	60.9 ± 21.9	11.6 ± 7.9*	39.9 ± 26.1
12 months	22	62.8 ± 21.3	9.4 ± 6.6*	49.6 ± 27.2
18 months	17	65.0 ± 19.8	7.3 ± 4.6*	62.2 ± 19.8
24 months	13	66.1 ± 16.0	6.8 ± 5.0*	63.6 ± 20.7

*$p < .01$ compared with enrollment period.

MTX. This patient is a 58-year-old man with a history of asthma since age 5 and corticosteroid dependency since 1985. He had been started on MTX when his prednisone dose was 22.5 mg; on MTX it was possible to reduce his prednisone dose to 12.5 mg. His past medical history was significant for corticosteroid-induced hyperglycemia, osteopenia, cataracts, and hypertension. He presented to clinic with right-sided pleuritic chest pain; a chest x-ray documented a right upper lobe cavitary lesion and infiltrate. Computed tomography (CT) of the chest revealed prominent central bronchiectasis with typical "railroad tracks." The diagnosis of ABPA was confirmed with fulfillment of the major criteria (eosinophilia 12%, a positive immediate and later aspergillus skin test response, total serum IgE of 907 ng/ml, and precipitating antibodies to aspergillus). This patient was successfully treated with a burst of oral prednisone and subsequent tapering back to 12.5 mg without flare of either his asthma or ABPA. MTX has subsequently been discontinued in this patient.

Several other clinical observations were noted during this 24-month study. All 25 study patients have required a burst of oral prednisone on at least one occasion. Prednisone intervention therapy has been in association with upper respiratory viral infections, sinusitis, or prophylaxis for a surgical procedure. Three of the 25 patients developed recurrence of nasal polyps, as their oral corticosteroid therapy was being reduced. These three patients maintained asthma stability. One of the three patients has been able to discontinue prednisone, but has required sinus surgery, including polypectomies, due to incomplete control of his sinus disease with topical nasal corticosteroids. Eight of the 25 study patients have developed eosinophilia $\geq 5\%$ of their leukocyte differential count as their oral corticosteroid dose has reduced, in spite of maintenance of pulmonary function test stability. All patients who have completed 24 months of MTX therapy, with consequent corticosteroid dose reduction, had a weight reduction. The average weight reduction has been 15 pounds. Four patients were able to reduce or discontinue antihypertensive and/or oral hypoglycemic drug regimens.

Our study group has also reported the results of a 36-month analysis, which focused on the effects of MTX discontinuation in the previously reported corticosteroid-dependent adult asthma patients (50). Of the originally enrolled 25 patients, 16 have discontinued MTX. Reasons for MTX discontinuation were lack of further benefit (six), MTX toxicity (four), noncompliance with follow-up visits (one), exceeding a cumulative MTX dose of 1500 mg (one), and use of alternative therapy (four). At the time of MTX discontinuation, the mean cumulative MTX dose was 1472.5 ($\pm$ 334.5) mg and the average duration of MTX was 29.3 ($\pm$ 6.0) months. For these 16 patients, the average dose of prednisone at enrollment was 19.2 ($\pm$ 6.6) mg; at 12 months of MTX treatment, this dose was reduced to 9.9 ($\pm$ 7.3) mg ($p <.001$). At the time of MTX discontinuation, the prednisone dose was 9.5 ($\pm$ 4.9) mg ($p <.001$). Three months after MTX discontinuation, the mean prednisone dose had increased to 15.2 (± 6.1) mg. MTX toxicity resulting in patient discontinuation of treatment included leukopenia/thrombocytopenia (one), pneumonitis (one), and liver biopsy changes (two). These biopsies changes were mild to moderate in nature, but consistent with MTX toxicity.

This 36-month prospective open-label study of MTX in corticosteroid-dependent adult asthma have allowed us to make several observations and conclusions. MTX corticosteroid-sparing effects appear to plateau after 12 to 18 months of treatment. When MTX therapy is stopped, the need for corticosteroid use increases. There is a predictable toxicity profile experienced especially with long-term MTX therapy. MTX is efficacious in some patients with corticosteroid-dependent asthma, and may be an acceptable alternative for oral corticosteroids when the commitment is made for careful MTX monitoring. However, MTX appears to be principally a corticosteroid-sparing agent and does not appear to offer permanent reduction in corticosteroid use in asthma or to prevent exacerbations of this disease.

The toxicity profile of MTX in asthma is similar to that observed in the treatment of other chronic inflammatory diseases, such as rheumatoid arthritis (51). In approximately one-third of patients given MTX, treatment was discontinued due to adverse effects, less than 1% of which were life-threatening. Commonly occurring side effects include gastrointestinal problems (10%), stomatitis (6%), reversible hematologic effects (3%), and reversible alopecia (1%). The rare but serious side effects included hepatotoxicity and pneumonitis.

The extent to which low-dose MTX causes liver damage is still uncertain. Cited risk factors for the development of hepatotoxicity include diabetes, obesity, continued alcohol intake, preexisting liver disease, older age, and renal insufficiency. It is unclear how patients taking MTX should be monitored for possible liver damage. Persistently increased serum liver enzyme levels, particularly late in a course of therapy, or decreasing serum albumin levels may indicate liver damage (52). Unfortunately, serum enzyme abnormalities correlate poorly with histologic changes, and liver biopsy is the only reliable way to monitor for liver toxicity in patients taking MTX. Although the incidence of clinically significant complications from liver biopsy is small (0.2%), severe postbiopsy bleeding can occur, and the procedure has some risks. There has been extensive debate over the timing and frequency of liver biopsies in patients receiving MTX. Some authors suggest that there is no need for liver biopsies (52), while others recommend that a routine biopsy be done after every 1,500 to 2,500 mg of MTX (53,54).

Although several investigators use liver biopsies to assess the hepatotoxicity of low-dose pulse MTX therapy, no single study provides sufficient data to determine the value of liver biopsies in monitoring MTX-associated liver damage. Consequently, Whiting-O'Keefe et al. (55) performed a meta-analysis of 15 studies (n = 636 patients) examining the relationship between long-term, low-dose MTX administration (10–30 mg/week) and biopsy evidence of liver fibrosis. The incidence of progression of liver disease (defined as worsening of at least one grade on Roenigk's histologic classification) was 27.9% (95% confidence intervals 24.3 to 31.6). The rate of progression of liver disease in the 15 studies was associated with the cumulative dose of MTX ($p = .01$). On average, patients had a 6.7% (95% confidence intervals 2.1 to 11.4) chance of progressing at least one histologic grade on liver biopsy for each gram of MTX taken. The overall incidence of advanced histologic changes was 5.0%; these changes were not associated with cumulative MTX dose ($p = .08$). Patients with a history of heavy drinking (≥ 100 g alcohol per week) were more likely to have advanced changes on liver biopsy ($p = .003$) and to show histologic progression ($p = .0002$). Patients with psoriasis were more likely than patients with rheumatoid arthritis to have advanced changes and histologic progression.

From our limited experience, we concur with these conclusions that risk increases with total MTX cumulative dose and with heavy consumption of alcohol. Corticosteroid-dependent asthma patients who are being considered for MTX should be requested to abstain from alcohol. Liver biopsies should be done periodically to monitor for the occurrence of liver toxicity, especially in light of the investigational nature of this therapy in asthma.

MTX-associated pneumonitis is well documented, with a mortality of less than 1%. Risk factors for development of this toxicity include use of the drug in combination with other cytotoxic therapy (such as cyclophosphamide), increased frequency of administration, and tapering of corticosteroids or previous adrenalectomy. Clinical features consist of headache, myalgias, chills, cough and dyspnea. Chest x-ray findings include bilateral reticular infiltrates, acinar infiltrates, nodular shadows, and pleural effusion. Reduced diffusing capacity is seen. Histopathologic changes of note are mononuclear inflammatory cell infiltrate and rare granuloma formation and occasional tissue eosinophilia. Patient rechallenge does not always result in recurrence of symptoms, which speaks against a hypersensitivity reaction. Preferential concentration of the drug in the lung has also been documented. It is recommended that patients have baseline chest x-rays and DL_{CO}s, prior to initiation of MTX therapy.

In summary, three randomized, double-blind, placebo-controlled trials of 12 to 24 weeks' duration have demonstrated the ability of MTX to reduce prednisone requirements. One controlled trial of 13 weeks' duration showed no differences with MTX when compared to placebo. Open-label safety data from Mullarkey and colleagues and our own study group have suggested that MTX toxicities in patients with corticosteroid-dependent asthma are consistent with those reported in other population groups and that MTX is generally well-tolerated when carefully monitored. MTX appears to be corticosteroid-sparing and not remission-inducing in the asthma population. The precise role of MTX in the spectrum of current and future therapies for asthma needs refinement and can best be accomplished by a multicenter, randomized, double-blind, placebo-controlled trial of at least 12 months' duration. Mechanistic issues, as well as a temporal analysis of bronchial responsiveness to methacholine, should be incorporated into this trial.

CONCLUSIONS

The use of alternative anti-inflammatory agents in the treatment of corticosteroid-dependent asthma has been reviewed. At present, auranofin and MTX have been most extensively and rigorously evaluated and, therefore, should be considered first choices for carefully selected populations of corticosteroid-dependent asthma. The clinical decision to initiate such a trial commits the patient to compliance with medication usage and laboratory monitoring and the prescriber to careful follow-up and periodic reevaluation of the risk/benefit of these agents in the patient corticosteroid-dependent asthma.

REFERENCES

1. Djukanovic R, Roche WR, Wilson JW, Beasley CRW, Howarth PH, Holgate ST. Mucosal inflammation in asthma. *Am Rev Respir Dis* 1990;142:434–457.
2. Research Subcommittee of the Empire Rheumatism Council. Gold therapy in rheumatoid arthritis: report of a multicenter controlled trial. *Ann Rheum Dis* 1960;19:95–119.
3. Penney NS. Gold therapy: dermatological uses and toxicities. *J Am Acad Dermatol* 1979;1:315–320.
4. Penney NS, Liboh V, Gottlieb NL, et al. Inhibition of prostaglandin synthesis and human epidermal enzymes by aurothiomalate in vitro: possible actions of gold in pemphigus. *J Invest Dermatol* 1974;63:356.
5. Lipsky PE, Liff M. Inhibition of antigen- and mitogen-induced human lymphocyte proliferation by gold compounds. *J Clin Invest* 1977;59:455.
6. Suzuki S, Yamauchi N, Miyamoto T, Muranaka M. Gold-induced reduction in reactivity to histamine in isolated guinea pig tracheal rings. *J Allergy Clin Immunol* 1983;72:469–474.
7. Suzuki S, Yamauchi N, Miyamoto T, Muranaka M. Gold-induced reduction in reactivity to histamine in isolated guinea pig tracheal rings. *J Allergy Clin Immunol* 1983;72:469–474.
8. Gordon DA. Gold compounds. In: Kelley WN, Harris Ed, Ruddy S, et al., eds. *Textbook of rheumatology,* 3rd ed. Philadelphia: Saunders 1989;804–820.
9. Blodgett RC. Auranofin: experience to date. *Am J Med* 1983;75:86.
10. Walz DT, DeMartino MJ, Griswold DE, Intoccia AP, Flanagan TL. Biological actions and pharmacokinetic studies of auranofin. *Am J Med* 1983;75 (6A):90–108.
11. Malo PE, Wasserman M, Parris D, Pfeiffer D. Inhibition by auranofin of pharmacologic and antigen-induced contractions of the isolated guinea pig trachea. *J Allergy Clin Immunol* 1986;77:371–376.
12. Wojtecka-Lukasik EW, Supata I, Maslinski S. Auranofin modulates mast cell histamine and polymorphonuclear leukocyte collagenase release. *Agents Actions* 1986;18:68–70.
13. Marione G, Columbo M, Galeone D, et al. Modulation of the release of histamine and arachidonic acid metabolites from human basophils and mast cells by auranofin. *Agents Actions* 1986;18:100–102.

14. Muranaka M, Miyamoto T, Shida T, et al. Gold salt in the treatment of bronchial asthma: a double-blind study. *Ann Allergy* 1978;40:132–137.
15. Muranaka M, Nakajima K, Suzuki S. Bronchial responsiveness to acetylcholine in patients with bronchial asthma after long-term treatment with gold salt. *J Allergy Clin Immunol* 1981;67:350–356.
16. Klaustermeyer WB, Noritake DT, Kwong FK. Chrysotherapy in the treatment of corticosteroid-dependent asthma. *J Allergy Clin Immunol* 1987;79(5):720–725.
17. Bernstein DI, Bernstein IL, Bodenheimer SS, Pietrusko RG. An open study of auranofin in the treatment of steroid-dependent asthma. *J Allergy Clin Immunol* 1988; 81:6–16.
18. Berlow BA, Liebhaber MI, Dyer Z, et al. The effect of dapsone in steroid-dependent asthma. *J Allergy Clin Immunol* 1991;87:710–715.
19. Graham W. Adverse effects of dapsone. *Int J Dermatol* 1975;14:494–500.
20. Charous BL. Open study of hydroxychloroquine in the treatment of severe symptomatic or corticosteroid-dependent asthma. *Ann Allergy* 1990;65:53–58.
21. Calderon E, et al. Is there a role for cyclosporine in asthma? *J Allergy Clin Immunol* 1992;89(2):629–636.
22. Alexander AG, Barnes NC, Kay AB. Trial of cyclosporin in corticosteroid-dependent chronic severe asthma. *Lancet* 1992;339:324–328.
23. Szceklik A, Nizankowska E, Dworski R, Domagala B, Pinis G. Cyclosporin for steroid-dependent asthma. *Allergy* 1991;46:312–315.
24. Stiehm ER, Ashida E, Kim K, et al. Intravenous immunoglobulins as therapeutic agents [Clinical Conference]. *Ann Intern Med* 1987;107:367–382.
25. Ochs HD, Fischer SH, Wedgewood RJ. Modified immune globulin: its use in the prophylactic treatment of patients with immune deficiency. *J Clin Immunol* 1982;2(suppl 2):22s–30s.
26. Soovill JF. Reactions to immunoglobulin. *Medical Research Council Special Report Series* 1971;310:106.
27. Hammarstrom L, Person MAA, Smith CIE. Anti-IgA selective IgA deficiency. *Scand J Immunol* 1983;18:509.
28. Wells JV, Buckley RH, Schanfield MS, et al. Anaphylactic reactions to plasma infusions in patients with hypogammaglobulinemia and anti-IgA bodies. *Clin Immunol Immunopathol* 1971;8:265–268.
29. Huston DP, Kavanaugh AF, Rohane PW, et al. Immunoglobulin deficiency syndromes and therapy. *J Allergy Clin Immunol* 1991;87:1–17.
30. Buckley RH, Schiff RI. The use of intravenous immune globulin in immunodeficiency diseases. *N Engl J Med* 1991;325:110–117.
31. Kawada K, Terasaki PI. Evidence of immunosuppression by high-dose gamma globulin. *Exp Hematol* 1987;15:133–136.
32. Stohl W. Cellular mechanisms in the in vitro inhibition of pokeweed mitogen-induced B-cell differentiation by immunoglobulin for intravenous use. *J Immunol* 1986;126:4407–4413.
33. Sultan Y, Kazatchkine MD, Maisoneuve P, Nydegger UE. Anti-idiotype suppression of autoantibodies to factor VIII (anti-hemophilic factor) by high-dose intravenous gamma globulin. *Lancet* 1984;2:765–768.
34. Hahn BH, Ebking RM. Suppression of murine lupus nephritis by administration of anti-idiotype antibody to anti-DNA. *Hum Immunol* 1984;132:187–190.
35. Blaser K, de Weck AL. Regulation of the IgE antibody response by idiotype-anti-idiotype network. *Prog Allergy* 1982;32:203–264.
36. Leung DYM. Immunomodulation by intravenous immune globulin in Kawasaki disease (symposium). *J Allergy Clin Immunol* 1989;84:588–594.
37. Mazer BD, Gelfand EW. An open-label study of high-dose intravenous immunoglobulin in severe childhood asthma. *J Allergy Clin Immunol* 1991;87(5):976–983.
38. Cream JJ, Pole DS. The effect of methotrexate and hydroxyurea on neutrophil chemotaxis. *Br J Dermatol* 1980;120:557.
39. Suarez CR, Pickett WC, Bell DH, et al. Effect of low dose methotrexate in neutrophil chemotaxis induced by leukotriene B4 and complement C5a. *J Rheumatol* 1987;14:9.
40. Ternowitz T, Bjerring P, Andersen PH, et al. Methotrexate inhibits the human C5a-induced skin response in patient with psoriasis. *J Dermatol* 1987;89:192.

41. Van De Kerkhof PCM, Bauer FW, Maasen DE, et al. Methotrexate inhibits the leukotriene B4 induced intradermal accumulation of polymorphonuclear leukocytes. *Br J Dermatol* 1985;113:25a.
42. Johnson HD, Summersgill JT, Raff MJ. The in vitro effects of methotrexate on the phagocytosis and intracellular killing of Staphylococcus aureus by human neutrophils. *Cancer* 1986;57:23–43.
43. Wilkens RF. Reappraisal of the use of methotrexate in rheumatic disease. *Ann J Med* 1983;75(suppl 4B):19–25.
44. Mullarkey MF, Blumenstein BA, Andrade WP, et al. Methotrexate in the treatment of corticosteroid-dependent asthma: a double-blind crossover study. *N Engl J Med* 1988;318:603–607.
45. Mullarkey MF, Lammert JK, Blumenstein BA. Long-term methotrexate treatment in corticosteroid-dependent asthma. *Ann Intern Med* 1990;112:577–581.
46. Erzurum SC, Leff JA, Cochran JE, et al. Lack of benefit of methotrexate in severe, steroid-dependent asthma: a double-blind, placebo-controlled study. *Ann Intern Med* 1991;114:353–360.
47. Shiner RJ, Nunn AJ, Chung KF, et al. Randomised, double-blind, placebo-controlled trial of methotrexate in steroid-dependent asthma. *Lancet* 1990;336:137–140.
48. Dyer PD, Vaughan TR, Weber RW. Methotrexate in the treatment of steroid-dependent asthma. *J Allergy Clin Immunol* 1991;88:208–212.
49. Sorkness CA, Busse WW, Bush RK. Use of oral methotrexate in corticosteroid-dependent adult asthma: a twenty-four month analysis (abstract). *J Allergy Clin Immunol* 1991;87(1, Part 2):298.
50. Sorkness CA, Joseph JC, Busse WW, et al. The effect of oral methotrexate discontinuation in corticosteroid-dependent adult asthma: a 36 month analysis (abstract). *J Allergy Clin Immunol* 1992;89(1, Part 2):286.
51. Methotrexate in rheumatoid arthritis. Health and Public Policy Committee, American College of Physicians. *Ann Intern Med* 1987;107:418–419.
52. Bridges SL, Alarcon GS, Koopman WJ. MTX-induced liver abnormalities in RA. *J Rheumatol* 1989;16:1180–1183.
53. Furst DE, Kremer JM. Methotrexate in rheumatoid arthritis. *Arthritis Rheum* 1988;31:305–314.
54. Groff GD, Shenberger KN, Wilke WS, et al. Low dose oral methotrexate in rheumatoid arthritis: an uncontrolled trial and review of the literature. *Semin Arthritis Rheum* 1983;12:333–347.
55. Whiting-O'Keefe QE, Fye KH, Sack KD. Methotrexate and histologic hepatic abnormalities: a meta-analysis. *Am J Med* 1991;90:711–716.

Drugs and the Lung,
edited by C.P. Page and W.J. Metzger.
Raven Press, Ltd., New York © 1994

8

Chemotherapy in Lung Cancer

*Charlotte Rayner and †Stephen G. Spiro

*Royal Brompton National Heart and Lung Hospital, SW3 6LR,† Department of
Thoracic Medicine, University College Hospital and Middlesex Hospital,
London W1N 8AA, United Kingdom

Lung cancer is the commonest malignancy in the Western world, and its incidence is steadily increasing in Third World countries. It is now responsible for approximately 180,000 deaths per year in the United States and 40,000 deaths per year in Great Britain. Until 1980, there had been a continued increase in incidence with mortality rates in men, rising from 4.9 per 100,000 in 1930 to 71.6 per 100,000 in 1980. Mortality rates in the United States have been higher among whites than nonwhites, although over the last 15 years there has been a reversal in this trend. The most recent incidence data show that the age adjusted lung cancer incidence in white American men has started to fall. This supports the British data that during the 1980s, the incidence in men has plateaued and is now beginning to fall slowly (1,2).

Unfortunately, the incidence of lung cancer in women continues to increase; the male to female ratio a decade ago was 10:1 and is now 2:1. In the United States 34,000 women die each year from lung cancer, which is now about to overtake breast cancer as the commonest cause for cancer-related deaths in women. Age-specific mortality in Great Britain shows that there is a cohort of elderly patients in the population with a high incidence of lung cancer, but in the younger age groups there is a welcome decrease in the mortality rates (Fig. 1).

The most important factor in the etiology of lung cancer is cigarette consumption. The risk of bronchial carcinoma is related to the number of cigarettes smoked and the age at which smoking started. The increasing incidence of lung cancer in women reflects their persisting smoking habits and the overall increase in smoking in the developing countries will cause an epidemic of lung cancer within the next two decades. Sadly, despite aggressive medical and surgical therapy, prospects for cure remain bleak in a primarily preventable disease.

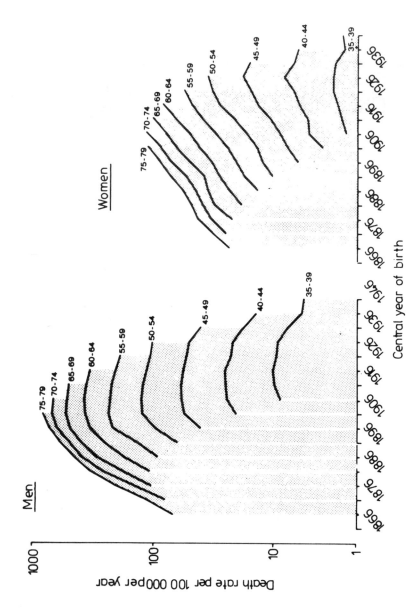

FIG. 1. Age-specific mortality from lung cancer in England and Wales during 1941–1980 plotted against central year of birth. From ref. 3, with permission.

CELL TYPES

The most important factors influencing choice of therapy are the histological cell type of the tumor and the clinical stage of disease.

Histological Cell Type

Lung cancer is divided into non–small cell (NSCLC) and small cell (SCLC) types. Small cell lung cancer comprises approximately 20% of all lung cancer and non–small cell cancer 80%, of which 50% are squamous and 20% adenocarcinomas. The growth rate of a tumor is the most important factor determining its natural history and the chance of long-term survival. Squamous cell cancers tend to be slow growing and remain localized, and therefore carry a reasonable prognosis. However, small cell carcinoma has a rapid growth rate, with a volume doubling time of 30 days, disseminates widely, and is seldom amenable to surgery.

The approach to treatment of lung cancer is based on the cell types–an essential parameter to diagnose as it is a cornerstone in planning treatment. NSCLC can be cured by surgery, but only about 20% of all new cases are operable after clinical staging. Of these a number will be unresectable because of poor lung function or significant coexistent medical illness. However, of those undergoing a so-called curative resection, 75% will relapse either within the thorax or with distant metastases within 5 years—leaving an overall 5-year survival rate of 25% (or 5% of all new patients presenting with the disease). Thus systemic therapy is relevant to the great majority of patients with NSCLC at some stage. The value of cytotoxic chemotherapy and radiotherapy (as a local treatment) will be assessed below.

For SCLC the role of surgery is minimal as the disease is staged to be inoperable at diagnosis in almost all cases. A tiny proportion of patients (less than 5%) are considered operable on their presenting radiographs and scans. Perhaps a third of this small population will go to surgery, and only those with hilar and mediastinal nodes free of disease at pathological staging stand an acceptable chance of long-term survival. Therefore, chemotherapy (with or without radiotherapy) forms the mainstay of the approach to SCLC.

CHEMOTHERAPEUTIC AGENTS USED IN LUNG CANCER

Alkylating Agents

Alkylating agents exert their cytotoxic effects by the formation of covalent linkages (alkylation) with components of DNA. As a result, there is major disruption to the DNA molecule resulting in disturbed cell growth, mitotic activity, cellular differentiation, and function. They are most cyto-toxic to rapidly proliferating tissue.

Cyclophosphamide

This alkylating agent is a nitrogen mustard. The clinical spectrum for use of cyclophosphamide is broad, including its use as an immunosuppressive as well as a cytotoxic agent. It was initially developed by modifying the chemical structure of mechlorethylene with the aim of achieving a greater selectivity for neoplastic tissue. Cyclophosphamide is inactive until metabolized by the P-450 mixed function oxidase system, producing an inactive metabolite, and through a nonenzymatic pathway to produce toxic metabolites known as phosforamide mustard and acrolein. The nonenzymatic pathway may occur within the liver or at other sites within the circulatory system, which therefore minimizes hepatic damage. Cyclophosphamide is well absorbed orally, and when used as an immunosuppressant is often given by this route. In the treatment of lung cancer, it is given as an intravenous slow bolus injection, at a dose usually between 700 and 1000 mg/m^2. When used in combination therapy, depending on the frequency of administration and the other agents being given, the dose may be lower. The side effects of cyclophosphamide are numerous. Nausea and vomiting are common and treatment is symptomatic. The bone marrow is very susceptible to the effect of alkylating agents. Myelosuppression is the dose-limiting factor, and changes may be seen within the bone marrow 8 h after administration. Following conventional intravenous therapy, the white cell nadir occurs at approximately 7 to 10 days with full recovery expected by 21 days. The frequency of dosing is therefore limited to approximately every 3 weeks. Alopecia is more pronounced with cyclophosphamide than with other nitrogen mustards, but hair regrows following cessation of therapy. Mucosal ulceration, nail changes, pigmentation, and postural dizziness have been reported. Acrolein can cause inflammation of the epithelium of the urinary tract. With higher dose therapy, hemorrhagic cystitis is common and if this occurs the dosage should be reduced. However, cystitis can now be prevented by intravenous administration of sulfur hydral compounds such as 2-mercaptoethane sulfonate (MESNA), which binds to acrolein, preventing its effects on the bladder. It is important to keep the patient well hydrated when administering cyclophosphamide.

Interstitial pulmonary fibrosis is rarely a complication of cyclophosphamide in patients with lung cancer, possibly because of the relatively short duration of therapy and short survival. Symptoms can develop 2 weeks after dosage, causing dyspnea, low-grade fever, pleuritic chest pain, and occasionally a hypersensitivity reaction. Findings include pyrexia, bilateral basal crackles with associated basal shadowing on chest x-ray, or occasionally pulmonary edema. This reaction normally responds to steroid therapy, but progression to death has been reported. The lung is also more sensitive to the development of a radiation pneumonitis following cyclophosphamide therapy.

Ifosfamide

Ifosfamide is related to cyclophosphamide. It does not demonstrate cross-resistance with other alkylating agents apart from cyclophosphamide. Its side effects are similar to those of cyclophosphamide, but the dose given is larger (two to three times), and MESNA is given routinely to prevent hemorrhagic cystitis.

Lomustine (CCNU)

Lomustine is a lipid-soluble alkylating agent that is both rapidly absorbed and metabolized completely. The metabolites produced have a half-life ranging between 16 and 48 h. Because of the high lipid solubility, the drug and its metabolites cross the blood-brain barrier and appear in significant concentrations within the cerebrospinal fluid. Clinical toxicity includes bone marrow suppression, nausea and vomiting, and, at high dose, nephrotoxicity.

Antimetabolites

Methotrexate

This antimetabolite acts by competitive inhibition of dihydrofolate reductase. In normal cellular function, folate is reduced by dihydrofolate reductase and becomes an essential component in the synthesis of purines and pyrimidines. Methotrexate inhibits purine ring synthesis by competitive inhibition and prevents the production of ribonucleotides and deoxyribonucleotides. Methotrexate is absorbed orally, but at higher doses this can be unpredictable. There is a direct relationship between dose and plasma concentration. Metabolism is in a triphasic fashion: phase I is due to distribution into body fluids with a half-life of 45 min, phase II reflects renal clearance with a half-life of 2 h, and phase III has a half-life of nearly 7 h. If methotrexate enters expanded body spaces, particularly pleural effusions or ascites, storage of the drug occurs with slow release into the systemic circulation, causing prolonged elevation of plasma drug levels and severe bone marrow suppression. Methotrexate is bound to plasma proteins, and between 50% and 90% of each dose is excreted unchanged into the urine by a combination of filtration and active tubular secretion. With impaired renal function, or when used with other drugs that are also actively secreted, excretion may fall and increased toxicity is possible.

Other side effects include mucosal ulceration, diarrhea, a hemorrhagic enteritis that may progress to interstinal perforation, alopecia, dermatitis, and neuro- nephrotoxicity. An interstitial pneumonitis may occur. With higher-dose therapy, folinic acid may be given 24 h after the methotrexate to reduce toxicity.

Natural Products

Vinca Alkaloids

The periwinkle plant vinca rosa has long been known to have beneficial properties. Initially it was thought to be active in diabetes mellitus. In 1958 Noble and coworkers (4) observed that it produced bone marrow suppression in animals. Alkaloidal fractions were isolated, and Johnson (5) produced four active alkaloids. Of these, vincristine (and to a lesser extent vinblastine and vindesine), have become important in the treatment of lung cancer. The mode of action is thought to be by specific binding to the protein tubulin. By binding to tubulin, there is disruption of microtubules, which are an essential component of the mitotic process. Cell division is arrested at metaphase, chromosomes are not segregated, and cell death occurs. Other functions of the microtubules including phagocytosis are also affected (6). Vinca alkaloids have an unpredictable oral absorption, and they are therefore administered intravenously. Vinblastine and vincristine bind to plasma proteins and are then concentrated in platelets, leukocytes, and erythrocytes. Vinblastine is metabolized within the liver to an active derivative. Vincristine is also metabolized by the liver but there is no active metabolite produced. The standard dose of vincristine is 1.4 mg/m^2 with a maximum dose of 2 mg. Vindesine is given as a slow intravenous bolus at a maximal dose of 5 mg/m^2. These agents do not demonstrate cross-resistance despite similarity of chemical structure.

The most important side effect of vincristine is neurotoxicity, which is the dose-limiting factor. Demyelination and axonal degeneration occur. This is rarely seen in children and increases in incidence with the age of the patient. It begins with distal paresthesia followed by weakness and loss of reflexes, and later by ataxia, muscle cramps, and pain. Neurological studies have shown that in asymptomatic patients the ankle jerk becomes suppressed as the earliest and most consistent sign of the neuropathy. If the patient develops paresthesiae, treatment should be halved and if symptoms progress the drug is stopped. Muscular weakness involving the larynx and the extrinsic muscles can develop, as can autonomic neuropathy, leading to constipation, urinary retention, and hypotension.

Bone marrow suppression is the major toxic effect of vinblastine, with a leukocyte nadir occurring between 4 and 10 days. Other side effects include nausea, vomiting, inappropriate antidiuretic hormone (ADH) secretion, and cardiac toxicity. Vindesine's major toxic manifestations include both bone marrow suppression and neurotoxicity. The dose should be reduced by 50% at the onset of symptoms.

Podophyllotoxins

Podophyllotoxin was extracted from the mandrake plant (mayapple). It was initially used by the American Indian as an emetic and for its cathartic actions. Two semisynthetic derivatives have been produced—Etoposide (VP16-213) and Tenoposide (VM-26). Etoposide has become an important drug in the therapy of SCLC. The mode of action is by the formation of a DNA enzyme complex by interaction with topoisomerase II and DNA. The drug may be given either as an oral preparation or intravenously. The oral dose is approximately 50% of the intravenous dose, although absorption can be variable both within an individual and between individuals. There is a biphasic pattern of clearance with half-lives of 3 and 12 h. The drug is partially metabolized by the liver and approximately 45% of the dose is excreted in the urine, two-thirds of this in an unchanged form and one-third as a metabolite. The usual intravenous dose is between 100 and 200 mg/m^2 daily. The dose schedule is important; efficacy is improved when given as repeated daily doses over 3 or 5 days when compared with a large dose on a single day. It is administered over 30 to 60 min because if given more rapidly hypotension and bronchospasm may occur. The oral preparation is in capsule form of 50 or 100 mg, but because of its variable absorption, the efficacy is less predictable than when the drug is given intravenously. Etoposide is marrow suppressive with leukopenia being its main dose-limiting effect. The white cell nadir occurs at 10 to 14 days and there is full recovery usually by 3 weeks. Approximately 15% of all patients will develop nausea, vomiting, and diarrhea when the drug is given intravenously, and when given orally this may increase to 55%. Other side effects include alopecia, fever, dermatitis, and a mild hepatic toxicity. A peripheral neuropathy may develop and if given with vincristine, this can be severe (7).

Antibiotics

Adriamycin is an anthracycline antibiotic produced by the fungus *Streptomyces pancetius,* initially identified in 1969. It has a very similar structure to daunorubicin, the chemical structure differing by a single hydroxyl group. Initial concentration occurs in the cell nuclei, binding with DNA causing an interruption of both DNA and RNA synthesis with breakage of single and

double strands and failure of sister chromatid exchange. There is also production of free radicals when Adriamycin reacts with the microsomal cytochrome P-450 reductase. An intermediate radical then reacts with oxygen to
produce superoxide and iron radicals. As a result cell destruction occurs
with disruption of the lipid membrane of the cell walls (8).

Adriamycin is administered intravenously as an infusion, at a dose of
about 50 mg/m^2. There is a multiphasic pattern of clearance. Sixty percent
of hepatic blood flow is initially cleared of drug, and the active metabolite
Adriamycinol is produced in the liver. Further metabolism is by conjugation
and excretion into the bile. Only 10% is renally excreted, and this occurs in
the first 6 h after a dose, turning the urine red for up to 2 days. The dose
must be reduced if there is hepatic dysfunction or if patients have hyperbi-
lirubinemia. Myelosuppression occurs with a white cell count nadir occurring at 10 to 14 days. A similar pattern is seen in the platelets and erythrocyte cell lines. Recovery occurs by 21 to 28 days. Other side effects include
alopecia, stomatitis, diarrhea, and vomiting. Myocardial toxicity is a major
feature limiting the use of Adriamycin. Two types of cardiomyopathy are
recognized, an acute form and a chronic cumulative dose-related form. The
acute type is characterized by arrhythmias and repolarization changes in the
ECG. If more severe, a pericarditis/myocarditis syndrome may develop with
severe impairment of cardiac function. The more chronic dose-related type
of toxicity presents as progressive biventricular failure, with cardiac dilatation and pulmonary vascular congestion seen on the chest x-ray. The mechanism of toxicity appears related to the binding of the drug to DNA in nuclei
and mitochondria. The drug is only slowly liberated from cells, and there is
inhibition of protein synthesis interfering with normal protein regeneration.
Myocardial interstitial fibrosis occurs with loss of contractile substance and
mitochondrial swelling with distortion seen on electron microscopy. The
mortality rate from this condition is over 50%. However, the frequency of
serious cardiomyopathy is low provided the cumulative dose of Adriamycin
is kept below 500 mg/m^2. Cyclophosphamide, or the administration of other
anthrocycline antibiotics, will potentiate cardiotoxicity and there is synergy
between irradiation and Adriamycin in causing cardiotoxicity and also pneumonitis. If there is underlying hepatic dysfunction, the dose causing cardiotoxicity will be even less (9,10).

Platinum Containing Compounds

The cytotoxic action of these compounds were discovered in 1965 (11).
Cisdiaminedichloroplatinum (*cis*-platinum) is the most active of these compounds, penetrating cells by diffusion, its chloride atoms are then displaced
and the platinum complex produced reacts with DNA forming cross-links
with DNA during DNA synthesis. There is also a reaction with nucleophils,
and these reactions are thought to be responsible for its toxic effects, partic-

ularly nephrotoxicity, ototoxicity, and intense nausea and vomiting. The drug is inactive orally and is usually given at a dose of 30 to 60 mg/m^2 by infusion over 1 h with the patient being kept well hydrated. Approximately 90% of the platinum will be bound to plasma proteins following nonenzymatic conversion to an inactive metabolite. High concentrations of *cis*-platinum occur in the liver, kidneys, and intestine with only minimal uptake by the CNS. The drug is slowly excreted by the kidneys and it should not be given if the creatinine clearance is reduced to 75% of the predicted glomerular filtration rate (GFR).

Following administration, the patient is kept well hydrated and a diuresis is maintained for 24 h. Side effects include cumulative dose-related nephrotoxicity, ototoxicity with hearing impairment and tinnitus, and intense emesis. Myelosuppression will occur, but the severity of this is influenced by which other agents are being used concomitantly. Rarer side effects include peripheral neuropathy, convulsions, and cardiac toxicity.

Control of the nausea and vomiting produced by platinum containing compounds is essential. High dose of infused metaclopramide is given with dexamethasone. If this fails a 5-hydroxytryptamine (5-HT) antagonist, e.g., Ondanestrone, can be used with excellent effect.

Carboplatin is as effective as *cis*-platinum with less nephrotoxicity and less emesis. Unfortunately, its expense prohibits its routine use.

CHEMOTHERAPY IN SMALL CELL LUNG CANCER

Single Agents

Small cell lung cancer is responsive to most cytotoxic agents; a list of response rates in summarized in Table 1.

TABLE 1. *Single-agent response rates in previously untreated patients with small cell lung cancer (SCLC)*

Agent	Response rate (%)[a]
Carboplatin	65
Ifosfamide	60
Cisplatin	55
Etoposide	45
Nitrogen mustard	40
Cyclophosphamide	40
Methotrexate	35
Vincristine	30
Vinblastine	30
Adriamycin	30
Carmustine (BCNU)	25
Lomustine (CCNU)	15

[a]Complete and partial responses only.

Response is judged to be complete (CR) if all evaluable disease clears clinically, on x-rays and (if applicable) computed tomography (CT) or ultrasound scans. It is rarely achieved with single-agent chemotherapy. A partial response (PR) is a reduction in measurable tumor by at least 50%, measured in two perpendicular diameters. Anything less than a 50% response is taken as a lesser response, and grouped into the category of stable disease for purposes of analysis. The median survival of SCLC with single agents (3–6 months), is better than the untreated natural history (1–3 months) and approximates the median survival of patients treated with radiotherapy alone to the primary tumor site.

Combination Chemotherapy

The major step in improving the median survival of patients with SCLC has been their greatly increased response rates to combinations of cytotoxic agents. Most chemotherapy regimens include three drugs, often four, and occasionally more. However, the improvements, first documented late in the 1970s, have not escalated, despite huge efforts and innumberable clinical trials. The active newer agents (etoposide, ifosfamide, cisplatin) have replaced some of the original agents (methotrexate, CCNU, and the vinca alkaloids), but have not substantially improved survival. Yet the newer drugs, particularly *cis*-platinum and etoposide, are more toxic and have to be given with due care and knowledge. Several regimes have become established as approximately equipotent in the treatment of SCLC and are summarized in Table 2. Until new agents with entirely different modes of action become available, it is unlikely that the prognosis for SCLC will change. Nevertheless, there has been considerable progress during the last 10 years in rationalizing chemotherapy in terms of whom to treat, the optimal duration of treatment, the value of maintenance treatment, high dose or intensive chemotherapy, alternating or nonalternating regimens, and the place of radiotherapy. All of these will be discussed in some detail.

In all regimes response rates are highest in patients presenting with limited disease, i.e., disease confined to the hemithorax, including the mediastinum and the ipsilateral supraclavicular fossa. A complete response in 50% of patients presenting with limited disease (LD) is common. The response rates for those with extensive disease (ED) at diagnosis are lower. Extensive disease includes spread outside the hemithorax and the ipsilateral supraclavicular fossa. Approximately 30% of new patients with SCLC have limited disease at presentation. The overall median survival for LD patients treated with chemotherapy is 15 to 18 months, and for those with extensive disease is 6 to 12 months (12,13).

TABLE 2. *Common drug schedules in the treatment of SCLC*

1.	A.	Cisplatin	60 mg/m^2	day 1
		Etoposide	120 mg/m^2	days 1, 2, 3
		Alternating every 21 days with		
	B.	Cyclophosphamide	600 mg/m^2	
		Adriamycin	50 mg/m^2	
		Vincristine	2 mg	
2.		Cyclophosphamide	750 mg/m^2	
		Adriamycin	40 mg/m^2	
		Vincristine	2 mg	
		Every 21 days		
3.		Adriamycin	40 mg/m^2	
		Cyclophosphamide	500 mg/m^2	
		Vincristine	2 mg	
		Etoposide	60 mg/m^2	days 1, 2, 3
		Every 21 days		

Duration of Chemotherapy

As combination chemotherapy became established, it was advocated to treat for 1 year once a CR was obtained. However, in those not achieving a CR (the majority in the 1970s), treatment was continued until relapse. This was therefore a prolonged period of cyclical chemotherapy with ever-increasing morbidity, to say little of the uncertainty facing the patient enduring this process. It has become clear, however, that the response to chemotherapy is rapid and usually maximal by three to four cycles. Studies have evaluated the minimal effective duration of chemotherapy without obvious disadvantage to overall survival. Further, the role of maintenance chemotherapy (either the same cyclical chemotherapy or a modified form of chemotherapy) has been evaluated in several recently published studies.

In a London Lung Cancer Group study (14), 616 patients were randomized to receive either four or eight courses of chemotherapy. There was also a further randomization at relapse, when patients received either symptomatic treatment or further chemotherapy using different agents than those during initial treatment. Patients allocated to receive four courses of chemotherapy with no further chemotherapy at relapse had a median survival of 30 weeks. The other three treatment arms had similar median survivals of 39 to 42 weeks. It was concluded that if only four courses of chemotherapy were given initially there was a poorer median survival, which was improved if patients received chemotherapy at relapse. If patients received eight courses initially, then no further advantage was obtained from further chemotherapy at relapse. The disadvantage of four courses only with no therapy on relapse was even greater for the responding patients.

The Medical Research Council (15) gave 497 patients six cycles of a four-drug regimen, with mediastinal radiotherapy between course 2 and 3 in responding patients with limited disease. After the initial six cycles, patients whose disease remained controlled were randomized to receive either no further chemotherapy or six further courses of the same drugs, but at the longer interval of 4 weeks instead of 3. The overall response rate was 66%, similar to the London group with 61% (14) and a median survival of 39 weeks. There was no improvement in survival for patients who received maintenance treatment, although for the 97 patients who were complete responders after the initial six courses of chemotherapy, there was a hint of longer survival with maintenance treatment. This was 42 weeks compared with 30 for those without maintenance treatment. An attempt was also made to assess quality of life during chemotherapy. The toxicity of maintenance therapy led to a poorer quality of life as judged by both the physician and patient.

A similar study from France looked at the possible survival advantages for complete responders continuing with a further six courses of chemotherapy, compared with just an initial six. There was no survival advantage for those receiving a total of 12 courses of chemotherapy (16).

The European Organization for Research and Treatment of Cancer (EORTC) treated 426 patients with five cycles of induction chemotherapy consisting of cyclophosphamide, Adriamycin, and etoposide (17). The patients who responded during induction therapy were randomized to seven further chemotherapy cycles or no treatment. The time to relapse was prolonged by further treatment, but there was no overall survival advantage with maintenance therapy.

The National Cancer Institute (NCI) of Canada Lung Cancer Group performed two studies sequentially. In the first study patients received three cycles of cyclophosphamide, Adriamycin, and vincristine (CAV) with thoracic irradiation. This was then followed by a 1-year maintenance program consisting of lomustine, procarbazine, and methotrexate (18). In the second study a similar group of patients were treated with six cycles of CAV alone. No significant differences were noted in the survival of the two groups. In the latter study, the median survival was 49 weeks for limited disease and 34 weeks for extensive disease.

The cancer and acute leukemic group B (CALGB) (19) performed a randomized trial that presented further support for the nonmaintenance approach. Patients who achieved a remission with combination chemotherapy were randomized to receive further chemotherapy or no additional elective treatment. Maintenance therapy increased the survival in a subset of patients with limited disease who achieved a complete response. In all other groups, no prolongation of remission was seen. In 1986 another randomized trial of 300 patients specifically addressed the question of duration of chemotherapy. Patients with clearly demonstrable residual disease, i.e., partial remission or less, were excluded. Limited and extensive stage CR patients were randomized separately. In extensive disease there was no significant prolongation of survival with maintenance treatment, but unfortunately for limited disease the numbers were inadequate to provide any conclusions (20).

It now seems reasonable to limit chemotherapy to six courses for new cases of SCLC. The question remains, however, as to whether patients presenting with limited disease and a good prognosis (see below), i.e., those who present with the highest prognostic factor score for good survival, should be treated more aggressively. The answer to this is not yet known.

Alternating Chemotherapy

Alternating cycles of combination chemotherapy allows patients to receive all or most of the drugs active against SCLC. The concept is logical and attractive, also attempting to expose the tumor to chemotherapy in its different stages of cell division rendering it, in theory, more vulnerable to death from chemotherapy. Unfortunately there is no evidence that alternating cycles of treatment enhances the overall survival, although some regimens increase overall response rates. Since most of the cytotoxic agents are marrow toxic, alternating cycles lessen the temptation of giving two or three drugs with similar toxicity within the same combination cycle, and these drugs can be separated, e.g., cyclophosphamide from etoposide, and mixed with drugs of differing toxicity, hence minimizing serious side effects to the patient.

Most studies incorporate five or six drugs given in two or three drug cycles. For example Osterlind et al. (21), gave cyclophosphamide, Adriamycin, and vincristine alternately with *cis*-platinum, etoposide, and methotrexate to 76 patients. The overall response rate was 82% with 47% of limited-disease patients achieving a complete response, and 38% of ED patients. The median survivals were 16.6 and 11.4 months, respectively, but this was considered to be no better than most nonalternating regimens.

More recent studies have compared the addition of an extra drug to a standard regimen, for example CAV with or without etoposide. In one such study (22), there was no advantage for the patients given etoposide in addition, but toxicity was greater.

Studies of standard chemotherapy versus alternating regimens showed similar overall response rates with a higher CR rate for the alternating regimen (23). However, the increased remission rates with alternating chemotherapy did not turn into a survival advantage.

A similar type of study confined to limited disease patients, comparing an alternating and nonalternating regimen, randomized 400 patients. This showed a median survival of 15.1 and 16.5 months for the nonalternating and alternating regimens, respectively (24). However, both treatments were considered equally effective.

Dose Escalation

In the late 1970s studies showed that dose escalations of cyclophosphamide, methotrexate, and CCNU improved both response rate and survival. However by increasing the dose there was greater toxicity. Studies that increased the dose of CAV did not improve response rate but observed increasing toxicity, particularly bone marrow suppression. To circumvent this side effect, prior bone marrow harvest followed by high-dose chemotherapy and reinfusion of the bone marrow has been evaluated. Souhami et al. (25) gave cyclophosphamide at 160 to 200 mg/kg to patients with small-volume limited-disease SCLC and showed an improved response rate increasing from 30% with conventional doses to 85% with high-dose treatment; 58% of patients had a complete response. This study also showed a marked reduction in tumor mass on CT scan after a single course of the cyclophosphamide therapy. A second similarly designed study gave two identical cycles of high-dose cyclophosphamide achieving a response rate of 91% after the two cycles, but similar to the 85% achieved with one cycle in the first study. This suggested that there remained a population of cyclophosphamide-resistant cells that made cure impossible with this regimen, despite a very high CR rate (26,27).

Etoposide also demonstrates a steep dose-response curve. A study in 13 patients with extensive SCLC treated with etoposide at 1.2 g/m^2 over 3 days for two cycles showed a response in eight patients, which was complete in four. Additional treatment with cyclophosphamide, vincristine, and Adriamycin did not improve the response rate (28). These observations prompted further studies of etoposide alone and in combination with high-dose cyclophosphamide and *cis*-platinum as induction therapy for patients with extensive disease. Both with single and high-dose etoposide, and also when combined with cyclophosphamide, the complete response rate was only 30% and there was no survival benefit (29). With the addition of *cis* platinum to high-dose etoposide and cyclophosphamide the complete response increased to 65%. This was measured by CT assessment and bronchoscopy. Unfortunately the median survival and response duration was unchanged when compared to historical controls. Toxicity produced was severe with myelosuppression leukopenia and thrombocytopenia lasting up to 10 days. Autologous bone marrow transplantation was not performed (30).

Despite the high complete response rate achieved by dose escalation, it is disappointing that the median survival and response duration remained unchanged.

Reinduction or Late Intensification

Another approach to overcome the problem of relapse from residual disease is to treat the remaining small tumor burden following an initial response. The assumption is that with a small residual tumor mass, cure may be possible and cross-resistance would be minimal. Aggressive treatment following an initial response to chemotherapy is unsuitable for patients with progressive disease or for those with a deteriorating performance status. Despite the fact that the majority of studies treated mainly good responders in good physical condition, the results have been disappointing. Both single and multiple drug regimens have been used. Results suggest that useful dose-response relationships do not exist in previously treated patients. Unfortunately most of the trials include only small numbers of patients, and are not controlled. In a typical study 77 patients with SCLC were given induction chemotherapy of cyclophosphamide, Adriamycin, and vincristine every 21 days for four to six cycles. The overall response rate was 72%. The 26 patients who achieved complete remission received intensification with two further cycles of ifosfamide 5 g/m^2, methotrexate 30 mg/m^2, and etoposide 100 mg/m^2 per day (IME) for 3 days. Six of the patients in partial remission achieved a complete remission on IME. Median survival in the limited disease group was 11 months compared with 7 months in the extensive disease patients, and four of the patients were alive at 2 years. There was no significant prolongation of the median survival in the patients in complete remission following induction chemotherapy. Although this sequential six-drug regimen produced higher response rates, median survival was unchanged (31). It is unlikely that benefit will be seen in patients who achieve a CR and then receive late intensification chemotherapy.

Another approach recently examined, is to change the cycling of chemotherapy administration (32). The London Lung Cancer Group gave a weekly regimen of *cis*-platinum and etoposide, alternating with CAV, to 70 patients (33). The overall response was 91% with a CR rate of 50%. Median survival for the whole group was 54 weeks—58 weeks for limited disease and 42 for extensive disease patients. Toxicity was tolerable and mainly hematological. These results were considered promising, and a randomized study of 12 courses of weekly chemotherapy versus six courses of chemotherapy given every 3 weeks has just been concluded.

PROGNOSTIC FACTORS

Although the great majority of patients with SCLC initially respond to chemotherapy, it is certain that only a small number are potentially curable. Thus, if these patients could be identified early and selected out for standard, or even more intensive chemotherapy, the remaining majority could be treated in a more appropriate way, as they appear doomed to die some months following an initial response to drug treatment. It can be argued that these patients should be given a minimum of treatment, and this philosophy is currently being investigated in several studies, and clear guidelines are emerging.

Recently, attention has focused on the condition of the patient at presentation, and a prognostic index established from simple clinical and biochemical measurements. Early studies identified performance status and weight loss as important prognostic factors, but other variables including simple biochemical and hematological parameters have been evaluated. In a multivariate analysis performance status, serum albumin, sodium, and alkaline phosphatase were identified as important prognostic parameters (34). When these four variables were evaluated in a group of 366 patients presenting with SCLC treated with chemotherapy, the patients could be divided into a good prognosis group with a high performance status and normal serum albumin, sodium, and alkaline phosphatase; a poor prognosis group with a low performance status and a low serum albumin or increased sodium or alkaline phosphatase; and an intermediate prognosis group with at least one variable abnormal. There was a clear-cut difference in survival between the groups (Fig. 2). When the more complicated staging criteria for limited and extensive disease were included in the analysis (e.g., CT brain, thorax and abdomen, and bone scans), and compared with the four simple prognostic factors previously identified, no additional information of prognostic value was obtained (Fig. 3). Other studies have confirmed these findings and other factors have also been identified, such as being female in a Danish study

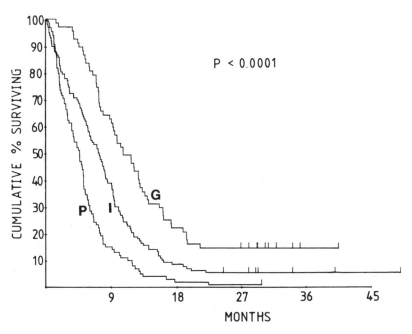

FIG. 2. Survival related to prognostic category. G, good; I; intermediate; P, poor.

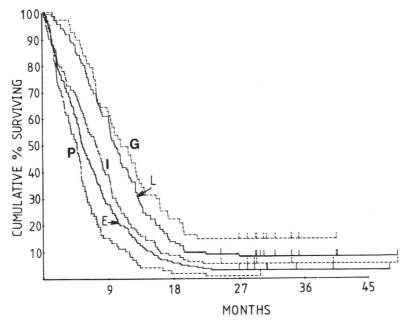

FIG. 3. Survival related to prognostic category and disease extent. G, good; I, intermediate; P, poor; E, extensive; L, limited disease.

(35). Another review of determinants of improved outcome in an analysis of 2,580 patients also identified performance status, female sex, age less than 70, and normal lactate dehydrogenase as favorable independent predictors (36).

These assessments made at the time of diagnosis are now being used as determinants for therapy. Poor and intermediate prognosis patients are best advised to be given 3, 4, or 6 months of chemotherapy in randomized studies to ascertain whether short-course chemotherapy confers any survival disadvantage on these patients. The challenge is for the good-prognosis patients. To date there is no evidence that short-course chemotherapy is a disadvantage for good-prognosis patients, but at the same time the question remains open as to whether intensifying chemotherapy for good-prognosis patients might improve their long-term survival. Long-term survival in good-prognosis patients remains the most important challenge in trying to improve overall survival in SCLC.

LONG-TERM SURVIVAL

Despite attempts either to intensify initial chemotherapy or prolong therapy with or without the addition of radiotherapy, the likelihood for patients

TABLE 3. A summary of studies reporting long-term survivors of treatment for small cell carcinoma of the lung (>24 months)

Reference	Treatment and duration	Long-term survivors							
		LD		ED		Total			
		No.	(%)	No.	(%)	No.	(%)		
Einhom et al. (37)	CAV/RT 24 months	5/19	(26)	1/39	(3)	6/58	(10)		
Smith et al. (38)	CVPAM RT Prolonged to tolerance	4/17	(24)	1/25	(4)	5/42	(12)		
Livingstone et al. (39)	CAV/RT 24 months	12/102	(12)	5/271	(2)	17/373	(5)		
Ginsberg et al. (40)	C,CCNU,V + A,hex/RT 18 months	7/36	(19)	1/36	(3)	8/72	(11)		
Maurer and Pajak (41)	C + M or MV,RT 6 months vs. indefinite	9/108	(8)	1/103	(1)	10/211	(5)		
Hansen et al. (42)	CMC + V + TR CMCV + RT CMC + AV 18 months	11/166	(7)	3/171	(2)	14/337	(4)		
Minna et al. (43)	VAC + RT CMC + VAPr + RT 4 months 12 months 24 months	16/69	(23)	4/99	(4)	20/168	(12)		
Natale and Wittes (44)	VP16/CISpl CAV/RT 4 months LD	5/24	(21)	2/20	(10)	7/44	(16)		
Aisner et al. (45)	CA VP16 + MER 24 months	3/14	(21)	0/24	(0)	3/38	(8)		
Souhami et al. (27)	CV VP16 +/− RT 9 months	12/130	(9)	7/241	(3)	19/371	(5)		

LD, limited disease; ED, extensive disease; C, cyclophosphamide; A, Adriamycin; V, vincristine; P, prednisolone; M, methotrexate; CCNU, lomustine; hex, hexamethylmelamine; CISpl, cis-platinum; VP16, epipodophyllotoxin; Pr, procabazine; MER, methanol-extracted residue of BCG; RT, radiotherapy.

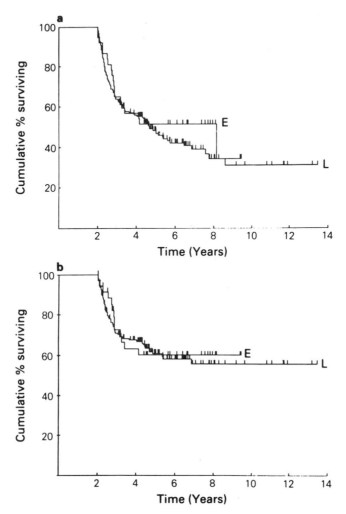

FIG. 4. Long-term survival in small cell lung cancer. **a:** Survival curve showing effects of deaths from all causes. **b:** Survival curves; deaths only from small cell lung cancer. From ref. 13, with permission. E, extensive disease; L, limited disease.

presenting with limited disease being alive at 2 years is less than 10%, and for extensive disease about 2% (13). Table 3 summarizes long-term survival data for some recent studies, and shows typical chemotherapy regimens used and the 2-year survival.

Most long-term follow-up studies show that 40% of survivors are either able to return to work or to the level of activity enjoyed before diagnosis. There have, however, been reports of cerebral problems developing in some survivors, namely memory loss and deteriorating scores on psychometric testing. In most of these patients prophylactic cerebral irradiation had been given after chemotherapy, and this may have been in part responsible.

A review of 2,500 patients entered into clinical trials in the United Kingdom has shown that the overall 2-year survival is 5.8%. Patients with limited disease had an 8% incidence of 2-year survival and extensive disease patients 2% (13). The chances of dying of SCLC continued between 2 and 5 years after treatment, but there were very few deaths from SCLC after 5 years (Fig. 4). However, patients continued to die of other causes unrelated to SCLC, including NSCLC and other cancers (13). In this retrospective study long-term survival was not affected by the addition of radiotherapy to the mediastinum after chemotherapy, or by sex, age or prognostic factor status at diagnosis.

In another study, 874 patients treated in Denmark produced 72 patients who were disease free 18 months after beginning treatment (47). The 5-year survival was 24% for these 72 patients, with a tenfold greater subsequent mortality than expected for age-matched controls. The risk of late relapse was greatest in patients who had presented with metastatic disease, particularly liver or bone marrow involvement. Radiotherapy to the primary tumor site and mediastinum again did not appear to confer a survival advantage. The risk of relapsing from SCLC fell considerably if the patients were still disease free at 3 years. Again second cancers developed in several of these long-term survivors and the cumulative risk of this rose to 32%, the latest occurring 5.4 years after diagnosis of the original small cell tumor.

NEWER CONCEPTS FOR CYTOTOXIC CHEMOTHERAPY

Low-Dose Etoposide

It is clear that for those patients with poor prognostic factors for survival (low performance status, or abnormal sodium, albumin, or liver function tests), the response to conventional chemotherapy has been clearly defined but will only prolong median survival for 6 to 9 months. For these patients, and also older patients, it may appear logical to attempt to obtain their remission with potentially less toxic therapy.

Etoposide, when given as a single agent, can produce acceptably high response rates. However, it has the disadvantage of having an unpredictable absorption profile, and in some studies up to 10% of patients suffered significant bone marrow toxicity. Recently the scheduling of etoposide has been shown to be important in influencing maximum response rates. Slevin et al. (48) compared 500 mg/m^2 i.v. over 24 h with 100 mg/m^2 over 2 h i.v. on 5 consecutive days, both regimens given every 3 weeks. In the 24-h arm of the study, there was a 10% partial response rate, but in the 5-day schedule the response rate was 89% (in 16 patients).

The value of etoposide as an oral agent was first shown in a study of a single-day intravenous regimen with a 20% response rate versus a 3-day oral regimen with a 65% response rate (49). Several studies have now shown oral etoposide to be generally very well tolerated, and is as likely to produce a response as any other regimen. In 22 relapsed patients given single-agent oral etoposide 50 mg/m² per day for 21 consecutive days, a CR or PR was seen in 45% of patients despite previous chemotherapy, which in 18 patients included etoposide (50). Studies are now evaluating low-dose oral etoposide in elderly and poorer prognostic patients with 14- or 21-day cycles, and high response rates are recorded with minimal gastrointestinal or marrow toxicity.

Colony Growth Stimulation Factors (G-CSF)

Hemopoietic growth factors are at the center of considerable clinical activity in a wide range of malignant and nonmalignant diseases, including solid tumors, hemopoietic malignancies, aplasetic anemia, AIDS, and idiopathic neutropenias.

Studies in lung cancer have centered on granulocyte CSF, given together with conventional cytotoxic chemotherapy. In a study from Manchester (51), the addition of G-GSF was extremely effective in reducing the extent and duration of neutropenia by 80%. Life-threatening infections occurred during chemotherapy with no G-GSF, and these infections resulted in 30 extra days in hospital for i.v. antibiotics.

A large study of G-CSF versus placebo given during six courses of combination chemotherapy in SCLC showed a 40% incidence of neutropenia for patients receiving G-CSF compared with 77% for those on placebo. The number of days of treatment with intravenous antibiotics, days in hospital, and incidence of confirmed infections, fell by 50% with G-CSF (52).

These growth factors will allow a more rapid recovery of the bone marrow, with less toxicity, and could allow either dose intensification of cytotoxic chemotherapy and/or more frequent application of cytotoxic schedules (53). This may provide a possible way forward for more intensive chemotherapy in SCLC.

New Drugs for SCLC

The most active newer agents assessed in phase II trials include epirubicin, interleukin-2, teniposide, mitozolomide, and CPT 11 (a camptothecin analogue) all recently reviewed by Talbot and Smith (54) and summarized in Table 4. All these agents have been evaluated in only a small number of patients and their true activity is not yet clearly known.

TABLE 4. *Response rates for new single agents in SCLC*

Drug	Dosage/schedule	No. of patients	Response (%)
Epirubicin	120 g/m² i.v. q 21 days	71	48
Interleukin-2	4.5 × 106 MU/m² i.v. over 96 h q 7 days × 4	10	30
Teniposide	120–140 mg/m² i.v. day 1,3,5 q 21	44	34
Mitozolomide	70–90 mg/m² po q 42 days	18	28
CPT-11	100 mg/m² i.v. q 7 days	35	37

From Talbot and Smith (54).

Camptothecin is a plant alkaloid isolated from the Asian tree *Camptotheca acuminata,* but its clinical use is limited by severe hemorrhagic cystitis and low response rates (55). CPT 11 has, however, more encouraging preclinical and antitumor activity, and in man is better tolerated than its parent compound (56).

Epirubicin has been in clinical use for some years, but interest has recently focused on possible dose escalation, which has achieved objective response rates of 50% but adverse effects include myelosuppression, alopecia, nausea, and vomiting, but no cardiotoxicity (57,58).

Of the podophyllins, etoposide remains the most effective member of this class of cytotoxic agents. Teniposide has not, as yet, seriously challenged the place of etoposide.

Biological response modifiers represent a new approach in cancer treatment. Patients treated with interleukin-2, usually in combination with or following chemotherapy, show an encouraging objective response rate. However, toxic effects discontinued treatment in 10% of patients. Dose-limiting toxicity includes hypotension, hemolysis, renal failure, hepatic dysfunction, and allergy.

The role of interferon-γ as maintenance treatment is currently being evaluated in patients achieving a complete response to conventional chemotherapy.

THE ROLE OF RADIOTHERAPY IN SMALL CELL LUNG CANCER

Combined Modality Treatment (Chemotherapy and Radiotherapy)

One of the earliest studies in SCLC compared radiotherapy with surgery in 1962. Of 73 patients treated with radiotherapy, 62 completed treatment, and of 71 randomized to surgery, 24 were inoperable at thoracotomy. Results after 10 years showed a slight superiority for radiotherapy, with four patients being alive, all of whom had received radiotherapy. A second Medical Research Council study in 1979 compared the effect of radiotherapy to the primary tumor site with chemotherapy and radiotherapy. After combined modality therapy, the median survival was 43 weeks compared with 25 weeks with radiotherapy alone. At 1 year 57% of patients who received combined therapy had developed metastases compared with 79% in those who received just radiotherapy (59). It was evident that chemotherapy both controlled the primary site and delayed the appearances of metastatic disease. Radiotherapy, however, remains an integral part of treatment, although its role in combined modality therapy is still under investigation. A study in 1984 randomized patients to 12 courses of combination chemotherapy, with half receiving radiotherapy (40 Gy over 20 days) after the fourth course of chemotherapy, and then completing 12 courses, provided a response was maintained. There was no difference in survival between the two treatment groups. When the results were analyzed for disease stage, no advantage was seen for the addition of radiotherapy for either limited or extensive disease patients apart from a small reduction in local recurrence rate (60). A recent meta-analysis of all randomized studies of chemotherapy versus chemotherapy and radiotherapy has shown an advantage for the combined treatment for 3 years survival of 5%. Thus radiotherapy should be given to the mediastinum and primary tumor site in all patients who show a major response following chemotherapy. However, the best time during chemotherapy for the administration of radiotherapy remains uncertain.

Some studies have looked at sequential, alternating, or concurrent radiotherapy with chemotherapy. The Eastern Cooperative Oncology Group (ECOG) has studied 34 patients with alternating chemotherapy and hyperfraction radiation therapy in limited stage SCLC, giving *cis*-platinum and etoposide every 3 weeks, with radiation administered twice daily to a total dose of 45 Gy. Sixty-two percent of patients had a complete response and eight a partial response (61). A second study with only 23 patients used concurrent *cis*-platinum and etoposide chemotherapy with twice daily radiation therapy to a total of 45 Gy over 3 weeks. The overall response rate was 91% with a median follow-up of 22 months. Median survival has not yet been reported. Toxicity in the form of esophagitis occurred in 73% of patients (62). A similar regimen was studied at the National Cancer Institute in 25 patients who received etoposide 80 mg/m^2 on days 1, 2, 3, 27, 28, and 29 with *cis*-platinum 80 mg/m^2 on days 1 and 27 with concurrent chest radiotherapy twice a day from days 6 to 24. Seventy-two percent of patients had a complete response and seven a partial response. Survival was 63% at 2 years (63). Another pilot study included 40 patients who received 1.5 Gy twice daily for 3 weeks to a total of 45 Gy with concurrent *cis*-platinum and etoposide, followed by six maintainance cycles of this regimen, alternating with cyclophosphamide, Adriamycin, and vincristine. A complete response occurred in 78% of patients with partial response in 18%—an overall response of 95%. Toxicity included myelosuppression and esophagitis, and four deaths were related to toxicity, including two cases of pulmonary fibrosis. One-year survival was 67% and 2-year 36% (64). It can be seen from these small pilot studies that there is very good control of local disease, but larger randomized studies are required (65).

Palliation

It must be emphasized that for relapsed SCLC, radiotherapy is an excellent palliative tool for superior vena caval obstruction, bone pain, recurrent hemoptysis, recurrent infection secondary to local relapse, and breathlessness.

Prophylactic Cranial Irradiation (PCI)

The brain is a common site for metastases in SCLC, with an incidence of 13% to 67% at autopsy. The role of PCI remains controversial. It has been documented that brain metastases respond to chemotherapy in similar fashion to metastatic disease elsewhere. Studies giving cranial irradiation to asymptomatic patients upon completion of chemotherapy for controlling their primary disease report a considerably lower incidence of relapse within the brain. However, there is no evidence that PCI prolongs survival, although by reducing the incidence of brain relapse it prevents patients developing a complication associated with high morbidity. There is still debate as to whether PCI has a survival impact in patients who achieve a CR with initial chemotherapy. A randomized study organized by the British Medical Research Council (MRC) is currently in progress to resolve this question. Other groups that have administered PCI reported a deterioration of higher cerebral function in a percentage of patients.

QUALITY OF LIFE

There are only a few studies evaluating quality of life during treatment of lung cancer. The treatment of SCLC revolves around chemotherapy and the balance of duration and intensity of therapy, with the resultant effect on quality of life. The obvious drawbacks are the toxic side effects of treatment, and the necessity for hospital admission to administer and monitor chemotherapy. There is also considerable psychological morbidity associated with a diagnostic label of cancer and with apprehension about chemotherapy.

Other factors involved in assessing the appropriateness of chemotherapy include social circumstances and cultural and religious beliefs. There are a number of assessment scales of quality of life that have been well validated. These include the Karnofsky performance scale (66), which is simple and widely used. A more complex assessment is the EORTC questionnaire (67), and other measures include a daily diary card system. The diary card is sensitive to short-term changes in quality of life and useful for comparing the effects of therapy during the treatment periods. In one of the London lung cancer group studies, prophylactic cranial irradiation was associated with an increase in nausea and vomiting and sickness, and related variables worsened as chemotherapy continued (68). Chemotherapy is, however, an important specific symptomatic treatment. For example, in 100 consecutive patients receiving chemotherapy, specific symptomatic treatment was given throughout, and symptoms were assessed every 3 weeks by two independent observers. In patients who completed four courses of chemotherapy, most had an improvement in symptoms, although a few complained of increasing anorexia. Eighty percent had noted a marked improvement in pain control resulting in cessation or reduction of analgesia (69). About four-fifths of patients presenting with SCLC respond to chemotherapy and as a result have their life prolonged, and the control of symptoms improves their quality of life, at least in the short term.

NON–SMALL CELL LUNG CANCER

Surgery

Surgery remains the best prospect for cure. The chances of long-term survival are greatest if the tumor is small (less than 3 cm), squamous, in the periphery of the lung, and if the hilar and mediastinal nodes are not involved by metastases. Survival rates drop progressively with increasing size of the primary tumor, the size of resection (lobectomy or pneumonectomy), and the presence of nodal metastases. Five-year survival for a peripheral squamous tumor is 70%, but with hilar nodal involvement it drops to about 30%. Once the mediastinum is involved, the survival prospects are poor. Radiologically obvious mediastinal nodal enlargement is certain to be due to tumor and the patient irresectable. For large nodes (greater than 1 cm in diameter) not visible on the chest radiographs and only identified with CT scanning, mediastinoscopy must be performed to confirm whether they contain tumor, which will render the disease unresectable. There is a probable salvage rate for surgery in patients whose mediastinal nodal disease is only discovered at thoracotomy after a negative mediastinoscopy (up to 15% of cases going to thoracotomy) (70), and this is better still if the involvement is microscopic and only found at postoperative pathological staging (up to 40% 5-year survival in some series, especially if squamous cell).

However, surgical survival rates will not increase as most failures are due to relapse of disease not identified at preoperative staging. Better, more sensitive staging may develop to exclude more patients from surgery in the future.

Radiotherapy

Radiotherapy can be given at several points during the course of NSCLC: preoperatively, instead of surgery, postresection, to inoperable patients with limited disease in radical dosage, and to inoperable patients as palliative therapy, either to the primary tumor or to symptomatic metastases.

Preoperative Radiotherapy

Preoperative radiotherapy has been attempted in a few uncontrolled studies to sterilize or reduce the bulk of the primary tumor mass, often including the mediastinum. However, the postoperative survival data are no better than for surgery alone, and this approach has now been abandoned. Early studies of superior sulcus tumors suggested that survival was improved by preoperative irradiation as compared to surgery alone. However, subsequent studies failed to confirm this advantage.

Alternative Therapy to Surgery

Irradiation of primary tumors that appeared operable, but were not resected because of either medical contraindications or patient refusal, appeared to do just as well with radiotherapy as with surgery in a study of Smart and Hilton (71) in 1956. This study with carefully selected cases contained only squamous cell cancers, and achieved a 5-year survival rate of 22.5%. However, subsequent trials have failed to equal these results. Deeley's (72) study in 1967, which was larger, achieved a 1-year survival figure of 36%, with only 6% of patients alive at 5 years. A further controlled study of 58 patients randomized to radical radiotherapy or surgery found a 7% 5-year survival for the radiotherapy group, and 23% for surgery.

Postoperative Radiotherapy

The role of postoperative irradiation has for long been uncertain. Uncontrolled studies in the 1970s indicated that there may be a survival advantage to all non–small cell types for post/resection irradiation, even if the resection appeared curative. However, two recent large randomized studies firmly refute this. A European study randomized 175 patients undergoing curative resection, with no tumor extension beyond the lung, and no involvement of lymph nodes, to either just follow-up or 60 Gy radiotherapy in 6 weeks, beginning 3 to 4 weeks postoperatively (73). The patients comprised all cell types, although the majority were squamous. There was no increase in survival in the irradiated group. For the squamous cancers the analysis showed a possible detrimental survival effect of radiation therapy, although this was not statistically significant. However, irradiation decreased the rate of local relapse and most relapses (85%) were extrathoracic, although this had no effect on overall survival.

A further detailed study on squamous cell tumors in 1986 chose a dose of 50 Gy, given 28 days postsurgery in the active arm of the study, which involved 210 eligible patients (74). The two groups were well matched, both anthropometrically and for tumor stage. There was no evidence that radiotherapy improved survival and, although the local recurrence rates were somewhat reduced in the radiotherapy arm, the decrease was not significant.

Postoperative irradiation to patients known to have undergone a noncurative resection also failed to achieve a survival advantage. Results show only a 5% to 8% 5-year survival rate.

Radical Radiotherapy for Locally Inoperable Disease

In otherwise fit patients with a small volume of intrathoracic disease that is not resectable, usually because of mediastinal lymph node involvement, it is common practice to attempt curative therapy with irradiation. This requires doses of up to 60 Gy, but has produced disappointing results, with 5-year survival figures ranging from 3% to 17% (Table 5).

Some still refute the claims that radical radiotherapy confers no definite short- or long-term survival advantage to patients, but most accept the high

TABLE 5. *Survival after radical radiotherapy for inoperable non–small cell lung cancer (NSCLC)*

Reference	No. of patients	Survival (%)	
		1 year	5 years
Deeley and Singh (1967) (75)	513	36	6
Caldwell and Bagshawe (1968) (76)	284	30	6
Perez-Tamayow and Soberon (1969) (77)	277	30	6
Guttman (1971) (78)	103	59	9
Lee (1974) (79)	180	37	3
Cox and Kennelly (1980) (80)	141	57	10
Edinburgh Lung Cancer group (1986) (81)	42	–	17

risk of failure because of occult extrathoracic disease, and also imperfect control of the local intrathoracic tumor bulk. In most unselected studies, the 5-year survival rate with radical radiotherapy up to 60 Gy is about 5%. Earlier randomized studies of radiotherapy versus conservative therapy in the United States (82) and in Oxford, which gave between 40 and 50 Gy, failed to show any advantage for treatment. These studies have been criticized for including some small cell tumors and using older orthrovoltage radiation equipment, and for failing to show that the two groups in each study were perfectly matched. However, it is very unlikely that radical doses of conventional irradiation will make an impact on survival in locally inoperable NSCLC.

Attempts to improve the effectiveness of radiotherapy with hyperbaric oxygen and various radiosensitizing drugs such as misonidazole and small doses of cisplatin have failed to establish a clear-cut advantage. Currently the most interesting possibility is hyperfractionation, in which intensive treatment is given three times a day for 2 to 3 weeks instead of conventional daily dosages. This is the subject of a controlled randomized study in the United Kingdom at present, comparing hyperfractionation to conventional dose radical radiotherapy.

Palliative Radiotherapy

The value of radiotherapy in palliating certain distressing symptoms is beyond dispute. Relief of symptoms will improve the quality of life for most of these patients for a useful period of time in both NSCLC and SCLC.

Hemoptysis and cough, the most common and perhaps most disturbing symptoms, are easily controlled by radiotherapy in up to 80% of sufferers. Dyspnea caused by bronchial obstruction can be relieved in about half the patients, and dysphagia in 80% if due to lymph node compression. The syndrome of superior vena cava obstruction is improved in 60% of sufferers at least in relieving symptoms, although the distended neck veins and collaterals may continue to remain visible. Pain, due to bony metastases, is totally relieved in 50% and partially in a further 30% of sufferers. Numerous dose schedules for the relief of bone pain are available, including 30 Gy in ten fractions over 2 weeks, 20 Gy in five fractions over 5 days, or single fractions of 7.5 to 10 Gy to the symptomatic area. The administration of a single large fraction to a painful bone is particularly effective, and saves much traveling and hospital time, which would be necessary for longer courses of treatment. Recent multicenter studies have shown that a single fraction of 7.5 Gy is as effective as a longer course of irradiation for controlling bone pain.

Brain metastases tend to respond relatively poorly to radiotherapy. Initial treatment should be with oral dexamethasone 4 mg times a day for 48 h, which resolves the edema around the metastasis. If acceptable improvement occurs, then radiotherapy can consolidate this and the steroids may be withdrawn. However, if the steroid trial makes little difference to the neurological deficit, then radiotherapy is unlikely to have an additional effect (83). Spinal cord compression is relatively common in lung cancer, and accounts for 1% to 2% of all cases of this presentation. Pain or bony tenderness often precedes the syndrome and may help to localize the site of compression. Treatment must be prompt and preceded by a myelogram if there is any doubts as to the lower level of the lesion. Responses to radiotherapy are usually incomplete and disappointing.

Chemotherapy

The response rate of NSCLC to cytotoxic agents is much lower than for SCLC (Table 6). There have been hundreds of studies comparing different regimens, usually with no control group data, and often with poorly categorized patients as regards age, cell type, disease stage, and performance status. However, chemotherapy has been evaluated reasonably carefully in some circumstances (84).

Adjuvant Chemotherapy Prior to Resection

There have been several pilot studies of combinations of chemotherapy given to patients with inoperable NSCLC because of mediastinal nodal involvement, in whom response rates to chemotherapy have been up to 55%. Most of the chemotherapy regimens contain mitomycin C and cisplatin. These have been recently reviewed. Following two to four courses of chemotherapy, if there is a radiological response, patients have gone to thoracotomy and resection has been possible in up to 70% of cases. In some instances, there was no histological evidence of tumor at the time of resection (89). However, most of the resections were radical, i.e., involving complete

TABLE 6. *Objective average response to single agent chemotherapy in lung cancer*

Drug	Small cell[a]	Squamous[b]	Adeno[b]	Large[b]
Ifosfamide	63	27[c]	23[c]	36[c]
Vincristine	42	10	23	0
Epipodophyllotoxin	40	25	12	0
Cyclophosphamide	33	20	20	23
Methotrexate	30	25	30	12
Adriamycin	30	20	15	25
CCNU	15	30	20	17
Cis-platinum	35	20	12	13

[a]Hanson and Rorth (1980) (84)
[b]Souhami R (1984) (87) and Bakowski and Crouch (1983) (88)
[c]Constanzi (1982) (85); Harrison (1982) (86)

nodal dissection within the mediastinum. To date there is no good evidence that this approach prolongs survival. The patients chosen for combined modality treatment have been young, fit, and highly motivated. Nevertheless the median survival varies from 10 to 32 months with 3- and 4-year survival rates of 34% and 40%, respectively. This is considerably greater than one might expect with a nonsurgical approach, i.e., radical radiotherapy with or without chemotherapy. Long-term results of larger randomized controlled studies are awaited.

Chemotherapy in Advanced Non–Small Cell Lung Cancer

Despite many studies of different chemotherapy regimens in inoperable advanced disease, there are only a handful of controlled studies. These show no important clinical advantage of combination chemotherapy in patients with metastatic intra- and extrathoracic disease (90). A study by Cellarino et al. (91) randomized 128 patients to cyclophosphamide, Adriamycin, and cis-platinum, alternating with methotrexate, etoposide, and CCNU versus best supportive care. The response rate to chemotherapy was 21% and these were partial responses only. The median survivals were 34 weeks with chemotherapy and 21 weeks without, but the difference was not significant.

A Canadian study (92) compared two chemotherapy regimens to best supportive care, and showed a small but significant survival benefit for the treated groups despite responses of only 16% and 25% to the two chemotherapy regimens in the study. The median survivals were 33, 25, and 18 weeks—the latter for best supportive care. The dilemma is that within these patient groups, treatment undoubtedly benefits some patients as the 1-year survival rate was double (20%) for the chemotherapy-treated patients; however, the negative side is the exposure to potentially lethal toxicity for those doomed to do badly (93).

It is recommended that chemotherapy for advanced disease be withheld outside controlled clinical trials.

Chemotherapy for Localized Inoperable Disease

Another area of research is the possible role of chemotherapy in patients whose disease would usually be considered suitable for radical radiotherapy. Mitomycin C, ifosfamide, and cisplatin have been shown to be a very active regimen in good performance status patients with small volume NSCLC, producing a 45% response rate (94). A recent American study (95) compared cis platinum and vindesine followed by radiotherapy versus radiotherapy alone, and showed a 5-month advantage in median survival for the combined approach (13.8 vs. 9.7 months). The role of chemotherapy in addition to radiotherapy in localized disease is now being evaluated.

NEW DRUGS IN NON–SMALL CELL LUNG CANCER

The response rate of newer agents, as for the most established drugs, is lower for NSCLC than for SCLC (Table 7). There are some phase II studies of newer agents and Table 7 summarizes those trials that have recorded a response rate of about 30% or greater.

Camptothecin analogues showed considerable activity in early trials. A Japanese study had a response rate of 41%, but based on only 22 evaluable patients. Leukopenia, nausea, vomiting, and diarrhea occurred in about half the subjects (96).

Navelbine is a semi-synthetic vinca alkaloid with a long terminal half-life compared with the other vincas and a large volume of distribution, suggesting high tissue uptake, which is most striking in the lung. A 33% response rate was seen in 69 previously untreated patients and similar response was noted for squamous and adenocarcinomas (97). Of importance, the incidence of neuropathy (7%) was lower than with vincristine of vindesine. The dose-limiting toxicity was neutropenia. These early results are encouraging.

Zeniplatin is a water-soluble third-generation platinum analogue. In preclinical studies it has a superior therapeutic dose ratio to that of cisplatin. When given to 29 previously untreated patients with advanced NSCLC, six achieved a response.

At least three new antimetabolites have activity as single agents—10 EDAM (a mcthrotrcxatc analogue), trimetrexate (a lipophilic antifolate), and gemcitabine (an analogue of cytosine arabinoside). All have activity recorded of up to 25%, but less in most phase II studies.

Of three new alkalating agents fotemustine has moderate activity only, but probably not more than a response rate of 15% (98).

Studies on biological response modifiers are also disappointing. In a small trial of 12 evaluable patients, a 33% response rate was seen with a combination of interleukin-2 and tumor necrosis factor alpha (99,100).

TABLE 7. *Response rates for new single-agent drugs in NSCLC*

Drug	Dose and schedule	No. evaluated	Response (%)
Interleukin-2	1×10^6 cetus $MU/m^2/24$ h i.v. q 21	12	33
+			
Tumor necrosis factor	25–100 μg/m^2/d d 1–5 q 21		
Navelbine	30 mg/m^2 i.v. q 21 days	69	33
Zeniplatin	145 g/m^2 i.v. q 21 days	18	33
CPT-11	100 mg/m^2 i.v. q 7 days	22	41

From Talbot and Smith (54).

PARANEOPLASTIC SYNDROMES

All types of lung cancer are associated with paraneoplastic syndromes, causing morbidity and mortality if left untreated. These syndromes occur more frequently and with a broader spectrum in SCLC.

Hypercalcemia

This most commonly occurs in squamous cell carcinoma and is due either to bony metastases or to the production of parathormone from the primary tumor. Symptoms include anorexia, vomiting, polydipsia, polyuria, abdominal pain, constipation, weight loss, and bone pain. If the condition is left untreated, the patient becomes confused and can progress to coma and death. Initial therapy is with intravenous hydration with normal saline. Up to 6 L per day may be necessary, depending on the degree of dehydration and the cardiovascular status. A loop diuretic may be added to promote calcium excretion. It is essential to maintain hydration if diuretics are used. Prednisolone at 40 mg daily or hydrocortisone 100 mg four times a day are often added to further reduce serum calcium levels. Its action, although effective, is usually short lived. Once initial therapy has been given, assessment of the cause of hypercalcemia is made. If this is secondary to parathormone production, a reduction in tumor mass, either by resection, radiotherapy, or chemotherapy as appropriate, may be effective. If metastatic disease is the cause, radiotherapy can be given to a specific area, but often the metastases are widespread and systemic therapy may be necessary. Intravenous diphosphonates at 7.5 mg/kg per day may be given, with dose reduction if renal impairment is present. The recent development of oral etidronate means that treatment can be continued following cessation of i.v. therapy. The recommended dose is 20 mg/kg per day for a maximum of 30 days. This may also improve bone pain. The most common side effect is gastrointestinal disturbances, including diarrhea and nausea. Calcitonin has been used to treat hypercalcemia, either as a subcutaneous or intravenous infusion, but its effect is short lived. Mithromycin, a cytotoxic drug, rapidly reduces hypercalcemia when given as an infusion at 25 μg/kg. Its toxicity includes myelosuppression, limiting the frequency with which it can be used to approximately every 21 days.

The Syndrome of Inappropriate Antidiuretic Hormone Secretion (SIADH)

In 1938 Winkler and Cranshaw described a case of hyponatremia associated with carcinoma of the lung. The syndrome of inappropriate ADH was then fully described in two separate series of patients (101,102). This is the most frequently detected paraneoplastic syndrome in patients with SCLC. The cardinal features are a dilutional hyponatremia, urine osmolality greater than plasma osmolality, and a persisting urinary sodium excretion greater than 20 mmol/L with normal renal function. SIADH may also be induced by cyclophosphamide and vincristine, which are commonly used chemotherapeutic agents in SCLC, although this is rare (103). Patients with SIADH can be asymptomatic; however, most complain of weakness, nausea, anorexia, and confusion. Water deprivation was the treatment of choice, but demeclocycline at a dose of 300 to 600 mg per day makes fluid restriction unnecessary. Demeclocycline antagonizes the action of ADH by competing for renal tubular binding sites. Treatment of the primary tumor, either with radiotherapy or chemotherapy, will often correct the electrolyte balance by reducing tumor mass and the secretion of antidiuretic hormone.

Ectopic ACTH

Small cell lung cancer is the most frequent cause of ectopic adrenocorticotropic hormone (ACTH) secretion. The classic Cushing syndrome is rarely seen as the physical changes take time to appear, and SCLC overwhelms the patient rapidly. The usual abnormalities are proximal muscle weakness in association with hypokalemia, glucose intolerance, mild hypertension, hyperpigmentation, and hirsutism. Physiological or metabolic changes are seen in approximately 2% to 7% of SCLC sufferers (104). Although the syndrome is not common, abnormalities of cortisol metabolism are seen in up to 47% of patients presenting with SCLC. Treatment directed at the underlying tumor may effectively reduce ACTH production.

Hypertrophic Pulmonary Osteoarthropathy

This is most commonly seen with squamous cell carcinoma; its pathogenesis remains unexplained. Periostitis develops at the distal ends of the tibia, fibular, radius, and ulnar, and causes pain, heat, and swelling. In most cases clubbing is also present. Treatment to the primary tumor may cause resolution and other therapies such as vagotomy may occasionally help. Often the changes persist and control of symptoms requires nonsteroidal antiinflammatory drugs.

Lambert-Eaton Syndrome

This occurs almost exclusively in SCLC. The characteristic features are of a progressive proximal muscle weakness with wasting, dryness of the mouth, and difficulty in swallowing. The syndrome may precede the presentation of tumor by several months but the onset of symptoms can be rapid. Clinical examination shows weakness, although muscle power can increase after brief exercise. Reflexes may be absent at rest and transiently return following exercise. Electromyogram (EMG) analysis shows posttetanic potentiation. Symptoms can be improved with guanadine hydrochloride and the treatment of choice is 3/4 amidopyridine at 10 to 20 μg four to six times per day. Steroids may also improve muscle strength, but the major control of symptoms is by chemotherapy or radiotherapy to reduce the tumor bulk.

Other neuromyopathies occur with lung carcinoma, including peripheral neuropathy, subacute cerebellar degeneration, and amyotrophic lateral sclerosis. Myopathies such as polymyositis and dermatomyositis also occur. Brain stem syndromes and cerebellar degeneration occasionally respond to a reduction in primary tumor mass.

SYMPTOM CONTROL

The majority of patients with lung cancer die from the disease within a year of diagnosis. Maintenance of the quality of life with good symptom control is important. Supportive care is essential both within the hospital and in the community.

Dyspnea

Dyspnea is a subjective symptom. Anxiety may increase its severity. Dyspnea due to obstruction of a major airway can be treated by radiotherapy, and also sometimes by endobronchial laser therapy. Pleural effusions are common and should be drained if symptomatic. It is likely that the pleural effusion will recur following drainage, and therefore pleurodesis is advisable with instillation of 3g of tetracycline powder. Chemical pleurodesis can be painful and 10 ml of 1% lignocaine should be mixed with the pleurodesing agent. Pain and fever can occur for 24 h following the instillation but nonsteroidal anti-inflammatory drugs should be avoided as they may hinder pleurodesis. If the lung does not reexpand following aspiration of an effusion, then a chemical pleurodesis is not possible. A surgical pleurectomy can be considered but if at surgery the lung cannot expand because of pleurally based tumor, the pleural cavity can be permanently drained by inserting a shunt to the peritoneal cavity with excellent control of symptoms, and surprisingly little prospect of metastatic disease affecting the abdominal cavity.

Cough

This is common and distressing. Suppression can be best achieved with codeine linctus or linctus methadone. Bubivocaine 0.25% via a nebulizer can be helpful to suppress cough arising anywhere in the large airways (105). Oral morphine (as linctus methadone) becomes valuable if the cough persists, particularly at night. Steroids can sometimes reduce cough, particularly if secondary to pleural, pericardial, or diaphragmatic inflammation secondary to the carcinoma.

Hemoptysis

Major hemoptysis occurs rarely but can be life threatening. Blood-stained sputum, however, is much more common. Treatment with radiotherapy to the primary tumor is usually effective. Laser therapy via a bronchoscope is also effective, but laser is only of value if there is major airway obstruction. However, as hemoptysis is common with central tumors, the burning off of tumor tissue will resolve the hemoptysis in most cases.

Nausea and Vomiting

Usually these symptoms are related to therapy, either cytotoxic agents or opiates. During chemotherapy, antiemetics should be given both prior to and following chemotherapy. Metaclopramide may be given orally, as an injection or in high dose intravenously. Haloperidol is also effective. Odansetron is the first of a new class of 5-HT receptor antagonists and is a most effective antiemetic. For most regimens 8 mg i.v. given with chemotherapy followed by 8 mg po b.d. for 3 days is effective. The drug is expensive and one policy is to use this agent if metoclopramide fails. Nausea induced by opiates should always be anticipated, and each opiate dose should be accompanied by an antiemetic such as prochlorperazine, haloperidol, or cyclizine. Other causes of vomiting include constipation, raised intracranial pressure, and anxiety.

Pain

Pain is one of the major symptoms in patients with lung cancer. There are many therapeutic strategies available to treat pain, and it is important to emphasize to patients and their relatives that pain can be controlled. The choice of treatment depends on the cause of the pain. Whatever method is used analgesics should be given on a regular basis in titrated doses so that pain is well controlled. Regular reassessment is essential. In addition to analgesics, radiotherapy is excellent for localized bone pain. Nerve block for root and in particular brachial plexus pain can be effective. Where possible, analgesics should be given orally. If pain control is inadequate, the dosage should be increased or a more potent analgesic chosen. If the drugs cannot be given orally, then subcutaneous infusions are a useful alternative. With acute severe pain, morphine elixir given every 4 h controls symptoms rapidly. Once this has been achieved, then the patient can be converted to a sustained release morphine preparation given twice daily. The major side effect of opiates are nausea, vomiting, and constipation. Prophylactic laxatives must be given to all patients receiving opiates. Prophylactic antiemetics are also necessary but their requirement tends to fall after about 10 days of opiate therapy. Corticosteroids are often used as coanalgesics, and nonsteroidal anti-inflammatory drugs should be given regularly with opiates as they enhance pain control, particularly if pain is from the liver or bones.

Superior Vena Cava Obstruction

Dexamethasone can improve symptoms occasionally. However, radiotherapy is the treatment of choice in NSCLC or relapsed SCLC. Ten percent of new cases of SCLC present with superior vena caval obstruction, and in an undiagnosed patient the diagnosis of the type of underlying cancer must be made by bronchoscopy, node aspiration (if a palpable node is present), or mediastinoscopy. Chemotherapy is the correct treatment of superior vena cava obstruction if it is due to SCLC. If there is a further relapse radiotherapy may be helpful, or the insertion of a stent into the superior vena cava, under radiological control, can be most successful, giving instant symptomatic relief.

REFERENCES

1. Spiro SG. Lung tumours. In: Brewis RAL, Gibson GJ, Geddes DM, eds. *Textbook of respiratory medicine*. Sussex: Bailliere Tindall 1990;832–879.
2. Spiro SG. Lung cancer—presentation and treatment. *Med Int* 1991;91:3798–3805.
3. Coggon D, Acheson ED. Trends in lung cancer mortality. *Thorax* 1983;38:721–723.
4. Noble RL, Beer CT, Cutts JH. Further biological activities of vincaleukoblastine—an alkaloid isolated from vincarosea. *Bio Chem Pharmacol* 1958;1:347–348.
5. Johnson IS. Plant alkaloids. In: Holland JF, Frei E III, eds. *Cancer medicine;* 2nd ed. Philadelphia: Lea & Febiger, 1982;910–919.
6. Creasey WA. Plant alkaloids. In: Becker FF, ed. *Cancer, vol 5: A comprehensive treatise*. New York: Plenum Press, 1977;379–425.
7. Slevin ML, Clark PI, Osborne RJ, et al. A randomised trial to evaluate the effect of schedule in the activity of etoposide in small cell lung cancer. *Proc Am Soc Clin Oncol* 1986;5:175.
8. Tritten TR, Murphee SA, Sartorelli AC. Adriamycin: a proposal on the specificity of drug action. *Biochem Biophys Res Commun* 1978;84:802–808.
9. Editorial. Daunorubicin and the heart. *Br Med J* 1974;4:431–432.

10. Freidman MA, Bordech MJ, Billingham ME, Rider AK. Doxorubicin cardiotoxicity. Serial endomyocardial biopsies and systolic time intervals. *JAMA* 1978;240:1603–1606.
11. Rosenberg B, VanCamp L, Trasko JE, Manseur VH. Platinum compounds: a new class of potent anti-tumour agents. *Nature* 1969;222:385–386.
12. Bunn PA, Ihde DC. Small cell brochogenic carcinoma: a review of therapeutic results. In: Livingston RB, ed. *Lung cancer,* vol 1, The Hague, Boston, London: Martinus Nijhoff, 1981;169–208.
13. Souhami RL, Law K. Longevity in small cell lung cancer. *Br J Cancer* 1990;61:584–589.
14. Spiro SG, Souhami RL, Geddes DM, Ash CM, Quinn H, Harper P, Tobias JS, Partridge M, Eraut D. Duration of chemotherapy in small cell lung cancer: a Cancer Research Campaign trial. *Br J Cancer* 1989;59:578–583.
15. Medical Research Council Lung Cancer Working Party. Controlled trial of twelve versus six courses of chemotherapy in the treatment of small cell lung cancer. *Br J Cancer* 1989;59:584–590.
16. Lebeau B, Chastang C, Allard P, Migueres J, Boita F, Fichet D, and the Petites Cellules Group. Six versus twelve cycles for complete responders to chemotherapy in SCLC: definitive months of a randomised clinical trial. *Eur Resp J* 1992;5:286–290.
17. Splinter TAW. EORTC 08825: induction vs induction plus maintenance chemotherapy (CT) in small cell lung cancer (SCLC). Definitive evaluation. (Abstract). *Lung Cancer* 1988;4:A100.
18. Feld R, Evans WK, DeBoer G, Quirt IC, Shepherd FA, Yeoh JL, Pringle JF, Payne DG, Herman JG, Chamberlain D. Combined modality induction therapy without maintenance chemotherapy for small cell carcinoma of the lung. *J Clin Oncol* 1984;2:294–301.
19. Maurer LH, Tulloch M, Weiss RB, Bloom J, Leone L, Glidewell O, Pajak TF. A randomised combined modality trial in small cell carcinoma of the lung. Comparison of combination chemotherapy–radiation therapy versus cyclophosphamide–radiation therapy. Effects of maintenance chemotherapy and prophylactic whole brain irradiation. *Cancer* 1980;45:30–39.
20. Cullen M, Morgan D, Gregory W, Robinson M, Cox D, McGivern D, Ward M, Richards M, Stableforth D, Macfarlane J et al., and the Midlands Small Cell Lung Cancer Group. Maintenance chemotherapy for anaplastic small cell carcinoma of the bronchus: a randomised controlled trial. *Cancer Chemother Pharmacol* 1986;17:157–160.
21. Osterlind K, Hansen M, Hirsch FR, Dombernowsky P, Sorenson S, Pedersen AG, Hansen HH. Combination chemotherapy of limited-stage small cell lung cancer. A controlled trial on 221 patients comparing two alternating regimens. *Ann Oncol* 1991;2:41–46.
22. Jett JR, Everson L, Therneau TM, Krook JE, Dalton RJ, Marschke RF Jr, Veeder MH, Brunk SF, Mailliard JA, Twito DI. Treatment of limited stage small cell lung cancer with cyclophosphamide, dixirubicin and vincristine with or without etoposide: a randomised trial of the North Central Cancer Treatment Group. *J Clin Oncol* 1990;8:33–38.
23. Ettinger DS, Finkelstein DM, Abeloff MD, Ruckdeschel JC, Aisner SC, Eggleston JC. A randomised comparison of standard vs alternating chemotherapy and maintenance versus no maintenance therapy for extensive stage small cell lung cancer: a phase III study of the Eastern Co-operative Oncology Group. *J Clin Oncol* 1990;8:230–240.
24. Goodman GE, Crowley JJ, Blasko JC, Livingston RB, Beck TM, Demattia MD, Budowski RM. Treatment of limited small cell lung cancer with etoposide and cisplatin alternating with vincristine, doxorubicin and cyclophosphamide versus concurrent etoposide, vincristine, doxorubicin and cyclophosphamide and chest radiotherapy. A Southern Oncology Group study. *J Clin Oncol* 1990;8:39–47.
25. Souhami RL, Finn GP, Gregory WP, Birkhead B, Buckman RA, Harper PG, Edwards D, Goldstone AH, Spiro SG, Geddes DM. High dose cyclophosphamide in small cell lung cancer. *J Clin Oncol* 1985;3:958–963.
26. Souhami RL, Harper PG, Linch D, Trask C, Goldstone AM, Tobias J, Spiro SG, Geddes DM, Guimaraes M, Fearon F, Smyth JF. High dose cyclophosphamide with autologous bone marrow transplantation as initial treatment for small cell carcinoma of the bronchus. *Cancer Chemother Pharmacol* 1982;8:31–34.

27. Souhami RL, Harper PG, Linch D, Trask C, Goldstone AH, Tobias JS, Spiro SG, Geddes DM, Richards JDM. High dose cyclophosphamide with autologous bone marrow transplantation for small cell carcinoma of the bronchus. *Cancer Chemother Pharmacol* 1983;10:205–207.
28. Wolff SN, Johnson DH, Hande KR. High dose etoposide as single agent chemotherapy for small cell carcinoma of the lung. *Cancer Treat Rep* 1983;67:957–958.
29. Johnson DH, Wolff SN, Hainsworth JD, Porter LL, Grosh WW, Hande KR, Greco FA. Extensive stage small cell bronchogenic carcinoma: intensive induction with high dose cyclophosphamide plus high dose etoposide. *J Clin Oncol* 1985;3:170–175.
30. Johnson DH, Deleo MS, Hande KR, Wolff SN, Hainsworth JD, Greco FA. High dose induction chemotherapy with cyclophosphamide, etoposide and cisplatin for extensive stage small cell lung cancer. *J Clin Oncol* 1987;5:703–709.
31. Hardman DD, Green JA, Errington RD, Myint S, Warenius HM. Treatment of small cell lung cancer with induction chemotherapy followed by late intensification. *Med Oncol Tumour Pharmacol* 1989;6:227–232.
32. Cohen MH, Ihde DC, Bunn PA, Fossieck BE, Mathews MJ, Shackney SE, Johnson-Easty A, Makuch R, Minna JD. Cyclic alternating combination chemotherapy for small cell bronchogenic carcinoma. *Cancer Treat Rep* 1979;63:163–170.
33. Miles DW, Earl HM, Souhami RL, Harper PG, Rudd R, Ash CM, James L, Trask CW, Tobias JS, Spiro SG. Intensive weekly chemotherapy for good prognosis patients with small cell lung cancer. *J Clin Oncol* 1991;9:280–285.
34. Souhami RL, Bradbury J, Geddes DM, Spiro SG, Harper P, Tobias JS. Prognostic significance of laboratory parameters measured at diagnosis in small cell carcinoma of the lung. *Cancer Res* 1985;45:2872–7882.
35. Osterlind K, Hansen HH, Hansen M, Dombernowsky P, Anderson PK. Long term disease free survival in small cell carcinoma of the lung. A study of clinical determinants. *J Clin Oncol* 1986;4:1307–1313.
36. Albain KS, Crowley JJ, Leblanc M, Livingstone RB. Determinants of improved outcome in small cell lung cancer. An analysis of 2,580 patients. Southwest Oncology Group Database. *J Clin Oncol* 1990;8:1563–1574.
37. Einhorn LH, Bond WH, Hornback N, Beng-Tek Joe BT. Long term results in combined modality treatment of small cell carcinoma of the lung. *Semin Oncol* 1978;5:307–313.
38. Smith IE, Sappino AP, Bondy PK, Gilby ED. Long-term survival five years or more after combination chemotherapy and radiotherapy for small cell lung carcinoma. *Eur J Cancer Clin Oncol* 1981;17:1249–1253.
39. Livingston RB, Trauth CJ, Greenstreet RL. Small cell carcinoma: clinical manifestations and behaviour with treatment. In: Greco FA, Oldham RK, Bunn PA, eds. *Small Cell Lung Cancer.* New York: Grune & Stratton, 1981;285.
40. Ginsberg SJ, Comis RL, Gottlieb AJ, King GB, Goldberg J, Zamkoff K, Elbadawi A, Meyer JA. Long-term survivorship in small cell anaplastic lung carcinoma. *Cancer Treat Rep* 1979;63:1347–1349.
41. Maurer LH and Pajak TF. Prognostic factors in small cell carcinoma of the lung. A cancer and leukaemia Group B study. *Cancer Treat Rep* 1981;65:767–774.
42. Hansen M, Hansen HH, Dombernowsky P. Long-term survival in small cell carcinoma of the lung. *J Am Med Assoc* 1980;244:247–250.
43. Minna JD, Bunn PA Jr, Carney DN, et al. Experience of the National Cancer Institute (USA) in the treatment and biology of small cell lung cancer. *Bull Cancer* (Paris) 1982;69–83.
44. Natale RB, Wittes RE. Combination cis-platinum and etoposide in small cell lung cancer. *Cancer Treat Rep* 1982;9(suppl):91.
45. Aisner J, Whitacre M, Van Echo DA, Wesley M, Wiernik PH. Doxorubicin, cyclophosphamide and VP16-213 (ACE) in the treatment of small cell lung cancer. *Cancer Chemother Pharmacol* 1982;7:187–193.
46. Morstyn G, Ihde DC, Lichter AS, Bunn PA, Carney DN, Glatstein E, Minna JD. Small cell lung cancer 1973–1983: early prognosis and recent obstacles. *Int J Radiat Oncol Biol Phys* 1984;4:515–539.
47. Osterlind K, Hansen M and Dombernowsky P. Mortality and morbidity in long term

surviving patients treated with chemotherapy with or without irradiation for small cell lung cancer. *J Clin Oncol* 1986;4:1044–1052.

48. Slevin ML, Clark PI, Joel SP. A randomised trial to evaluate the effect of schedule on the activity of Etoposide in small cell lung cancer. *J Clin Oncol* 1989;7:1333–1340.

49. Cavalli F, Sonntag RW, Junji F. VP-16-213 monotherapy for remission induction of small cell lung cancer. A randomised trial using three dosage schedules. *Cancer Treatment Reports* 1979;62:473–475.

50. Johnson DH, Greco FA, Strupp J, Hande KR, Hainsworth JD. Prolonged administration of oral etoposide in patients with relapsed or refractory small cell lung cancer: a Phase II trial. *J Clin Oncol* 1990;8:1613–1617.

51. Bronchud MH, Scarffe JH, Thatcher N. Phase I/II study of recombinate granulocyte colony stimulation factor in patients receiving intensive chemotherapy for small cell lung cancer. *Brit J Cancer* 1987;56:809–813.

52. Crawford J, Ozer H, Stroller R, et al. Reduction by granulocyte colony stimulation factor of fever and neutropenia induced by chemotherapy in small cell lung cancer. *New Eng J Med* 1991;325:164–170.

53. Drings P, Fischer JR. Biology and clinical use of GM-CSF in lung cancer. *Lung* 1990;168(suppl):1059–1068.

54. Talbot DC, Smith IE. New drugs in lung cancer. *Thorax* 1992;47:188–194.

55. Ohono R, Okada K, Masoka T, et al. An early phase II study of CPT 11: a new derivative of camptothecin in the treatment of leukaemia and lymphoma. *J Clin Oncol* 1990;8:1907–1912.

56. Negoro S, Fukuoka M, Niitani H, et al. Phase II study of CPT 11; new camptothecin derivative in small cell lung cancer. *Proc Am Soc Clin Oncol* 1991;10:241.

57. Eckhardt S, Kolaria K, Vukas D, et al. Phase II study of 4 epi-doxorubicin in patients with untreated small cell lung cancer. South-eastern European Oncology Group. *Med Oncol Tumour Pharmacother* 1990;7:19–23.

58. Blackstein M, Eisenhauer EA, Wierzbick R, Yoshida S. Epirubicin in extensive small cell lung cancer. A phase II study in previously untreated patients: a National Cancer Institute of Canada Clinical Trials Group Study. *J Clin Oncol* 1990;8:385–389.

59. Medical Research Council Lung Cancer Working Party. Radiotherapy alone or with chemotherapy in the treatment of small cell carcinoma of the lung. *Brit J Cancer* 1979;40:1–10.

60. Souhami RL, Geddes DM, Spiro SG, et al. A controlled trial of radiotherapy in small cell lung cancer treated by combination chemotherapy. *Brit Med J* 1984;288:1643–1646.

61. Johnson D. *Personal communication.* Eastern Cooperative Oncology Group, 1988.

62. Turrisi AT, Glover DJ, Mason BA. A preliminary report: Concurrent twice daily radiotherapy plus platinum-etoposide chemotherapy for limited small cell lung cancer. *Int J Radiol Oncol Biol Phys* 1988;15:183–187.

63. Johnson B, Grayson J, Woods E. Limited stage small cell lung cancer treated with concurrent etoposide/cisplatin and twice daily chest irradiation. *Sixth International Conference on the Adjuvant Therapy of Cancer,* Tucson, Arizona 1990.

64. Turrisi A, Wagner H, Glover D, Mason B, Oken M, Baromi P. Limited small cell lung cancer: Concurrent bid thoracic radiotherapy with platinum-etoposide an ECOG study. *Proc Am Soc Clin Oncol* 1990; 9:247.

65. Looney WB, Hopkins HA. Rationale for different chemotherapeutic and radiation therapy strategies in cancer management. *Cancer* 1991;67:1471–1483.

66. Karnofsky D, Burchenal JK. Clinical evaluation of chemotherapeutic agents in cancer. In: McLeod CM, ed. *Evaluation of Chemotherapeutic Agents.* New York: Columbia University Press, 1949;199–205.

67. Coates A, Abraham S, Kaye SB, Sowerbutts T, Frewin C, Fox RM, Tattersall MH. European organisation for research on treatment of cancer. Proceedings of the EORTC Quality of Life Workshop (May 1981, November 1981, June 1982). *Eur J Cancer and Clin Oncol* 1983;19:203–208.

68. Geddes DM, Dones L, Hill E, Law K, Harper PG, Spiro SG, Tobias JS, Souhami RL. Quality of life during chemotherapy for small cell lung cancer: assessment and use of a daily diary card in a randomised trial. *Euro J Cancer* 1990;26:484–492.

69. Geddes DM. Quality of life. Small cell lung cancer. *Clinics in Oncology* 1985;4:1.

70. Naruke T, Goya T, Tsuchiya R, Suemasu K. The importance of surgery to non-small cell carcinoma of lung with mediastinal lymph node metastases. *Ann Thoracic Surg* 1988;46:609–610.
71. Smart J, Hilton G. Radiotherapy of cancer of the lung: results in a selected group of cases. *Lancet* 1956;i:880–881.
72. Deeley TJ. The treatment of carcinoma of the bronchus by megavoltage x-rays. *Br J Radiol* 1967;40:801–822.
73. Van Houtte P, Rochmans P, Smets P, Goffin JC, Lustman-Marechal J, Vanderhaeft P, Henry J. Postoperative radiation therapy in lung cancer: a controlled trial after resection of curative disease. *Int J Radiat Oncol Biol Phys* 1980;6:983–986.
74. The Lung Cancer Study Group. Effects of postoperative mediastinal radiation on completely resected Stage II and Stage III epidermoid cancer of the lung. *N Eng J Med* 1986;315:1377–1381.
75. Deeley TM, Singh SP. Treatment of inoperable carcinoma of the bronchus by megavoltage x-rays. *Thorax* 1967;22:562–565.
76. Caldwell WL, Bagshawe MA. Indications for and results of irradiation of carcinoma of the lung. *Cancer* 1968;22:999–1004.
77. Perez-Tamayow R, Soberon M. The place of radiotherapy in the treatment of bronchogenic carcinoma. *Mol Med* 1969;66:876–880.
78. Guttman RJ. Radical supervoltage therapy in inoperable carcinoma of the lung. In: Deelev RJ, ed. *Modern Radiotherapy for Carcinoma of the Bronchus*. London: Butterworths. 1971:181.
79. Lee RE. Radiotherapy of bronchogenic carcinoma. *Semin Oncol* 1974;3:245.
80. Coy P, Kennelly GM. The role of curative radiotherapy in the treatment of lung cancer. *Cancer* 1980;45:698–702.
81. Edinburgh Lung Cancer Group. Patients presenting with lung cancer in South East Scotland. *Thorax* 1987;42:853–857.
82. Roswit B, Patno ME, Rapp R. The survival of patients with inoperable lung cancer: A large scale randomised study of radiation therapy versus placebo. *Radiology* 1968;90:688–697.
83. Felletti R, Souhami RL, Spiro SG, et al. Social consequences of brain or liver relapse in small cell carcinoma of the bronchus. *Radiother Oncol* 1985;4:335–339.
84. Hansen RR, Rorth M. Lung Cancer. In: Pinedo HM, ed. *The EORTC Cancer and Chemotherapy Annual 2*. Amsterdam and Oxford: Excerpta Medica, 1980;267–283.
85. Constanzi JJ, Morgan LR, Hokanson J. Ifosfamide in the treatment of extensive non-oat cell carcinoma of the lung. *Seminars in Oncology* 1982;9(4)(suppl 1):61–65.
86. Harrison EF, Hawke JE, Hunter HL. Single-dose ifosfamide: efficacy studies in non-small cell lung cancer. *Seminars in Oncology* 1982;9(4)(suppl 1):56–60.
87. Souhami RL. The management of advanced non small cell carcinoma of the bronchus. In: Smyth JF, ed. *The management of lung cancer*. London: Edward Arnold, 132–149.
88. Bakowski MT, Crouch JC. Chemotherapy of non-small cell lung cancer: a reappraisal and a look to the future. *Cancer Treat Rep* 1983;10:159–172.
89. Faber LP, Bonomi PD. *Seminars in surgical oncology* 1990;6:225–262.
90. Gralla RJ, Kris MG. Chemotherapy in non small cell lung cancer: results of recent trials. *Semin Oncol* 1988;15(suppl 4):2–5.
91. Cellerino R, Tummarella D, Guidi F, Isodori P, Raspujl M, Biscontini B, Fatali G. A randomised trial of alternating chemotherapy versus best supportive care in advanced non small cell lung cancer. *J Clin Oncol* 1991;9:1453–1461.
92. Rapp E, Pater JL, Willan A, et al. Chemotherapy can prolong survival in patients with advanced non-small cell lung cancer. Report of a Canadian multicenter randomised trial. *J Clin Oncol* 1988;6:633–641.
93. O'Connell JP, Kris MG, Gralla RJ, et al. J Clin Oncol 1986;4:1604–14.
94. Cullen MH, Jashi R, Chetiyawardana AD, Woodroffe CM. Mitomycin, ifosfamide and cisplatin in non small cell lung cancer: good enough to compare. *Br J Cancer* 1988;58:359–361.
95. Dillman RO, Seargren SL, Propert KJ, et al. A randomised trial of induction chemotherapy plus high dose radiation versus radiation alone in stage III non small cell lung cancer. *N Engl J Med* 1990;323:940–945.

96. Fukuoka M, Negoro S, Niitani H, Taguchi T. A phase II study of a new camptothecin derivative, CPT-11 in previously untreated non small cell lung cancer (abstract). *Pro Am Soc Clin Oncol* 1990;9:226.
97. Depierre A, Lemaine E, Daubouis G, Garnier G, Jacoulet P, Dalphin JC. Efficacy of navelbine in non small cell lung cancer. *Semin Oncol* 1989;16:26–29.
98. Monnier A, Pugol JL, Cerrina ML, et al. Fotemustine in non small cell lung cancer: phase II study in 32 patients with poor prognostic factors. *Proc Am Soc Clin Oncol* 1991;10:248.
99. Krigel R, Lynch E, Kucuk O, et al. Interleukin 2 therapies prolong survival in metastatic non small cell lung cancer. *Proc Am Soc Clin Oncol* 1991;10:246.
100. Yang SC, Owen-Schaub L, Mendiguren-Rodrigue A, Grimm EA, Hong WK, Roth JA. Combination immunotherapy for non small cell lung cancer. Results with interleukin-2 and tumour necrosis factor alpha. *J Thoracic Cardiovascular Surg* 1990;99:8–12.
101. Schwartz WB, Bennett W, Curelop S, Bartter FC. A syndrome of renal sodium loss and hyponatraemia probably resulting from inappropriate secretion of antidiuretic hormone. *Am J Med* 1957;98:129–134.
102. Amatrude TT, Merlow PJ, Gallagher JC, Sawyer WH. Carcinoma of the lung with inappropriate antidiuresis demonstration of anti-diuretic hormone like activity in tumour extract. *New Engl J Med* 1963;269:544–549.
103. North WG, Maurer LH, O'Donnell JF. The neurophysins in small cell lung cancer. In: Greco FA, ed. *Biology and management of lung cancer.* Boston: Martinus Nighoff, 143–164.
104. Bondy PK, Gilby ED. Endocrine function in small cell undifferentiated carcinoma of the lung. *Cancer* 1982;50:2147–2153.
105. Heyse-Moore L. *Respiratory symptoms in the management of terminal disease, 2nd ed.* London: Edward Arnold, 1984;113–119.

Drugs and the Lung,
edited by C.P. Page and W.J. Metzger.
Raven Press, Ltd., New York © 1994

9

Antibiotics and the Lung

Robert Wilson and Kenneth W. T. Tsang

Host Defence Unit, Department of Thoracic Medicine, Royal Brompton National Heart and Lung Institute, London SW3 6LR, United Kingdom

The number of different microorganisms that infect the lung and bacterial antibiotic resistance have both increased, which means that familiar antibiotics may no longer always be effective. Some new infections have been recognized, and bacteria that were once considered of low virulence, viruses, and fungi now cause severe infections in immunocompromised patients. New antibiotics have been developed, but because of their rapid generation time and thus greater opportunity to evolve, bacteria will continue to present difficult clinical challenges. In this chapter we will deal generally with antibiotics used to treat lung infections, but only cover in detail management of bacterial infections of the bronchial tree and community acquired pneumonia in immunocompetent patients. We will not consider treatment of nosocomial infections or antituberculous chemotherapy.

Antibiotics affect both host and microorganism, and can have both beneficial and adverse effects. To choose an antibiotic, one should know the infecting organism, or, failing this, the organisms that are commonly implicated in a particular clinical presentation. It is also critical to know the distribution of antibiotic-resistant strains likely to be encountered. Successful outcome of treatment will depend upon the type of infection, the virulence and antibiotic sensitivity of the pathogen, the status of the host defenses, the presence or absence of preexisting disease of the lung or other part of the body, and the choice of antibiotic therapy (1,2).

PATHOGENESIS

The function of the lung is gas exchange and we therefore inhale potential infective agents from our environment continually during life. However, because of efficient multilayered defense mechanisms (Table 1) the healthy

TABLE 1. *The multilayered defense mechanisms of the respiratory tract against infection*

Mechanical:	upper respiratory tract filtration, mucociliary clearance, cough, surfactant, epithelial barrier
Local:	bronchus associated lymphoid tissue, secretory IgA, lysozyme, transferrin, antiproteinases, alveolar macrophages
Systemic:	neutrophil polymorphonuclear leukocytes, complement, immunoglobulins

lung is sterile from the first bronchial division. If the "first-line" defenses such as mucociliary clearance and the alveolar macrophage are overcome, systemic defenses can be mobilized, such as influx of neutrophils from the circulation.

Bronchial infections usually occur in the context of weakened host defenses, and are caused by relatively avirulent bacteria that often form part of the normal upper respiratory tract commensal flora: nontypeable *Haemophilus influenzae, Streptococcus pneumoniae,* and *Moraxella catarrhalis.* Deficiencies of the host defenses may be congenital, e.g., cystic fibrosis or primary ciliary dyskinesia, or acquired, e.g., viral infection or cigarette smoking. When the host defenses are impaired the clearance of inhaled bacteria, often from the commensal flora in the nasopharynx, is delayed. The bacteria can then utilize numerous mechanisms (Table 2) to avoid those defenses that remain and multiply and spread contiguously (3) within the airways. It is tempting to speculate that the reason that a few species are responsible for most bronchial infections is because they possess these properties, while other species that do not infect the lung do not. Some bacterial factors damage the airway mucosa (4), while others further impair the host defenses (5). Most of the bacteria are intraluminally associated with the secretions, although some may adhere to the epithelial surface, particularly in areas of epithelial damage (4). If the host response to the infection is successful, or if effective antibiotic treatment is given, then bacteria are eliminated and the acute infection resolves. However, if bacterial colonization of the lower respiratory tract persists, which will be influenced by both host and bacterial determinants, then the infection can become chronic. This leads to a host inflammatory response that can be damaging (6). Large numbers of neutrophils traffic into the bronchial tree (7) and may cause damage

TABLE 2. *Bacterial strategies to impair clearance from the airways*

Impair ciliary function
Stimulate mucus production
Affect ion transport across epithelium
Break down local immunoglobulin
Alter phagocyte function
Alter lymphocyte function
Damage epithelium
Adhere to damaged epithelium and collagen

by spilling proteinase enzymes and reactive oxygen radicals (8). This damage further disables the host defenses, and thus facilitates further bacterial colonization. A self-perpetuating vicious circle (Fig. 1) of host- and bacterial-derived lung damage can insidiously occur (6).

Conversely, although pneumonia can also occur in patients with weakened host defenses, the bacteria involved are usually more virulent and may infect individuals with intact host defenses. They reach the alveoli by aspiration from the pharynx, or inhalation from the environment via fomites or droplet spread, or by contiguous spread through the bronchial tree. Once the bacteria have reached the alveoli the development of pneumonia will depend upon the pathogenic potential of the strain involved, together with host factors including lack of recent exposure to the particular serotype involved. For example, the pneumococcal capsule protects the bacterium against most of the acute-phase hose defenses. Components of the cell wall (9) and bacterial toxins (10) generate a florid inflammatory response. The bacteria are invasive and the infection may spread in the bloodstream to cause disease at sites distant from the lung. If the disease is uncontrolled rapid death may ensue. The bacteriology of pneumonia is very different depending on whether the infection is community or hospital acquired (Table 3).

The antibiotic treatment of chronic bronchial infections, for example, bronchiectasis and cystic fibrosis, may be complicated by barriers to penetration of antibiotic to the site of infection, such as scarring of the airway and plentiful mucus that may harbor millions of bacteria. These barriers are

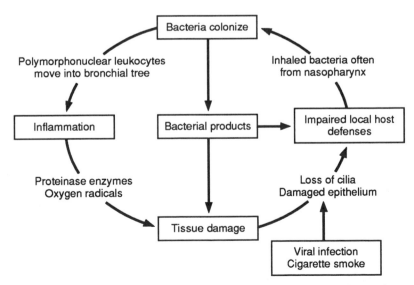

FIG. 1. A self-perpetuating vicious circle of host- and bacterial-mediated lung damage in chronic bronchial sepsis.

TABLE 3. *Bacteria causing community-acquired and hospital-acquired pneumonia*

Community-acquired
  Common
    Streptococcus pneumoniae
    Mycoplasma pneumoniae
    Chlamydia pneumoniae (TWAR)
    Haemophilus influenzae
    Legionella pneumophila
  Uncommon
    Klebsiella pneumoniae
    Staphylococcus aureus
    Moraxella catarrhalis
    Chlamydia psittaci
    Coxiella burnetti
    Gram-negative bacteria
Hospital-acquired
  Pseudomonas aeruginosa
  Staphylococcus aureus
  Klebsiella sp.
  Enterobacter sp.
  Escherichia coli
  Serratia marcescens
  Proteus sp.
  Acinetobacter sp.
  Citrobacter sp.

not present in pneumonia, and because the patient has often been previously well the lung's host defenses may be comparatively intact.

ANTIBIOTIC CLASSES

Penicillins

Gram-positive bacteria, such as streptococci and staphylococci, have only capsular material and peptidoglycan external to their cytoplasmic membrane. These components afford little shielding and agents with targets on the outer surface of the cytoplasmic membrane, e.g., beta-lactams, have relatively unhindered target access. Antibiotics with cytoplasmic or ribosomal targets, however, must cross the cytoplasmic membrane, usually by active transport. Gram-negative bacteria have an outer lipopolysaccharide layer external to the peptidoglycan layer and cytoplasmic membrane. Being hydrophilic, most antibiotics cross this outer wall by passive diffusion through pores created by porin proteins. Uptake varies with the drug's charge, size, and hydrophobicity, and also with the number of pores. Once across the outer layer the antibiotics have access to the cytoplasmic membrane, which must be crossed by those with ribosomal and cytoplasmic targets.

All beta-lactam antibiotics (penicillins, cephalosporins, carbapenems, and monobactams) interfere with the biosynthesis of the peptidoglycan structure of the cell wall of actively dividing bacteria, which leads to lysis. They bind to transpeptidase and carboxypeptidase enzymes called penicillin binding proteins (PBPs), located beneath the cell wall outside the cytoplasmic membrane, and interfere with their function. Beta-lactams also activate the autolysis system of bacteria, which disrupts the structural integrity of the cell wall (11,12). Penicillins generally have a short half-life. They are divided into groups depending on their structure and pharmacological properties (Table 4), and because of their broad spectrum of activity are commonly used to treat pneumonia and bronchial infections. Although most of the penicillins are excreted in the urine in an active form, the ureidopenicillins have a dual mode of excretion—through the biliary tree (20–30%) and the urinary tract. This means that in patients with renal failure the serum half-life is not increased proportionally.

Bacterial resistance to penicillins and other beta-lactam antibiotics arises either due to release of enzymes that break down the antibiotic, or due to changes in the PBPs, or due to failure of the antibiotic to penetrate through the outer wall porin channels. The most common group of beta-lactamases produced by clinical isolates are the plasmid-mediated TEM enzymes that exist in many Enterobacteriaceae, *H. influenzae,* and *Neisseria* species. Development of new beta-lactam antimicrobial agents during the past decades has resulted in a number of drugs with increased, albeit not total, resistance to beta-lactamases. Another pharmacological approach has been the development of beta-lactamase inhibitors that can be used in combination with a beta-lactam drug to overcome the beta-lactamase–mediated resistance (13).

Clavulanic acid is currently combined with amoxycillin as Augmentin and ticarcillin as Timentin. Although it has a low level of antibacterial action itself, it inhibits beta-lactamases of numerous pathogenic gram-positive and gram-negative bacteria by forming a stable inactive complex, but not the chromosomally mediated enzymes produced by some Enterobacteriaceae and *Pseudomonas aeruginosa* (13). Sulbactam is another beta-lactamase inhibitor used clinically that resembles clavulanic acid.

Allergic reactions to penicillin and its synthetic analogues are quite common (3–5% of general population) but true immunoglobulin E (IgE)-dependent anaphylaxis is rare. It has an incidence of about 0.05% and a mortality of 0.0002% (14,15). Most anaphylactic responses follow the drug being given parenterally, and there is no association with atopy. As many as 85% of patients who are allergic to penicillin can tolerate the drug when given it again so sensitization may only be temporary. Confirmation of IgE-related sensitization may be obtained by standard skin prick testing with a derivative of a penicilloyl determinant. Anaphylactic reactions almost never occur except in patients who give a positive response (14–16). Almost all beta-lactam antibiotics show some cross-sensitization, although it happens little

TABLE 4. *The penicillins*

Category	Examples	Comment
Natural penicillins	Benzyl penicillin (parenteral only as broken down by gastric acid) Penicillin V (oral)	Penicillinase sensitive
Penicillinase resistant penicillins	Flucloxacillin Methicillin (not used as associated with interstitial nephritis)	Semisynthetic penicillins with acyl side chain; developed to treat penicillinase producing staphylococci
Amino penicillins	Ampicillin Amoxycillin (more completely absorbed)	Oral and parenteral; active against a wider variety of bacteria including *E. coli*, *P. mirabilis*, *H. influenzae*, salmonella, shigella and listeria
Carboxy penicillins	Carbenicillin (large sodium load) Ticarcillin (greater activity against *Pseudomonas*; cf. carbenicillin) Temocillin (6 alpha-methoxy substitution gives long half-life and more resistance against beta-lactamase enzymes)	Parenteral; also active against *P. aeruginosa*, Enterobacteriaceae
Ureido and piperazine penicillins	Azlocillin (acyl derivative of urea as side chain) Piperacillin (piperazine side chain)	Parenteral; better penetration gives increased activity against a number of species, especially *P. aeruginosa* and *Klebsiella*; more susceptible to beta-lactamases c.f. carboxy penicillins

with cephalosporins and almost never with the new beta-lactam antibiotics such as aztreonam and imipenem (14,16). Patients who have a strong history of penicillin anaphylaxis and need penicillin for a serious infection can be desensitized, but in practice an alternative antibiotic can usually be chosen.

Cephalosporins

Cephalosporins are classified as first- (e.g., cephradine, cephalexin), second- (e.g., cefaclor, cefuroxime), or third-generation (e.g., cefotaxime, ceftriaxone, ceftazidime, moxalactam) antibiotics (17,18). The second-generation cephalosporins extended the antibacterial spectrum of the first generation, not only against Enterobacteriaceae, but also *H. influenzae*. The third generation is represented by a very diverse group of potent antibiotics with a broader spectrum and with much more stability against beta-lactamase enzymes. Coagulopathy and disulfiram (antabuse)-like reactions have been observed with several cephalosporins, particularly moxalactam, that possess an *N*-methylthiotetrazole group at the 3 position of the dihydrothiazine ring. Risk factors for bleeding include serious illness, malnutrition, and hepatic disease—all of which may be present in patients with cystic fibrosis. Patients should receive prophylactic vitamin K and be monitored for prolonged bleeding time (19).

Cephalosporins are a remarkably safe class of antibiotic (20). Anaphylactic reactions are very rare in spite of their structural similarity to penicillin. The incidence of skin rash, fever, or late-onset urticaria with a third-generation cephalosporin such as cefotaxime is on the order of 2%. A serum sickness–like illness does occur, albeit very infrequently, in patients treated orally with cefaclor. Some cephalosporins are potent inducers of chromosomally mediated beta-lactamases and can cause resistance to many agents by this mechanism (17,21). Linked to this inducibility is the ability of the bacteria to undergo mutation to high-level constitutive beta-lactamase production.

Cefixime and cefuroxime-axetil (an orally absorbed ester preparation of cefuroxime) are two newly available oral cephalosporins with greater resistance to hydrolysis by a broad array of beta-lactamases, but they are much less well absorbed from the gastrointestinal tract than older agents such as cefaclor (22,23).

Carbapenems

Thienamycin is the only currently available antibiotic of the new carbapenem class; it is unstable and causes renal toxicity and inadequate urinary levels when used alone (17). Cilastatin is an inhibitor of the renal enzyme responsible for this problem. The combination, thienamycin plus cilastatin, is called imipenem and has very good activity against all categories of pathogenic bacteria. For the lung it is used most commonly to treat either nosocomial infections or patients with chronic bronchial sepsis; it might be considered as monotherapy in severe nosocomial respiratory infections instead of the commonly used combination of a beta-lactam plus aminoglycoside.

Monobactams

Aztreonam is the first synthetic monobactam (17,24) and has a narrow spectrum of action. It has a high affinity for PBP-3 of susceptible gram-negative bacteria (including *P. aeruginosa*) but does not bind to the essential PBPs of gram-positive and anaerobic bacteria. Most nonaeruginosa pseudomonads such as *P. maltophilia* and *P. cepacia* are not inhibited. Because aztreonam lacks the bicyclic nucleus of the penicillins and cephalosporins, cross-reactivity is rare. Superinfections by gram-positive organisms, especially enterococci and staphylococci, have occurred in patients treated with aztreonam alone.

Macrolides

Macrolides are so called because they possess a macrocyclic lactone nucleus. They inhibit protein synthesis of susceptible organisms by reversible binding to the 50S ribosomal subunit (25,26). Resurgence of interest in this class has occurred with recognition of respiratory diseases caused by mycoplasma, legionella, and chlamydia species. A number of 14-, 15-, and 16-membered macrolides have been synthesized in recent years with the goal of overcoming some of the problems of the older erythromycin agents, such as variable activity of erythromycin against *H. influenzae,* gastrointestinal side effects, and the need to administer the drug four times a day (27).

Erythromycin inhibits most hemolytic streptococci and *M. catarrhalis.* It also inhibits *M. pneumoniae, L. pneumophila,* and chlamydia species including *C. pneumoniae.* Activity against *H. influenzae* is variable and many strains require 4 mg/L. Activity against anaerobic species is extremely variable (25,26).

Resistance to macrolides can be either chromosomal or plasmid mediated, and be inducible or constitutively expressed. The biochemical basis is by methylation of adenine residues, which prevents binding of erythromycin to the binding site (28). Resistance of *S. pneumoniae* has remained low in most countries, although the multiply resistant (including penicillin) strains first described in South Africa are resistant. Resistance of *M. pneumoniae* and *L. pneumophila* has not been noted.

The first of the new macrolides to become available was the oxime derivative roxithromycin. This antibiotic has an improved pharmacokinetic profile but little extra activity against *H. influenzae* (29). Clarithromycin is a derivative of erythromycin with an alkylated hydroxyl group at C6. It has improved activity against legionella and chlamydia, but similar activity to erythromycin for *M. catarrhalis* and *H. influenzae* (27,29). However its 14-OH metabolite is also active against *H. influenzae,* and the effects of the parent antibiotic and the metabolite are additive so that overall action is superior (27,29–31). Clarithromycin is rapidly absorbed from the gastrointestinal tract and the half-lives of the parent compound and the 14-OH metabolite are 5 and 7h, respectively, allowing twice daily dosing. Liver impairment alters the pharmacokinetics of clarithromycin and its metabolite so that less metabolite is formed. Metabolism to the 14-OH metabolite is saturable so that after an 800-mg dose there is minimally more metabolite than after a 250-mg dose (30). There has been very recent interest in the activity of clarithromycin against *Mycobacterium avium intracellulare.*

Another new macrolide is azithromycin. This antibiotic rapidly penetrates into tissues and body fluids and the highest concentrations are found in the intracellular environment (32,33). This might be an advantage when treating intracellular pathogens such as legionella and chlamydia, but clinical evidence is lacking. High tissue concentrations persist for up to 5 days after a single oral dose. Azithromycin need only be administered once daily and because of the long tissue half-life it has been recommended to be given for only 3 days to treat infective bronchitis. However, little data are available on relapse following such short courses. There must also be some concern whether low serum levels of antibiotic could deal with potential bacteremic illness caused for example by pneumococci.

Because they are more potent and have improved pharmacokinetics the newer macrolides can be taken less frequently at lower dosage and have a much improved gastrointestinal side-effect profile (27,34). Macrolides may result in alteration of hepatic enzyme systems, and may therefore interact with drugs such as theophylline. However, not all studies have demonstrated a reduction in theophylline clearance with erythromycin (35).

Quinolones

Uniquely among antimicrobials in clinical use, the primary bacterial target of fluoroquinolones is DNA gyrase, an enzyme that introduces negative supercoiling into DNA and separates interlocked DNA molecules. They therefore damage DNA, and interfere with DNA replication, segregation of bacterial chromosomes, transcription, and other cellular processes (36). However, the critical lethal event involved in quinolone action remains to be determined (36,37). It is interesting that killing by quinolones is reduced, paradoxically, by increasing the quinolone concentration over a certain level and is also markedly inhibited by rifampicin or chloramphenicol. These observations have in common inhibition of protein synthesis, which might suggest that quinolone killing of bacteria is associated with new protein synthesis (38).

In general, quinolones have good activity against most Enterobacteriaceae, fastidious gram-negative bacilli including *H. influenzae,* and gram-negative cocci such as *M. catarrhalis.* They are active against *P. aeruginosa,* but less so against other pseudomonas species. They have good activity against *S. aureus,* but are less active against streptococci and enterococci, and have minimal activity against anaerobes (37). They are active *in vitro* against chlamydia, mycoplasma, and legionella species (37,39,40), and they also have some activity against mycobacterial species (41), but clinical data are lacking.

The development of quinolones is probably the most exciting recent advance in the antibiotic management of respiratory infections, although their role has proved to be contentious (37,42), not least with respect to their efficacy in pneumococcal infection (37,42,43). It has been suggested that persistence of pneumococci in sputum despite treatment may delay clinical response or be associated with early relapse. Pneumococcal bacteremia has occurred in some patients during treatment with oral ciprofloxacin (44), although quinolones have been used successfully to treat both nosocomial and community-acquired pneumonia requiring hospitalization, including patients with pneumococcal bacteremia (45,46).

Two mechanisms of quinolone resistance have been identified: alteration in the target enzyme DNA gyrase and decreased drug permeation (47). Only chromosomal-mediated quinolone resistance has been found so far, and single-step mutation to high-level resistance is very rare, but high-level resistance can be selected by serial exposure of bacteria to increasing drug concentrations. In certain clinical settings the emergence of resistance has been problematic, and *P. aeruginosa* and *S. aureus* have been particularly troublesome (47).

The common interactions and side effects of quinolones are given in Table 5. Temafloxacin is a new quinolone antibiotic with improved activity against *S. pneumoniae.* However, this antibiotic had to be withdrawn soon after launch as a result of reported serious adverse reactions. These included symptoms of severe hypoglycemia, hepatic dysfunction, hemolytic anemia and renal dysfunction, requiring dialysis in some instances, and anaphylaxis and death.

Tetracyclines

Tetracyclines are broad-spectrum oral antibiotics that work by binding to the bacterial 30S ribosomal subunit and inhibiting protein synthesis (25,54). Their use in respiratory infections has been limited by emergence of pneu-

TABLE 5. *Interactions and side effects associated with fluoroquinolones*

Side effect/interaction	Comment
Delayed theophylline clearance	Partly cytochrome P-450 inhibition
Reduced oral absorption if given with magnesium and aluminium-containing antacids, sucralfate that contains aluminium, iron-containing preparations	Mechanism is chelation; therefore no interaction with H_2 antagonists
Possible cartilage damage	Only demonstrated in high dosage in animal studies, no human evidence
Central nervous system	For example, insomnia, dizziness, confusion, anxiety (all relatively common), fits very rare, possible GABA receptor interaction
Gastrointestinal	Incidence about 15%, nausea most common
Lens opacities	Only demonstrated in high dosage in animal studies
Crystalluria	Poor solubility of quinolones in alkaline urine, not reported as causing nephrotoxicity in patients
Skin rash	Low frequency, photosensitization variable
Nonsteroidal anti-inflammatory drugs	Increased frequency of convulsions in patients taking enoxacin and fenbufen

From refs. 37, 48–53.

mococcal resistance (55). The semisynthetic newer tetracyclines such as doxycycline and minocycline have advantages in that they have a much longer half-life in serum, which allows once daily dosage, and they are more lipophilic which allows them to pass directly through the lipid bilayer and not depend on porins. Plasmids impart resistance by coding for proteins that interfere with active transport through the cytoplasmic membrane (25).

Gastrointestinal irritation is the most frequent side effect, although this can be reduced if the medication is administered with food—but not milk or other dairy products, which reduce absorption. They pose a special danger to pregnant women because fatal reactions due to hepatotoxicity have occurred. With the exception of doxycycline, which is excreted in the feces largely as an inactive conjugate, they increase uremia in patients with chronic renal failure. They cause brown discoloration of the teeth and may retard growth of bone in the human fetus and in children (25,54).

Chloramphenicol

Chloramphenicol is unique among antimicrobial agents in that it contains a nitrobenzine moiety and is a derivative of dichloroacetic acid (25,54). It inhibits bacterial protein synthesis by binding reversibly to the 50S ribosomal subunit. The antibiotic is well absorbed, penetrates into tissues, and has good activity against common respiratory pathogens such as *H. influ-*

enzae and *S. pneumoniae* and many anaerobic bacteria. However, its use is severely curtailed by its potential to cause bone marrow toxicity. This occurs in two forms, first dose-related bone marrow suppression, which usually begins 5 to 7 days after initiation of treatment and is reversible, and second, idiosyncratic aplastic anemia, which is very rare and unrelated to dose. Resistance to chloramphenicol occurs via plasmid-mediated acetylation, which prevents binding to the ribosome.

Trimethoprim-Sulfamethoxazole

This antibiotic combination acts synergistically by inhibiting sequential steps in the bacterial pathway generating folate cofactors that function as one carbon donors in the synthesis of nucleic acids (56). The antibiotic combination is commonly used to treat community-acquired respiratory infections, although most relevant pathogens are resistant to the sulfonamide component, and trimethoprim resistance has increased particularly in *M. catarrhalis* and *S. pneumoniae*. The commonest mechanism of trimethoprim resistance is plasmid mediated and involves dihydrofolate reductase with reduced affinity for trimethoprim. The antibiotic is now the first-choice treatment of *Pneumocystis carinii* infection in immune compromised hosts such as AIDS patients. It is not recommended for infants under 2 months of age because of the risk of kernicterus, or for pregnant or lactating women. Serious side effects are not common, but the sulfonamide component can lead to hypersensitivity reactions such as rash, vasculitis, erythema nodosum, erythema multiforme, and Stevens-Johnson syndrome (56).

Aminoglycosides

Aminoglycosides consist of two or more aminosugars that via a glycosidal bond are bound to a central hexose or aminocyclitol molecule (57). Several derivatives have been synthesized to enhance the antimicrobial range, reduce toxicity, and protect against bacterial enzymes responsible for mediating resistance. Their spectrum is broad, and they are particularly active against aerobic gram-negative rods. For lung infections they are usually used in combination with a beta-lactam to treat chronic bronchial sepsis or nosocomial infections.

Aminoglycosides act at the ribosomal level to inhibit bacterial protein synthesis, and as they are not absorbed from the intestines can only be given parenterally. Their bactericidal effect is greatly concentration dependent, and peak concentrations in serum correlate with clinical and bacteriological response (58), while low concentrations contribute little to efficacy but do increase the risk of accumulation and therefore toxicity. Because of interpatient variability the dosage and frequency of administration should be adjusted individually from peak and trough serum measurements.

Resistance to aminoglycosides can result from alterations in cellular permeability or the ribosomal target, but most commonly is due to enzymes that modify aminoglycoside structure (e.g., acetylation, adenylation, or phosphorylation), which may be carried on plasmids, transposons, or the chromosome (59). The toxicity of aminoglycosides is based on accumulation and the major side effects involve the kidney and ear (57). Reduced glomerular filtration and proteinuria both usually show gradual recovery after discontinuation of therapy. Cochlear ototoxicity is caused by permanent degeneration of hair cells in the organ of Corti, starting in the high-pitch region of the basilar membrane. Vestibular damage also occurs, but because the patient can compensate for this disturbance it is usually less serious.

PHARMACOKINETICS OF ANTIBIOTICS IN THE LUNG

During bronchial infections bacteria are associated with the epithelium and its secretions; during pneumonia they are in the alveoli associated with phagocytes and exudate, while some such as legionella and chlamydia are intracellular pathogens. The concentration of antibiotic in the lung may be markedly different from that observed in serum as there are significant barriers to antibiotic penetration to these sites of infection (60–62). In the presence of inflammation, the partitioning of antibiotics in tissue compartments may be altered due to increased membrane permeability. Thus for drugs such as beta-lactams that do not cross membranes easily, penetration increases in the presence of inflammation. Conversely during resolution antibiotic concentrations at the site of infection may fall, which at least theoretically could allow bacterial persistence and predispose to relapse (63,64). However, the situation will be complicated as infection, particularly if it is chronic, may change tissue anatomy and physiology in various ways. For example, blood flow to the site of infection may be increased due to vasodilatation, or conversely may be reduced by poor blood supply of damaged, scarred airways.

Clinical efficacy may be directly related to concentrations of antibiotic at the site of infection in the lung. At other sites in the body there is a clear relation between local concentrations and clinical efficacy. For example, antimicrobials, which concentrate in the urine, are known to be effective, even when serum concentrations would predict a clinical failure (65). However, in the lung conclusive evidence is lacking. The efficacy of antituberculous chemotherapy has been linked to effective entry into phagocytes (66), and cephalosporins despite their ability to kill legionella *in vitro,* are ineffective in treating infections because they do not penetrate into infected cells to kill the pathogen (67). The *in vivo* activity of azithromycin seems to relate more closely to its tissue concentration than to its serum concentration, which is low (68). A study of amoxycillin in the treatment of pneumonia and severe acute exacerbations of chronic bronchitis showed that clinical response to treatment occurred more rapidly in those patients with sputum levels of 0.25 μg/ml or above (64). A similar prediction of clinical outcome from sputum concentrations was found with bacampicillin, an ester preparation of ampicillin that increases gastrointestinal absorption (69).

Measurement of Antibiotic Concentration at Sites of Infection

Blood

The site of infection is often difficult to define and sample, particularly on repeated occasions or in ill patients. Therefore, blood, which is easily accessible, is commonly used. There are three serum pharmacokinetic parameters that are likely to influence clinical outcome. The first is peak concentration, the second is the area under the serum concentration curve produced by repeated measurements after a single dosage, and the third is the duration of time the serum concentration curve remains above the mean inhibitory concentration (MIC) of an antibiotic for the bacterium. For beta-lactam antibiotics studies suggest that duration of time above MIC is most important (70,71), while for aminoglycosides it is peak drug concentration (71–73).

Whole Lung Tissue

This measurement usually involves tissue taken at thoracotomy after previous "timed" antibiotic administration. This is a crude measure of antibiotic penetration into the site of infection because lung tissue consists of many different components. Interstitial fluid concentrations of antibiotics probably equate with those of serum because the capillary endothelium is relatively permeable (60–62).

Bronchial Mucosa

Bronchial mucosa biopsies are usually obtained at bronchoscopy and have the advantage over whole lung biopsies in that there are less constituent tissue types, and that they are more clinically relevant to bronchial infections (60,74). Baldwin et al. (75) studied multiple bronchial biopsies taken from ten subjects. Ciliated epithelium occupied 22.3% of the biopsy, submucosa 53.4%, muscle 17.6%, and glandular tissue 7%. There was no difference between second- and fourth-generation bronchi, but there was considerable variation between samples from the same subject, which means that multiple biopsies should be taken. Over half the tissue was usually submucosa composed largely of acellular material. The effect of disease, for example, goblet cell hyperplasia in chronic bronchitis, on antibiotic concentration of mucosal biopsies has not been investigated.

Epithelial Lining Fluid

Epithelial lining fluid (ELF) concentrations of antibiotic can be measured in samples obtained by bronchoscopic bronchoalveolar lavage. Concentrations of constituents of ELF can be given as percentages of protein or albumin. Urea can be used as a reference marker to calculate ELF volume (76). By virtue of its small molecular weight and relatively nonpolar nature, it travels across membranes easily, and therefore exists in the same concentration in the lining fluid as in blood. However, this can overestimate the lining fluid volume, as with longer lavage dwell times urea diffuses from interstitium and blood. In conventional lavage, up to 200 ml has to be instilled to reach the alveoli and provide an adequate distal airway sample, but unfortunately this volume necessitates longer dwell times. Microlavage tries to overcome this problem by using a plastic catheter inserted via the bronchoscope to get further distal into the bronchial tree, which allows smaller lavage volumes and shorter dwell times (77). The total cell counts in microlavage samples are less than those obtained by conventional lavage, which means that the technique cannot be used for sampling both ELF and alveolar cells.

Sputum

The largest number of bacteria in bronchial infections are intraluminal bacteria associated with secretions (3,4,78), rather than being attached to the epithelium or within the bronchial wall. Penetration of antibiotics into secretions is generally poor, so it is an important site to measure concentration. Although results have been widely reported, there are considerable methodological difficulties in obtaining accurate information, including pooling of secretions in the bronchial tree, which causes major variation between samples, and contamination with blood or saliva (60,61). For example, erythromycin sputum levels have been reported to be 5% or 85% of serum levels (60) in different studies.

Phagocytes

Antibiotic penetration into phagocytes can be studied *ex vivo* (e.g., in macrophages obtained by bronchoalveolar lavage) or *in vitro*. The most popular *in vitro* method is to incubate cells with the antibiotic, then wash the cells rapidly and measure the amount of antibiotic associated with the cell pellet (79). There are a number of difficulties with this methodology; for example, the antibiotic may be bound to the surface of the cell, or may rapidly leak out of the cell during washing or centrifugation (in a few minutes with fluoroquinolones and erythromycin), or it may be inactivated by metabolism or binding to inner cell membranes.

The entry of an antibiotic into cells does not guarantee its efficacy against intracellular pathogens (80). There may be several reasons for this: the level of intracellular antibiotic achieved relative to the MIC of the pathogen, the mechanism of action of the drug (e.g., a beta-lactam would depend upon bacteria dividing for its action), the intracellular distribution of pathogen and antibiotic may be different, and the antibiotic may be inactivated by the intracellular microenvironment (e.g., pH). The bioactivity of intracellular antibiotic can be assessed by an increase in the intracellular killing of phagocytosed bacteria (81).

Several authors have speculated that accumulation of antibiotics within cells may result not only in the killing of intracellular pathogens, but also in the transport and subsequent release of antibiotic in areas of infection by phagocytes following chemotactic gradients.

TREATMENT OF LUNG INFECTIONS

Chronic Bronchitis

Chronic bronchitis causes cough or recurrent cough with excess sputum production, and is strictly defined as cough and sputum that has persisted for a total of 3 months in the previous 2 years. In the United Kingdom the Clean Air Acts of 1956 and 1968 reduced air pollution, and cigarette smoke is now the major etiological factor, although the level of air pollution may still exacerbate the condition. Some patients with chronic bronchitis may have other associated respiratory conditions, such as airflow obstruction, which may be partly reversible, and emphysema.

The cause of an acute exacerbation of respiratory symptoms associated with chronic bronchitis is frequently either viral infection or inhalation of airborne irritants, or sometimes allergy, rather than bacterial infection (82,83). However, bacterial infection commonly supervenes, signaled by the change in color of the sputum from mucoid to purulent. The three main bacterial pathogens are nontypeable *H. influenzae*, *S. pneumoniae*, and *M. catarrhalis* (82,84,85). A number of trials have suggested that there is no benefit from antibiotic treatment of acute exacerbations of chronic bronchitis (86). In one prospective double-blind study of 40 patients who had symptoms severe enough to require hospital admission, but no evidence of pneumonia, tetracycline 500 mg four times daily was no better than placebo as assessed by improvement in spirometry, arterial blood gases, and physician assessment (87). However, most of the trials can be criticized because of patient selection criteria, lack of controls, or the use of only subjective assessments.

A recent large study has helped answer this controversial question (88). This was a community-based study in which exacerbations were monitored in 173 patients with chronic bronchitis over a 3½ year period. Treatment included antibiotic (amoxycillin 40%, trimethoprim/sulfamethoxazole 40%, doxycycline 20%) or placebo administered in a randomized double-blind crossover fashion. Three levels of severity of exacerbation were recognized: the most severe grade had worsening dyspnea, increased sputum volume, and purulence; a lesser grade was any two of these symptoms; and the least severe grade was any one of the symptoms together with evidence of fever or an upper respiratory tract infection. Success was judged by resolution of symptoms after 21 days. The results showed that placebo appeared to be as good as antibiotic in the least severe category of exacerbation, but antibiotic was superior in the most severe group, with failure rates of 53% and 34% for placebo and antibiotic, respectively. This study strongly suggests that antibiotics are useful in the more severely affected patient with purulent sputum and dyspnea.

One criticism of this study (88) was that bacteriology was not performed. However, the bacteriology of sputum in chronic bronchitis is difficult to interpret because the bacteria involved are part of the normal upper respiratory tract flora and may therefore contaminate expectorated sputum. Pathogenic organisms may be cultured much of the time and results do not correlate with symptoms (89). Sputum culture should not be performed routinely, but when it is performed well on a freshly expectorated sample it can give useful information for difficult clinical cases, epidemiological studies, and antibiotic trials. Gram stains of sputum should be performed, together with culture and sensitivity, to assess neutrophilia and to ensure that the secretions are from the tracheobronchial tree as judged by absence of squamous cells.

A major consideration when treating bronchial infections is how to achieve effective antibiotic levels at the site of infection (60). Recent studies have indicated that the two important sites of infection are mucus and the respiratory epithelium (3,4,78). Antibiotics generally penetrate poorly into mucus. In patients with frequent bronchial infections, barriers to penetration of the antibiotic to the sites of infection develop. The bronchial tree is damaged and less well supplied by the circulation. The mucosa is thickened and scarred, and the lumen contains an abundance of thick purulent secretions, sometimes harboring millions of bacteria.

When considering antibiotic therapy it is important to appreciate that antibiotics do not achieve a satisfactory clinical response by killing all the bacteria in the airways. Instead, they control the level of infection by reducing bacterial numbers, and the host defenses are then able to complete the clearance. Patients with more severe respiratory disease have compromised host defenses that are less able to do this. This may also be true of elderly patients, or those with other medical conditions such as heart failure. When an exacerbation has resolved, the host defenses may have been further impaired, for example, by loss of ciliated epithelium due to epithelial damage caused by the infection, predisposing the patient to a second infection until the defenses have recovered. This will be particularly true if bacterial clearance is incomplete as rapid relapse may occur when the antibiotic is stopped. During the winter months some patients may suffer repeated infections for these reasons.

The bacterial species implicated in bronchial infections are now more commonly resistant to frequently prescribed antibiotics such as amoxycillin, ampicillin, tetracycline, erythromycin, and trimethoprim (82,85,90). At present, amoxycillin and ampicillin are the most commonly prescribed antibiotics in the United Kingdom, and there has been a gradual increase in the frequency of resistant nontypeable *H. influenzae* both here (90) and in other parts of the world (91). In the majority of cases this is due to beta-lactamases, but it can also be caused by altered PBPs (90). Beta-lactamase production by *M. catarrhalis* is estimated in some studies to be over 70% (90). The incidence of resistant strains is higher in patients who have received repeated courses of antibiotics.

It may be helpful when deciding on antibiotic prescription for airway infection to divide patients into groups based on clinical criteria (88,92,93) as shown in Table 6. The most important criterion should be production of mucopurulent or purulent sputum (88), although one must be wary of the clinical "catch" of an asthmatic patient masquerading as a bronchitic in whom the sputum may be yellow due to the presence of eosinophils. Patients in group 1 are previously healthy subjects who, usually because of prior viral infection, get a secondary bacterial tracheobronchitis. They are unlikely to have received recent antibiotics and therefore the incidence of infection by resistant strains is lower. These patients do not have difficult barriers to prevent the antibiotic reaching the bacteria and their host defenses are relatively intact and able to augment the action of the antibiotic. Patients in group 2 have chronic bronchitis due to cigarette smoking and no associated medical problems; usually they have one or two infective exacerbations every winter. Patients in group 3 can be termed "chronic bronchitis plus." They have more extensive bronchitis and frequently have associated respiratory conditions such as airflow obstruction or emphysema. They are often elderly and may suffer from unrelated medical conditions. These patients have more frequent exacerbations and have therefore had repeated courses of antibiotics. The incidence of resistant bacterial strains is thus higher. Because their bronchial disease is more severe their host defenses are more disabled, and there are barriers to penetration of the antibiotic to the site of infection. Group 4 patients have daily purulent sputum production, and when investigated they are frequently found to have bronchiectasis, usually of the cylindrical type (94).

TABLE 6. *Categories of patients with bronchial infections and antibiotic prescription*

Category	Clinical problem	Choice of oral antibiotic	Notes
Group 1 Previously healthy patients with postviral tracheobronchitis Group 2 Chronic bronchitis	Mucopurulent or purulent sputum indicates need for antibiotic	Amoxycillin Ampicillin Trimethoprim Erythromycin Tetracycline	Course of 5 or 7 days usually sufficient
Group 3 Chronic bronchitis plus Group 4 Chronic bronchial sepsis	More severe respiratory disease, other medical problems, elderly; barriers to antibiotic penetration; increased frequency of resistant bacteria; increased morbidity and mortality	Consider beta-lactamase–stable cephalosporins, e.g., cefaclor, cefixime; Quinolones, e.g., ciprofloxacin, ofloxacin; Amoxycillin/clavulanate	Length of course dictated by patient's recovery and return of sputum to mucoid; need to reassess patient

The choice of antibiotic in groups 1 and 2 is not critical, and is influenced by cost and side-effect profile as well as efficacy. Indeed, because their host defenses are relatively intact, most will clear the infection without antibiotic treatment at all. This may explain some of the trial results that have demonstrated equivalent results for antibiotic and placebo (86,88). The patient may of course clear the infection more quickly if given an antibiotic.

For patients in group 3 the choice of antibiotic may be more important, but there is no convincing evidence to support the notion that new (more expensive) antibiotics should be used. There may be plausible reasons why some new antibiotics might be more effective than older agents, including beta-lactamase stability, increased potency, or increased penetration into the bronchial mucosa, but clinical trials have usually shown equivalent results. It may be that to demonstrate differences between antibiotics, stricter criteria to judge efficacy, other than subjective clinical response after the course of antibiotics, will need to be used when treating more seriously ill (i.e., group 3) patients.

Chronic Bronchial Sepsis

A general framework for management of patients with chronic bronchial sepsis (94), whatever the cause (e.g., cystic fibrosis, ciliary dyskinesia, hypogammaglobulinemia, but in over 60% of cases idiopathic), is shown in Table 7. When most patients are investigated by thin-section high-resolution computed tomography (CT) scanning, they are found to have bronchiectasis.

TABLE 7. *Framework for management of established bronchiectasis*

Specific treatment for any cause identified (e.g., aspiration, hypogammaglobulinemia)
Physiotherapy techniques to enhance mucus clearance
Management of the bronchiectasis
    Curative surgical resection of localized disease with no underlying cause or
    Palliative surgical resection of a "sump" of pus defying medical treatment
    Control symptoms medically (e.g., antibiotics) to prevent disease progression
    In the future there may be ways to reduce "vicious circle" (Fig. 1) mediated inflammatory
        lung damage, e.g., nebulized recombinant α-1-antitrypsin
Management of associated disease (e.g., purulent rhinosinusitis, airflow obstruction)
Monitor control of inflammatory activity of disease, e.g., by indium-111-labeled white cell
    scan
Follow-up of the patient to detect
    Increase in severity of symptoms
    Increase in severity of bronchiectasis, i.e., spread of bronchiectasis to new parts of the
        lung, or appearance of it for first time in a patient with previous purulent sputum but no
        imageable bronchiectasis
    Deterioration in lung or heart function
    Other complications
Revision of treatment according to disease activity
If deterioration defies treatment, consider lung transplantation
Follow up transplanted patient to detect recurrence of disease in the graft

The florid, suppurative type of saccular bronchiectasis, which was localized and usually followed a severe lung infection is now quite rare (94). However, an insidiously progressive cylindrical type of bronchiectasis is more common and well described (94). This type of bronchiectasis may be underrecognized because such patients are often not investigated, particularly if they also smoke.

The bacteriology of patients with chronic bronchial sepsis is similar to chronic bronchitis, but may include other species such as *P. aeruginosa,* and sputum culture may frequently show a mixed growth of bacteria. Production of enzymes such as beta-lactamases by one species may protect another otherwise-sensitive species, which is the so-called indirect pathogenicity (95).

The short-, medium-, and long-term outcomes of antimicrobial therapy warrant consideration. Only the most severely affected patients (e.g., those with cystic fibrosis) will not respond to antibiotics by clearing of purulent secretions in the first instance. Antibiotics may need to be given by the intravenous route, both to achieve bactericidal concentrations in the bronchial mucosa, and to deal with resistant bacteria such as *P. aeruginosa.* An intravenous carboxy, ureido, or piperazine penicillin plus an aminoglycoside is commonly used. Quinolone antibiotics have given us the opportunity for the first time to treat *P. aeruginosa* infection orally.

Initial clearance of infected secretions may have one of several outcomes, each requiring a different strategy of treatment. These outcomes probably depend largely on how capable residual host defenses are of maintaining the bronchial tree "sterile," although it has to be appreciated that even in remission such patients are colonized by bacteria (96). Where damage is less severe, host defenses may maintain the patient infection-free until typically the next viral infection causes recurrence. Where damage is more severe sputum often becomes purulent again over several weeks, and where serious damage is present purulent sputum may recur literally a few hours after discontinuing antibiotics. So in these varying circumstances antibiotic strategy has to be tailored to the patient. At one end of the spectrum antibiotics may be needed only for use after infective exacerbations associated with purulent sputum production, but may be required continuously where damage is severe and recurrence of infection is rapid (97). Gradual recurrence of infection over several weeks, signaled by increase in volume and purulence of sputum, makes it necessary to decide when to treat (98). Pulsed intravenous therapy, for example for 2 weeks every 6 weeks, may be one answer (99). However, the outcome of such an approach would need to be carefully monitored as outlined in Table 7.

Because concentration of antibiotic at the site of airway infection is important, the idea of delivering the antibiotic directly onto the mucosa by inhalation is appealing. Five placebo controlled trials (100–104) have been conducted on the use of long-term nebulized antipseudomonal therapy to reduce colonization by *P. aeruginosa* and improve patient lung function. Stead et al. (103) compared ceftazidime therapy with gentamicin plus carbenicillin and placebo. There was no significant difference between the antibiotic regimens but both significantly improved lung function, body weight, and sputum production in comparison with placebo. Moreover, hospital admissions were significantly reduced during the 8-month period on active treatment in comparison with the pretreatment period. Only one trial (104) failed to show any benefit, and this used a smaller dose of nebulized gentamicin than was used in the other trials.

Nebulized delivery can certainly increase the antibiotic concentration in secretions. For example, aminoglycosides administered systemically do not penetrate well into bronchial secretions and concentrations may be well below the MIC for the infecting organism. Following administration of gentamicin 2 mg/kg intramuscularly to tracheotomized patients, the mean peak serum concentration was 6.75 μg/ml but the mean peak concentration in bronchial secretions was 1.83 μg/ml. In contrast, intratracheal or aerosol administration of gentamicin resulted in low serum concentrations and high local levels. Endotracheal administration of 10 ml gentamicin 2 mg/kg in 0.9% saline given over 5 min resulted in a mean serum concentration a half-hour following administration of 1.04 μg/ml compared with a mean sputum concentration at the same time of >400 μg/ml. Sputum concentrations declined rapidly but remained high, with a mean concentration at 4 h of 43.4 μg/ml and 13.8 μg/ml at 6 h (105).

Aerodynamic diameter of the droplets is the most important property governing pulmonary deposition. Particles in the range of 5 to 10 μm are deposited mainly in the large conducting airways and oropharynx. Conversely, particles in the range of 1 to 4.9 μm are deposited primarily in the small conducting airways and alveoli (106). A maximum of 50% alveolar deposition has been measured in healthy volunteers for monodispersed 3-μm particles. Droplets are generally deposited either by inertial impaction or gravitational sedimentation (107). Inertial impaction occurs particularly when airflow is rapid and results in deposition in the oropharynx, trachea, or on airway walls particularly at bifurcations. Gravitational sedimentation is the major mechanism responsible for deposition in the small conducting airways and alveoli where airflow is reduced. Peripheral deposition is enhanced by slow steady breathing, increasing the inhaled volume, and having a period of breath holding between inhalations (108).

Penetration of aerosols into the respiratory tract is influenced by airflow obstruction and the presence of secretions. Central deposition in the large airways by impaction is more common in patients with asthma, bronchitis, or bronchiectasis, and thus the antibiotic may not reach the smaller airways where much of the infection is located (78). Altered breathing patterns, such as occur with airflow obstruction, also tend to lead to central deposition (108). Inhaled antibiotics might be used in a number of ways: as prophylaxis, for example, to prevent gram-negative colonization on the intensive care unit, or to prevent *P. aeruginosa* colonization in cystic fibrosis; to treat an acute exacerbation; or to reduce bacterial numbers in patients chronically colonized and thus indirectly reduce airway inflammation. It is for this latter indication that there is the most convincing evidence of success.

Community-Acquired Pneumonia

The morbidity and mortality of community-acquired pneumonia remains significant, particularly in patients with well-documented negative prognostic features such as advanced age and preexisting illness (109,110), despite the use of potent antimicrobial agents and intensive care facilities. *S. pneumoniae* is the most frequent pathogen causing community-acquired pneumonia (110). In a prospective study of the causes of community-acquired pneumonia in Nottingham, United Kingdom, which utilized countercurrent immunoelectrophoresis to identify pneumococcal antigen and serological evidence of other infective agents in paired samples of serum, a pathogen was implicated in 97% of 127 cases and *S. pneumoniae* accounted for 76% (110). The other bacterial causes of community-acquired pneumonia are shown in Table 3. The bacteriology is very different from nosocomial pneumonia in which gram-negative bacilli arc the predominant organisms, although the pneumococcus is still quite frequently isolated (111). Epidemics of *Mycoplasma pneumoniae* occur about every 4 years (112). Spread within families is very common, and the outcome of infection may be pneumonia, tracheobronchitis, or pharyngitis alone, or it may be asymptomatic. Legionnaire's disease, which occurs in association with water systems and cooling towers, may cause serious illness. cases may occur sporadically or as outbreaks, and usually occur in or near buildings with contaminated water supplies. *Chlamydia pneumoniae* respiratory infections have recently been described (113) and their real incidence has not yet been determined.

Several studies have made unsuccessful attempts to identify pathogens on the basis of presenting clinical features. Results from culture of blood and secretions take 24 h, and serological diagnosis of atypical infections are retrospective. For these reasons a combination of a beta-lactam antibiotic (e.g., amoxycillin or cefuroxime) and a macrolide (e.g., erythromycin) is recommended for seriously ill patients with community-acquired pneumonia (114,115). The macrolide antibiotic will deal with the atypical infections such as mycoplasma, legionella, and chlamydia. Cefuroxime might be preferred to amoxycillin because it is not broken down by the beta-lactamase enzymes of *H. influenzae* and *M. catarrhalis*. When pneumonia occurs following an influenza infection, *S. aureus* should be considered as a possible etiological agent and flucloxacillin included in the antibiotic regimen.

In hospital series, mortality rates have varied between 5.7% (116) and 33% (117). Prognostic indicators for mortality include increasing age, preexisting illness, confusion, apyrexia, tachypnea, hypotension, raised blood urea, and a markedly abnormal white blood cell count (118). When pneumonia is managed in the community, amoxycillin or ampicillin are commonly given. However, during a year in which mycoplasma infections are frequent a macrolide should probably be used. Clarithromycin 250 mg twice daily is as effective as erythromycin 500 mg four times daily and is better tolerated with less gastrointestinal side effects (34). Macrolide antibiotics are effective against *S. pneumoniae,* but resistance of *H. influenzae* is quite frequent. *H. influenzae* is probably a commoner pathogen in the elderly (116).

Penicillins have been widely used for many years but pneumococci have remained very susceptible with an MIC for benzylpenicillin of less than 0.06 mg/L. The first report of penicillin-resistant pneumococci was from Australia in 1967 (119). Over the next decade similar strains became widespread in New Guinea and were occasionally found elsewhere (120). The majority of these isolates had a low level of resistance to penicillin, with MICs between 0.1 and 1 mg/L. However, by 1978 strains with high-level resistance to penicillin (MIC $\geq$2 mg/L), often associated with resistance to several other classes of antibiotic, had been isolated, firstly in South Africa (121,122) and subsequently elsewhere. In Spain particularly, nasopharyngeal carriage and invasive disease due to multiresistant pneumococci are very prevalent (123,124).

Penicillin resistance arises by evolution of penicillin resistant forms of the PBPs (125). Whether penicillin resistance should influence treatment of pneumococcal infections largely depends on the degree of resistance and the site of infection. Meningitis caused by pneumococci with any degree of penicillin insensitivity is associated with a poor response and a high mortality even with high-dose penicillin therapy (126). The relevance of pneumococcal resistance to the treatment of pneumonia and bacteremia is less obvious because parenteral administration produces peak serum levels above the MIC of even highly resistant pneumococci, although this might not be the case if patients are treated with oral therapy at home. A recent retrospective survey in Spain addressed this question (127). When pneumonia was caused by a low-level penicillin-resistant strain, intravenous penicillin or another beta-lactam in high dosage was usually successful. However, two patients with organisms with high-level resistance, 4 and 8 mg/L, respectively, did not respond to penicillin therapy. At the moment penicillin-resistant strains, particularly of the high-level variety, are very infrequent in the United Kingdom (128), and the guidelines for antibiotic therapy outlined above need not be adjusted yet. Resistance to penicillin is linked to that for other antibiotics, and various patterns of resistance have been described—the most resistant isolates being resistant to all beta-lactam antibiotics, chloramphenicol, erythromycin, tetracycline, clindamycin, and rifampicin (129). Vancomycin might be considered as first-line therapy should these strains become more prevalent in the United Kingdom, or for a patient with pneumonia returning from holiday in Spain.

CLINICAL TRIALS

The properties one might consider ideal for an antibiotic are given in Table 8. It is possible to try to assess how closely a particular antibiotic comes to achieving some of these ideals. For example, *in vitro* activity against relevant pathogens can be measured and the pharmacokinetics can be assessed. Similarly, the side-effect profile can be carefully monitored. However, when it comes to judging clinical efficacy there are difficulties, for both airway infections and pneumonia.

Chronic Bronchitis

Most antibiotic trials are conducted with the aim of obtaining registration of a compound with a licensing body, and are required to demonstrate safety and equivalence with other antibiotics currently available for a particular clinical indication. It is not surprising therefore that most trials show that antibiotics are equally good. For ethical reasons a placebo group is rarely used, despite the paucity of good evidence to justify antibiotic use in exacerbations of chronic bronchitis. The trial conducted by Anthonisen et al. (88) demonstrated that in order to show that antibiotics are a useful part of management of bronchial infections, more severely ill patients need to be studied, and production of purulent sputum is a prerequisite. Patients fulfilling these more rigorous criteria are less numerous and therefore such trials are more difficult to conduct. An example of one such trial showed superiority of ofloxacin compared with amoxycillin in treating infective exacerbations of airway disease (130), and another superior clearing of bacterial pathogens from sputum by ciprofloxacin compared with ampicillin (131). It is probably also important, in order to demonstrate differences between antibiotics, to judge them by criteria other than subjective clinical recovery from the acute

TABLE 8. *Properities of an ideal oral antibiotic for lower respiratory tract infections*

Spectrum to cover all likely pathogens
Complete absorption from gut
Good penetration into bronchial mucosa and secretions
Maintain adequate serum levels to deal with bacteremia
No side effects
Once daily administration

TABLE 9. *Criteria for oral antibiotic trials in patients with bronchial infections*

Reasonably seriously ill
Clinical recovery (including sputum purulent to mucoid)
Lung function, e.g., supply patient with peak flow meter
Pathogen eradication from sputum (at end of course and 1-week follow-up)
Need for subsequent therapy
Time until next infective exacerbation
Prevention of hospital admission
Quality of life, including speed of recovery

event. Some suggestions are given in Table 9. Although short-term bacterial eradication is a valuable end point for clinical trials, long-term clinical evaluation may be a more valid criterion for antibiotic comparisons (96). If bacteriology is to be used then it is difficult to understand why a sputum culture after a modest follow-up of perhaps a week is not universally applied, as is routine for antibiotic studies in the urinary tract (132).

Pneumonia

Diagnosis of pneumonia is clinically less straightforward (133). Objective evidence of pneumonia must be obtained in the form of a new pulmonary infiltrate on chest x-ray. Chest radiographs can suggest pneumonia but also be compatible with other diagnoses such as heart failure, old scarring, pulmonary embolus, tumor, etc. Determination of the etiologic agent may be difficult, and in some cases, e.g., mycoplasma, can only be obtained retrospectively. Pneumonia is a serious illness from which people die. Large trials demonstrating good efficacy of a particular antibiotic, but no patient deaths, are open to questions about the severity of illness of the patients enrolled (34). Pneumonia trials should attempt to stratify for severity of illness to allow interpretation, and to decrease the possibility that severely ill patients with a corresponding poor prognosis would be disproportionately randomized to one arm of the study. For example, a scoring system might be designed from the important clinical observations and laboratory results (118). The end point for classification of cure should be explicit, and might be defined as resolution of presenting symptoms and signs (including chest radiograph) after a fixed time following discontinuation of the test antibiotic.

EFFECTS OF ANTIBIOTICS OTHER THAN BACTERIAL KILLING

The Effects of Sub-MIC of Antibiotics

It has been known for over 50 years that bacteria are affected by growth in the presence of low concentrations of antibiotics (134). It has also been recognized that antibiotic concentrations significantly below those that prevent bacterial multiplication can be effective in the treatment of infections (135). Exposure to sub-MIC of antibiotics has previously been shown to alter toxin production by bacteria (136), their adherence to host cells (137) and mucin (138), bacterial morphology, which may in turn effect phagocytosis and bacterial adherence (139–141), and phagocytosis by other mechanisms (142–144).

Bacterial adherence to mucosal surfaces is thought to be an important part of their pathogenesis. Sublethal concentrations of antibiotics may exert their antiadhesive properties in at least four ways (140): altering the overall shape of the bacterium and in so doing modifying its approach to receptors located on the surface of eukaryotic cells; promoting the release of an adhesin from the bacterial cell surface; inducing formation of functionally deficient adhesins; and suppressing synthesis or secretion of surface located adhesins. These effects have been shown for most antibiotic classes, and the mechanisms underlying them may be complex; for example, the antibiotic may interfere with the mechanism of export or assembly of adhesins as well as their synthesis.

Numerically most bacteria infecting the airways are intraluminally associated with secretions. Antibiotics generally penetrate poorly into secretions, and it is likely that for at least part of the time (145) bacteria are exposed to sub-MIC of antibiotic. *H. influenzae* infection of respiratory tissue organ culture causes slowing of ciliary beat and damage to epithelium (4). Tsang et al. (146) have recently demonstrated that the presence of sub-MIC of either a beta-lactam or quinolone antibiotic with the infected organ culture did not affect bacterial growth but did preserve ciliary beat and reduce damage. These observations suggest that antibiotics might in some way disable bacteria without necessarily killing them, thus protecting local host defenses from damage and in this way enhancing bacterial clearance.

There is conflicting evidence as to whether exposure to sub-MIC of antibiotics select for resistant strains (147,148). Certainly beta-lactam antibiotics can induce the synthesis of novel PBPs or alter the balance of existing PBPs (149), and many antibiotic-resistance mechanisms (particularly those encoded by plasmids) are inducible (147).

Postantibiotic Effect

The term *postantibiotic effect* (PAE) refers to a period of time after complete removal of antibiotic during which there is no growth of the target organism (150). This is a feature of many antimicrobial agents and has been documented with a variety of common bacterial pathogens. Several factors influence the presence or duration of the PAE, including the type of organism, type of antibiotic, concentration of antibiotic, duration of antibiotic exposure, and antibiotic combinations (150). *In vitro* beta-lactam antibiotics demonstrate a PAE against gram-positive cocci but, with the exception of imipenem (150,151), fail to produce a PAE with gram-negative bacilli. Antibiotics that inhibit RNA or protein synthesis, and quinolone antibiotics, produce an *in vitro* PAE against both gram-positive and gram-negative bacteria.

It is proposed that the two most likely mechanisms of PAE are drug-induced nonlethal damage and persistence of antibiotic at the bacterial binding site. The most important clinical relevance is probably in determining dosage regimens. For example, the long PAE produced by aminoglycosides permits them to be dosed infrequently (150).

The Effect of Antibiotics on Neutrophil Function and Mucus Secretion

Prolonged courses of erythromycin are commonly used in Japan to treat diffuse panbronchiolitis and other forms of chronic bronchial sepsis (152). How they might work is obscure because the bacteria that infect these patients, such as *P. aeruginosa,* are resistant to the antibiotic. Two recent observations might be relevant. First, erythromycin has anti-inflammatory actions such as inhibition of both chemotaxis and random migration of neutrophils (153), and inhibition of their generation of reactive oxygen species (154). These effects might be expected to protect lung tissue from damage caused by a chronic host inflammatory response stimulated by persistent airway infection (3,6,155). Second, erythromycin is a strong inhibitor of mucus secretion *in vitro* (156) and possibly *in vivo* (157). Erythromycin, similar to glucocorticoids, inhibits the synthesis and secretion of a mucus secretagogue derived from human pulmonary macrophages (158). A major problem in patients with chronic bronchial sepsis is excess production of secretions that are difficult to clear, so erythromycin may benefit patients in this way.

The Effect of Antibiotics on the Normal Commensal Flora

Antibiotics given to treat lower respiratory tract infections will have profound effects on the normal commensal flora of the upper respiratory (159) and gastrointestinal tracts (160), sometimes with adverse consequences. Nasopharyngeal colonization of the upper respiratory tract with resistant gram-negative bacteria and yeasts commonly occurs when seriously ill hospitalized patients are given broad-spectrum antibiotics. Antibiotic combinations, usually given to broaden the spectrum until the causative pathogen is identified (161), increase this risk. Superinfection or nosocomial pneumonia caused by antibiotic-resistant strains may result.

The bacteria comprising the intestinal flora are mostly strict anaerobes. The balance of this ecosystem prevents colonization by exogenous bacteria and the emergence of certain species of bacteria that are always present in the normal flora, but can become pathogenic if their numbers increase. This protection afforded by the normal flora has been termed colonization resistance. Disturbance of the balance by broad-spectrum antibiotics might lead to simple diarrhea, or in the most severe circumstances pseudomembranous colitis due to *Clostridium difficile* (162). The effect of an oral antibiotic on the intestinal flora depends mainly upon its spectrum, its absorption, and the presence or absence of biliary secretion.

REFERENCES

1. Neu HC. General concepts on the chemotherapy of infectious diseases. *Med Clin North Am* 1987;71:1051–1064.
2. Pennington JE. Penetration of antibiotics into respiratory secretions. *Rev Infect Dis* 1981;3:67–73.
3. Wilson R. Infections of the airways. *Curr Opin (Infect Dis)* 1991;4:166–175.
4. Read RC, Wilson R, Rutman A, Lund V, Todd HC, Brain APR, Jeffery PK, Cole PJ. Interaction of non-typable *Haemophilus influenzae* with human respiratory mucosa *in vitro. J Infect Dis* 1991;163:549–558.
5. Wilson R, Pitt T, Taylor G, Watson D, Macdermot J, Sykes D, Roberts D, Cole PJ. Pyocyanin and 1-hydroxyphenazine produced by *Pseudomonas aeruginosa* inhibit human ciliary beating *in vitro. J Clin Invest* 1987;79:221–229.
6. Cole P, Wilson R. Host-microbial interrelationships in respiratory infection. *Chest* 1989;95(suppl):217S–221S.
7. Currie DC, Peters AM, Garbett ND, George P, Strickland B, Lavender JP, Cole PJ. Indium-III labelled granulocyte scanning to detect inflammation in the lungs of patients with chronic sputum expectoration. *Thorax* 1990;45:541–544.
8. Amitani R, Wilson R, Rutman A, Read R, Ward C, Burnett D, Stockley R, Cole PJ. Effects of human neutrophil elastase and *Pseudomonas aeruginosa* proteinases on human respiratory epithelium. *Am J Respir Cell Mol Biol* 1991;4:26–32.
9. Tuomanen E, Rich R, Zach O. Induction of pulmonary inflammation by components of the pneumococcal cell wall. *Am Rev Respir Dis* 1987;135:869–874.
10. Feldman C, Munro NC, Jeffery PK, Mitchell TJ, Andrew PW, Boulnois GJ, Guerreiro D, Rohde JAL, Todd HC, Cole PJ, Wilson R. Pneumolysin induces the salient histological features of pneumococcal infection in the rat lung *in vitro. Am J Respir Cell Mol Biol* 1991;5:416–423.
11. Wright AJ, Wilkowske CJ. The penicillins. *Mayo Clin Proc* 1987;62:806–820.
12. Tomasz A. From penicillin-binding proteins to the lysis and death of bacteria: a 1979 review. *Rev Infect Dis* 1979;1:434–467.
13. Parker RH, Eggleston M. Beta lactamase inhibitors: another approach to overcoming antimicrobial resistance. *Infect Control* 1987;8:36–40.
14. Holgate ST. Penicillin allergy: how to diagnose and when to treat. *Br Med J* 1988;296:1213–1214.
15. Petz LD. Immunologic cross-reactivity between penicillins and cephalosporins: a review. *J Infect Dis* 1978;137:s74–s79.
16. Saxon A, Beall GN, Rohr AS, Adelman DC. Immediate hypersensitivity reactions to beta lactam antibiotics. *Ann Intern Med* 1987;107:204–215.
17. Thompson RL. Cephalosporin, carbapenem, and monobactam antibiotics. *Mayo Clin Proc* 1987;62:821–834.
18. Goldberg DM. The cephalosporins. *Med Clin North Am* 1987;71:1113–1133.
19. Andrassy K, Bechtold H, Ritz E. Hypoprothrombinemia caused by cephalosporins. *J Antimicrob Chemother* 1985;15:133–136.
20. Neu HC. Third generation cephalosporins: safety profiles after 10 years of clinical use. *J Clin Pharmacol* 1990;30:396–403.
21. Pechere JC. Resistance to third generation cephalosporins: the current situation. *Infection* 1989;17:333–337.

22. Baldwin DR, Andrews JM, Ashby JP, Wise R, Honeybourne D. Concentrations of cefixime in bronchial mucosa and sputum after three oral multiple dose regimens. *Thorax* 1990;45:401–402.

23. Sanders CS. Beta lactamase stability and *in vitro* activity of oral cephalosporins against strains possessing well characterised mechanisms of resistance. *Antimicrob Agents Chemother* 1989;33:1313–1317.

24. Westley-Horton E, Koestner JA. Aztreonam: a review of the first monobactam. *Am J Med Sci* 1991;302:46–49.

25. Wilson WR, Cockerill FR. Tetracyclines, chloramphenicol, erythromycin, and clindamycin. *Mayo Clin Proc* 1987;62:906–915.

26. Washington JE, Wilson WR. Erythromycin: a microbiological and clinical perspective after 30 years of clinical use. *Mayo Clin Proc* 1985;60:189–203.

27. Neu HC. The development of macrolides: clarithromycin in perspective. *J Antimicrob Chemother* 1991;27(a):1–9.

28. Horiouchi S, Weisblum B. Post transcriptional modification of mRNA conformation: mechanism that regulates erythromycin-induced resistance. *Proc Nat Acad Sci USA* 1980;77:7079–7083.

29. Hardy DJ, Hensey DM, Beyer JM, Vojtko C, McDonald EJ, Fernandes PB. Comparative *in vitro* activities of new 14, 15, and 16 membered macrolides. *Antimicrob Agents Chemother* 1988;32:1710–1719.

30. Hardy DJ, Swanson RN, Rode RA, Marsh K, Shipkowitz NL, Clement JJ. Enhancement of the *in vitro* and *in vivo* activities of clarithromycin against *Haemophilus influenzae* by 14 hydroxy clarithromycin, its major metabolite in humans. *Antimicrob Agents Chemother* 1990;34:1407–1413.

31. Olsson-Liljequist B, Hoffman BM. *In vitro* activity of clarithromycin combined with its 14 hydroxy metabolite a-62671 against *Haemophilus influenzae*. *J Antimicrob Chemother* 1991;27(a):11–17.

32. Cooper MA, Nye K, Andrews JM, Wise R. Pharmacokinetics and inflammatory fluid penetration of orally administered azithromycin. *J Antimicrob Chemother* 1990;26: 533–538.

33. Baldwin DR, Wise R, Andrews JM, Ashby JP, Honeybourne D. Azithromycin concentrations at the sites of pulmonary infection. *Eur Respir J* 1990;3:886–890.

34. Anderson G, Esmonde TS, Coles S, Macklin J, Carnegie C. A comparative safety and efficacy study of clarithromycin and erythromycin stearate in community acquired pneumonia. *J Antimicrob Chemother* 1991;27:(suppl A):117–124.

35. Zitelli BJ, Howrie DL, Altman H, Maroon TJ. Erythromycin-induced drug interactions. *Clin Pediatr* 1987;26:117–119.

36. Hooper DC, Wolfson JS. Mode of action of the quinolone antimicrobial agents: review of recent information. *Rev Infect Dis* 1989;11(suppl 5):S902–S911.

37. Hooper DC, Wolfson JS. Fluoroquinolone antimicrobial agents. *N Engl J Med* 1991;324:384–394.

38. Furet YX, Pechere JC. Usual and unusual antibacterial effects of quinolones. *J Antimicrob Chemother* 1990;26(suppl B):7–15.

39. Lipsky BA, Tack KJ, Kuo C, Wang SP, Grayston JT. Ofloxacin treatment of *Chlamydia pneumoniae* (strain TWAR) lower respiratory tract infections. *Am J Med* 1990;89:722–724.

40. Saito A, Sawatari K, Fukuda Y, Nagasawa M, Koga H, Tomonaga A, Nakazato H, Fujita K, Shigeno Y, Suzuyama Y, et al. Susceptibility of *Legionella pneumophila* to ofloxacin *in vitro* and in experimental legionella pneumonia in guinea pigs. *Antimicrob Agents Chemother* 1985;28:15–20.

41. Leysen DC, Haemers A, Pattyn SR. Mycobacteria and the new quinolones. *Antimicrob Agents Chemother* 1989;33:1–5.

42. Ball P. Overview of experience with ofloxacin in respiratory tract infection. *Scand J Infect Dis* 1990;Suppl 68:56–63.

43. Daves BI, Maesen FP, Baur C. Ciprofloxacin in the treatment of acute exacerbations of chronic bronchitis. *Eur J Clin Microbiol* 1986;5:226–231.

44. Cooper B, Lawlor M. Pneumococcal bacteraemia during ciprofloxacin therapy for pneumococcal pneumonia. *Am J Med* 1989;87:475.

45. Gentry LO, Rodriguez-Gomez G, Kohler RB, Khan FA, Rytel MW. Parenteral fol-

lowed by oral ofloxacin for nosocomial pneumonia and community acquired pneumonia requiring hospitalisation. *Am Rev Respir Dis* 1992;145:31–35.
46. Khan FA, Basir R. Sequential intravenous-oral administration of ciprofloxacin versus ceftazidime in serious bacterial respiratory tract infections. *Chest* 1989;96:528–537.
47. Wolfson JS, Hooper DC. Bacterial resistance to quinolones: mechanisms and clinical importance. *Rev Infect Dis* 1989;11(suppl 5):S960–S968.
48. Wijnands WJA, Vree TB, Van Heerwarden CLA. The influence of quinolone derivatives on theophylline clearance. *Br J Clin Pharmacol* 1986;22:677–683.
49. Hooper DC, Wolfson JS. Adverse effects of quinolone antimicrobial agents. In: Wolfson JS, Hooper DC, eds. *Quinolone antimicrobial agents*. Washington, DC: American Society for Microbiology, 1988;249–271.
50. Okazazi O, Kurata T, Tachizawa H. Effect of new quinolones on drug metabolising enzyme system of rat hepatic microsomes. *Chemotherapy* 1988;34:149–154.
51. Wolfson JS, Hooper DC. Pharmacokinetics of quinolones: newer aspects. *Eur J Clin Microbiol Infect Dis* 1991;10:267–274.
52. Norrby SR. Side effects of quinolones: comparisons between quinolones and other antibiotics. *Eur J Clin Microbiol Infect Dis* 1991;10:378–383.
53. Adam D. Use of quinolones in paediatrics. *Rev Infect Dis* 1989;11:(suppl 5):1113–1116.
54. Francke EL, Neu HC. Chloramphenicol and tetracyclines. *Med Clin North Am* 1987;71:1155–1168.
55. Gopalakrishna KV, Lerner PI. Tetracycline-resistant pneumococci: increasing incidence and cross resistance to newer tetracyclines. *Am Rev Respir Dis* 1973;108:1007–1010.
56. Foltzer MA, Reese RE. Trimethoprim-sulfamethoxazole and other sulfonamides. *Med Clin North Am* 1987;71:1177–1193.
57. Horrevorts AM, Driessen OMJ, Michel MF, Kerrebijn KF. Pharmacokinetics of antimicrobial drugs in cystic fibrosis. Aminoglycoside antibiotics. *Chest* 1988;94(suppl): 1205–1255.
58. Laskin OL, Longstreth JA, Smith CR, Lietman PS. Netilmicin and gentamicin multidose kinetics in normal subjects. *Clin Pharmacol Ther* 1983;34:644–650.
59. Mayer KH. Review of epidemic aminoglycoside resistance worldwide. *Am J Med* 1986;80(suppl 6B):56–64.
60. Baldwin DR, Honeybourne D, Wise R. Pulmonary disposition of antimicrobial agents: *in vivo* observations and clinical relevance. *Antimicrob Agents Chemother* 1992;36: 1176–1180.
61. Bergogne-Berezin E. Pharmacokinetics of antibiotics in respiratory secretions. In: Penington JE, ed. Respiratory infections: *diagnosis and management*, 2nd ed. New York: Raven Press, 1989;608–631.
62. Valcke Y, Pauwels R, Van Der Straeten M. Pharmacokinetics of antibiotics in lungs. *Eur Respir J* 1990;3:715–722.
63. Law MR, Holt HA, Reeves DS, Hodson ME. Cefaclor and amoxycillin in the treatment of infective exacerbations of chronic bronchitis. *J Antimicrob Chemother* 1983;11: 83–88.
64. Stewart SM, Anderson IME, Jones GR, Calder MA. Amoxycillin levels in sputum, serum and saliva. *Thorax* 1974;29:110–114.
65. Bailey RR, Roberts AP, Gower PE, De Wardener HE. Prevention of urinary tract infection with low dose nitrofurantoin. *Lancet* 1971;2:1112–1114.
66. Mackaness GB, Smith N. The action of isoniazid (isonicotinic acid hydrazide) on intracellular tubercle bacilli. *Am Rev Tuberc* 1952;66:125–133.
67. Miller MF, Martin JR, Johnson P, et al. Erythromycin uptake and accumulation by human polymorphonuclear leukocytes and efficacy of erythromycin in killing ingested legionella pneumophila. *J Infect Dis* 1984;149:714.
68. Davies BI, Maesen FPV, Gubbelman S. Azithromycin (CP-62,993) in acute exacerbations of chronic bronchitis: an open clinical, microbiological and pharmokinetic study. *J Antimicrob Chemother* 1989;23:743–751.
69. Maesen FPV, Beeuwkes H, Davies BI, Buytendijk HJ, Brombacher PJ, Weeman J. Bacampicillin in acute exacerbations of chronic bronchitis—a dose range study. *J Antimicrob Chemother* 1976;2:279–285.
70. Frimodt-Moller N, Bentzon MW, Thomsen VF. Experimental infection with *Strep-*

tococcus pneumoniae in mice: correlation of *in vitro* activity and pharmacokinetic parameters with *in vivo* effect for 14 cephalosporins. *J Infect Dis* 1986;154:511–517.

71. Schentag JJ. Correlation of pharmacokinetic parameters to efficacy of antibiotics: relationships between serum concentrations, mic values, and bacterial eradication in patients with gram negative pneumonia. *Scand J Infect Dis* 1991;74:218–234.

72. Moore RD, Smith CR, Lietman PS. Association of aminoglycoside plasma levels with therapeutic outcome in gram negative pneumonia. *Am J Med 1984;77:657–662.*

73. Moore RD, Smith CR, Lietman PS. The association of aminoglycoside plasma levels with mortality in patients with gram negative bacteraemia. *J Infect Dis* 1984;149:443–448.

74. Honeybourne D, Andrews JM, Ashby JP, Lodwick R, Wise R. Evaluation of the penetration of ciprofloxacin and amoxycillin into the bronchial mucosa. *Thorax* 1988;43:715–719.

75. Baldwin DR, Wise R, Andrews JM, Honeybourne D. Quantitative morphology and water distribution of bronchial biopsies. *Thorax* 1992;47:504–507.

76. Rennard SI, Basset G, Lacossier D, O'Donnell KM, Pinkston P, Martin G, Crystal RG. Estimation of epithelial lining fluid recovered by lavage using urea as a marker of dilution. *J Appl Physiol* 1986;60:532–538.

77. Baldwin DR, Wise R, Andrews JM, Honeybourne D. Microlavage—a technique for detecting the volume of epithelial lining fluid. *Thorax* 1991;46:658–662.

78. Baltimore RS, Christie CDC, Walker Smith GJ. Immunohistopathologic localisation of *Pseudomonas aeruginosa* in lungs from patients with cystic fibrosis. *Am Rev Respir Dis* 1989;140:1650–1661.

79. Van Der Auwera P, Matsumoto T, Husson M. Intraphagocytic penetration of antibiotics. *J Antimicrob Chemother* 1988;22:185–192.

80. Hand WL, King-Thompson NL. Contrasts between phagocyte antibiotic uptake and subsequent intracellular bactericidal activity. *Antimicrob Agents Chemother* 1986;29:135.

81. Easmon CSF, Crane JP. Uptake of ciprofloxacin by human neutrophils. *J Antimicrob Chemother* 1985;16:67–73.

82. Chodosh S. Treatment of acute exacerbations of chronic bronchitis: state of the art. *Am J Med* 1991;91(suppl 6A):87S–92S.

83. Gump DW, Phillips CA, Forsyth BR, et al. Role of infection in chronic bronchitis. *Am Rev Respir Dis* 1976;113:465–474.

84. May JR. The bacteriology and chemotherapy of chronic bronchitis. *Br J Dis Chest* 1965;59:57–65.

85. Hager H, Verghese A, Alvarez S, Berk SL. *Branhamella catarrhalis* respiratory infections. *Rev Infect Dis* 1987;9:1140–1149.

86. Anonymous. Antibiotics for exacerbations of chronic bronchitis? *Lancet* 1987;2:23–24.

87. Nacotra MD, Rivera M, Awe RJ. Antibiotic therapy of acute exacerbations of chronic bronchitis. A controlled study using tetracycline. *Ann Intern Med* 1982;97:18–21.

88. Anthonisen NR, Manfreda J, Warren CPW, Hershfield ES, Harding GKM, Nelson NA. Antibiotic therapy in exacerbations of chronic obstructive pulmonary disease. *Ann Intern Med* 1987;106:196–204.

89. Ellis DA, Anderson IME, Stewart SM, Calder J, Crofton JW. Exacerbations of chronic bronchitis: exogenous or endogenous infection? *Br J Dis Chest* 1978;72:115–121.

90. Powell M, McVey D, Kassim MH, Chen HY, Williams JD. Antimicrobial susceptibility of *Streptococcus pneumoniae*, *Haemophilus influenzae* and *Moraxella (Branhamella) catarrhalis* isolated in the UK from sputa. *J Antimicrob Chemother* 1991;28:249–259.

91. Wilson R. Cefaclor. *Int J Antimicrobial Agents* 1993;2:185–198.

92. Wilson R. The pathogenesis and management of bronchial infections: the vicious circle of respiratory decline. *Rev Contemp Pharmacother* 1992;3:103–112.

93. Lohde H. Respiratory tract infections: when is antibiotic therapy indicated? *Clin Ther* 1991;13:149–156.

94. Cole PJ. Bronchiectasis. In: Brewis RAL, Gibson GJ, Geddes DM, eds. *Textbook of respiratory medicine*. London: Bailliere Tindall, 1990;726–759.

95. Dragicevic P, Hill SL, Burnett D, Merrikin D, Stockley RA. Activities and sources of

beta lactamase in sputum from patients with bronchiectasis. *J Clin Microbiol* 1989;27:1055–1061.

96. Groeneveld K, Van Alphen L, Eijk PP, Visschers G, Jansen HM, Zanen HC. Endogenous and exogenous reinfections with *Haemophilus influenzae* in patients with chronic obstructive pulmonary disease: the effect of antibiotic treatment on persistence. *J Infect Dis* 1990;161:512–517.

97. Currie DC, Garbett ND, Chan KL, Higgs E, Todd H, Chadwick MV, Gaya H, Nunn AJ, Darbyshire JH, Cole PJ. Double blind randomised study of prolonged higher dose oral amoxycillin in purulent bronchiectasis. *Q J Med* 1990;76:799–816.

98. Regelmann WE, Elliott GR, Warwick WJ, Clawson CC. Reduction of sputum *Pseudomonas aeruginosa* density by antibiotics improves lung function in cystic fibrosis more than do bronchodilators and chest physiotherapy alone. *Am Rev Respir Dis* 1990;141:914–921.

99. Pedersen SS, Jensen T, Hoiby N, Koch C, Flensborg EG. Management of *Pseudomonas aeruginosa* lung infection in Danish cystic fibrosis patients. *Acta Paediatr Scand* 1987;76:955–961.

100. Carswell F, Ward C, Cook DA, Speller DCE. A controlled trial of nebulised aminoglycoside and oral flucloxacillin versus placebo in the outpatient management of children with cystic fibrosis. *Br J Dis Chest* 1987;81:356–360.

101. Hodson ME, Penketh ARL, Batten JC. Aerosol carbenicillin and gentamicin treatment of *Pseudomonas aeruginosa* infection in patients with cystic fibrosis. *Lancet* 1981; 2:1137–1139.

102. Jensen T, Pedersen SS, Garne S, Heilmann C, Hoiby N, Koch C. Colistin inhalation therapy in cystic fibrosis patients with chronic *Pseudomonas aeruginosa* lung infection. *J Antimicrob Chemother* 1987;19:831–838.

103. Stead RJ, Hodson ME, Batten JC. Inhaled ceftazidime compared with gentamicin and carbenicillin in older patients with cystic fibrosis infected with *Pseudomonas aeruginosa*. *Br J Dis Chest* 1987;81:272–279.

104. Kun P, Landau LI, Phelan PD. Nebulised gentamicin in children and adolescents with cystic fibrosis. *Aust Paediatr J* 1984;20:43–45.

105. Odio W, Vanlaer E, Klastersky J. Concentrations of gentamicin in bronchial secretions after intramuscular and endotracheal administration. *J Clin Pharmacol* 1975;15:518–524.

106. Stahlofen W, Gebhart J, Heyder J. Experimental determination of the regional deposition of aerosol particles in the human respiratory tract. *Am Ind Hyg Assoc J* 1980;41:385–398.

107. Stuart BO. Deposition of inhaled aerosols. *Arch Intern Med* 1973;131:60–73.

108. Newman SP, Clarke SW. Therapeutic aerosols 1—physical and practical considerations. *Thorax* 1983;38:881–886.

109. Austrian R. Pneumococcal pneumonia. Diagnostic, epidemiologic, therapeutic and prophylactic considerations. *Chest* 1986;90:738–743.

110. British Thoracic Society. Community acquired pneumonia in adults in British hospitals in 1982–1983: a survey of aetiology, mortality factors and outcome. *Q J Med* 1987;62:195–220.

111. Bartlett JG, O'Keefe P, Tolly FP, Louie TJ, Gobach SL. Bacteriology of hospital acquired pneumonia. *Arch Intern Med* 1986;146:868–871.

112. MacFarlane JT, Finch RG, Ward MJ, MacRae AD. Hospital study of adult community acquired pneumonia. *Lancet* 1982;2:255–258.

113. Grayston JT, Campbell LA, Kuo CC, Mordhorst CH, Saikku P, Thom DH, Wang SP. A new respiratory tract pathogen: *Chlamydia pneumoniae* strain TWAR. *J Infect Dis* 1990;161:618–625.

114. Torres A, Serra-Batlles J, Ferrer A, Jimenez P, Celis R, Cobo E, Rodriguez-Roisin R. Severe community acquired pneumonia: epidemiology and prognostic factors. *Am Rev Respir Dis* 1991;144:312–318.

115. Woodhead MA, MacFarlane JT, Rodgers FG, Laverick A, Pilkinton R, MacRae AD. Aetiology and outcome of severe community acquired pneumonia. *J Infect* 1985; 10:204–210.

116. Ortqvist A, Kalin M, Lejdebron L, Lundberg B. Diagnostic fibreoptic bronchoscopy and protected brush culture in patients with community acquired pneumonia. *Chest* 1990;97:576–582.

117. Venkatesan P, Gladman J, MacFarlane JT, Barker D, Berman P, Kinnear W, Finch RG. A hospital study of community acquired pneumonia in the elderly. *Thorax* 1990;45:254–258.
118. Venkatesan P, MacFarlane JT. Epidemiology, pathogenesis, and prevention of pneumonia. *Curr Opin Infect Dis* 1991;4:145–149.
119. Hansman D, Bullen MM. A resistant pneumococcus. *Lancet* 1967;2:264–265.
120. Appelbaum PC. Worldwide development of antibiotic resistance in pneumococci. *Eur J Clin Microbiol* 1987;6:367–377.
121. Appelbaum PC, Bhamjee A, Scragg NJ, Hallett AF, Bowen AJ, Cooper RC. *Streptococcus pneumoniae* resistant to penicillin and chloramphenicol. *Lancet* 1978;2:995–997.
122. Jacobs MR, Koornhof HJ, Robins-Browne RM, Stevenson CM, Vermaak ZA, Freiman I, Miller GB, Witcomb MA, Isaacson M, Wards JI, Austrian R. Emergence of multiply resistant pneumococci. *N Engl J Med* 1978;299:735–740.
123. Linares J, Garau J, Dominguez C, Perez JL. Antibiotic resistance and serotypes of *Streptococcus pneumoniae* from patients with community acquired pneumococcal disease. *Antimicrob Agents Chemother* 1983;23:545–547.
124. Latorre C, Juncosa T, Sanfeliu I. Antibiotic resistance and serotypes of 100 *Streptococcus pneumoniae* strains isolated in a children's hospital in Barcelona, Spain. *Antimicrob Agents Chemother* 1985;28:357–359.
125. Dowson CG, Hutchison A, Brannigan JA, George RC, Dansman D, Linares J, Tomasz A, Maynard Smith J, Spratt BG. Horizontal transfer of penicillin binding protein genes in penicillin resistant clinical isolates of *Streptococcus pneumoniae*. *Proc Natl Acad Sci USA* 1989;86:8842–8846.
126. Radetsky MS, Istre GR, Johansen TL, Parmelee SW, Lauer BA, Wiesenthal AM, Glode MP. Multiply resistant pneumococcus causing meningitis: its epidemiology within a day care centre. *Lancet* 1981;2:771–773.
127. Pallares R, Gudiol F, Linares J, Ariza J, Rufi G, Murgui L, Dorca J, Viladrich PF. Risk factors and response to antibiotic therapy in adults with bacteraemic pneumonia caused by penicillin resistant pneumococci. *N Engl J Med* 1987;317:18–22.
128. Nair P. Incidence of decreased penicillin sensitivity of *Streptococcus pneumoniae* from clinical isolates. *J Clin Pathol* 1988;41:720–721.
129. Zighelboim S, Tomasz A. Multiple antibiotic resistance in South African strains of *Streptococcus pneumoniae:* mechanism of resistance to beta lactam antibiotics. *Rev Infect Dis* 1981;3:267–276.
130. Lam WK, Chau PY, So SY, Leung YK, Chan JCK, Ip M, Sham MK. Ofloxacin compared with amoxycillin in treating infective exacerbations in bronchiectasis. *Respir Med* 1988;83:299–303.
131. Chodosh S, Tuck J, Stottmeier KD, Pizzuto D. Comparison of ciprofloxacin with ampicillin in acute infectious exacerbations of chronic bronchitis. *Am J Med* 1989;87(S5A):107–112.
132. Brumfitt W, Hamilton-Miller JMT. Augmentin plus clavulanic acid in the treatment of recurrent urinary tract infections. *Antimicrob Agents Chemother* 1984;25:276–278.
133. Chow JW, Yu VL. Antibiotic studies in pneumonia. *Chest* 1989;96:453–456.
134. Gardner AD. Morphological effects of penicillin on bacteria. *Nature* 1940;146:837–838.
135. O'Grady F. Antibiotics in the 1980's. In: Sarner M, ed. *Advanced medicine,* vol 18. London: Pitman Medical, 19xx;55–71.
136. Grimwood K, To M, Rabin HR, Woods DE. Inhibition of *Pseudomonas aeruginosa* exoenzyme expression by subinhibitory antibiotic concentrations. *Antimicrob Agents Chemother* 1989;33:41–47.
137. Chopra I, Linton A. The antibacterial effects of low concentrations of antibiotics. *Adv Microb Physiol* 1986;28:211–259.
138. Vishwanath S, Guay CM, Ramphal R. Effects of subminimal inhibitory concentrations of antibiotics on the adherence of *Pseudomonas aeruginosa* to tracheobronchial mucin. *J Antimicrob Chemother* 1987;19:579–583.
139. Lorian V, Atkinson B. Abnormal forms of bacteria produced by antibiotics. *Am J Clin Pathol* 1975;64:678–688.
140. Chopra I. Antibiotics and bacterial adhesion. *J Antimicrob Chemother* 1986;18:553–556.

141. Stephens DS, Krebs JW, McGee ZA. Loss of pili and decreased attachment to human cells by *Neisseria meningitidis* and *Neisseria gonorrhoeae* exposed to subinhibitory concentrations of antibiotics. *Infect Immunol* 1984;46:507–513.

142. Veringa EM, Verhoef J. Clindamycin at subinhibitory concentrations enhances antibody- and complement-dependent phagocytosis by human polymorphonuclear leukocytes of *Staphylococcus aureus*. *Chemotherapy* 1987;33:243–249.

143. Desnottes JF, Diallo N, Loubeyre C, Moreau N. Effect of perfloxacin on microorganism: host cells interaction. *J Antimicrob Chemother* 1990;20(suppl B):17–26.

144. Keller N, Raponi G, Hoepelman IM, Rozenberg-Arska M, Verhoef J. Effects of subinhibitory concentrations of ciprofloxacin and fleroxacin on the opsonization and phagocytosis of bacteria. *Rev Infect Dis* 1989;2(suppl 5):S1067.

145. Mandell LA, Afnan M. Mechanisms of interaction among subinhibitory concentrations of antibiotics, human polymorphonuclear neutrophils, and gram-negative bacilli. *Antimicrob Agents Chemother* 1991;35:1291–1297.

146. Tsang K, Rutman A, Lund V, Roberts D, Cole PJ, Wilson R. Interaction of non-typable *Haemophilus influenzae* with human adenoid organ culture in the presence of subMIC concentrations of amoxycillin, loracarbef and ciprofloxacin. *Am Rev Respir Dis* 1992;145:A548.

147. Tomich PK, An FY, Clewell DB. Properties of erythromycin-inducible transposon Tn917 in *Streptococcus fecalis*. *J Bacteriol* 1980;141:1366–1374.

148. Grassi GG. Drug-inactivating enzymes of bacteria grown in subminimal inhibitory concentrations of antibiotics. *Rev Infect Dis* 1979;1:852–857.

149. Rossi L, Tonin E, Cheng YR, Fontana R. Regulation of penicillin-binding protein activity: description of a methicillin-inducible penicillin binding protein in *Staphylococcus aureus*. *Antimicrob Agents Chemother* 1985;27:823–831.

150. Zhanel GG, Hoban DJ, Harding GKM. The post antibiotic effect: a review of *in vitro* and *in vivo* data. *Ann Pharmacother* 1991;25:153–163.

151. Bustamante CI, Drusano GL, Tatem BA, Standiford HC. Post antibiotic effect of imipenem on *Pseudomonas aeruginosa*. *Antimicrob Agents Chemother* 1984;26:678–682.

152. Kudoh S, Uetake T, Hagiwara K, Hirayama M, Hus LH, Kimura H, Sugiyama Y. Clinical effects of low dose long-term erythromycin chemotherapy on diffuse panbronchiolitis. *Nappon Kyobu Shikkan Gakkai Zasshi* 1987;25:632–642.

153. Esterley NB, Furey NL, Flanagan LE. The effect of antimicrobial agents on leukocyte chemotaxis. *J Invest Dermatol* 1978;70:51–55.

154. Eyraud A, Desnotes J, Lombard JY, Laschi-Loquerie A, Tachon P, Veysseyre C, Evreux JC. Effects of erythromycin, josamycin and spiramycin on rat polymorphonuclear leukocyte chemotaxis. *Chemotherapy* 1986;32:379–382.

155. Ras GJ, Anderson R, Taylor GW, Savage JE, Van Niekerk E, Joone G, Koornhof HG, Saunders J, Wilson R, Cole PJ. Clindamycin, erythromycin and roxithromycin inhibit the proinflammatory interactions of *Pseudomonas aeruginosa* pigments with human neutrophils *in vitro*. *Antimicrob Agents Chemother* 1992;36:1236–1240.

156. Goswami SK, Kivity S, Marom Z. Erythromycin inhibits respiratory glycoconjugate secretion from human airways in vitro. *Am Rev Respir Dis* 1990;141:72–78.

157. Suez D, Szefler S. Excessive accumulation of mucus in children with asthma: a potential role for erythromycin? A case discussion. *J Allergy Clin Immunol* 1986;77:330–334.

158. Marom Z, Goswami SK. Erythromycin inhibits mucus secretion from human airways *in vitro* by affecting macrophage mucus secretagogue. *Am Rev Respir Dis* 1988;137:6.

159. Trigg CJ, Wilks M, Herdman MJ, Clague JE, Tabaqchali S, Davies RJ. A double blind comparison of the effects of cefaclor and amoxycillin on respiratory tract and oropharyngeal flora and clinical response in acute exacerbations of bronchitis. *Respir Med* 1991;85:301–308.

160. Hooker KD, Dipiro JT. Effect of antimicrobial therapy on bowel flora. *Clin Pharmacol* 1988;7:878–888.

161. Allan JD. Antibiotic combinations. *Med Clin North Am* 1987;71:1079–1090.

162. Bartlett JG. *Clostridium difficile*: clinical considerations. *Rev Infect Dis* 1992;12(suppl 2):S243–S251.

Drugs and the Lung,
edited by C.P. Page and W.J. Metzger.
Raven Press, Ltd., New York © 1994

10

Potassium Channel Openers

John Morley

Haldane Research, Ltd., Kew TW9 5JG, United Kingdom

Potassium channels are small pores that allow potassium and homologous ions (e.g., $^{86}Rb^+$) to traverse the lipid layers that comprise the plasmalemma of eukaryocytes. Since mammalian cells contain K^+ at substantially higher concentration (about 150 mM) than that in extracellular fluid (about 5 mM), it follows that such pores will usually have a greater probability of being closed than open and thereby will avoid nullifying the K^+ gradient that is generated by the K^+/Na^+-adenosine triphosphatase (ATPase) transposer in the plasmalemma.

Of interest therefore was the observation that, in cardiac cells, plasmalemmal ion channels that were selective for K^+ developed a higher probability of opening when the intracellular concentration of adenosine triphosphate (ATP) was lowered (1). From this finding has stemmed an extensive literature describing the distribution, electrophysiology, and pharmacology of channels described variously as ATP-sensitive, ATP-regulated, or ATP-dependent and abbreviated as K_{ATP}. The extensive literature in this field is being followed by reviewers, which allows nonspecialists to keep abreast of this topic. It is recommended that readers consult such literature for detailed information pertaining to cell biology, electrophysiology, and smooth muscle pharmacology of K_{ATP} channels (2–5), as well as the broader issue of describing the properties of such channels in airway smooth muscle by comparison with the nine or more additional K^+ channels whose properties also influence the transportation of K^+ across cell membranes (6). A recent book (7) is timely, for it focuses upon a modulation of K^+ channels by drugs, and, by covering general pharmacology, is helpful in placing this drug category in perspective.

It is the capacity of certain substances to modify K^+ channels that has led to the considerable interest of pharmacologists in this research area. Initial interest arose following the finding that such channels are present in insulin secreting cells (8), for such channels exhibited a higher probability of being closed in the presence of sulfonylureas, such as glibenclamide (9). This finding provided a cellular mechanism to account for hypoglycemic actions of glibenclamide and, of greater import to the pharmacologist, provided a simple method for recognizing which pharmacological or physiological phenomena might be secondary to opening of K_{ATP} channels. Commercial interest, however, has stemmed from the finding that drugs known to affect the cardiovascular system did so as a direct consequence of the opening of K^+ channels. Thus, the coronary vasodilator nicorandil, the antihypertensive cyanoguanidines, and the antihypertensives minoxidil and diazoxide all share the capacity to open K^+ channels (4). Hence, the various benzopyrans that have been selected by reference to opening of K^+ channels (e.g., cromokalim and bimakalim) have been selected and developed primarily as antihypertensive drugs.

Against this background, it is not surprising that research publications have given considerable prominence to projected use of K^+ channel openers in cardiovascular therapy. By way of contrast, asthma is usually consigned to the status of a minor option, vying for publication or presentation space with urogenital pharmacology. Unusually, the pharmacology of the (now abandoned) benzopyran SDZ PCO 400 was investigated with the specific objective of assessing therapeutic potential as an anti-asthma therapy. Certain unexpected findings made during that analysis indicate that the therapeutic potential for K^+ channel opening drugs in asthma may be greater than has been suggested either in reviews directed to asthma pharmacology or to the pharmacology of K^+ channels. Furthermore, delineation of the effects of drugs that open K^+ channels upon intact airways in laboratory animals has contributed to the evidence dissociating acute changes of airway hyperreactivity from inflammatory events (10–12).

AIRWAY OBSTRUCTION AND AIRWAY HYPERREACTIVITY

Understanding of airway pharmacology has been retarded by a repeated failure to differentiate between airway obstruction and airway hyperreactivity. Over the last two decades, those interested in experimental medicine and in the selection of novel anti-asthma drugs have directed inordinate attention to identification of airway spasmogens (and their antagonists). By selecting this research option, investigators reveal a failure to comprehend that, unless airway obstruction in asthma could be attributed predominantly to a single spasmogen, study of the mechanism of changed responsivity in asthmatic airways would be preferred as a basis for drug selection; thus, anti-hyperreactivity drugs would seem more likely to have a profile that is not spasmogen selective and thereby be effective in a wider range of clinical circumstances than would selective antagonists of airway spasmogens. This failure in research direction is not easily excused since, in the context of spasmolysis of airway smooth muscle, the corresponding advantage of sympathomimetics over selective antagonists is clearly perceived. The parallel between nonselective, physiological inhibition of contraction of airway smooth muscle (by existing anti-asthma drugs) and nonselective, physiological inhibition of expression of airway hyperreactivity (whether by existing anti-asthma drugs or by compounds currently in development) should be obvious (11–13), but only to those who have perceived that airway obstruction is an *indicator* rather than a *manifestation* of airway hyperreactivity. Since the same process (airway obstruction) is used to detect and quantify both obstruction and hyperreactivity of the airways, it has been usual for the pharmacology of the two processes to be presumed similar or, worse, not to be differentiated with clarity by persons who purport to comprehend the distinction. These comments are of direct relevance to the pharmacology of drugs that open K^+ channels, since an understanding of the pharmacology of these substances and their unusual potential as anti-asthma therapies hinges upon acceptance and understanding of the distinction between airway hyperreactivity and airway obstruction.

SPASMOLYTIC EFFECTS OF DRUGS THAT OPEN K^+ CHANNELS

The membrane potential of smooth muscle cells lies in the range of -50 to -60mV, which is substantially less than the equilibrium potential for K^+ (-85 mV). Consequently, opening of K^+ channels in physiological circumstances (i.e., low extracellular concentration of K^+) will lead to hyperpolarization. This effect of compounds that open K^+ channels can be measured directly in isolated trachealis cells by use of microelectrodes and the increased efflux of ions may be detected using either $^{42}K^+$ or $^{86}Rb^+$ (6). In consequence of this hyperpolarization, the opening of voltage sensitive channels that permit ingress of Ca^{2+} will be impaired, so that smooth muscle activation by stimuli that use this channel as a transducer is diminished. Addition of compounds that open K^+ channels to isolated airway smooth muscle causes relaxation for a wide range of agonists, but this effect is not accounted for fully by impaired opening of channels for Ca^{2+}, since drugs that close these channels (e.g., nifedipine and verapamil) have relatively little effect upon airway smooth muscle when contraction is due to endogenous agencies (i.e., spontaneous tone); furthermore, the maximal spasmolytic effect of drugs that inhibit the opening of Ca^{2+} channels can be augmented by addition of compounds that open K^+ channels (6). In this respect, airway smooth muscle may resemble vascular smooth muscle since opening of voltage-sensitive plasmalemmal channels to Ca^{2+} cannot account for relaxation in response to compounds that open K^+ channels in the absence of depolarization or external Ca^{2+}, as has been observed in certain isolated preparations of vascular smooth muscle (4). To account for these

TABLE 1. *Median effective concentration (EC_{50}) estimates (μM) from cumulative dose-effect relationships[a]*

Compound	Basal tone	
	Human	Guinea pig
rac-Isoprenaline	0.048	0.005
	(0.035–0.067)	(0.004–0.006)
rac-Fenoterol	0.26	0.0035
	(0.19–0.35)	(0.003–0.0041)
rac-Formoterol	0.27	0.0005
	(0.17–0.43)	(0.0004–0.0006)
rac-Adrenaline	0.35	0.089
	(0.26–0.49)	(0.076–0.10)
MKS 492	1.19	1.30
	(0.91–1.57)	(1.02–1.68)
rac-Terbutaline	1.30	0.063
	(0.97–1.64)	(0.05–0.08)
PCO 400	1.74	1.79
	(1.45–2.08)	(1.16–2.88)
rac-Trimethoquinol	3.25	0.0025
	(2.37–4.44)	(0.0021–0.0031)
AH 21-132	4.39	4.09
	(3.72–5.17)	(3.23–5.15)
rac-Salbutamol	7.39	0.013
	(5.57–9.76)	(0.01–0.015)
rac-Salmeterol	8.3	0.15
	(3.63–35.13)	(0.12–0.17)
Aminophylline	158	130
	(118–208)	(122–138)

[a]Defined for a range of spasmolytic agents on addition to isolated airway smooth muscle (human bronchus and guinea pig trachea), which had been contacted by endogenous agencies (spontaneous tone); $n = 10$ or more in each instance (unpublished observations).

anomalies, evidence has been presented in favor of mobilization of Ca^{2+} from intracellular stores or even indirect mechanisms, such as activation of endothelium to produce relaxant materials. Not surprisingly, the biochemical mechanism underlying opening of K^+ channels is unknown, but readers may find the model proposed for K_{ATP} channels by Edwards and Weston (2) conceptually useful. By comparison with other spasmolytic agents acting on airway smooth muscle, and more particularly guinea pig trachea, compounds that open K^+ channels are not especially potent spasmolytic agents (Table 1).

SUPPRESSION OF AIRWAY HYPERREACTIVITY BY SDZ PCO 400

A variety of substances have been shown to induce changed reactivity of the guinea pig airways to injected spasmogens, including platelet-activating factor (PAF) (14), immune complexes (15), endotoxin (16), antigen (17),

($\pm$)isoprenaline (18), ($\pm$)salbutamol (19), and ozone (20). Using anesthe-tized ventilated animals, it is possible to define dose-effect relationships to histamine before, and immediately after, intravenous infusion of PAF, ($\pm$)iso-prenaline, or repetitive injection of immune complexes over a period of 1 h. Coincident infusion of SDZ PCO 400 (0.1 or 1.0 mg/kg/h) during the infusion period caused a dose-related inhibition of the hyperreactivity to his-tamine, with efficacy of SDZ PCO 400 being greatest for hyperreactivity due to immune complexes, than to PAF, and than to ($\pm$)isoprenaline (21). Suppression of airway hyperreactivity due to PAF or acute allergic reactions has been reported for other anti-asthma drugs in the guinea pig (22,23). Solely on the basis of these studies, it cannot be presumed that such drugs prevent the development of airway hyperreactivity, although the capacity of ketotifen to influence airway hyperreactivity due to PAF was not detected if administration of ketotifen was delayed until after exposure to PAF (un-published observations).

To define the effects of SDZ PCO 400 upon airway hyperreactivity in a reaction that corresponded closely to those used in clinical pharmacology, acute allergic reactions were studied. Quite unexpectedly, it was observed that insufflation of SDZ PCO 400 could wholly abolish the acute airway obstruction due to intravenous injection of antigen and, moreover, abolish expression of airway hyperreactivity 24 h later. Such a profile of action is reminiscent of the characteristics of cromoglycate in allergic asthma, prompting consideration of whether the anti-allergic profile might be asso-ciated with activation of mast cells or diminished accumulation of inflam-matory leukocytes within the airway lumen. However, in marked contrast to *in vivo* findings, Schultz-Dale reactions in passively sensitized airway tis-sue were unaffected even by very high concentrations of SDZ PCO 400, while leukocyte influx into the airways was undiminished, even at dose lev-els that were supramaximal for suppression of airway hyperreactivity.

These findings raised the possibility that SDZ PCO 400 might be capable of suppressing established hyerreactivity and that efficacy of SDZ PCO 400 in this respect might be greater than, and distinct from, spasmolytic efficacy. Therefore, conditions were selected that allowed demonstration of a mar-ginal and transient reduction of airway obstruction due to histamine when SDZ PCO 400 was infused intravenously in normal (isoreactive) animals. A comparable experiment was performed, but using a lower dose of histamine in animals made hyperreactive by infusion of PAF or immune complexes, when suppression by the *same dose* of SDZ PCO 400 was much more pro-nounced and persistent (Fig. 1). The inference can be made that SDZ PCO 400 has inhibited expression of airway hyperreactivity by a mechanism other than spasmolysis.

No mechanism has been established to account for this unexpected prop-erty of SDZ PCO 400. However, it was possible to demonstrate that the protective effect during an acute allergic reaction was wholly abrogated by

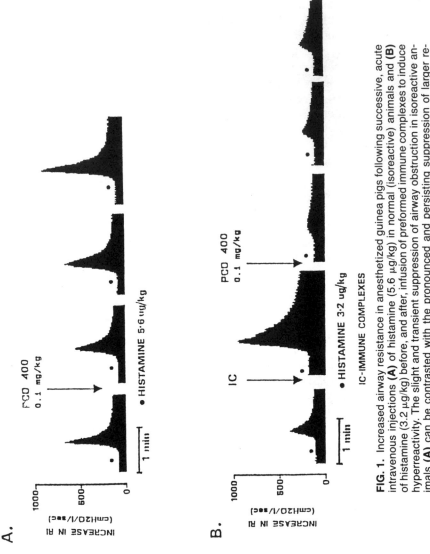

FIG. 1. Increased airway resistance in anesthetized guinea pigs following successive, acute intravenous injections (**A**) of histamine (5.6 µg/kg) in normal (isoreactive) animals and (**B**) of histamine (3.2 µg/kg) before, and after, infusion of preformed immune complexes to induce hyperreactivity. The slight and transient suppression of airway obstruction in isoreactive animals (**A**) can be contrasted with the pronounced and persisting suppression of larger responses in hyperreactive animals (**B**) [See Chapman et al. (21) for detailed methodology].

bilateral vagal section, suggesting that the locus of action might lie in nerve tissue. There were *in vitro* findings to indicate that openers of K^+ channels could impair ganglionic transmission in the vagus nerve and reduce the release of acetylcholine (24,25) in the guinea pig, but differentiation between neural and spasmolytic effects was clarified when Ichinose and Barnes (26) studied nonadrenergic, noncholinergic bronchoconstrictor responses to vagal stimulation and showed cromakalim to be more effective as an inhibitor of bronchoconstrictor responses to nerve stimulation than of comparable bronchoconstriction induced by intravenous injection of substance P. A mechanistic explanation is suggested by the finding that sympathomimetics, isoquinolines, and xanthines, like SDZ PCO 400, also appear to be more potent in hyperreactive than in isoreactive animals (27). In the case of ($\pm$)isoprenaline, there is evidence that hyperpolarization of smooth muscle cells is associated with increased membrane conductance and an equilibrium potential near to the equilibrium potential for K^+; hence, it has been suggested

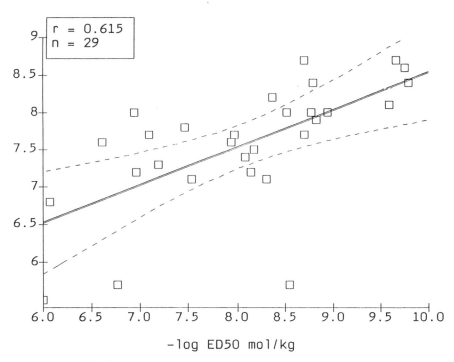

FIG. 2. Correlation between relaxation of isolated rat portal vein (p IC_{50}) (ordinate) and suppression of established airway hyperreactivity of the type depicted in Fig. 1 (abscissa). All 29 compounds were inhibitors of K^+ channels and while the majority (17) lie within the 95% confidence limits (*dashed lines*), there are 12 outliers, including compounds with proportionately greater activity as inhibitors of expression of established airway hyperreactivity (unpublished observations).

(28) that elevation of intracellular adenosine $3',5'$-cyclic monophosphate (cAMP) and activation of protein kinase A cause phosphorylation of some critical element of the membrane components that control channel closure (2) to open a different population of K^+ channels, the large Ca^{2+}-dependent K^+ channels. It might reasonably be expected that highly potent selective phosphodiesterase (PDE) isoenzyme inhibitors will share this property with sympathomimetics and that therefore all three categories of drug (potassium channel openers, sympathomimetics, PDE isoenzyme inhibitors) will impair the expression of airway hyperreactivity.

The practical consequence of distinguishing spasmolytic effects of substances that open K^+ on airway (or other) smooth muscle from suppression of airway hyperreactivity by an action on neural tissue is the prospect of selecting compounds that impair expression of airway hyperreactivity without spasmolysis, thereby avoiding cardiovascular side effects. That this prospect might be realized is indicated by the occurrence of outliers from the line of identity when suppression of airway hyperreactivity and spasmolysis are compared for a series of compounds known to inhibit opening of K^+ channels in vitro (Fig. 2). BRL 55836 has been proposed as having selectivity for K^+ channels (29), but it will be appreciated that this differentiation has been based upon spasmolysis, a further example of the failure of pharmacologists to recognize the critical role of hyperreactivity in airway pharmacology. By reference to Fig. 2, it can reasonably be expected that compounds will be disclosed with considerably greater potency than levcromakalim or SDZ PCO 400 on tests relating to airway hyperreactivity and with proportionately lesser actions on vascular or other smooth muscles.

POSITIONING OF K^+ OPENING DRUGS IN AIRWAY PHARMACOLOGY

As there is now every likelihood that K_{ATP} opening compounds will be developed for use in clinical asthma per se, it is appropriate to consider what place such drugs might have in the pharmacological armamentarium. To make such assessment, it is necessary to compare the pharmacological profile of compounds that open K^+ channels with anti-asthma drugs that are already available (Table 2). Reference to this table indicates that drugs that open K^+ channels fall into a category that is already occupied by sympathomimetics, and that anti-asthma activities already defined for these compounds are shared by selective PDE isoenzyme inhibitors, compounds that additionally exhibit the capacity to impair leukocyte recruitment into the pulmonary airways (11–13). Current recommendations for asthma management give emphasis to early use of drugs that will diminish the inflammatory events that are characteristic of asthma, reserving spasmolytic therapy for control of intermittent symptoms (30). If the recommendations of clinical experts are able to predominate over commercial promotion, the progressive

TABLE 2. *Reclassification of anti-asthma drugs by reference to pharmacological profiles*

Category	Classification		Mechanism
	Existing	Proposed	
Parasympatholytics	Bronchodilator	Spasmolytic (I)	Spasmogen antagonism
Histamine (H_1) antagonists	Anti-allergic	Spasmolytic (I)	Spasmogen antagonism
Leukotriene antagonists	Anti-allergic	Spasmolytic (I)	Spasmogen antagonism
β-adrenoceptor agonists	Bronchodilator	Antihyperreactivity (II)	Presynaptic inhibition
Xanthines	Bronchodilator	Antihyperreactivity (II)	Presynaptic inhibition
K^+ channel openers	Bronchodilator	Antihyperreactivity (II)	Presynaptic inhibition
Cromones	Anti-allergic	Pulmonary eosinophilopenia (III)	Reduced priming of eosinophils Bronchoconstrictor reflex inhibition
Ketotifen	Anti-allergic	Pulmonary eosinophilopenia (III)	Reduced priming of eosinophils Abrogation of sympathomimetic hyperreactivity
Glucocorticosteroids	Anti-inflammatory	Pulmonary leukopenia (IV)	Reduced priming of leukocytes/impaired secretion by leukocytes
Cyclosporin A	Immunosuppressive	Pulmonary leukopenia (IV)	Reduced priming of leukocytes
Selective PDE isozyme inhibitors	Bronchodilator	Antihyperreactivity/pulmonary leukopenia (II and IV)	Presynaptic inhibition/suppression of leukocyte motility

From ref. 13.

expansion of the market for sympathomimetics will be halted and might reasonably be expected to decline, if only in money terms, since generic formulations of existing sympathomimetics will be a proven and inexpensive rescue therapy. Evolution of sympathomimetics into long-acting forms such as ($\pm$)salmeterol and ($\pm$)formoterol are less appropriate to this objective, being more expensive and, by virtue of the persisting symptom relief, liable to compromise attempts to establish anti-inflammatory therapy as a primary objective in patient care. On the basis of disclosed information, drugs that open K^+ channels will therefore have to compete with existing sympathomimetics and projected PDE isoenzyme inhibitors as drugs for symptom control.

IS THERE A NEED FOR K^+ OPENING DRUGS IN ASTHMA?

It is not unusual to hear, publicly or privately, the opinion that use of inhaled steroids, supplemented with inhaled sympathomimetics for symptom control, is perfectly adequate for asthma therapy. Given the increased incidence and severity of asthma in industrialized societies, such therapeutic strategy may be regarded as palliative, so that such complacency is not warranted. Nevertheless, if it is accepted that existing therapy is adequate, the issue arises as to whether anything is to be gained by attempting to substitute compounds into either drug category.

Long-term administration of inhaled steroids, especially as doses are increased, may reasonably give cause for concern (31). Compounds that open K^+ channels do not influence recruitment of inflammatory cells into the lung during an acute allergic reaction and will have no direct influence upon the site of action of steroids as inhibitors of inflammatory cell accumulation within intrapulmonary airways. It is known that low doses of steroids suffice to impair inflammatory cell accumulation in asthmatic lungs (32), yet there is a tendency to employ steroids at higher doses with the objective of diminishing airway hyperreactivity (33). Given the capacity of K^+ channel openers to so markedly affect expression of airway hyperreactivity in clinical circumstances (34), it might be argued that use of drugs that open K^+ channels as therapy for symptom control might help in the objective of keeping regular doses of inhaled steroids to a minimum. For such argumentation to hold, it has to be presupposed that existing sympathomimetics cannot achieve such an objective.

Table 2 suggests that properties of drugs of the type currently proposed as K^+ channel openers offer no advantage over existing sympathomimetics. For acute administration, this cannot be contested, since acute administration of single doses of sympathomimetics are strikingly impressive inhibitors of airway hyperreactivity both in the guinea pig (27) and in man (35). However, during regular administration of sympathomimetics, bronchodilator effects [elevated forced expiratory volume in 1 sec (FEV_1)] persist, whereas the capacity to protect patients from induced airway obstruction is progressively lost (36–38). In the guinea pig, it is relatively easy to demonstrate that the effects of sympathomimetics represent a summation of smooth muscle spasmolysis, suppression of hyperreactivity (most pronounced acutely), and induction of airway hyperreactivity (most pronounced on sustained exposure). Spasmolysis and suppression of airway of hyperreactivity can be accounted for by adrenoceptor occupancy, with opening of large Ca^{2+}-dependent K^+ channels accounting for the latter effect; however, induction of hyperreactivity is unrelated to adrenoceptors or adrenoceptor occupancy, being manifest by both enantiomers and, in contrast to spasmolytic effects of adrenoceptor occupancy, being abrogated by vagal section (39).

Thus, the extent to which drugs that open K^+ channels will supplant sympathomimetics will depend upon the relative value to the patient of bronchodilator effects over suppression of responses to provocation stimuli. There is some indication that loss of protection from provocation stimuli is perceived as a deficiency by the patient. Thus, it has long been appreciated that the practical consequence of this loss of protection is a shortening of the interval between successive inhalations when ($\pm$)salbutamol is used on demand (40). Whether the clear theoretical advantage of drugs that open K^+ channels over existing sympathomimetics will alone justify the increased medication cost would be doubtful, were it not for the minority of patients who use sympathomimetics excessively. If the cause of increased mortality in such patients (41) can be related to induction of airway hyperreactivity *per se* or loss of protection against clinically important stimuli of asthma exacerbation, some degree of therapeutic transfer would seem inevitable.

FUTURE DEVELOPMENTS

Two future developments merit mention, since the outcome of such studies will substantially influence the prospects of drugs selected for anti-asthma therapy as openers of K^+ channels.

First, it is now evident that airway hyperreactivity, both in the guinea pig and in asthmatics, is markedly heterogeneous, so that whether a procedure leads to airway hyperreactivity depends upon the spasmogen used for test purposes. The limited studies undertaken hitherto with SDZ PCO 400 and cromakalim have focused upon histamine and acetylcholine sensitivity (42). However, in allergic hyperreactivity in the guinea pig, spasmogens such as peptidoleukotrienes more readily reveal airway hyperreactivity and more probably determine lethal outcome in this species (19,23). It is already evident that SDZ PCO 400 was not uniformly effective as an inhibitor of expression of airway hyperreactivity; hence, it will be prudent to ascertain whether drugs that open K^+ channels are particularly effective against hyperreactivity that is revealed by constrictor response to spasmogens of particular importance in asthma and to make appropriate comparison with sympathomimetics and selective PDE isoenzyme inhibitors.

Second, it is likely that the first generation of drugs that open K^+ channels will have profound cardiovascular actions, if only because compounds were selected to achieve this particular objective. Delivery by inhalation may limit manifestation of this property, which must be considered an adverse effect in asthma therapy. However, a more productive approach will be to select compounds by reference to effects upon the airways, especially since there is a reasonable prospect of selecting compounds that are highly effective as inhibitors of manifestations of airway hyperreactivity, without having spasmolytic actions and hence cardiovascular side effects.

At present, the introduction into asthma therapy of drugs that open K^+ channels can be expected to help in clarifying the objective of rescue therapy. Whether drugs in this category supersede sympathomimetics will depend upon clinical confirmation of animal pharmacology and correct positioning of this drug category in therapy. It should not be forgotten that openers of K^+ channels will be contemporaries of selective PDE isoenzyme inhibitors, which should be positioned as once-daily oral therapies with a capacity to impair intrathoracic accumulation of inflammatory cells, effect bronchodilation, and impair the development or expression of airway hyperreactivity (11). Should PDE isoenzyme inhibitors with such a profile be introduced successfully, prospects for openers of K^+ channels may be slim.

ACKNOWLEDGMENTS

I am grateful to Dr. Ian Chapman for preparation of Table 1 and to Dr. Karl-Heinz Buckheit for preparation of Fig. 2.

REFERENCES

1. Noma A. ATP-regulated K^+ channels in cardiac muscle. *Nature* 1983;305:147–148.
2. Edwards G, Weston AH. The pharmacology of ATP-sensitive potassium channels. *Ann Rev Pharmacol Toxicol* 1993;33:597–637.
3. Evans JM, Longman SD. Potassium channel activators. *Ann Rep Med Chem* 1991; 26:73–82.
4. Quast U. Potassium channel openers: pharmacological and clinical aspects. *Fundam Clin Pharmacol* 1993;in press.
5. Small RC, Berry JL, Foster RW, Green KA, Murray MA. The pharmacology of potassium channel modulators in airway smooth muscle: relevance to airways disease. In: Weston AH, Hamilton TC, eds. *Potassium channel modulators*. London: Blackwell Scientific, 1992;442–461.
6. Small RC, Berry JL, Cook SJ, Foster RW, Green KA, Murray MA. Potassium channels in airways. In: Chung F, Barnes PJ, eds. *Pharmacology of the respiratory tract: clinical and experimental*. New York: Marcel Dekker, 1993;137–176.
7. Weston AH, Hamilton TC. *Potassium channel modulators*. London: Blackwell Scientific, 1992.

8. Cook DL, Hales CN. Intracellular ATP directly blocks K^+ channels in pancreatic beta-cells. *Nature* 1984;311:271–273.
9. Quast U, Cook NS. Moving together: K^+ channel openers and ATP-sensitive K^+ channels. *Trends Pharmacol Sci* 1989;10:431–435.
10. Chapman ID, Foster A, Morley J. The relationship between inflammation and hyperreactivity of the airways in asthma. *Clin Exp Immunol* 1993;23:168–171.
11. Morley J. New drug developments for asthma. In: Morley J, ed. *Preventive therapy in asthma*. London: Academic Press, 1991;254–273.
12. Morley J. Immunopharmacology of asthma. *Trends Pharmacol Sci/Immunol Today* 1993;14:208–213, 317–322.
13. Morley J. Comments on the nomenclature and classification of anti-asthma drugs. *Pulmon Pharmacol* 1993;6:11–14.
14. Mazzoni L, Morley J, Page CP, Sanjar S. Induction of hyperreactivity by platelet activating factor in the guinea-pig. *J Physiol* 1985;365:107P.
15. Sanjar S, Colditz IG, Aoki S, Boubekeur K, Morley J. Pharmacological modulation of eosinophil accumulation in the guinea-pig. In: Morley J, Colditz IG, eds. *Eosinophils in Asthma*. London: Academic Press, 1988;4:201–212.
16. Chapman ID, Hoshiko K, Mazzoni L, Morley J. Characteristics of airway hyperreactivity following intravenous infusion of endotoxin in the guinea-pig. *Br J Pharmacol* 1993;108:210P.
17. Hoshiko K, Morley J. Allergic bronchospasm and airway hyperreactivity in the guinea-pig. *Jpn J Pharmacol* 1993;63(in press).
18. Sanjar S, Kristersson A, Mazzoni L, Morley J, Schaeublin E. Increased airway reactivity in the guinea-pig follows exposure to intravenous isoprenaline. *J Physiol* 1990;425:43–54.
19. Hoshiko K, Morley J. Exaccerbation of airway hyperreactivity by ($\pm$)salubtamol in sensitized guinea-pigs. *Jpn J Pharmacol* 1993;63(in press).
20. Murlas CG, Roum JH. Sequence of pathologic changes in the airway mucosa of guinea-pigs during ozone-induced bronchial hyperreactivity. *Am Rev Respir Dis* 1985;131:314–320.
21. Chapman ID, Kristersson A, Mathelin G, Schaeublin E, Mazzoni L, Boubekeur K, Murphy N, Morley J. Effects of a potassium channel opener (SDZ PCO 400) on guinea-pig and human pulmonary airways. *Br J Pharmacol* 1992;106:423–429.
22. Sanjar S, Mazzoni L, Schaeublin E, Smith D, Morley J. The effect of prophylactic anti-asthma drugs on PAF-induced airway hyperreactivity. *Jpn J Pharmacol* 1989;51:151–160.
23. Hoskiko K, Kristersson A, Morley J. Ketotifen inhibits exacerbation of allergic airway hyperreactivity by racemic-salbutamol in the guinea-pig. *J Allergy Clin Immunol* 1992;91:909–916.
24. Hall AK, MacLagan J. Effect of cromakalim on cholinergic neurotransmission in the guinea-pig trachea. *Br J Pharmacol* 1988;92:792P.
25. McCaig DJ, de Jonckheere B. Effect of cromakalim on bronchoconstriction evoked by cholinergic nerve stimulation in guinea-pig isolated trachea. *Br J Pharmacol* 1989;98:662–668.
26. Ichinose M, Barnes PJ. A potassium channel activator modulates both excitatory non-cholinergic and cholinergic neurotransmission in guinea pig airways. *J Pharmacol Exp Ther* 1990;252:1207–1212.
27. Foster A, Chapman ID, Mazzoni L, Morley J. Resolution of airway obstruction by reduction of airway hyperreactivity. *Br J Pharmacol* 1992;106:3P.
28. Kume H, Takai A, Tokuno H, Tomita T. Regulation of Ca^{2+}-dependent K^+-channel activity in tracheal myocytes by phosphorylation. *Nature* 1989;341:152–154.
29. Bowring NE, Arch JRS, Buckle DR, Taylor JF. Comparison of the airways relaxant and hypotensive potencies of the potassium channel activators BRL 55834 and levcromakalim (BRL 38227) in vivo in guinea-pig and rat. *Br J Pharmacol* 1993;in press.
30. Sheffer AL. Guidelines for the diagnosis and management of asthma. *J Allergy Clin Immunol* 1991;88:427–534.
31. Toogood JH. Complications of topical steroid therapy for asthma. *Am Rev Respir Dis* 1990;141:S89–S96.
32. Lundgren R, Soderberg M, Horstedt P, Stenling R. Morphological studies of bronchial

mucosal biopsies from asthmatics before and after ten years of treatment with inhaled steroids. *Eur Respir J* 1988;1:883–889.

33. Woolcock AJ, Jenkins CR. Clinical responses to corticosteroids. In: Kaliner MA, Barnes PJ, Persson CGA, eds. *Asthma; its pathology and treatment*. New York: Marcel Dekker, 1991;633–666.
34. Williams AJ, Lee TH, Cochrane GM, Hopkirk A, Vyse T, Chiew F, Lavender E, Richards DH, Owen S, Stone P, Church S, Woodcock AA. Attenuation of nocturnal asthma by cromakalim. *Lancet* 1990;336:334–335.
35. Magnussen H, Rabe KF. Low dose fenoterol aerosol protects against histamine-induced bronchoconstriction in mild asthmatics: a dose response study. *Clin Exp Allergy* 1992;22:690–693.
36. Jenne JW, Ahrens RC. Pharmacokinetics of beta-adrenergic compounds. In: Jenne JW, Murphy S, eds. *Drug therapy for asthma: research and clinical practice*. New York, Basel: Marcel Dekker, 1987;31:213–258.
37. Cheung D, Timmers AC, Zwinderman AH, Bel AH, Dijkman JH, Sterk PJ. Long-term effects of a long-acting beta$_2$-adrenoceptor agonist, salmeterol, on airway hyperresponsiveness in patients with mild asthma. *N Engl J Med* 1992;327:1198–1203.
38. O'Connor BJ, Aikman SL, Barnes PJ. Tolerance to the nonbronchodilator effects of inhaled beta$_2$-agonists in asthma. *N Engl J Med* 1992;327:1204–1208.
39. Morley J. Adverse reactions to sympathomimetics in laboratory animals. In: Costello JF, Mann RD, eds. *Beta agonists and the treatment of asthma*. Carnforth, UK: Parthenon Press, 1992;55–65.
40. Conolly ME, Hui KK, Borst SE, Jenne JW. Beta-adrenergic tachyphylaxis (desensitisation) and functional antagonism. In: Jenne JW, Murphy S, eds. *Drug therapy for asthma*. New York: Marcel Dekker, 1987;259–296.
41. Spitzer WO, Suissa S, Ernst P, Horwitz RI, Habbick B, Cockcroft D, Boivin J-F, McNutt M, Buist AS, Rebuck AS. The use of beta-agonists and the risk of death and near death from asthma. *N Engl J Med* 1992;326:501–506.
42. Chapman ID, Mazzoni L, Morley J. Action of SDZ PCO 400 and Cromakalim on airway smooth muscle in vivo. *Agents Actions* 1991;34(suppl):53–62.

Drugs and the Lung,
edited by C.P. Page and W.J. Metzger.
Raven Press, Ltd., New York © 1994

11

Selective Phosphodiesterase Isozyme Inhibitors

Theodore J. Torphy, *Kenneth J. Murray and
*Jonathan R. S. Arch

*Department of Inflammation and Respiratory Pharmacology, SmithKline Beecham
Pharmaceuticals, King of Prussia, Pennsylvania 19406-0939; *Department of
Cellular Biochemistry, SmithKline Beecham Pharmaceuticals,
Welwyn, Herts AL6 9AR, United Kingdom*

Spurred by the recognition that airway inflammation plays a fundamental role in the pathophysiology of asthma (1,2), the focus of research related to discovering novel anti-asthmatic drugs has undergone a marked change. Whereas research once concentrated on bronchodilators, agents that provide acute symptomatic relief, the emphasis of most drug discovery efforts over the last decade has centered on novel anti-inflammatory drugs, agents that have the potential to alter the course of the disease. Although regulation of inflammatory and immune cell dysfunction is likely to remain the major focus of anti-asthmatic drug therapy for the foreseeable future, the recently reported link between the use of β-adrenoceptor agonists and diminished control of asthma (3–5) has renewed interest in discovering novel bronchodilators with unique molecular mechanisms of action. Thus, the inadequate control of both the acute and chronic manifestations of asthma provided by current therapies has lent substantial impetus to developing drugs with improved therapeutic profiles.

A considerable amount of interest has been generated in cyclic nucleotide phosphodiesterase (PDE) isozymes as molecular targets for novel bronchodilators and anti-inflammatory drugs (6–8). Several factors account for this interest. First, the second messengers cyclic 3',5'-adenosine monophosphate (cAMP) and cyclic 3',5'-guanosine monophosphate (cGMP) regulate the function of key cells involved in the pathophysiology of asthma. cAMP exerts a broad suppressant effect on the activity of immune and inflammatory cells (7,9–11), and both cAMP and cGMP mediate relaxation of airway smooth muscle (7,12,13). Obviously, then, inhibition of PDE activity and the consequent accumulation of cyclic nucleotides in the appropriate tissues should be of benefit in the therapy of asthma. The second factor that has led to increased interest in PDE inhibitors as anti-asthmatic agents is the recognition that at least five families of PDE isozymes exist, with each family having a somewhat distinct tissue or cellular distribution (6,7,14,15). Thus, cyclic nucleotide levels in different cells are often regulated by a different PDE isozyme or set of isozymes. The ability to target novel, isozyme-selective PDE inhibitors for specific cells or tissues of interest is a key factor in improving the side-effect profile of these compounds vis-à-vis standard, non-selective PDE inhibitors (e.g., theophylline). Finally, the ability to synthesize molecules with a remarkable degree of isozyme selectivity has been demonstrated (6,16–18). Collectively, these factors provide a compelling rationale for exploring the potential utility of isozyme-selective PDE inhibitors in the treatment of asthma.

Because the idea that isozyme-selective PDE inhibitors may be useful in the treatment of asthma is relatively new, little supportive information from the clinic is available. Consequently, most of this chapter focuses on the preclinical data that support this concept. Particular emphasis is placed on the characteristics of PDE isozymes, the role of various isozymes in the regulation of airway smooth muscle and inflammatory cell function, and factors that can alter the activity of PDEs in cells that are pertinent to the pathophysiology of asthma. Finally, the limited clinical data available are reviewed and key issues related to the development of therapeutically useful compounds are discussed.

PHOSPHODIESTERASE ISOZYMES

Nomenclature and Characteristics

PDEs inactivate cyclic nucleotides by catalyzing the hydrolysis of their 3′-phosphoester bonds to form inactive 5′-nucleotide products. At least five different families of PDE isozymes have been identified (14,15). These isozymes can be distinguished by several characteristics, including their primary amino acid sequence, kinetic behavior, substrate preference, subunit organization, regulatory properties, susceptibility to phosphorylation, and sensitivity to synthetic inhibitors. The PDE isozyme classification and nomenclature most widely accepted is detailed in Table 1. Listed in Table 2 are examples of archetypical isozyme-selective PDE inhibitors.

PDE isozymes that are stimulated by Ca^{2+}/calmodulin belong to a family designated PDE I. Ca^{2+}/calmodulin allosterically interacts with this PDE to markedly increase catalytic activity. The increased catalytic activity in response to Ca^{2+}/calmodulin results from a decreased K_m and an increased V_{max} (40,41). Based upon biochemical characteristics at least two subtypes of this isozyme exist, one of which (PDE I_α) hydrolyzes cGMP ($K_m \sim 3$

TABLE 1. *Characteristics of phosphodiesterase isozymes[a]*

Family	Isozyme	K_m (μM)[b]	
		cAMP	cGMP
I_α[c]	Ca^{2+}/CaM-stimulated	30	3
I_β[c]	Ca^{2+}/CaM-stimulated	1	2
II	cGMP-stimulated	10	30
III	cGMP-inhibited	0.2	0.2
IV	cAMP-specific	3	>3000
V	cGMP-specific	150	1

[a]Nomenclature and values are from refs. 7,14,15,17.

[b]Kinetic values are approximate and vary depending on species, tissue, isolation procedure, and enzyme purity. The existence of multiple subtypes within a single isozyme family can also contribute to kinetic heterogeneity.

[c]Kinetically distinct subtypes of PDE I are arbitrarily designated PDE I_α and PDE I_β.

TABLE 2. *Examples of isozyme-selective PDE inhibitors*

Isozyme	Selective inhibitors	IC_{50} or [K_i] (μM)[a]	Reference
PDE I_α	Trifluoperazine[b]	1	19
	Vinpocetine	[14]	20
	8-Methoxymethyl-IBMX[c]	4	21
PDE I_β	Trifluoperazine[b,d]	1	19
PDE II	None		
PDE III	Cilostamide	[0.005]	22
	Enoximone	3	23
	Imazodan	8	24
	Milrinone	[0.3]	25
	Org 9935	0.15	26
	Siguazodan	0.8	27
	SK&F 94120	[7]	28
	SK&F 95654	0.7	29
	Trequinsin	0.0003	30
PDE IV	Denbufylline	[0.8]	31
	Nitraquazone	2	32
	Rolipram	[0.9]	33
	Ro 20-1724	5	33
	Tibenelast	15	34
PDE III/IV	Benzafentrine	[0.3]/[0.5][e]	35
	Org 30029	24/16[e]	36
	Zardaverine	0.6/0.8[e]	37
PDE V	MY-5445	[0.5]	22
	SK&F 96231	[2]	38
	Zaprinast	0.4	39

[a]IC_{50}s determined in the presence of $\sim$ 1 μM cAMP or cGMP.

[b]Trifluoperazine and other phenothiazines act as noncompetitive inhibitors by antagonizing calmodulin.

[c]IBMX, 3-isobutyl-1-methylxanthine.

[d]Effects of vinpocetine and 8-methoxymethyl-3-isobutyl-1-methylxanthine on PDE I_β are unknown.

[e]The first number represents IC_{50} or K_i for PDE III and the second number represents the IC_{50} for PDE IV.

μmol/L) with a greater affinity than cAMP ($K_m \sim$ 40 μmol/L) (41), whereas a second form (PDE I_β) displays little substrate preference ($K_m \sim$ 2 μmol/L for both cAMP and cGMP) (42). Two compounds, vinpocetine and 8-methoxymethyl-3-isobutyl-1-methylxanthine, have been reported to be selective inhibitors of PDE I (Table 2). In addition, trifluoperazine and other calmodulin antagonists inhibit the Ca^{2+}/calmodulin-dependent component of PDE I activity.

PDE II has a high K_m for both cAMP and cGMP ($K_m \sim$ 10–30 μmol/L) and is alloserically activated by low concentrations of cGMP (43). In the absence of cGMP, PDE II displays positive cooperativity with respect to cAMP hydrolysis. In the presence of low concentrations of cGMP (0.1–1 μmol/L), the degree of cooperativity is reduced along with the apparent K_m for cAMP. Inhibitors of PDE II with substantial isozyme selectivity have yet to be reported.

PDE III hydrolyzes both cAMP and cGMP with low K_m ($\sim$ 0.2 μmol/L), but its V_{max} for cAMP is at least tenfold greater than its V_{max} for cGMP (44,45). Cyclic GMP thus serves as a potent competitive inhibitor of PDE III–mediated cAMP hydrolysis, a characteristic that has resulted in this isozyme being named the cGMP-inhibited PDE. As discussed later, this isozyme is subject to phosphorylation by at least two protein kinases (46) and is selectively inhibited by a number of compounds, examples of which are listed in Table 2. Consistent with the important functional role of PDE III in the cardiovascular system and in platelets (6,16), several of these compounds are being developed as inotrope/vasodilators or anti-aggregatory agents.

As its name implies, the cAMP-specific PDE, or PDE IV, has a K_m for cAMP ($\sim$ 3 μmol/L) that is three orders of magnitude less than its K_m for cGMP (47,48). This enzyme also contains a high affinity binding site for the PDE IV-selective inhibitor, rolipram (47). Rolipram binds to this site with a K_d of 1 nmol/L, whereas it inhibits human recombinant PDE IV catalytic activity with an apparent K_i of 60 nmol/L. Moreover, the rank order of potency of various PDE inhibitors against PDE IV catalytic activity is distinct from that for competition with the high affinity rolipram-binding site. Thus, the functional relationship between the high affinity rolipram-binding site and PDE IV catalytic activity is not clear. It has been proposed, however, that this high affinity binding site could represent an allosteric site on PDE IV or could reflect high affinity binding of rolipram to the catalytic site of a distinct, noninterconvertable tertiary or quaternary conformation of the enzyme (47,49). In addition to rolipram, other PDE IV–selective inhibitors include denbufylline, nitraquazone, and Ro 20-1724 (Table 2).

PDE V, also called the cGMP-specific PDE, has a K_m for cAMP of 150 μmol/L and a K_m for cGMP of 1 μmol/L. PDE V is present in large amounts in the retina and is critically involved in phototransduction (14). PDE V subtypes are also found in other tissues, particularly smooth muscle, and this isozyme has recently been purified to homogeneity from bovine lung (50). Purified PDE V serves as a substrate for both cAMP-dependent and cGMP-dependent protein kinase (51), although the functional consequences of this phosphorylation are not clear. PDE V is selectively inhibited by zaprinast, MY-5445, and SK&F 96231 (Table 2).

In considering the therapeutic implications of the existence of multiple PDE isozymes, it is important to be mindful of a few key points. First, although there is a distinct tissue distribution of these isozymes, many tissues contain multiple PDEs. Consequently, the "tissue specificity" of the various isozymes tends to be relative rather than absolute. Second, as discussed below, multiple subtypes of each of the five isozymes are likely to exist. Thus, if these subtypes have a unique tissue distribution, the opportunities to design inhibitors that target individual tissues or cell types may extend far beyond those associated with broadly inhibiting all subtypes within one of the five families illustrated in Table 1. Finally, although some PDEs possess a degree of selectivity for either cAMP or cGMP, all isozymes will hydrolyze both cyclic nucleotides. Consequently, it is virtually impossible to gauge the functional importance of individual isozymes in tissues that contain multiple forms simply by identifying the PDEs present. Instead, detailed analyses must be carried out in which the biochemical and functional responses to isozyme-selective PDE inhibitors are evaluated in intact tissues.

Molecular Biology

Enormous progress has been made in the identification of genes and complementary deoxyribonucleic acids (cDNAs) that encode PDEs. In fact, it has become clear that different genes or families of genes encode the functionally distinct PDE isozymes described in Table 1. The discovery, evaluation, classification, and expression of these genes and cDNAs has been described in detail elsewhere (15,52) and no attempt will be made to duplicate this information. Instead, attention will be focused on how these differences may account for the unique catalytic and regulatory properties of individual PDE isozymes.

Amino acid sequences deduced from cDNA clones or direct sequencing of purified protein have yielded important information regarding enzyme structure and function (15,52). The most remarkable observation made from sequence analyses of various isozymes is the substantial homology among members of various PDE families over an internal sequence of ~ 270 amino acids (Fig. 1A). This region contains threonine, serine, and histidine residues that are invariant in a dozen PDE sequences. This suggests that this 270–amino acid region accounts for a key function common to all PDEs, e.g., catalytic activity. Indeed, analysis of the catalytic activity of various PDE IV mutants confirms this proposal and further indicates that one threonine

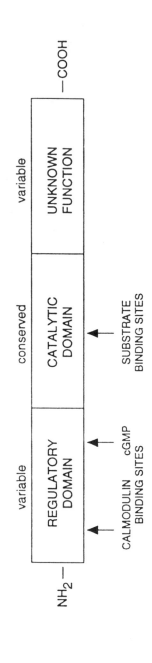

A

variable | conserved | variable

NH₂— | REGULATORY DOMAIN | CATALYTIC DOMAIN | UNKNOWN FUNCTION | —COOH

CALMODULIN BINDING SITES cGMP BINDING SITES SUBSTRATE BINDING SITES

B

```
205                                                                                                        260
hmPDEIV   LKKFRIPVDT MVTYMLTLED HYHADVAYHN SLHAADVLQS THVLLATPA. .......... ...LDAVFTD
rbPDEIV   ---H------ -MM------- ---------- ---------- ---------- .......... ...-------
hhPDEIII  FEA-K--IRE FMN-FHA--I G-R,-IP--- RIH-T---HA VWY-TTQ-IP GLSTVINDHG STSDSDSDSG FTHGHMGYVF SKTYNVTDDK YGC-SGNIPA
hrPDEV    VD--H--QEA L-RF-YS-SK G-R.KIT--- WRHGFNVG-T MFS--V-GK. .......... ..-KRY---

261                                                                                                        367
hmPDEIV   LEILAALFAA AIHDVDHPGV SNQFLINTNS ELALMYNDES VLENHHLAVG FKLL...QEY NCDIFQNLSK RQRQSLRKMV IDMVLATDMS KHMTLLADLK
rbPDEIV   ---------- ---------- ---------- ---------- ---------- ------...-E ---------- ---------- ---------- ----------
hhPDEIII  --LM-LYV-- -M-Y----R T-A--VA-SA PQ-VL---R- -----A-AA WN-FMSRPEY NF.LI--DH VEFKHF-FL- -EAI----LK --FDFV-KFN
hrPDEV    --A--MVT-- FC--I--R-T N-LYQMKSQN P--KLHGS.- I--R---EF- KT--...RDE SLN-----NR --HEHAIH-M DIAII---LA LYFKKRTMFQ

368                                                                                                        449
hmPDEIV   TMVETKKVTS SGVLLLDNYS DRIQVLRNMV H......CAD LSNPFKPLEL YRQWTDRIMA EFFQQGDRER ERGMEISP.M CDKHTA.SVE KSQVGFIDYI
rbPDEIV   ---------- ---------- ---------- ---------- ---------- ---------- ---------- ---------- ---------- ----------
hhPDEIII  GK-NDDVGI. ...DWT-EN --LL-CQMCI K.....L-- ING-A-CK-- HL---G-VN --YE---E-A SL-LP---.F M-RSAP.QLA NL-ES--SH-
hrPDEV    KIVDQSKTYE SEQE.WTQ-M MLE-TRKEI- MAMMMTAC.- --AI---W-V QS-VALLVA- --WE---L-- TVLQQNPIP- M-RNK-DELP -L------FV
```

and two histidine residues are critical for the expression of catalytic activity (53). Flanking the area of sequence homology are highly variable N-terminal and C-terminal extensions. These areas may represent regulatory domains that are targets for allosteric activators or inhibitors, or serve as substrates for phosphorylation by various protein kinases. Alternatively, these variable areas may be important for targeting newly synthesized enzymes to specific subcellular structures or organelles.

Because the catalytic regions possess a significant degree of homology, it is tempting to suggest that the structural information confering selectivity for various classes of inhibitors is contained within the N-terminal and C-terminal extensions. However, detailed sequence comparison of the catalytic domains of four PDEs reveals a more complex picture (Fig. 1B). While the catalytic domains of two subtypes of PDE IV, one from human monocyte and the other from rat brain, are nearly identical, the sequences of the catalytic domains of human PDE III and PDE V differ from each other as well as from PDE IV. Thus, inhibitor selectivity could result from either the substantial differences in the amino acid sequences of N-terminal and C-terminal extension, or more subtle differences in the sequences of catalytic domains.

It has been recognized recently that each isozyme class is composed of multiple subtypes (15). These subtypes can be encoded by distinct genes or can represent products of two or more alternately spliced mRNAs. Representative examples of cloned mammalian isozyme subtypes are listed in Table 3 and detailed discussions of these and other PDE family subtypes appear elsewhere (15,52). Sequence analyses of these PDE subtypes indicate a substantial homology among different members of the same isozyme class. For example, human recombinant PDE IV_A and PDE IV_B possess a 76% amino acid identity over the entire sequence and a 90% amino acid identity within the catalytic domain (61,62). Interestingly, human PDE IV_A and PDE IV_B have greater sequence homology with their rat counterparts than they have with each other (62). Thus, there appears to be a greater degree of sequence conservation between the same isozyme subtype from different species than among different subtypes from the same species.

FIG. 1. Structure of cyclic nucleotide PDEs. **(A)** The conserved region, corresponding to the putative catalytic domain (see text), is flanked by regions of variable length (not drawn to scale) and sequence. Binding sites for cyclic nucleotide substrates and allosteric regulators (calmodulin and cGMP) are indicated. **(B)** Alignment of the deduced primary amino acid sequence of the conserved regions of four cloned cyclic nucleotide PDEs: hmPDE IV (hPDE IV_A), a cAMP-specific PDE from human monocytes (61); rbPDE IV, a cAMP-specific PDE from rat brain (59); hhPDE III, a cGMP-inhibited cAMP PDE from human heart (57); hrPDE V, a cGMP-specific PDE from human retina (64). *Dashes* indicate identical amino acid sequences; *periods* indicate sequence gaps introduced to maximize alignment. Sequences are compared to part of the conserved domain (residues 205 to 449) of hmPDE IV (61). (From ref. 18.)

TABLE 3. *Cloned mammalian PDEs[a]*

Isozyme family	Species	Tissue source	References	Comments
I	Rat	Brain	53a	
	Bovine	Brain	54	
II	Bovine	Retina	55	
	Bovine	Adrenal cortex	56	
III	Human	Heart	57	
IV	Rat	Brain	58	
	Rat	Brain	59	
	Rat	Testis	60	4 cDNAs (2 correspond to rat brain clones)
	Human	Monocyte	61	
	Human	Brain	62	
V	Mouse	Retina	63	α and β subunits
	Bovine	Retina	64	α subunit
	Human	Retina	64	α subunit

[a]PDE isozyme families for which cDNA clones have been obtained are listed, along with the species and tissue source. Unless otherwise indicated (see text), the cDNA clones within isozyme families II, III, and IV represent distinct subtypes. cDNAs for PDE V α subunits from mouse, bovine, and human encode highly homologous proteins.

The existence of multiple subtypes within a single isozyme class holds an obvious implication for the design of enzyme inhibitors. Specifically, targeting a single subtype within a family of isozymes may result in a degree of tissue or cell selectivity that is even greater than that obtained with currently available isozyme-selective inhibitors. Although the possibility of improving cellular selectivity by targeting isozyme subtypes is supported by a recent report indicating a differential tissue distribution of human PDE IV_A versus PDE IV_B (62), it remains to be seen whether structural heterogeneity among isozyme subtypes can be exploited by rational drug design.

AIRWAY SMOOTH MUSCLE

Role of Cyclic Nucleotides

We now discuss the evidence that selective PDE inhibitors can act as direct relaxants of airway smooth muscle (ASM). Emphasis is given to the end physiological effect (i.e., relaxation) rather than to the molecular mechanisms that underlie the process, as the biochemical events that result in contraction or relaxation of ASM are not fully defined. Despite this, it is widely accepted that increasing the cAMP and/or cGMP content mediates relaxation of ASM (12,13) and this tenet provides a rationale for the use of PDE inhibitors as bronchodilators. The relaxant properties of cyclic nucleotides are largely derived from studies using β-adrenoceptor agonists and nitrovasodilators and it should be remembered that, as with these agents, the efficacy of PDE inhibitors can vary from species to species and due to the nature of the contractant used (65,66). Moreover, in spite of the virtually overwhelming evidence that both cAMP and cGMP can induce relaxation of smooth muscle, it should not be assumed that this is the only pathway by which cyclic nucleotide-elevating agonists elicit bronchodilation. For example, a recent study using human isolated ASM cells indicates that β-adrenoceptors are coupled directly to Ca^{2+}-dependent potassium channels via a stimulatory guanine nucleotide binding protein (67). Thus, it is possible that a portion of the bronchodilatory activity of β-adrenoceptor agonists results from a non-cAMP-mediated activation of potassium channels.

It is assumed, in common with striated muscle and other smooth muscle types, that contraction of airway smooth muscle is ultimately due to an increase in intracellular free Ca^{2+} ($[Ca^{2+}]_i$) (68). Therefore, there are only two broad mechanisms by which contraction can be modulated: (a) alteration in the levels of $[Ca^{2+}]_i$ and (b) changes in the sensitivity of the contractile apparatus to Ca^{2+}. Evidence exists suggesting that cyclic nucleotides can affect both of these processes.

The commonly held hypothesis of smooth muscle contraction is that Ca^{2+} by binding to calmodulin activates the enzyme myosin light chain kinase and that the subsequent phosphorylation of myosin light chains permits the cyclic interaction of the actin- and myosin-containing filaments. Although there is considerable evidence that contraction of tracheal muscle is determined by the degree of phosphorylation of myosin light chain (69), the presence of a second regulatory system is also suggested by experiments in which tension and myosin light chain phosphorylation are uncoupled (70,71). Although there are a limited number of studies with intact preparations that show that cAMP-mediated relaxation of ASM is due, at least in part, to effects on contractile proteins (72,73), the regulation of myosin light chain kinase by cAMP-dependent protein kinase is a widely invoked mechanism to describe the relaxant effects of cAMP (69). However, while this is an attractive hypothesis, experimental observations have cast doubt on whether it operates in intact ASM (74). Similarly, there are few reports indicating an effect of cGMP on contractile proteins (but see ref. 73).

There is more evidence that cAMP and cGMP can regulate $[Ca^{2+}]_i$ in ASM, although the precise mechanism remains to be determined (12,13,66). Agents that act through the cAMP pathway have been shown to reduce $[Ca^{2+}]_i$ in bovine ASM cells (73,74a,75) and in canine trachealis (76), although it appears that cGMP may also be more effective than cAMP in lowering $[Ca^{2+}]_i$ (73,74a). $[Ca^{2+}]_i$ may also be lowered due to effects on inositol metabolism and/or ion channels (13,65,77), and it is possible that the importance of each effect could vary depending on the species or the type of contractile agent used to induce tone.

Isozyme Profiles

As summarized in Table 4, "traditional" methods of analysis have been used to identify and characterize PDE isozymes in ASM from several spe-

TABLE 4. *Phosphodiesterase isozymes detected in airway smooth muscle and the functional effect of selective inhibitors*

Species	Isozymes present	References	Inhibitors evaluated	References
Bovine	I,II,(III)[a],IV[b],V	35, 78, 79	IV,III/IV,(III)[d],(V)	78, 79, 85, 88
Canine	I,II,III,IV,V	28	III,IV,(V)	65, 90
Guinea pig	III,IV[c]	80	III,IV,III/IV[e],V	38, 80, 91–94
Human	I[b],II,III,IV[b],V	81–84	III,IV,III/IV[e],V	81, 83, 84, 97

[a]Isozyme shown in parenthesis has not been detected or is present in low amounts.
[b]There is evidence for multiple forms of the isozyme.
[c]The conditions used would not have detected all isozymes (see text).
[d]Inhibitors of the isozymes shown in parenthesis have been shown to have little or no relaxant activity. It should be noted that the relaxant activity of any inhibitor may vary with the dose and the particular contractant used (see text for fuller details).
[e]The data suggest that a combined III/IV inhibitor is more effective than either a III or IV inhibitor alone.

cies. This involves separating activity by anion-exchange chromatography followed by determinating the kinetic properties and sensitivity of the resultant peaks to isozyme-selective inhibitors. However, there are some inherent limitations to this method, one of the most obvious being the usually heterogeneous nature of the tissue extract being evaluated. Studies using trachealis are no exception and, whereas most investigators take care to use the airway smooth muscle, it is likely that these preparations contain other cell types. The second major pitfall is related to analysis of peaks that contain more than one isozyme, as the results are often difficult to interpret and it is preferable to use further purification methods.

The supernatant fraction of a bovine tracheal smooth muscle extract contains greater than 95% of the total cellular PDE activity (78) and gives three major peaks of PDE activity on anion-exchange chromatography (35,78,79). When the first peak is subjected to calmodulin affinity-chromatography two activities are resolved. A Ca^{2+}/calmodulin–dependent PDE with high affinity and modest selectivity for cAMP remains bound to the column, whereas a cGMP-selective, zaprinast-inhibited activity is not retained, indicating that this peak contained both PDE I, probably the β subtype, and PDE V (78). The second peak can be identified as PDE II by virtue of the fact that the hydrolysis of cAMP is stimulated by cGMP. The third peak shows selectivity for cAMP over cGMP as a substrate and is inhibited by selective PDE IV inhibitors. However, cGMP and selective PDE III inhibitors cause a small (5–12%) decrease in hydrolysis of cAMP mediated by the activity in this peak. Therefore, the third peak appears to be a mixture of PDE III and IV, with the latter being the predominant activity (35,78,79). In addition, a further peak of rolipram-inhibited activity is detectable, suggesting the presence of multiple forms of PDE IV (78).

Characterization of the PDE isozymes from canine trachealis supernatants produces similar, although not identical, results to those described above (28). As with bovine trachealis, three major peaks of PDE activity can be resolved by anion-exchange chromatography. The first peak can be separated into PDE I and PDE V by calmodulin affinity-chromatography, the second peak contains PDE II, and the third peak contains both PDE III and PDE IV. However, as cGMP causes a marked inhibition of the third peak, it appears that canine trachea contains a relatively higher proportion of PDE III than does bovine trachea. Analysis of the PDE content of the particulate fraction from canine trachea shows it to contain PDE I, III, IV, and V (28).

Guinea pig trachea contains PDE III and IV (80), although this is unlikely to be a complete list as the assays conducted would not have revealed the presence of other isozymes.

As the PDE content of tissues may vary between species, reports on human airways are of particular relevance. These studies suggest that human ASM contains all five isozymes with multiple forms of PDE I (81) and PDE IV (82). Similarly, human peripheral airways contain all five isozymes (83,84) and again there is evidence for multiple forms of PDE I and of PDE IV (83).

In conclusion, ASM from a number of species, including human, has been shown to contain members of all five PDE isozyme families and in some cases may contain more than one form of PDE I and IV. PDE III does not give a distinct peak of activity, although it appears to be present in all studies. However, these biochemical analyses simply demonstrate the presence of a PDE isozyme in a tissue and give no information as to its physiological role. This aspect is discussed below.

Effects of Isozyme-Selective Inhibitors *In Vitro*

The effects of selective PDE inhibitors have been studied on bovine, canine, and guinea pig tracheal preparations and, in the main, the results reflect the differing PDE content of these species (see Table 4). There is agreement that PDE IV inhibitors are more effective relaxants of bovine trachealis than PDE III inhibitors, consistent with the small amount of PDE III in this tissue. In bovine trachealis strips precontracted with methacholine or histamine, the selective PDE III inhibitors, SK&F 94120, siguazodan (SK&F 94836), milrinone, and Org 9935 all fail to cause complete relaxation. In contrast, the PDE IV-selective inhibitor, rolipram, completely relaxes bovine trachealis with EC_{50} values in the range of 0.08 to 1 μmol/L (78,85). The dual PDE III/IV inhibitors, benzafentrine (AH 21-132) (79) and Org 30029 (78) are also effective relaxants, presumably due to their activity as PDE IV inhibitors. The biochemical effects of these inhibitors in intact tissues are compatible with their physiological effects: (a) benzafentrine raises cAMP levels and activates cAMP-dependent protein kinase (79) and (b) rolipram and SK&F 94120 increase cAMP and inhibit agonist-stimulated inositol triphosphate (IP_3) production (86,87). Despite the presence of PDE V in bovine trachealis, its selective inhibitor, zaprinast, has little or no relaxant action (78,85,88). However, there is evidence that zaprinast inhibits PDE V in intact bovine tracheal smooth muscle as it increases cGMP content by itself and causes a synergistic increase with sodium nitroprusside (88), although the possibility that high concentrations of zaprinast also inhibit PDE I should be considered (89).

Siguazodan has been shown to be an effective relaxant of canine trachealis in keeping with the relatively high proportion of PDE III activity in this tissue (28,65). Another report has shown a role for both PDE III and PDE IV in regulating the tone and cAMP content of canine trachealis (90). In this case, the protocol employed was to contract tissues with 1 or 3 μmol/L methacholine, conditions under which the PDE inhibitors, when used alone, cause no relaxation. Therefore, the ability of the PDE inhibitors to regulate cAMP metabolism was assessed by their ability to potentiate isoproterenol-induced relaxation and cAMP accumulation. Pretreatment with either a selective PDE III inhibitor (SK&F 94120) or a selective PDE IV inhibitor (Ro 20-01724) results in potentiation of both the physiological and biochemical response of the tissue to isoproterenol. The combination of SK&F 94120 and Ro 20-1724 produces an additive response that is not enhanced by the addition of the nonselective PDE inhibitor, 3-isobutyl-1-methylxanthine (IBMX). These results show that inhibition of either PDE III or PDE IV can decrease cAMP hydrolysis and that other PDEs (e.g., PDE I, II, and V) are unlikely to be involved. A similar approach was undertaken to study the effects of PDE inhibitors on sodium nitroprusside–induced relaxation and increases in cGMP content (90). Both IBMX and zaprinast, used singly, potentiate the response to sodium nitroprusside, and the combination of the two produces further potentiation. In contrast, neither siguazodan nor Ro 20-1724 alters responses to sodium nitroprusside. Collectively, these results suggest that PDE V and PDE I and/or PDE II are responsible for cGMP metabolism in canine trachealis (90).

Selective inhibitors of PDE III, IV, and V have all been shown to relax guinea pig tracheal preparations. A number of PDE III inhibitors including milrinone, CI-930, and SK&F 94120 will relax tissue precontracted with a variety of agonists (80,91–93). There are contrasting reports on the effects of cyclooxygenase inhibitors, as the relaxant action of milrinone is completely blocked by these agents (91), whereas they have little effect on SK&F 94120–induced relaxation (92,93). The PDE IV inhibitors, rolipram and Ro 20-1724, relax both histamine and carbachol-contracted preparations, but with increased potency against the former (80,93). In contrast to the results obtained with canine trachealis, combinations of PDE III and PDE IV inhibitors produce synergistic relaxation of guinea pig tracheal strips. As pretreatment with 3 μmol/L CI-930 (which had no effect by itself) reduces the EC_{50} value for rolipram-induced relaxation from 100 to 0.02 μmol/L (80), it is not surprising that the dual III/IV inhibitor benzafentrine is also an effective relaxant (94). Also in contrast to results from other species, relaxation of guinea pig trachea is obtained with the PDE V inhibitors, zaprinast (93), and SK&F 96231 (38), although zaprinast is ineffective when administered prior to spasmogen challenge in this species (95).

As with other species, the effects of selective PDE inhibitors on tone in human airways are dependent on the contractant. For example, rolipram and Org 9935 (PDE III inhibitor) relax with equal potency human bronchial preparations contracted with either histamine or methacholine (83). In contrast, zaprinast is more effective against histamine-contracted tissues and even in this case is considerably less potent than rolipram or Org 9935. Both rolipram and Org 9935 produce biphasic concentration-response curves indicating that dual inhibition of PDE III and IV may be the most effective mechanism for achieving relaxation in this tissue (83). A similar conclusion was drawn from another study in which it was found that the dual PDE III/IV inhibitor, zardaverine, is the most effective relaxant of inherent tone in rings of human peripheral airway (84). In this preparation, SK&F 94120 also causes complete relaxation, whereas only partial relaxation is observed with rolipram or zaprinast. Another III/IV inhibitor, benzafentrine, has also been shown to effectively reduce spontaneous tone in human bronchus (96). In human tracheal strips, rolipram is ineffective in reducing spontaneous tone, although another PDE IV inhibitor (denbufylline) as well as zaprinast and SK&F 94120 cause relaxation (97). However, when this preparation is contracted with a low concentration of methacholine, rolipram and SK&F 94120 are both more potent relaxants than either denbufylline or zaprinast. In primary cultures of human airway smooth muscle, rolipram, but not SK&F 94120, increases cAMP content (98).

Effects of Isozyme-Selective Inhibitors *In Vivo*

The PDE III inhibitors imazodan and CI-930 potently and completely reverse 5-hydroxytryptamine–induced bronchoconstriction in β-blocked anesthetized dogs (99). Another PDE III inhibitor, siguazodan, decreases pulmonary resistance, with a relatively smaller effect on dynamic lung compliance, in spontaneously breathing anesthetized dogs (38). Predictably, pronounced cardiovascular changes (increased cardiac contractility, decreased blood pressure) accompany these respiratory effects. A number of PDE III inhibitors have also been shown to be effective bronchodilators in various anesthetized guinea pig preparations (29,38,80,100).

In contrast to the effects of the PDE III inhibitors, the PDE IV inhibitors Ro 20-1724 and rolipram only partially reverse 5-hydroxytryptamine–induced bronchoconstriction in the dog, although there are no concomitant cardiovascular changes with these compounds (99). Similarly, these two agents (especially rolipram; $ED_{50} = 0.0008$ mg/kg) potently reverse histamine-induced bronchoconstriction in the guinea pig (80). The dual III/IV inhibitor benzafentrine is active against a variety of constrictors in the guinea pig (96), and the PDE V inhibitors zaprinast and SK&F 96231 reverse U46619 or histamine-induced bronchoconstriction in guinea pigs (38).

Overall, there is reasonable consensus that, of the presently available selective PDE inhibitors, only PDE IV inhibitors are effective relaxants of bovine trachea. In the dog, bronchodilatation can be elicited by both PDE III and IV inhibitors and, in the guinea pig, PDE III, IV, and V inhibitors have bronchodilatory effects. The question is which, if any, of these species is comparable to human airways. The data, at present, suggest that inhibitors of PDE III, IV, and possibly V have potential use as bronchodilators in man although the direct relaxant action of any selective PDE inhibitor has yet to be demonstrated unequivocally in large clinical trials (see below).

INFLAMMATORY CELLS

Role of Cyclic Nucleotides

There is abundant evidence that elevation of cAMP levels suppresses the activities of inflammatory cells (for reviews see 7,9,11,101). Every stage of the inflammatory process appears to be inhibited by cAMP, except that lymphocyte adherence to endothelial cells may be enhanced (Table 5). By inhibiting cellular proliferation, motility, and chemotaxis, cAMP may prevent proinflammatory cells from reaching a potential site of inflammation. Even if some cells do reach their target, the release of toxic proteins or proteases, reactive oxygen species, biogenic amines, and lipid inflammatory mediators will be suppressed by an elevation of cAMP, as will the effect of the inflammatory mediators on plasma extravasation. Furthermore, cAMP may prevent the release of cytokines from these cells, so that the recruitment and activation of further proinflammatory cells is suppressed.

The evidence for these roles of cAMP stems from studies with adenylyl cyclase activators (hormone mimics, forskolin, and cholera toxin), PDE inhibitors, and cAMP analogues, and will be outlined for each cell type in turn, except that discussion of studies involving isozyme selective PDE inhibitors is deferred until later in this section. The more rigorous studies have involved the measurement of cAMP levels, but in others it has been assumed that levels are increased. This is especially pertinent in the case of theophylline in view of the long-standing debate as to whether, at therapeutic doses, it acts via PDE inhibition or some other mechanism, such as adenosine receptor antagonism (10,102,103). Blockade of A_1 (but not A_2) adenosine receptors may, like PDE inhibition, lead to elevation of cAMP levels, and the dose levels employed in many animal studies are probably sufficient to cause a pronounced inhibition of all PDE isozymes (including those that hydrolyze cGMP), but other messenger systems may also be affected. As

TABLE 5. Relationships between inflammatory cell function and cyclic nucleotide levels

Cell type	Effect of cyclic nucleotide-elevating agents or cyclic nucleotide analogues		Association of cyclic nucleotide concentration changes with cell activation
	Cyclic AMP	**Cyclic GMP**	
Eosinophil	Number *in vivo* ↓ (111–124)		
	Chemotaxis ↓ (120,123,126)		
	Degranulation *in vivo* ↓ (109)		
	Degranulation *in vitro* → (116)		
	Reactive oxygen ↓ (132), (101,132,133,135,136)	Reactive oxygen ↑ (136)	
	TxA_2 ↓ (112,132,136,138)		
Neutrophil	Chemotaxis and chemokinesis ↓ (140,144,145)	Chemotaxis ↑ (144)	Cyclic AMP feedback role? ↑ (143,147)
	Aggregation ↓ (141,146)		
	Degranulation ↓ (140,146,147)	Degranulation ↑↓ (144,151)	
	Reactive oxygen ↓ (140,146,149–151)		
	PAF,LTB_4 ↓ (153)		
Mast cell/basophil	Histamine, LTC_4 ↓ (158–161)	Histamine ↑→ (7)	
	Degranulation ↓ (170,171)		
	Reactive oxygen and lipid mediators ↓ (166–171)		
Monocyte/macrophage	$TNF\alpha$ ↑↓ (165,167,170), (173,176)		Cyclic AMP ↑→ (160,162)
	IL-1 ↑↓ (177), (176)		
T lymphocyte	Activation and proliferation ↓ (180–184)		Cyclic AMP feedback role? ↑ (180)
	IL-2, $IFN\alpha$ ↓ (187)		
	IL-4 ↑ (187)		
B lymphocyte	Proliferation ↓ (191)	IL-5 ↑ (187)[a]	Cyclic GMP ↑ (180,181,184)
	Immune response ↑↓ (190)		
Platelet	Number *in vivo* ↓ (194,195)	Aggregation ↓ (16,242,243)	Cyclic GMP feedback role? ↑ (16)
	Aggregation ↓ (197)		
Endothelial cell	Lymphocyte adherence ↓ (202)		
	Permeability ↓ (198,200,204–209)		

↑, ↓, and → indicate an increase, decrease, or no effect on the function or the release of the molecule described. More than one arrow indicates conflicting reports. References are given in parentheses.

[a] Involvement of cyclic GMP rather than cyclic AMP speculative.

IL, interleukin; LT, leukotriene; PAF, platelet-activating factor; TNF, tumor necrosis factor; Tx, thromboxane.

discussed previously, it is also inappropriate to assume that all responses to β-adrenoceptor agonists are mediated by cAMP, since it is now recognized that these agents can activate ion channels directly via G proteins (104).

Much less is known about the involvement of cGMP than of cAMP in the regulation of inflammatory cell function. Elevation of either nucleotide often has a suppressant effect but in selected instances cGMP appears to oppose the suppressant effect of cAMP. However, because of the dearth of information on the role of cGMP, we will focus solely on the functional role of cAMP as well as the regulation of its metabolism in immune and inflammatory cells, except that selected references to the effects of cGMP-elevating agents on inflammatory cell function are given in Table 5.

Eosinophils

There is strong evidence that eosinophils play a pivotal role in lung inflammation in asthma (105–107). Eosinophils mature from precursors in the bone marrow and, after circulating briefly in the blood, adhere to the vascular endothelium before moving into the tissues, where they contribute to the inflammatory process by the exocytosis of toxic granule proteins as well as the release of reactive oxygen species and lipid inflammatory mediators, such as the leukotrienes and platelet-activating factor (108).

In vitro studies suggest that cAMP has a role in eosinophil chemotaxis, since this is inhibited by isoproterenol (109), and PDE inhibitors have been shown to inhibit granulopoiesis in general in cultured bone marrow (110). But it is studies on the effects of cAMP-elevating agents on blood and lung eosinophil levels *in vivo* that point most clearly to a role for cAMP in eosinophil production or distribution. A number of studies have shown that β-adrenoceptor agonists and theophylline or other xanthines can lower blood and tissue eosinophil numbers in normal or eosinophilic humans, and in animal models of eosinophilia. In humans, blood eosinopenia or a diminished eosinophilia is elicited by isoproterenol, epinephrine, salbutamol, terbutaline, aminophylline, and the xanthine PDE inhibitor diprophylline (111–117).

Unlike humans, normal rats respond to epinephrine with eosinophilia, but this is apparently due to contraction of the spleen resulting in cell mobilization. Thus after splenectomy, epinephrine elicits a propranolol-sensitive eosinopenia (113). Blood and lung eosinophilia can be induced in rats by intravenous injection of Sephadex beads, which embolize in the pulmonary vasculature. The blood eosinophilia is reduced by isoproterenol, salbutamol, and aminophylline; isoproterenol also reduces the number of eosinophils in bronchoalveolar lavage (BAL) fluids and in lung tissue (118,119). Antigen challenge can also induce BAL eosinophilia in rats, an effect that is inhibited by theophylline and salbutamol (120).

In guinea pigs, antigen-induced BAL eosinophilia can be inhibited by the β-adrenoceptor agonists fenoterol, SOM 1122 (121), and salmeterol (122), and also by theophylline (123,124). Some investigators have failed to reproduce all these findings, however (123,125,126). Platelet-activating factor–induced BAL eosinophilia can also be inhibited with aminophylline and salmeterol, but not salbutamol (127–129).

While these *in vivo* studies support a role for cAMP-elevating drugs in the control of eosinophilia, their relevance to asthma therapy may be questioned, since chronic administration with therapeutic concentrations of β-adrenoceptor agonists does not reduce eosinophilia. This may be because β-adrenoceptors on eosinophils or other targets are rapidly down-regulated or, as described later in this chapter, because cAMP PDE activity is up-regulated. Furthermore, these studies do not show whether such drugs inhibit eosinopoiesis, reduce eosinophil survival, or redistribute eosinophils away from the blood and lung, although the latter is suggested by the total rapid ($t_\frac{1}{2}$ = 2–5 h) eosinopenia elicited by theophylline in some patients (117), which contrasts with the plasma half-life of eosinophils in normal individuals of 8 to 12 h. These studies also fail to identify the primary cellular site of action, which could be eosinophils, eosinophil precursors, or cells that release cytokines that modulate eosinophil function. Indeed, it is possible that both xanthines and β-adrenoceptor agonists act in part by stimulating corticotrophin release and elevating glucocorticosteroid levels (130,131). However, in Sephadex-treated rats, the effect of dexamethasone is distinguished from that of the cAMP-elevating drugs by its ability to reduce the number of blood mononuclear cells (118).

Studies on human and guinea pig eosinophils *in vitro* demonstrate an involvement of cAMP in regulating the release of granule proteins, oxygen species, and lipid mediators (101), but there is little or no information on the role of cAMP in cytokine-induced priming of these cells.

Isoproterenol, salbutamol, theophylline, IBMX, cAMP analogues, prostaglandin E_2 (PGE_2) and cholera toxin inhibit secretory immunoglobulin (Ig)A and especially IgG-induced release of eosinophil-derived neurotoxin from human eosinophils. The effect of β-adrenoceptor agonists is enhanced by IBMX and that of PGE_2 is associated with an elevation of cAMP levels, implicating cAMP in these responses (132). Yukawa and colleagues (133) failed to find any effect of salbutamol on opsonized zymosan- or phorbol ester-induced eosinophil peroxidase release by human or guinea pig eosinophils, even though cAMP levels were raised. These discrepancies have been ascribed to differences in the time of preincubation with the β-adrenoceptor agonist since prolonged incubation leads to receptor desensitization (101).

The release of toxic oxygen species is suppressed in human or guinea pig eosinophils by β-adrenoceptor agonists, theophylline, IBMX, or cAMP analogues (101,132–136). The effect of theophylline occurs at concentrations that inhibit PDE and raise cAMP content of intact cells (101). Lower concentrations of theophylline increase superoxide generation, probably by antagonizing the stimulation of A_2 receptors by endogenous adenosine (135).

As with eosinophil peroxidase release, Yukawa et al. (133) failed to find an effect of salbutamol on superoxide release. Giembycz and Barnes (101) found such an effect of salbutamol but the concentration-response curve for salbutamol's effect on cAMP levels was to the left of that for respiratory burst inhibition, raising questions about the role of cAMP in this response.

Leukotriene (LT)B_4–induced thromboxane A_2 release from guinea pig eosinophils is inhibited by β-adrenoceptor agonists, theophylline, and cAMP analogues (132,134,136–138). Theophylline is effective at concentrations that inhibit PDE and elevate cellular cAMP content. In contrast to superoxide generation, low concentrations of theophylline do not stimulate thromboxane A_2 production (138).

Neutrophils

Neutrophils become activated after exercise-induced bronchospasm and allergen-induced early and late asthmatic responses, and, like eosinophils, they have the potential to produce airway damage and exacerbate inflammation by releasing reactive oxygen species, proteases, cationic proteins, and lipid inflammatory mediators. However, the evidence that they are involved in ongoing clinical asthma is weak and their role may be limited to the early stages of airways inflammation (106,139).

The role of cyclic nucleotides has been reviewed elsewhere (140). Most studies have been on human neutrophils. A variety of neutrophil chemotactic and activating agents elicit small and transient increases in cAMP levels. These responses appear to be indirect, since the activating agents f Met Leu Phe and the Ca^{2+} ionophore A23187 do not stimulate adenylyl cyclase in isolated membranes. Furthermore, depending on the stimulus, increases in cAMP levels are Ca^{2+}-dependent or -independent, and enhanced by or insensitive to PDE inhibition (140). It is probable that these elevations of cAMP levels serve a feedback role, with neutrophil activation being mediated by elevation of Ca^{2+} levels and activation of protein kinase C (141,142). This view is supported by the finding that the cAMP response to f Met Leu Phe is suppressed by a putative inhibitor of adenylyl cyclase without affecting superoxide generation (143). Moreover, agents that elevate cAMP and cAMP analogues generally suppress neutrophil activity, as outlined below.

Chemotaxis and chemokinesis of neutrophils are decreased by isoproterenol, epinephrine, PDE inhibitors, cAMP and analogues, and cholera toxin (140,144,145). However, the dose of cholera toxin required to decrease chemotaxis was much greater than that required to raise cAMP levels (140).

Neutrophil degranulation, assessed by the release of acid hydrolases or β-glucuronidase in response to zymosan, latex particles, immune complexes, or f Met Leu Phe, is inhibited by β-adrenoceptor agonists, PGE_1, histamine, theophylline, and cAMP analogues (140,146,147). A number of workers have failed to reproduce these effects with β-adrenoceptor agonists, but neither did they detect an elevation in cAMP levels. This is probably because these agonists cause a rapid desensitization of the receptors (148). As in the case of chemotactic responses in neutrophils, studies on cholera toxin have produced confusing results, since it raises cAMP levels in the absence or presence of a PDE inhibitor, but inhibits β-glucuronidase release only in the presence of a PDE inhibitor (140).

Superoxide anion generation, elicited in neutrophils by such agents as f Met Leu Phe and LTB_4, is inhibited by the cAMP-elevating agents forskolin, isoproterenol, PGE_1, histamine and H_2 agonists, theophylline, and enprofylline, as well as by dibutyryl cAMP (140,146,149,150). Low concentrations of theophylline enhance superoxide generation, but, as in eosinophils, this is apparently due to antagonism of endogenous adenosine at A_2 receptors (151). The biosynthesis of platelet-activating factor and LTB_4 in response to f Met Leu Phe and A23187 is inhibited by isoproterenol and IBMX (152). In addition, neutrophil aggregation is suppressed by a variety of cAMP-elevating agents (141,146).

A number of studies have addressed the effects of the xanthine PDE inhibitor pentoxifylline on neutrophil function. This agent inhibits neutrophil degranulation and adhesion to endothelium (153) and reduces neutrophil deformability (154), but it is not certain that elevation of cAMP levels mediates all these effects.

Mast Cells and Basophils

Human lung mast cells release histamine, LTC_4, PGD_2, platelet-activating factor, various chemotactic peptides, proteolytic enzymes, and proteoglycans. Basophils release a slightly different range of mediators, prostanoids being a notable omission. Some of these agents are bronchoconstrictors and most are proinflammatory. The important role played by mast cell–derived spasmogens in the immediate asthmatic response to inhaled allergens has long been recognized, but the failure of β-adrenoceptor agonists and a number of other mast cell stabilizers (not including disodium cromoglycate or nedocromil) to inhibit the late asthmatic response or demonstrate anti-inflammatory activity in asthma suggests that mast cells do not play a special role in chronic asthma (155). Recent evidence that mast cells and basophils elaborate interleukin (IL)-3, GM-CSF, and IL-5, which promote eosinophil production, chemotaxis, and activation, and IL-4, which induces the switch of B-cell immunoglobulin synthesis to IgE (156,157), has revitalized interest in these cells, but unless β-adrenoceptor agonists and those stabilizers that proved ineffective in asthma fail to inhibit the release of these cytokines from mast cells and basophils, the role of these cells in chronic asthma will remain unclear.

Many studies have shown that agents that elevate cAMP levels, including β-adrenoceptor agonists, PDE inhibitors, prostaglandins of the E series, cholera toxin, histamine H_2 agonists, vasoactive intestinal peptide, forskolin, and adenosine (acting via A_2 receptors), inhibit immunologically mediated release of mediators, notably histamine and LTC_4, from mast cells and basophils (158–161). The β-adrenoceptor agonists are especially potent inhibitors of mediator release from both types of cell. Desensitization of human lung mast cells to β-adrenoceptor agonists has been reported (162), but this takes place over hours, in contrast to the rapid desensitization that occurs when eosinophils or neutrophils are incubated with β-adrenoceptor agonists. Intriguingly, isoproterenol inhibits immunologically stimulated *de novo* synthesis of PGD_2 and LTC_4 in human lung mast cells at concentrations that fail to affect the release of performed histamine. Furthermore, isoproterenol abolishes A 23187-induced LTC_4 release, but does not affect histamine release in response to the same agent (163). Studies in a mouse mast cell line suggest that this might be because inhibition of histamine release requires an increase in cAMP-dependent protein kinase activity that is sufficient to prevent an increase in $[Ca^{2+}]_i$, whereas inhibition of eicosanoid and platelet-activating factor synthesis is mediated by smaller increases in protein kinase activity that do not affect $[Ca^{2+}]_i$ (164).

Although most evidence indicates that elevation of cAMP levels suppresses mediator release from mast cells and basophils, it was at one time suggested that elevation of cAMP levels is an essential biochemical event in IgE-mediated stimulus-secretion coupling. This was because immunologic activation of rat peritoneal mast cells using antigen, anti-IgE, concanavalin A, or antibody to the Fc_ε-receptor was found to cause a rapid rise in cAMP levels that preceded histamine release. It was nevertheless clear that a rise in cAMP levels was not an obligatory event for histamine secretion, because some agents (compound 48/80 and A 23187) actually provoke a rapid decrease in cAMP levels prior to histamine release (160,162). Furthermore, in contrast to rat peritoneal mast cells, immunologic stimulation of human basophils and lung mast cells fails to elicit any changes in cAMP levels (162). The relevance of the transient rise in cAMP levels in rat peritoneal mast cells in response to immunologic stimulation therefore remains a mystery.

Monocytes and Macrophages

Airway macrophages arise from circulating monocytes, which mature into macrophages during their residence within the airways. The airways of normal subjects as well as asthmatics are lined with macrophages, and in atopic subjects they respond to allergens by releasing potent eosinophil chemoattractants, such as platelet-activating factor, LTB_4, and cytokines, in addition to other lipid mediators, reactive oxygen species, and hydrolytic enzymes. It has therefore been proposed that the activation of macrophages triggers the influx of eosinophils and possibly other inflammatory cells into the lungs of asthmatics (165). This notion is supported by similarities between the pharmacology for inhibition of macrophage activity and inhibition of bronchial hyperreactivity in asthmatics.

The release of reactive oxygen species and lipid mediators from macrophages and monocytes in response to such agents as opsonized zymosan, f Met Leu Phe, or lipopolysaccharide, but not in response to protein kinase C activators or A 23187, is generally suppressed by agents that elevate cAMP levels, and by cAMP analogues (166–171). A notable exception is that whereas monocyte activation is inhibited by β_2-adrenoceptor agonists and adenosine (via A_2 receptors), these, and other agents that activate adenylyl cyclase via G proteins, have no effect in human mature alveolar macrophages (165,167,170). This suggests that PDE inhibitors, in contrast to β_2-adrenoceptor agonists, should exhibit anti-inflammatory activity in asthma if the release of reactive oxygen species and lipid mediators from macrophages plays an important role. Thus, nonselective PDE inhibitors, such as theophylline and enprofylline, appear to inhibit the release of reactive oxygen species and lipid mediators, although not the release of hydrolytic enzymes (170,171). Surprisingly, the effects of theophylline and forskolin are not synergistic in human aveolar macrophages and it has been suggested that they affect different pools of cAMP (171). It is also possible that the effect of theophylline is not mediated by cAMP. The latter conclusion was preferred as an explanation of why in human monocytes the selective PDE IV inhibitor rolipram caused a greater elevation of cAMP levels than theophylline, but was less able to inhibit f Met Leu Phe–stimulated superoxide generation (172).

Cyclic AMP–elevating agents and dibutyryl cAMP inhibit tumor necrosis factor-α (TNFα) production by human macrophages and by human and mouse monocytes (173–176). IL-1 synthesis by human monocytes, in contrast to TNFα production, is either enhanced by elevation of cAMP levels (177) or unchanged (176).

Lymphocytes

T lymphocytes probably play a role in all antigen-driven inflammatory responses as they are the only cells that directly recognize and respond to processed antigens. Since bronchial mucosal inflammation is an important feature of asthma, it is not surprising that evidence is accumulating that CD4 T lymphocytes are activated in the lungs of atopic asthmatics and following antigen challenge. The number of activated cells correlates with the severity of the asthma, and the T lymphocytes of steroid-resistant asthmatics are also steroid-resistant (178), further supporting the importance of these cells in asthma pathogenesis.

The T lymphocytes activated in atopic asthmatics belong to the T_{H2} subclass, which secrete IL-3, IL-4, IL-5, and GM-CSF (179). IL-5, possibly assisted by IL-3 and GM-CSF, promotes the differentiation, survival, chemotaxis, and activation of eosinophils. IL-3 and IL-4 promote the expansion and differentiation of mast cells in tissues, while IL-4 promotes the switching of B lymphocytes to IgE synthesis (178).

Several studies indicate that elevation of cAMP levels inhibits IL-2 and mitogen-induced T-lymphocyte activation and proliferation (180–184). The activity of cytotoxic T lymphocytes is similarly inhibited (185). Elevation of cAMP levels inhibits inositol triphosphate generation and Ca^{2+} mobilization elicited by perturbation of the T-cell receptor but not by activation of G proteins using guanosine triphosphate-γ (GTPγS) (183). Whether inhibition of phosphoinositide hydrolysis is the sole site of action of cAMP is unclear, as there is disagreement concerning whether cAMP inhibits T-cell activation elicited by phorbol esters or Ca^{2+} ionophores, which act downstream from phosphoinositide hydrolysis (181–183).

Apparently at odds with these findings (but reminiscent of findings in other inflammatory cells), the mitogen phytohemagglutinin raises cAMP levels in human peripheral blood lymphocytes. It now seems, however, that this is not an essential link in the mitogen signal and may be part of the mechanism by which high doses of mitogen inhibit lymphocyte proliferation (180).

The effects of cAMP in T_{H1} relative to T_{H2} cells are of particular interest in view of the evidence that T_{H2} cells are activated in asthmatics. Intriguingly, 8-bromo cAMP is a more potent inhibitor of IL-2 production by mouse T_{H1} clones than by T_{H2} clones, but a more potent inhibitor of IL-2–driven cellular proliferation in T_{H2} clones (186). PGE$_2$ inhibits IL-2 and to some extent interferon-γ production by human T-cell clones, but IL-4 production is unaffected and IL-5 production even stimulated by low concentrations of PGE$_2$ (187).

In vivo studies in man suggest that theophylline increases suppressor T-cell populations. Treatment with theophylline increases the proportion and number of T cells able to form E rosettes following incubation with theophylline *in vitro*. Such theophylline-sensitive cells suppress peripheral blood mononuclear cell proliferation (188). Aminophylline has been found to enhance renal transplantation survival rates, at the same time as raising the proportion of CD8 to CD4 expressing T cells (189).

B lymphocytes play a role in atopic asthma through their production of IgE. The role of cyclic nucleotides is less studied in these lymphocytes but there appears to be an inverse relationship between cAMP levels and immunoglobulin secretion (190). Regulation of human B-cell proliferation by cAMP is complex. Elevation of cAMP levels enhances proliferation driven by IL-4 but inhibits proliferation in response to IL-2 (191).

Platelets

Platelets have been suggested to contribute to lung inflammation in asthma by the release of cytotoxic oxygen species, platelet-derived growth factor (which may promote bronchial smooth muscle hypertrophy), and factors that are chemotactic for eosinophils. These substances may be released via activation of IgE receptors on platelets or, independently of IgE, by aspirin in sensitive subjects. The role of platelets in asthma remains controversial, but there is some evidence that they are activated in asthma (192,193).

Administration of β-adrenoceptor agonists to animals or humans lowers blood platelet numbers (194,195), while β-adrenoceptor antagonists have the opposite effect (196). There is also abundant evidence that elevation of cAMP levels inhibits platelet aggregation (197). The relevance of these findings to the inflammatory functions of platelets is dubious, however, since the aggregatory and inflammatory functions of platelets appear to be differentially regulated and there is little information on the involvement of cyclic nucleotides in the inflammatory responses.

Endothelial Cells

Endothelial cells provide an essential link in the process of lung inflammation since inflammatory cells must adhere to the vascular endothelium before passing between these cells into the lung tissue. Moreover, extravasation of plasma proteins, water, and solutes occurs when contraction of endothelial cells in the postcapillary venules of the tracheobronchial circulation creates pores between adjacent cells (198). This leads to edema and narrowing of the airways, epithelial shedding, the production of inflammatory mediators, an increased viscosity and quantity of airways mucus, and thus decreased mucociliary clearance (199,200). Links with thickening of the basement membrane and hypertrophy of smooth muscle have also been proposed (201).

Few studies have addressed the role of endothelial cell cyclic nucleotides in inflammatory cell adherence. Incubation of rat endothelial cells with dibutyryl cAMP enhances the subsequent adherence of lymphocytes, while the adenylyl cyclase inhibitor 2'5'-dideoxyadenosine decreases both the lymphocyte adherence and elevation of cAMP levels induced by IL-1 (202). This suggests that PDE inhibition might promote lymphocyte adhesion. There are no reports on the effects of cAMP-elevating drugs on adhesion molecule expression by endothelial cells, but forskolin, IBMX, pertussis toxin, and cholera toxin stimulate expression of the adhesion molecule ICAM-1 in a human glioma cell line. However, longer-term treatment (24 to 72 h) with these agents inhibits retinoic acid- and interferon-γ (IFNγ)-induced expression of ICAM-1 (203).

The effect of cAMP-elevating agents on the barrier function of endothelial cells and extravasation *in vivo* has been the subject of a number of studies. A variety of such agents reduce the permeability to proteins and low-density lipoproteins and increase electrical resistance in cultured endothelial cells (204,205). Studies with β-adrenoceptor agonists and other adenylyl cyclase activators *in vivo* have shown variable effects on extravasation in various vascular beds, including the lung. It appears that these agents reduce extravasation by relaxing endothelial cells, but this is opposed to various degrees by increases in venular hydrostatic pressure and the area of the vascular bed perfused (198,200,206–208). Most studies on xanthines show an inhibition of extravasation in the airways and other vascular beds (198,200,209).

Isozyme Profiles

As with ASM, isozyme profiles of inflammatory cells have been deduced from a combination of kinetic, pharmacological, and chromatographic techniques. PDE IV is the major isozyme in many inflammatory cells, but PDE III predominates in platelets and is present alongside PDE IV in T lymphocytes and probably in basophils as well. Furthermore, with the exception of eosinophils, monocytes, and possibly lymphocytes, inflammatory cells contain one of the main cGMP-hydrolyzing PDEs, i.e., PDEs I, II, or V. These profiles are summarized in Table 6.

Eosinophils

Two groups have characterized PDE isozymes in guinea pig eosinophils, obtaining similar results (136,210). Chromatographic separations were not conducted in these studies, but from the kinetics of cyclic nucleotide hydrolysis, the lack of sensitivity of cAMP hydrolysis to cGMP or Ca^{2+}/calmodulin, and the sensitivity to type IV isozyme inhibitors, it can be concluded that eosinophil PDEs are predominantly or exclusively PDE IV. Similar results are claimed for human blood eosinophils (211).

The majority of the cAMP PDE activity in guinea pig eosinophils is tightly membrane bound. Its kinetics can be resolved into two components, one with a K_m value typical of PDE IV (1–8 μmol/L), and another having a three- to nine-fold higher V_{max} and a much higher K_m value (31 or 368 μmol/L) (136,210). It is not known whether these values reflect the presence of different PDE isozymes or PDE IV subtypes, or simply arise artifactually though a physical change in the enzyme during the isolation procedure. Ro-

TABLE 6. *Phosphodiesterase isozymes detected in inflammatory cells*

Cell type	Isozymes detected	Species[a]	References
Eosinophil	**IV**	G,H	136, 210, 211
Neutrophil	**IV**	H	212–214
	V	H	212
	I or II	H	214
	I?	H	215, 216; cf. 212
Basophil	**IV**	H	217
	III	H	217
	V	H	217
Mast cell	**IV**	M	218
	II,III,V	R	219
Monocyte	**IV**	H	220–222
Macrophage	I,II,III, and/or IV	M	223
Lymphocyte	III	H	220, 224–226
	IV	H	225
	V?	H	220, 224–226
	non-I to V	H	225
Platelet	**III**	H	22, 228
	I	H	22, 227
	II	H	227
	V	H	22
Endothelial cell	II	P,O	229, 230
	IV	P,O	229, 230
	III	P	211

Predominant isozymes are given in bold type.
[a]H, human; G, guinea pig; M, mouse; R, rat; P, pig; O, ox.

lipram and denbufylline differ from other PDE inhibitors tested in displaying shallow concentration-inhibition curves, suggesting that these compounds inhibit two forms of PDE IV with different affinities. This may relate to the ability of rolipram and denbufylline to bind with nanomolar affinity to a proportion of the PDE IV isolated from certain tissue sources (47,49,211; K. A. Foster, J. R. S. Arch, and T. J. Torphy, unpublished). Whether rolipram and denbufylline differentially inhibit two catalytic forms of eosinophil PDE IV that have different K_m values for cAMP is not known since inhibitor concentration-response curves were conducted using only one concentration of cAMP (1 or 2 μmol/L).

Neutrophils

The characterization of human neutrophil PDE isozymes has been described in three recent papers. Schudt and coworkers (212), studying only the supernatant fraction, separated a PDE V and what appear to be two forms of PDE IV using Q-Sepharose chromatography. Only the major PDE IV peak was characterized using selective isozyme inhibitors, however. Low Hill coefficients (i.e., shallow concentration-response curves) were obtained for inhibition by rolipram, denbufylline, and Ro 20-1724. Nielson and colleagues (213), who also studied the supernatant fraction, identified only one PDE IV peak. Two minor peaks with greater cGMP- than cAMP-hydrolyzing activity (PDE I, II, or V) were also present. In another study it was determined that the particulate fraction of neutrophil homogenates contains 80% of total PDE activity (214). This activity appears to be PDE IV based upon its kinetics, its insensitivity to cGMP, and its sensitivity to PDE IV inhibitors (214). Two apparent K_m values were obtained (0.7 and 7.6 μmol/L). The soluble fraction exhibited similar activities for the hydrolysis of cAMP and cGMP, suggesting the presence of PDE I or II, but was not studied in detail.

Earlier studies (215,216) identified major peaks from ion exchange chromatography that were sensitive to Ca^{2+}/calmodulin (PDE I) in the human neutrophil supernatant fraction, together with peaks that were probably PDE II (216) and PDE IV (215). However, Schudt and colleagues (212) did not detect a Ca^{2+}/calmodulin-stimulated enzyme.

Mast Cells and Basophils

PDE isozymes have been characterized in human basophils and in mouse and rat mast cells. Chromatography of human basophil supernatants identified a minor PDE V peak and a major peak that appeared to be predominantly PDE IV with a minor contribution from PDE III (217). Studies on the effects of selective inhibitors and of cGMP on cAMP hydrolysis in whole homogenates also supported the presence of PDE IV with a minor PDE III component. The PDE III activity could be partly due to contamination of the basophils with lymphocytes, but since a selective PDE III inhibitor enhances the inhibition of histamine release by rolipram, it is probable that basophils contain some PDE III (217).

Mouse mast cells purified from bone marrow contain predominantly PDE IV, but a minor PDE I peak can also be identified by DEAE-Sepharose chromatography (218). However, previous work on the soluble fraction of rat peritoneal and thoracic mast cells did not clearly identify a PDE IV in this species (219). Three peaks were resolved by DEAE-Sephadex chromatography that, based on limited kinetic data and sensitivity to zaprinast, appear to have been PDEs V, II, and III.

Monocytes and Macrophages

Early work by Thompson and colleagues (220,221) demonstrated the presence of a cAMP-hydrolyzing PDE in human purified peripheral blood monocytes. The K_m value of approximately 1 μmol/L for cAMP and lack of cGMP-hydrolyzing activity (221) suggests that this enzyme is PDE IV. These kinetic values are consistent with those obtained using recombinant human monocyte PDE IV (47,61). A PDE IV from human monocytes (K_m = 1.6

μmol/L) has been identified more clearly recently and shown to be sensitive to rolipram and Ro 20-1724 (47,222).

Murine peritoneal macrophages contain both soluble and particulate cAMP PDEs (223). DEAE-cellulose chromatography of the soluble fraction appeared to resolve PDE I and III peaks, together with two peaks that showed properties associated with more than one isozyme (II and IV, and II, III, and IV).

Lymphocytes

Initial work identified only one kinetic form of cAMP PDE in mixed human lymphocytes, although enzymes of two different molecular weights could be separated (220). The low K_m value for cAMP (0.4 μmol/L) is consistent with the enzyme(s) being PDE III, but cGMP did not inhibit cAMP hydrolysis. By contrast, a subsequent study by Takemoto et al. (224) revealed that cAMP hydrolysis in homogentates of purified T cells could be inhibited by 80% by 10 μmol/L cGMP. More recently Robicsek and colleagues (225) failed to detect a peak of activity that was sensitive to CI 930 (PDE III-selective inhibitor) in the soluble fraction of platelet-free T lymphocytes. However, they identified an enzyme with a low K_m value (<1.0 μmol/L) for cAMP that was sensitive to neither CI 930 nor Ro 20-1724 (PDE IV-selective inhibitor), as well as two peaks that were sensitive to Ro 20-1724. Subsequently, the same group did detect a particulate PDE III activity in T lymphocytes as well as soluble PDE IV activity (226). Low levels of cGMP PDE activity (apparently PDE V) have been detected in one study (225) but not in another study (220).

Platelets

Peaks of activity with the properties of PDEs I, III, and V have been identified by DEAE-cellulose chromatography of human platelet supernatant (22). It has been suggested that PDE II is also present in these cells, since the Ca^{2+}/calmodulin-stimulated peak of activity (PDE I) is also stimulated by cGMP (227). Of the cAMP-hydrolyzing enzymes, PDE III is most abundant: more than 80% of the total low-K_m cAMP PDE in bovine and human platelets resides in a peak of activity that is inhibited by cGMP and selective PDE III inhibitors (228).

Endothelial Cells

Studies have been conducted on porcine (229) and bovine (230) aortic endothelial cells, but no information is available on postcapillary venular endothelial cells, which are the cells that control microvascular leakage. The majority of the cAMP and cGMP hydrolytic activity of both porcine and bovine endothelial cells resides in the soluble fraction of cell homogenates. PDE II and PDE IV are present in the soluble fraction from both species. Activity defined as PDE II isolated from the bovine, but not the porcine, source is peculiar in that it is inhibited by rolipram (IC_{50} = 3 µmol/L) when assayed using 0.25 µmol/L cAMP and in the absence of cGMP. PDE I is not present in either the particulate or soluble fractions. A PDE III activity in the particulate fraction of porcine pulmonary endothelial cells has also been identified (M.A. Giembycz, personal communication).

Effects of Isozyme-Selective Inhibitors

With a few notable exceptions, our knowledge concerning the effects of isozyme-selective PDE inhibitors on isolated immune and inflammatory cells has become available only over the last 5 years. This information is summarized in Table 7. Even today, little information is available with regard to the effects of isozyme-selective inhibitors on inflammatory processes *in vivo*. Because of this, *in vivo* anti-inflammatory effects of isozyme-selective inhibitors will not be discussed in a separate section, but rather will be discussed along with the *in vitro* information on the pertinent cell type.

Eosinophils

Rolipram and denbufylline are potent inhibitors of opsonized zymosan-stimulated H_2O_2 and basal superoxide generation in guinea pig eosinophils (136,210). Consistent with their effect on isolated eosinophil PDE IV activity, both compounds have shallow concentration-response curves for these functional effects. The PDE III-selective inhibitors SK&F 94120 and Org 9935 and the PDE V inhibitor zaprinast do not affect eosinophil function when studied at concentrations that are isozyme-selective (136,210).

Rolipram alone elicits a small but significant increase in cAMP levels and a marked increase in the cAMP-dependent protein kinase activity ratio in guinea pig eosinophils. Both rolipram and denbufylline markedly increase isoproterenol-stimulated cAMP accumulation (210). These data therefore support a dominant role for PDE IV in guinea pig eosinophils.

Very little is known about the effects of isozyme-selective PDE inhibitors in human eosinophils, although it has been stated that rolipram, but not SK&F 94120, inhibits H_2O_2 generation in human eosinophils (211). The PDE III/IV inhibitor zardaverine inhibits opsonized zymosan-stimulated superoxide production, but even in the presence of salbutamol its IC_{50} value (63 µmol/L) for this activity is well above its IC_{50} value (about 1 µmol/L) as an inhibitor of isolated PDE III and PDE IV (137).

In vivo studies in the rat have shown that denbufylline and rolipram reduce Sephadex-induced blood eosinophilia, together with the associated airway

TABLE 7. *Effects of isozyme-selective PDE inhibitors on inflammatory cell function*

Cell type	Species[a]	Function[b]	Isozyme-selectivity of inhibitors having:		References
			Effect	No effect	
Eosinophil	H	Reactive oxygen	IV	III	211
	G	BAL[c] eosinophilia	III and/or IV		123, 128, 232
	G	Reactive oxygen	IV	III, V	101, 136, 210
	R	Cyclic AMP	IV		210
	H	Blood eosinophilia	IV		231
Neutrophil	H	Reactive oxygen	IV	I, II, III	34, 212–214
		Enzyme	IV?		214; cf. 235
Basophil	H	Histamine, LTC$_4$	IV, III[d]	I, V	217, 236
		Cyclic AMP	I or V		236
Mast cell	H	Histamine, LTC$_4$	IV	III, V	7
	R	Histamine	V	IV	236
	M	Cyclic AMP, protein kinase, histamine	IV	III, V	7, 218
Macrophage	H	Reactive oxygen, LTB$_4$, TxB$_2$, enzyme		IV	167
	G	Reactive oxygen	IV		169
		Cyclic AMP	IV[e], III[e]	III	223
T Lymphocyte	H	Cytotoxicity, IL-2	IV		185, 237
		Blastogenesis	IV[f], III[f]		226
B Lymphocyte	H	Antibody	IV		238
Platelet	H	Ca, aggregation ATP, 5-HT, β-thromboglobulin	III	V[g], IV	227, 239, 240
Endothelial cell	G	Extravasation *in vivo*	IV, V	III, I	209
	P	Permeability	IV, III		205

[a] See footnote to Table 6 for code.

[b] Inhibition of the function described or inhibition of the release of the material specified (into cytosol for Ca), except for elevation of cyclic AMP levels and activation of cyclic AMP–dependent protein kinase.

[c] BAL, bronchoalveolar lavage.

[d] Potentiates effect of PDE IV inhibitor; no effect alone.

[e] Potentiates effect of PGE$_2$.

[f] PDE III and IV inhibition is synergistic.

[g] Trend to inhibition.

hyperresponsiveness *in vitro* and *in vivo* (231). Similarly, in guinea pigs, the PDE III/IV inhibitors zardaverine and benzafentrine suppress eosinophil accumulation in BAL fluids in response to antigen and, in the case of benzafentrine, in response to platelet-activating factor and IL-3 (123,128,232). The selective PDE IV inhibitors rolipram, Ro 20-1724, and nitraquazone also inhibit antigen-induced eosinophil accumulation in BAL fluid (233,234), but PDE III inhibitors are without effect (233).

Neutrophils

The f Met Leu Phe– or A 23187-evoked respiratory burst of human neutrophils is inhibited by the PDE IV inhibitors Ro 20-1724 and rolipram, and by the PDE III/IV inhibitor zardaverine, but not by ICI 74917 (PDE I–selective), zaprinast (PDE V–selective) or various PDE III inhibitors (34,212–214). These results are consistent with findings by the same workers that PDE IV is the dominant isozyme in human neutrophils.

The potency and efficacy of the PDE IV inhibitors (like that of β-adrenoceptor agonists) is dependent on the nature of the stimulus, since they are much less potent against superoxide production induced by complement fragment C5a than against superoxide production induced by f Met Leu Phe (214). Moreover, PDE IV inhibitors are almost inactive against the response to opsonized zymosan, despite causing similar elevations in cAMP levels in the presence of each stimulus (214). The efficacy of the PDE IV inhibitors also appears to be response-dependent, since these compounds have little effect on lysosomal enzyme release in response to f Met Leu Phe or opsonized zymosan (214). This finding, however, contrasts with an earlier report that Ro 20-1724 inhibits lysosomal enzyme release in response to complement-activated zymosan (235). It is also difficult to reconcile this lack of effect of PDE IV inhibition on lysozomal enzyme secretion with various reports that cAMP-elevating agents and cAMP analogues inhibit the release of acid hydrolases and β-glucuronidase (140,146,147), unless there is more than one cAMP pool that influences neutrophil degranulation or unless β-adrenoceptor agonists exert their inhibitory effect through a non-cAMP–mediated mechanism.

Mast Cells and Basophils

Data have been published on the effects of selective PDE isozyme inhibitors in human basophils (217,236) as well as mouse (218) and rat (236) mast cells. Results for human lung mast cells have also been described (7).

The human basophil data are consistent with the finding of a major PDE IV activity and minor PDE III and V activities (217). Thus rolipram and Ro 20-1724 inhibit antigen-induced histamine and LTC_4 release from human basophils (217,236), and rolipram potentiates the inhibitory effect of forskolin (217). Zaprinast, used at a concentration (100 μmol/L) that inhibits both PDE I and V, does not affect mediator release, even though cAMP levels are somewhat elevated. Zaprinast also fails to enhance the effect of rolipram on mediator release. This suggests that zaprinast elevates cAMP in a nonfunctional compartment. The selective PDE III inhibitor SK&F 95654 does not affect mediator release, but it potentiates the effect of rolipram (217). Similar synergies between PDE III and IV inhibitors have been reported for other tissues and cells (7).

PDE IV is also the major functional PDE isozyme in mouse bone marrow–derived mast cells, again consistent with isozyme chromatography data (218). Thus siguazodan (PDE III inhibitor) and zaprinast have no effect on basal or forskolin-stimulated cAMP-dependent protein kinase activity, whereas rolipram stimulates this activity, especially in the presence of forskolin. Parallel results are obtained for elevation of cAMP levels and inhibition of antigen-stimulated mediator release (7,218). Antigen-stimulated mediator release from human lung mast cells is similarly reduced by PDE IV inhibitors (rolipram, Ro 20-1724), whereas PDE III (SK&F 95654) and V (zaprinast) inhibitors have no effect (7).

Rat peritoneal mast cells seem to differ from human lung and mouse bone marrow-derived mast cells. Antigen-induced histamine release from the rat cells is inhibited by zaprinast but not by rolipram (236). This seems to be consistent with the isozyme profile of these cells (219), which, in retrospect, appears to include PDE V (as well as PDE II and III) but not PDE IV.

Monocytes and Macrophages

Only limited information is available on the effects of isozyme-selective PDE inhibitors on monocyte and macrophage function. In human monocytes, the PDE IV inhibitor rolipram produces only a modest (19%) inhibition of f Met Leu Phe–stimulated superoxide generation (172). In human macrophages, Ro 20-1724 has no effect on immunologically stimulated superoxide, LTB_4, thromboxane B_2, or N-acetyl-β-D-glucosamidase release, either when it is used alone or in the presence of isoproterenol (167). However, since isoproterenol alone is also ineffective, it would be useful to investigate the interaction of Ro 20-1724 with forskolin, which does inhibit the release of superoxide, LTB_4 and thromboxane B_2.

In contrast to the failure of Ro 20-1724 to affect human macrophage function, both Ro 20-1724 and rolipram inhibit f Met Leu Phe–stimulated superoxide generation by guinea pig macrophages. The PDE III inhibitor SK&F 94120, on the other hand, is ineffective (169). Ro 20-1724 and rolipram also enhance the elevation of cAMP levels induced by PGE_2 in mouse peritoneal macrophages (223). The PDE III inhibitors anagrelide and OPC 3689 also potentiate the PGE_2-induced rise in cAMP. These results for mouse macrophages seem consistent with chromatographic evidence for PDE III and PDE IV reported in the same article, but the isozymes have yet to be fully resolved.

Lymphocytes

The PDE IV inhibitor Ro 20-1724 suppresses the activity of human cytotoxic T lymphocytes (185) and IL-2 production by human T lymphocytes (237). Both Ro 20-1724 and CI-930, a PDE III inhibitor, inhibit blastogenesis in T lymphocytes and when used in combination their effects are synergistic (226). It thus appears that PDE III and PDE IV act in concert to regulate the cAMP concentrations in T lymphocytes.

Antibody production by B lymphocytes may also be inhibited by selective PDE IV inhibitors. Ro 20-1724 inhibits IgE production by peripheral blood mononuclear leukocytes and most, but not all, of this activity can be attributed to a direct effect on B cells (238).

Platelets

Consistent with the predominance of PDE III in human platelets, various PDE III inhibitors reduce agonist-induced Ca^{2+} mobilization and aggregation in these cells as well as inhibit the secretion of adenosine triphosphate (ATP), serotonin, and thromboglobulin (227,239,240). The effects of PDE III inhibitors on other proinflammatory activities of platelets have not been reported. Despite evidence for a PDE V activity in human platelets (22) and for an anti-aggregatory effect of cGMP-elevating agents (16,241–243), zaprinast has little anti-aggregatory effect. Rolipram has no effect, consistent with the lack of a PDE IV in human platelets (227).

Endothelial Cells and Extravasation

Consistent with reports that both PDE III and PDE IV are present in porcine endothelial cells, motapizone (PDE III inhibitor), rolipram (PDE IV inhibitor), and zardaverine (PDE III/IV inhibitor) each completely block hydrogen peroxide–induced increases in permeability of porcine endothelial cell monolayers (205). A somewhat different profile is obtained for inhibition of platelet-activating factor–induced extravasation in the airways of anesthetized guinea pigs (209). Rolipram is again effective *in vivo,* as is the PDE V inhibitor zaprinast (which was not evaluated in the porcine endothelial cell monolayers), but the PDE III inhibitor siguazodan is ineffective. Vinpocetine, a PDE I inhibitor, is also ineffective. There are no studies on the distribution of PDE isozymes in guinea pig endothelial cells to which these results can be related.

CELLULAR REGULATION OF PDE ACTIVITY

Changes in the absolute amount or activity of PDEs can markedly alter the sensitivity of cells to hormones, neurotransmitters, autocoids, and drugs. Two general mechanisms of PDE regulation have been documented (52). The first, designated "short-term" regulation, involves allosteric modulation of PDE activity via activating one or more second messenger pathways. The second type of PDE regulation, called "long-term" regulation, occurs through a change in the rate of enzyme synthesis or degradation.

Short-Term Regulation

Two PDE isozymes that are obvious targets for short-term allosteric regulation are PDE I and PDE II. Since PDE is allosterically activated by $Ca^{2+}/$ calmodulin, it stands to reason that an elevation in $[Ca^{2+}]_i$ could activate this isozyme, leading to a decrease in cellular cyclic nucleotide content. Indeed, studies with dog thyroid gland (244,245) and 1321N1 human astrocytoma cells (246,247) indicate that hormone-induced cAMP accumulation is reduced in the presence of agonists that stimulate Ca^{2+} mobilization, and that this effect is due to a Ca^{2+}-mediated activation of PDE I. Similarly, in bovine trachealis, neural stimulation or K^+-induced depolarization activates PDE I (248). The ability of contractile agonists to activate PDE I has also been demonstrated in porcine coronary arteries (249). With respect to PDE II, the activity of submicromolar concentrations of cGMP to increase markedly the ability of this isozyme against cAMP (43) suggests a mechanism by which increases in cGMP content could negatively affect cAMP levels in intact cells. In fact, recent studies indicate that in adrenal glomerulosa cells and pheochromocytoma cells, cAMP content is reduced in response to agents that stimulate guanylyl cyclase (250,251). The modulatory activity of guanylyl cyclase activators appears to be produced by a cGMP-mediated activation of PDE II.

Perhaps the most extensively studied form of short-term PDE regulation is the activation of PDE III via at least two separate phosphorylation pathways (46,52,252). These pathways are of major physiological importance in mediating the regulatory effects of hormones (e.g., insulin, glucagon, epinephrine) on lipid and carbohydrate metabolism. Phosphorylation of membrane-bound PDE III by cAMP-dependent protein kinase activates this isozyme in adipocytes (46), hepatocytes (253), and platelets (254). Similarly, PDE III is activated in adipocytes by insulin (46), although this activation is not mediated via cAMP-dependent protein kinase. Instead, insulin phosphorylates PDE III through a serine kinase that, in turn, is regulated through phosphorylation by the insulin receptor–associated tyrosine kinase (46). Indirect evidence suggests that adenylyl cyclase activators and insulin stimulate the phosphorylation of different serine residues on PDE III (46).

Another mechanism by which PDE III activity is subject to short-term regulation does not involve covalent modification through a phosphorylation cascade, but rather is based upon the ability of submicromolar concentrations of cGMP to inhibit competitively cAMP hydrolysis (25,45). In fact, considerable evidence exists suggesting that stimulation of guanylyl cyclase in platelets potentiates the anti-aggregatory activity of adenylyl cyclase activators (242,255,256). This potentiation apparently occurs because the cGMP formed in response to nitrovasodilators inhibits PDE III, thus leading to an increase in cAMP content (257). Evidence that such an interaction occurs in vascular smooth muscle also exists (256,258), although negative results using this tissue have been reported as well (259).

Information on the short-term regulation of PDE activity in airway smooth muscle or immunoinflammatory cells is woefully lacking. Although certain predictions can be made based upon our understanding of second messenger pathways in these cells as well as knowledge of their PDE isozyme profiles, definitive experimental results are not available.

Long-Term Regulation

Long-term regulation of PDE activity contrasts with that occurring via allosteric regulation in that it involves protein and mRNA synthesis, develops over hours of agonist treatment, and is only slowly reversible after agonist removal. Long-term PDE regulation has been observed in several cell lines, including C-6 glioma (260), neuroblastoma (261), hepatoma (262), lymphoma (263), and U937 monocytes (264), as well as fibroblasts (265) and Sertoli cells (266). Clearly, this phenomenon is not confined to a few selected cells, but instead appears to represent a general homeostatic mechanism by which target cells regulate their responsiveness to drugs, hormones, and autocoids that activate adenylyl cyclase. In most of the studies cited above the PDE isozyme being regulated was not identified unambiguously. Nonetheless, the kinetic characteristics of the induced enzyme are similar, if not identical, to those of PDE IV.

The nature of PDE IV up-regulation is exemplified by the actions of β-adrenoceptor agonists in U937 cells, a human monocytic cell line (264,267). Based upon standard biochemical characterization protocols, PDE IV is the most abundant isozyme present in U937 cells. Incubating intact U937 cells with salbutamol, a β-adrenoceptor agonist, produces a time- and concentration-dependent increase in PDE IV activity. This increase reaches a maximum within 4 h of agonist exposure and is sustained over a 24-h period. The ability of salbutamol to induce PVE IV is (a) reversible within 3 h of agonist removal, (b) abolished by cotreatment with inhibitors of protein or mRNA synthesis, (c) mimicked by prostaglandin E_2 and 8-bromo-cAMP, (d) preceded by a transient increase in cAMP content and cAMP-dependent protein kinase activity, and (e) potentiated by PDE IV inhibitors. The functional significance of PDE IV regulation in U937 cells is illustrated by the observation that salbutamol pretreatment produces a marked heterologous desensitization to the functional effects of other adenylyl cyclase activators (e.g., PGE_2) that do not act via the β-adrenoceptor (267).

Recent studies of Conti and colleagues suggest that a cAMP-dependent stimulation of gene transcription is responsible for agonist-induced up-regulation of PDE IV (268,269). In these studies, stimulating Sertoli cells with follicle-stimulating hormone was shown to produce a cAMP-dependent increase in the rate of transcription of two genes, ratPDE3 and ratPDE4, that encode two rat PDE IV subtypes. This results in an increase in mRNA levels for these subtypes and, subsequently, an increase in protein expression. Interestingly, different PDE IV genes that encode distinct isozyme subtypes are not equally susceptible to regulation. In Sertoli cells, for example, ratPDE3 mRNA levels are elevated by follicle-stimulating hormone to a much greater extent than are the levels of ratPDE4 mRNA (269). Thus, the degree to which cAMP can regulate PDE IV activity in different cells may vary depending on the PDE IV subtype that is expressed.

Regulation of PDE IV expression could have a substantial impact on the pathophysiology and treatment of asthma. Monocytes (270,271), lymphocytes (272), granulocytes (273), and mixed leukocytes (274) isolated from individuals with atopic disorders have a diminished functional responsiveness to β-adrenoceptor agonists. Furthermore, this reduced hormone sensitivity has been associated with an increase in the activity of a PDE with kinetic characteristics of PDE IV (275,276). Based upon this information, it has been proposed that elevated PDE activity is a fundamental biochemical defect that accounts for the depressed hormone sensitivity of leukocytes in atopic diseases (270,277).

Up-regulation of PDE IV activity in inflammatory cells may also occur as a consequence of the administration of β-adrenoceptor agonists for the treatment of asthma. Such up-regulation, if it indeed occurs in patients being treated with β-adrenoceptor agonists, could have a deleterious effect on airway function. Normally, endogenous activators of adenylyl cyclase such as epinephrine, prostaglandin E_2, and prostacyclin act as natural anti-inflammatory and bronchodilator agents (10,278). Theoretically, these homeostatic mechanisms would be compromised by a β-adrenoceptor agonist-induced up-regulation of PDE IV activity in immunoinflammatory cells and airway smooth muscle, thus allowing inflammatory processes and bronchoconstriction to proceed unchecked. To our knowledge, however, no clinical data are available to directly support this hypothesis.

CLINICAL RESULTS

Clinical studies on the effects of selective PDE inhibitors on respiratory function in humans are limited. The PDE III inhibitor enoximone was shown to decrease lung resistance and increase compliance in 11 spontaneously breathing and eight artificially ventilated patients with decompensated chronic obstructive pulmonary disease (279). Benzafentrine, a dual PDE III/ IV inhibitor, was assessed using whole-body plethysmography in 12 trained nonasthmatic human subjects, and evidence for bronchodilation was obtained when the compound was inhaled but not when it was administered intravenously or orally (94). Another PDE III/IV inhibitor, zardaverine, was devoid of bronchodilator activity when administered by inhalation to patients with chronic obstructive pulmonary disease (280). A preliminary report on the weak PDE IV inhibitor tibenelast showed that it slightly increased forced expiratory volume in 1 sec (FEV$_1$) in 40 asthmatic subjects, although this effect was not statistically significant (281). Two small clinical trials have been conducted with the PDE V inhibitor zaprinast. In adult asthmatics oral administration reduced exercise-induced bronchoconstriction but not histamine-induced bronchoconstriction (282), whereas no effects on exercise-induced bronchoconstriction were seen in a subsequent evaluation in asthmatic children (283).

Based upon the growing body of evidence from preclinical experiments supporting the bronchodilator and anti-inflammatory activity of isozyme-selective PDE inhibitors, the equivocal activity of compounds tested in the clinic thus far is somewhat surprising. Obviously, factors such as the use of compounds with insufficient potency or poor pharmacokinetic profiles could account for these results, as could employment of inappropriate patient populations or insufficient treatment durations, particularly with compounds that possess anti-inflammatory activity. Another potential problem relates to the therapeutic indices of the isozyme-selective PDE inhibitors examined to date. That is, the potential therapeutic efficacy of PDE isozyme inhibitors may not have been fully realized because of dose-limiting side effects of the compounds being evaluated. This problem may be particularly acute with systemic administration of compounds.

Although too few clinical studies have been conducted to fully describe the side-effect profiles for inhibitors of the various PDEs, tentative predictions can be made based upon the known pharmacology of representative isozyme-selective inhibitors as well as an understanding of the functional role of individual PDE isozymes in various tissues. For example, because of the importance of PDE III in regulating cAMP metabolism in the myocardium and in vascular smooth muscle, PDE III inhibitors increase cardiac contractility and induce vasodilation (284). A second concern with PDE III inhibitors is the potential arrhythmogenic activity of these compounds (285), particularly if this activity is due to PDE III inhibition per se rather than being a unique attribute of selected compounds. In addition to the known antidepressant activity of the PDE IV inhibitor rolipram, this compound produces a variety of gastrointestinal side effects, including nausea and vomiting (286), and has been shown to produce a large but transient change in plasma osmolality (287). Some or all of these adverse effects could be the result of PDE IV inhibition in the brain, gastrointestinal tract, and/or kidney. Finally, the role of cGMP as a second messenger mediating vasodilation, coupled with the importance of PDE V in regulating vascular cGMP content (288,289), suggests that inhibitors of this PDE have the potential to produce cardiovascular side effects. It should be stressed once again that with the possible exception of PDE III inhibitors, clinical experience with isozyme-selective PDE inhibitors is much too limited to make definitive conclusions regarding the potential impact, if any, that class-associated side effects will have on the utility of these agents as anti-asthmatics.

CONCLUSION

Interest in PDE inhibitors as anti-asthmatic agents has undergone a marked resurgence over the last 5 years. This renaissance has been fueled by the hope that targeting individual PDE isozymes in airway smooth muscle and inflammatory cells will improve the side-effect profile of nonselective PDE inhibitors. Preclinical studies employing animal models as well as human tissues and cells have provided compelling support for the proposal that isozyme-selective PDE inhibitors may have utility as bronchodilators, anti-inflammatory agents, or both. Overall, the data indicate that inhibition of either PDE III or PDE IV produces modest bronchodilator responses, whereas simultaneous inhibition of these isozymes produces a more profound bronchodilation. The potential bronchodilator activity of inhibitors selective for other isozymes (i.e., PDEs I, II, and V) has yet to be defined. With respect to anti-inflammatory activity, the preponderance of evidence supports PDE IV as the major molecular target.

It is becoming increasingly clear that the tissue distribution of PDE isozyme families is not absolute. That is, members of a single isozyme family are often present in more than one tissue or cell type. Consequently, while isozyme-selective PDE inhibitors may have improved therapeutic indices versus nonselective inhibitors, it is unlikely that the first generation of these compounds will be devoid of side effects stemming from inhibition of PDE isozymes in nontarget tissues. In the near term it is likely that most critical drug discovery efforts will center less on demonstrating the efficacy of isozyme-selective PDE inhibitors in various *in vitro* and *in vivo* settings, an area of investigation in which substantial knowledge now exists, and instead focus on improving the side-effect profile of these compounds. The application of molecular biology to identify additional PDE subtypes within individual PDE families, coupled with an understanding of the tissue distribution of these subtypes, represents a particularly attractive approach toward developing strategies to further improve the cell or tissue specificity of PDE inhibitors. In spite of the exciting preclinical data supporting the concept that isozyme-selective PDE inhibitors will be useful in the therapy of asthma, it is likely that the full potential of these compounds will not be known for many years.

ACKNOWLEDGMENT

The authors wish to thank Dr. Derek Buckle for his helpful suggestions and Ms. Dotti Lavan for her expert assistance and limitless patience in preparing this manuscript.

REFERENCES

1. Holgate ST. Inflammatory cells and their mediators in the pathogenesis of asthma. *Postgrad Med J* 1988;64:S82–S95.
2. Larsen GL. New concepts in the pathogenesis of asthma. *Clin Immunol Immunopathol* 1989;53:S107–S118.
3. Pearce N, Grainger J, Atkinson M, Burgess C, Culling C, Windom H, Beasley R. Case-control study of prescribed fenoterol and death from asthma in New Zealand: 1977–81. *Thorax* 1990;45:170–175.
4. Sears MR, Taylor DR, Print CG, Lake CD, Li Q, Flannery EM, Yates DM, Lucas MK, Herbiso GP. Regular inhaled beta-agonist treatment in bronchial asthma. *Lancet* 1990;336:1391–1396.
5. Spitzer WO, Suissa S, Ernst P, Horwitz RI, Habbick B, Cockroft D, Boivin J-F, McNutt M, Buist AS, Rebuck AS. The use of β-agonists and the risk of death or near death from asthma. *N Engl J Med* 1992;326:501–506.
6. Nicholson CD, Challiss RAJ, Shahid M. Differential modulation of tissue function and therapeutic potential of selective inhibitors of cyclic nucleotide phosphodiesterase iso-enzymes. *Trends Pharmacol Sci* 1991;12:19–27.
7. Torphy TJ, Undem BJ. Phosphodiesterase inhibitors: new opportunities for the treatment of asthma. *Thorax* 1991;46:512–523.
8. Giembycz MA, Dent G. Prospects for selective cyclic nucleotide phosphodiesterase inhibitors in the treatment of bronchial asthma. *Clin Exp Allergy* 1992;22:337–344.
9. Bourne HR, Lichtenstein LM, Melmon KL, Henney CS, Weinstein Y, Shearer GM. Modulation of inflammation and immunity by cyclic AMP. *Science* 1974;184:19–28.
10. Kuehl FA, Zanetti ME, Soderman DD, Miller DK, Ham EA. Cyclic AMP-dependent regulation of lipid mediators in white cells. A unifying concept for explaining the efficacy of theophylline in asthma. *Am Rev Respir Dis* 1987;136:210–213.
11. Kammer GM. The adenylate cyclase-cAMP-protein kinase A pathway and regulation of the immune response. *Immunol Today* 1988;9:222–229.
12. Torphy TJ. Biochemical regulation of airway smooth muscle tone: current knowledge and therapeutic implications. *Rev Clin Basic Pharm* 1987;6:61–103.
13. Giembycz MA, Raeburn D. Putative substrates for cyclic nucleotide-dependent protein kinases and the control of airway smooth muscle tone. *J Auton Pharmacol* 1991;11:365–398.
14. Beavo JA. Multiple isozymes of cyclic nucleotide phosphodiesterase. *Adv Second Messenger Phosphoprotein Res* 1988;22:1–30.
15. Beavo JA, Reifsnyder DH. Primary sequence of cyclic nucleotide phosphodiesterase isozymes and the design of selective inhibitors. *Trends Pharmacol Sci* 1990;1:150–155.
16. Weishaar RE, Cain MH, Bristol JA. A new generation of phosphodiesterase inhibitors: multiple molecular forms of phosphodiesterase and the potential for drug selectivity. *J Med Chem* 1985;28:537–545.
17. Thompson WJ. Cyclic nucleotide phosphodiesterases: pharmacology, biochemistry and function. *Pharmacol Ther* 1991;51:13–33.

18. Torphy TJ, Livi GP, Christensen SB IV. Novel phosphodiesterase inhibitors for the therapy of asthma. *Drug News Perspect* 1992;5:1993;6:203–214.
19. Levin RM, Weiss B. Binding of trifluoperazine to the calcium dependent activator of cyclic nucleotide phosphodiesterase. *Mol Pharmacol* 1977;13:690–697.
20. Hagiwara M, Endo T, Hidaka H. Effects of vinpocetine on cyclic nucleotide metabolism in vascular smooth muscle. *Biochem Pharmacol* 1984;33:453–457.
21. Lorenz KL, Wells JN. Potentiation of the effects of sodium nitroprusside and of isoproterenol by selective phosphodiesterase inhibitors. *Mol Pharmacol* 1983;23:424–430.
22. Hidaka H, Tanaka T, Itoh H. Selective inhibitors of three forms of cyclic nucleotide phosphodiesterases. *Trends Pharmacol Sci* 1984;5:237–239.
23. Kariya T, Dage RC. Tissue distribution and selective inhibition of subtypes of high affinity phosphodiesterase. *Biochem Pharmacol* 1988;37:3267–3270.
24. Moos WH, Humblet CC, Sircar I, Rithner C, Weishaar RE, Bristol JA, McPhail AT. Cardiotonic agents. 8. Selective inhibitors of adenosine 3',5'-cyclic phosphate phosphodiesterase III. Elaboration of a five-point model for positive inotropic activity. *J Med Chem* 1987;30:1963–1972.
25. Harrison SA, Reifsnyder DH, Gallis B, Cadd GG, Beavo JA. Isolation and characterization of bovine cardiac muscle cGMP-inhibited phosphodiesterase: a receptor for new cardiotonic drugs. *Mol Pharmacol* 1986;29:506–514.
26. Shahid M, Cottney JE, Walker GB, McIndewar I, Bruin JC, Spier I, Logan RT, Nicholson CD. Pharmacological and biochemical effects of Org 9935: a cardiotonic agent with positive inotropism, Ca sensitizing and vascular relaxant properties. *Br J Pharmacol* 1991;102:341P.
27. Murray KJ, England PJ, Hallam TJ, Maguire J, Moores K, Reeves ML, Simpson AWM, Rink TJ. The effects of siguazodan, a selective phosphodiesterase inhibitor, on human platelet function. *Br J Pharmacol* 1990;99:612–616.
28. Torphy TJ, Cieslinski LB. Characterization and selective inhibition of cyclic nucleotide phosphodiesterase isozymes in canine tracheal smooth muscle. *Mol Pharmacol* 1990;37:206–214.
29. Murray KJ, Eden RJ, Dolan JS, Grimsditch DC, Stutchbury CA, Patel B, Knowles A, Worby A, Lynham JA, Coates WJ. The effect of SK&F 95654, a novel phosphodiesterase inhibitor, on cardiovascular, respiratory and platelet function. *Br J Pharmacol* 1992;107:463–470.
30. Ruppert D, Weithman KU. HL 725, an extremely potent inhibitor of platelet phosphodiesterase and induced platelet aggregation in vitro. *Life Sci* 1982;31:2037–2043.
31. Nicholson CD, Jackman SA, Wilke R. The ability of denbufylline to inhibit cyclic nucleotide phosphodiesterase and its affinity for adenosine receptors and the adenosine re-uptake site. *Br J Pharmacol* 1898;97:889–897.
32. Glaser T, Traber J. TVX 2706—a new phosphodiesterase inhibitor with antiinflammatory action: biochemical characterization. *Agents Actions* 1984;15:341–348.
33. Némoz G, Moueqquit M, Prigent A-F, Pacheco H. Isolation of similar rolipram-inhibitable cyclic-AMP-specific phosphodiesterases from rat brain and heart. *Eur J Biochem* 1989;184:511–520.
34. Ho PPK, Wang LY, Towner RD, Hayes SJ, Pollock D, Bowling N, Wyss V, Ranetta JA. Cardiovascular effect and stimulus-dependent inhibition of superoxide generation from human neutrophils by tibenelast 5,6-diethoxybenzo(*b*)thiophene-2-carboxylic acid, sodium salt (LY186655). *Biochem Pharmacol* 1990;40:2085–2092.
35. Elliot KRF, Berry JL, Bate AJ, Foster RW, Small RC. The isoenzyme selectivity of AH 21-132 as an inhibitor of cyclic nucleotide phosphodiesterase activity. *J Enzyme Inhib* 1991;4:245–251.
36. Shahid M, Nicholson CD. Comparison of cyclic nucleotide phosphodiesterase isozymes in rat and rabbit ventricular myocardium: positive inotropic and phosphodiesterase inhibitory effects of Org 30029, milrinone and rolipram. *Naunyn Schmiedeberg's Arch Pharmacol* 1990;342:698–705.
37. Schudt C, Winder S, Muller B, Ukena D. Zardaverine as a selective inhibitor of phosphodiesterase isozymes. *Biochem Pharmacol* 1991;42:153–162.
38. Murray KJ, Eden RJ, England PJ, Dolan J, Grimsditch DC, Stutchbury CA, Patel B, Reeves ML, Worby A, Torphy TJ, Wood LM, Warrington BH, Coates WJ. Potential use of selective phosphodiesterase inhibitors in the treatment of asthma. *Agents Actions* 1991;34:S27–S46.

39. Lugnier C, Schoeffter P, LeBec A, Strouthou E, Stoclet JC. Selective inhibition of cyclic nucleotide phosphodiesterases of human, bovine and rat aorta. *Biochem Pharmacol* 1986;35:1743–1751.
40. Sharma RK, Wang JH. Regulation of cAMP concentration by calmodulin-dependent cyclic nucleotide phosphodiesterase. *Biochem Cell Biol* 1986;64:1072–1080.
41. Sharma RK, Wang JH. Purification and characterization of bovine lung calmodulin-dependent cyclic nucleotide phosphodiesterase. An enzyme containing calmodulin as a subunit. *J Biol Chem* 1986;261:14160–14166.
42. Rossi P, Giorgi M, Geremia R, Kincaid RL. Testis-specific calmodulin-dependent phosphodiesterase. A distinct high affinity cAMP isoenzyme immunologically related to brain calmodulin-dependent cGMP phosphodiesterase. *J Biol Chem* 1988;263:15521–15527.
43. Martins TJ, Mumby MC, Beavo JA. Purification and characterization of a cyclic GMP-stimulated cyclic nucleotide phosphodiesterase from bovine tissues. *J Biol Chem* 1982;257:1973–1979.
44. Grant PG, Colman RW. Purification and characterization of a human platelet cyclic nucleotide phosphodiesterase. *Biochemistry* 1984;23:1801–1807.
45. Degerman E, Belfrage P, Newman AH, Rice KC, Manganiello VC. Purification of the putative hormone-sensitive cyclic AMP phosphodiesterase from rat adipose tissue using a derivative of cilostamide as a novel affinity ligand. *J Biol Chem* 1987;262:5797–5807.
46. Manganiello VC, Degerman E, Smith CJ, Vasta V, Tornqvist H, Belfarge P. Mechanisms for activation of the rat adipocyte particulate cyclic-GMP-inhibited cyclic AMP phosphodiesterase and its importance in the antilipolytic action of insulin. *Adv Second Messenger Phosphoprotein Res* 1992;25:147–164.
47. Torphy TJ, Stadel JM, Burman M, Cieslinski LB, McLaughlin MM, White JR, Livi GP. Coexpression of human cAMP-specific phosphodiesterase activity and high affinity rolipram binding in yeast. *J Biol Chem* 1992;267:1798–1804.
48. Green DW, Cieslinski LB, Fisher SM, McLaughlin M, Livi GP, Torphy TJ. Kinetic and structural characterization of purified monocyte cAMP-specific phosphodiesterase. *Biochem J* 1993;submitted.
49. Torphy TJ, DeWolf WE Jr., Green DW, Livi GP. Biochemical characteristics and cellular regulation of phosphodiesterase IV. *Agents Actions* 1993;43:51–71.
50. Thomas MK, Francis SH, Corbin JD. Characterization of a purified bovine lung cGMP-binding cGMP phosphodiesterase. *J Biol Chem* 1990;265:14964–14970.
51. Thomas MK, Francis SH, Corbin JD. Substrate- and kinase-directed regulation of phosphorylation of a cGMP-binding phosphodiesterase by cGMP. *J Biol Chem* 1990;265:14971–14978.
52. Conti M, Jin SLC, Monaco L, Repaske DR, Swinnen JV. Hormonal regulation of cyclic nucleotide phosphodiesterases. *Endocr Rev* 1991;12:218–234.
53. Jin S-L, Swinnen JV, Conti M. Characterization of the structure of a low K_m, rolipram-sensitive cAMP phosphodiesterase. Mapping of the catalytic domain. *J Biol Chem* 1992;267:18929–18939.
53a.Repaske DR, Swinnen JV, Jin SLC, VanWyk JJ, Conti M. A polymerase chain reaction strategy to identify and clone cyclic nucleotide phosphodiesterase cDNAs. Molecular cloning of the cDNA encoding the 63-kDa calmodulin-dependent phosphodiesterase. *J Biol Chem* 1992;267:18683–18688.
54. Bentley JK, Kadlecek A, Sherbert CH, Seger D, Sonnenburg WK, Charbonneau H, Novack JP, Beavo JA. Molecular cloning of cDNA encoding a "63"-kDa calmodulin-stimulated phosphodiesterase from bovine brain. *J Biol Chem* 1992;267:18676–18682.
55. Li T, Volpp K, Applebury ML. Bovine cone photoreceptor cGMP phosphodiesterase structure deduced from a cDNA clone. *Proc Natl Acad Sci USA* 1990;87:293–297.
56. Sonnenburg WK, Mullaney PJ, Beavo JA. Molecular cloning of a cyclic GMP-stimulated cyclic nucleotide phosphodiesterase cDNA. Identification and distribution of isozyme variants. *J Biol Chem* 1991;266:17655–17661.
57. Meacci E, Taira M, Moos M, Smith CJ, Movsesian MA, Degerman E, Belfrage P, Manganiello V. Molecular cloning and expression of human myocardial cGMP-inhibited cAMP phosphodiesterase. *Proc Natl Acad Sci USA* 1992;89:3721–3725.
58. Colicelli J, Birchmeier C, Michaeli T, O'Neill K, Riggs M, Wigler M. Isolation and

characterization of a mammalian gene encoding a high-affinity cAMP phosphodiesterase. *Proc Natl Acad Sci USA* 1989;86:3599–3603.

59. Davis RL, Takaysasu H, Eberwine M, Myres J. Cloning and characterization of mammalian homologs of the *Drosophila* dunce+ gene. *Proc Natl Acad Sci USA* 1989; 86:3604–3608.
60. Swinnen JV, Joseph DR, Conti M. Molecular cloning of rat homologues of the *Drosophila melanogaster* dunce cAMP phosphodiesterase: evidence for a family of genes. *Proc Natl Acad Sci USA* 1989;86:5325–5329.
61. Livi GP, Kmetz P, McHale M, Cieslinski L, Sathe GM, Taylor DJ, Davis RL, Torphy T, Balcarek JM. Cloning and expression of cDNA for a human low-K$_m$, rolipram-sensitive cAMP phosphodiesterase. *Mol Cell Biol* 1990;10:2678–2686.
62. McLaughlin MM, Cieslinski LB, Burman M, Torphy TJ, Livi GP. A low-K$_m$, rolipram-sensitive, cAMP-specific phosphodiesterase from human brain. Cloning and expression of cDNA, biochemical characterization of recombinant protein and tissue distribution of mRNA. *J Biol Chem* 1993;268:6470–6476.
63. Baehr W, Champagne MS, Lee AK, Pittler SJ. Complete cDNA sequences of mouse rod photoreceptor cGMP phosphodiesterase alpha- and beta-subunits, and identification of beta-prime, a putative beta-subunit isozyme produced by alternative splicing of the beta-subunit. *FEBS Lett* 1991;278:107–114.
64. Pittler SJ, Baehr W, Wasmuth JJ, McConnell DG, Champagne MS, vanTuinen P, Ledbetter D, Davis RL. Molecular characterization of human and bovine rod photoreceptor cGMP phosphodiesterase a-subunit and chromosomal localization of the human gene. *Genomics* 1990;6:272–283.
65. Torphy TJ, Burman M, Huang LBF, Tucker SS. Inhibition of the low K$_m$ cyclic AMP phosphodiesterase in intact canine trachaelis by SK&F 94836: mechanical and biochemical responses. *J Pharmacol Exp Ther* 1988;246:843–850.
66. Rasmussen H, Kelley G, Douglas JS. Interactions between Ca^{2+} and cAMP messenger system in regulation of airway smooth muscle contraction. *Am J Physiol* 1990; 258:L279–L288.
67. Kume H, Kotlikoff MI. K$_{ca}$ in tracheal smooth muscle cells are activated by the α subunit of the stimulatory G protein, G$_s$. *Am Rev Respir Dis* 1992;145:A204.
68. Hartshorne DJ, Kawamura T. Regulation of contraction-relaxation in smooth muscle. *News Physiol Sci* 1992;7:59–64.
69. de Lanerolle P, Paul RJ. Myosin phosphorylation/dephosphorylation and regulation of airway smooth muscle contractility. *Am J Physiol* 1991;261:L1–L14.
70. Gerthoffer WT. Dissociation of myosin phosphorylation and active tension during muscarinic stimulation of tracheal smooth muscle. *J Pharmacol Exp Ther* 1987;24:8–15.
71. Gerthoffer WT. Regulation of the contractile element of airway smooth muscle. *Am J Physiol* 1991;261:L15–L28.
72. Sparrow MP, Pfitzer G, Gagelmann M, Ruegg JC. Effect of calmodulin Ca^{2+}, and cAMP protein kinase on skinned tracheal smooth muscle. *Am J Physiol* 1984;246: C308–C314.
73. Taylor DA, Bowman BF, Stull JT. Cytoplasmic Ca^{2+} is a primary determinant for myosin phosphorylation in smooth muscle cells. *J Biol Chem* 1989;264:6207–6213.
74. Stull JT, Hsu LC, Tansey MG, Kamm KE. Myosin light chain phosphorylation in tracheal smooth muscle. *J Biol Chem* 1990;265:16683–16690.
74a. Felbel J, Trockur B, Ecker T, Landgraf W, Hofmann F. Regulation of cytosolic calcium by cAMP and cGMP in freshly isolated smooth muscle cells from bovine trachea. *J Biol Chem* 1988;263:16764–16771.
75. Takuwa Y, Takuwa N, Rasmussen H. The effects of isoproterenol on intracellular calcium concentration. *J Biol Chem* 1988;263:762–768.
76. Gunst SJ, Bandyopadhyay S. Contractile force and intracellular Ca^{2+} during relaxation of canine tracheal smooth muscle. *Am J Physiol* 1989;257:C355–364.
77. Kume H, Takai A, Tokuno H, Tomita T. Regulation of Ca^{2+}-dependent K$^+$-channel activity in tracheal myocytes by phosphorylation. *Nature* 1989;341:152–154.
78. Shahid M, Van Amsterdam RGM, de Boer J, ten Berge RD, Nicholson CD, Zaagsma J. The presence of five cyclic nucleotide phosphodiesterase isoenzyme activities in bovine tracheal smooth muscle and the functional effects of selective inhibitors. *Br J Pharmacol* 1991;104:471–477.

79. Giembycz MA, Barnes PJ. Selective inhibition of a high affinity type IV cyclic AMP phosphodiesterase in bovine trachealis by AH 21-132. *Biochem Pharmacol* 1991; 42:663–677.
80. Harris AL, Lemp BM, Bentley RG, Perrone MH, Hamel LT, Silver PJ. Phosphodiesterase isozyme inhibition and the potentiation by zaprinast of endothelium-derived relaxing factor and guanylate cyclase stimulating agents in vascular smooth muscle. *J Pharmacol Exp Ther* 1989;249:394–400.
81. Torphy TJ, Undem BJ, Cieslinski LB, Luttman MA, Reeves MK, Hay DWP. Identification, characterization and functional role of phosphodiesterase isozymes in human airway smooth muscle. *J Pharmacol Exp Ther* 1993;265:1213–1223.
82. Giembycz MA, Belvisi MG, Miura M, Perkins RS, Kelly J, Tadjkarimi S, Yacoub MH, Giembycz MA, Barnes PJ. Soluble cyclic nucleotide phosphodiesterase isoenzymes from human tracheal smooth muscle. *Br J Pharmacol* 1992;107:52P.
83. de Boer J, Philpott AJ, van Amsterdam RGM, Shahid M, Zaagsma J, Nicholson CD. Human bronchial cyclic nucleotide phosphodiesterase isoenzymes: biochemical and pharmacological analysis using selective inhibitors. *Br J Pharmacol* 1992;106:1028–1034.
84. Rabe KF, Tenor H, Dent G, Schudt C, Liebig S, Magnussen H. Functional and biochemical characterisation of PDE isoenzymes regulating inherent tone in human peripheral airways. *Br J Pharmacol* 1992;107:54P.
85. Hall IP, Hill SJ. Effects of isozyme selective phosphodiesterase inhibitors on bovine tracheal smooth muscle tone. *Biochem Pharmacol* 1992;43:15–17.
86. Hall IP, Donaldson J, Hill SJ. Inhibition of histamine-stimulated inositol phospholipid hydrolysis by agents which increase cyclic AMP levels in bovine tracheal smooth muscle. *Br J Pharmacol* 1989;97:603–616.
87. Hall IP, Donaldson J, Hill SJ. Modulation of carbachol-induced inositol phosphate formation in bovine tracheal smooth muscle by cyclic AMP phosphodiesterase inhibitors. *Biochem Pharmacol* 1990;39:1357–1363.
88. Chilvers ER, Giembycz MA, Challis RAJ, Barnes PJ, Nahorski SR. Lack of effect of zaprinast on methacholine-induced contraction and inositol 1,4,5-trisphosphate accumulation in bovine tracheal smooth muscle. *Br J Pharmacol* 1991;103:1119–1125.
89. Murray KJ. PDE V_A inhibitors. *Drug News Perspect* 1993;6:150–156.
90. Torphy TJ, Zhou HL, Burman M, Huang LBF. Role of cyclic nucleotide phosphodiesterase isozymes in intact canine trachealis. *Mol Pharmacol* 1991;39:376–384.
91. Rossing TH, Drazen JM. Effects of milrinone on contactile responses of guinea-pig trachea, lung parenchyma and pulmonary artery. *J Pharmacol Exp Ther* 1986;238:874–897.
92. Bryson SE, Rodger IW. Effects of phosphodiesterase inhibitors on normal and chemically-skinned isolated airway smooth muscle. *Br J Pharmacol* 1987;92:673–681.
93. Hughes B, Gozzard N, Higgs G. Differential effects of phosphodiesterase isoenzyme inhibitors in reversing induced tone in guinea-pig trachea. *Br J Pharmacol* 1992; 105:185P.
94. Small RC, Foster RW, Berry JL, Chapman ID, Elliot KRF. The bronchodilator action of AH 21-132. *Agents Actions* 1991;34:S3–S26.
95. Langlands JM, Rodger IW, Diamond J. The effect of M&B 22948 on methacholine- and histamine-induced contraction and inositol 1,4,5-trisphosphate levels in guinea-pig tracheal tissue. *Br J Pharmacol* 1989;98:336–338.
96. Bewley JS, Chapman ID. AH21-132: a novel relaxant of airway smooth muscle. *Br J Pharmacol* 1988;93:52P.
97. Belvisi MG, Miura M, Peters MJ, Ward JK, Tadjkarimi S, Yacoub MH, Giembycz MA, Barnes PJ. Effect of isoenzyme-selective cyclic nucleotide phosphodiesterase inhibitors on human tracheal smooth muscle tone. *Br J Pharmacol* 1992;107:53P.
98. Hall IP, Townsend P, Daykin K, Widdop S. Control of tissue cyclic AMP content in primary cultures of human airway smooth muscle cells. *Br J Pharmacol* 1992;105:71P.
99. Heaslip RJ, Buckley SK, Sickels BD, Grimes D. Bronchial vs. cardiovascular activities of selective phosphodiesterase inhibitors in the anesthetized beta-blocked dog. *J Pharmacol Exp Ther* 1991;257:741–747.
100. Gristwood RW, Sampford KA. Inhibition of histamine-induced bronchoconstriction by SK&F 94836, salbutamol and theophylline in anaesthetised guinea-pigs. *Br J Pharmacol* 1987;92:631P.

101. Giembycz MA, Barnes PJ. Stimulus-response coupling in eosinophils: receptors, signal transduction and pharmacological modulation. In: Smith H, Cook RM, eds. *Immunopharmacology of eosinophils*. London: Academic Press, 1993;91–118.

102. Nielson CP, Crowley JJ, Morgan ME, Vestal RA. Polymorphonuclear leukocyte inhibition by therapeutic concentrations of theophylline is mediated by cyclic-3',5'-adenosine monophosphate. *Am Rev Respir Dis* 1988;137:25–30.

103. Krzanowski JJ, Polson JB. Mechanism of action of methylxanthines in asthma. *J Allergy Clin Immunol* 1988;82:143–145.

104. Stadel JM. β-Adrenoceptor signal transduction. In: Ruffolo RR, ed. β-*Adrenoceptors: molecular biology, biochemistry and pharmacology*. Progress in Basic and Clinical Pharmacology (Lomax P, Vesell ES, eds.), vol 7. Basel: S. Karger, 1991;67–104.

105. Busse WW, Sedgwick JB. Eosinophils in asthma. *Ann Allergy* 1992;68:286–290.

106. Kay AB, Corrigan CJ. Eosinophils and neutrophils. *Br Med Bull* 1992;48:51–64.

107. Smith H. Asthma, inflammation, eosinophils and bronchial hyperresponsiveness. *Clin Exp Allergy* 1992;22:187–197.

108. Weller PF. The immunobiology of eosinophils. *N Engl J Med* 1991;324:1110–1118.

109. Masuyama K, Ishikawa T. Direct interaction of guinea-pig eosinophils and adrenergic agents. *Int Arch Allergy Appl Immunol* 1985;78:243–248.

110. Gardner RV, Tebbi CK, Ambrus JL. The comparison of in vitro and in vivo effects of phosphodiesterase inhibitors—prostaglandin I_2 releasers on granulopoiesis. *J Med* 1980;11:361–376.

111. Koch-Weser J. Beta adrenergic blockade and circulating eosinophils. *Arch Intern Med* 1968;121:255–258.

112. Makino S, Ouellette JJ, Reed CE, Fishel C. Correlation between increased bronchial response to acetylcholine and diminished metabolic and eosinopenic responses to epinephrine in asthma. *J Allergy* 1970;46:178–189.

113. Reed CE, Cohen M, Enta T. Reduced effect of epinephrine on circulating eosinophils in asthma and after beta-adrenergic blockade or Bordetella pertussis vaccine. *J Allergy* 1970;46:90–102.

114. Gayard P, Gayard A, Charpin J. Effects des bronchodilateurs sur les test cutanés d'allergic. *Rev Fr Allergol* 1972;12:219–229.

115. Ohman JL, Laurence M, Lowell FC. Effect of propranolol on the eosinopenic responses of cortisol, isoproterenol and aminophylline. *J Allergy Clin Immunol* 1972;50:151–156.

116. Dahl R, Venge P. Blood eosinophil leukocyte and eosinophil cationic protein. *Scand J Respir Dis* 1978;59:319–322.

117. Braat MCP, Jonkers RE, Bel EH, Van Boxtel CJ. Qualification of theophylline-induced eosinopenia and hypokalaemia in healthy volunteers. *Clin Pharmacokinet* 1992;22:231–237.

118. Spicer BA, Baker RC, Hatt PA, Laycock SM, Smith H. The effects of drugs on Sephadex-induced eosinophilia and lung hyper-responsiveness in the rat. *Br J Pharmacol* 1990;101:821–828.

119. Cook RM, Musgrove NJR, Smith H. Eosinophils and the granulomatous reaction in rats injected with Sephadex particles. *Pulmon Pharmacol* 1989;2:185–190.

120. Tarayre JP, Aliaga M, Barbara M, Tisseyre N, Vieu S, Tisne-Versaille J. Model of bronchial allergic inflammation in the Brown Norway rat: pharmacological modulation. *Int J Immunopharmacol* 1992;14:847–855.f

121. Fügner A. Formation of oedema and accumulation of eosinophils in the guinea pig lung. *Int Arch Allergy Appl Immunol* 1989;88:225–227.

122. Sanjar S, McCabe PJ, Reynolds LH, Johnson M. Salmeterol inhibits antigen-induced eosinophil accumulation in the guinea-pig lung. *Fundam Clin Pharmacol* 1991;5:402.

123. Sanjar S, Aoki S, Kristerson A, Smith D, Morley J. Antigen challenge induced pulmonary airway eosinophil accumulation and airway hyperreactivity in sensitized guinea-pigs: the effect of anti-asthma drugs. *Br J Pharmacol* 1990;99:679–686.

124. Tarayre JP, Aliaga M, Barbara M, Tisseyre N, Vieu S, Tisne-Versailles J. Pharmacological modulation of a model of bronchial inflammation after aerosol-induced active anaphylactic shock in conscious guinea-pigs. *Int J Immunopharmacol* 1991;13:349–356.

125. Chand N, Harrison J, Rooney S, et al. Therapeutic approach for the evaluation of

antiasthma compounds in allergic bronchial inflammation in guinea pigs. *Am Res Respir Dis* 1991;143:A633.

126. Boubekur K, Marguin V, Bouhelal R, Morley J. Failure of long-acting beta-adrenoceptor agonists to diminish allergic eosinophilia of the airways in guinea-pigs. *Fundam Clin Pharmacol* 1991;5:402.

127. Sanjar S, Aoki S, Boubekeur K, Burrows L, Colditz I, Chapman I, Morley J. Inhibition of PAF-induced eosinophil accumulation in pulmonary airways of guinea-pigs by antiasthma drugs. *Jpn J Pharmacol* 1989;51:167–172.

128. Sanjar S, Aoki K, Boubekeur K, Chapman ID, Smith D, Kings MA, Morley J. Eosinophil accumulation in pulmonary airways of guinea-pigs induced by exposure to an aerosol of platelet-activating factor: effect of anti-asthma drugs. *Br J Pharmacol* 1990;99:267–272.

129. Whelan CJ, Johnson M. Inhibition by salmeterol of increased vascular permeability and granulocyte accumulation in guinea-pig lung and skin. *Br J Pharmacol* 1992; 105:831–838.

130. Szczeklik A, Podolec Z. Central regulation of blood eosinophilia by the beta adrenergic system in rats. *Int Arch Allergy* 1976;50:329–340.

131. Okyayuz GI, Ventura MA, Gardey C, Rey E, Thiroux G. Studies on methyl xanthines in intact and hypophysectomised rats: differences in pharmacokinetics and adrenocortical response. *Life Sci* 1985;37:1201–1211.

132. Kita H, Abu-Ghazaleh RI, Gleich GJ, Abraham RT. Regulation of Ig-induced eosinophil degranulation by adenosine 3′,5′ cyclic monophosphate. *J Immunol* 1991;146: 2712–2718.

133. Yukawa T, Ukena D, Kroegel C. Beta$_2$-adrenergic receptors on eosinophils. Binding and functional studies. *Am Rev Respir Dis* 1990;141:1446–1452.

134. Rabe KF, Giembycz MA, Dent G, Barnes PJ. β$_2$-adrenoceptor agonists and respiratory burst activity in guinea-pig and human eosinophils. *Fundam Clin Pharmacol* 1991; 5:402.

135. Yukawa T, Kroegel C, Chanez P, Dent G, Ukena D, Chung KF, Barnes PJ. Effect of theophylline and adenosine on eosinophil function. *Am Rev Respir Dis* 1989;140:327–333.

136. Dent G, Giembycz MA, Rabe KF, Barnes PJ. Inhibition of eosinophil cyclic nucleotide PDE activity and opsonised zymosan-induced respiratory burst by "type IV"-selective PDE inhibitors. *Br J Pharmacol* 1991;103:1339–1346.

137. Dent G, Evans PM, Chung KF, Barnes PJ. Zardaverine inhibits respiratory burst activity in human eosinophils. *Am Rev Respir Dis* 1990;161:A392.

138. Souness JE, Villamil ME, Scott LC, Tomkinson A, Giembycz, Raeburn D. Possible role of cyclic AMP phosphodiesterases in the actions of ibudulast on eosinophil thromboxane generation and airways smooth muscle tone. *Brit J Pharmacol* 1994;111: in press.

139. Boschetto P, Mapp CE, Picotti G, Fabbri LM. Neutrophils and asthma. *Eur Resp J* 1989;6:456S–459S.

140. Reibman J, Haines K, Weissmann G. Alterations in cyclic nucleotides and the activation of neutrophils. In: *Current topics in membranes and transport,* vol 35. New York: Academic Press, 1990;399–424.

141. Hopkins NK, Lin AH, Gorman RA. Evidence for mediation of acetyl glyceryl ether phosphorylcholine stimulation of adenosine 3′,5′ (cyclic) monophosphate levels in human polymorphonuclear leukocytes by leukotriene B$_4$. *Biochim Biophys Acta* 1983;763:276–283.

142. Korchak HM. Signaling mechanisms of neutrophil activation. In: Gilman SC, Rogers TG, eds. *Immunopharmacology.* Caldwell, NJ: Telford Press, 1989;65–88.

143. Simchowitz L, Spilber I, Atkinson JP. Evidence that the functional responses of human neutrophils occur independently of transient elevations in cyclic AMP levels. *J Cyclic Nucleotide Protein Phosphorylation Res* 1983;9:35–47.

144. Rivkin I, Neutze JA. Influence of cyclic nucleotides and phosphodiesterase inhibitor on in vitro human blood neutrophil chemotaxis. *Arch Int Pharmacodyn* 1977;228:196–204.

145. Harvath L, Robbins JD, Russell AA, Seamon KB. cAMP and human neutrophil chemotaxis. Elevation of cAMP differentially affects chemotactic responsiveness. *J Immunol* 1991;146:224–232.

146. Burde R, Seifert R, Buschauer A, Schultz G. Histamine inhibits activation of human neutrophils and HL-60 leukemic cells via H_2-receptors. *Naunyn Schmiedebergs Arch Pharmacol* 1989;360:671–678.
147. Wenzel-Seifert K, Ervens J, Seifert R. Differential inhibition and potentiation by cell-permeant analogues of cyclic AMP and cyclic GMP and NO-containing compounds of exocytosis in human neutrophils. *Naunyn Schmiedebergs Arch Pharmacol* 1991; 344:396–402.
148. Tecoma ES, Motulsky HJ, Traynor AE, Omann GM, Muller H, Sklar LA. Transient catecholamine modulation of neutrophil activation: kinetic and intracellular aspects of isoproterenol action. *J Leukocyte Biol* 1986;40:629–644.
149. Furui H, Suzuki K, Takagi K, Satake T. Effect of colforsin on human neutrophil superoxide production and intracellular calcium mobilization. *Clin Exp Pharmacol Physiol* 1989;16:199–209.
150. Kaneko M, Suzuki K, Furui H, Takagi K, Satake T. Comparison of theophylline and enprofylline effects on human neutrophil superoxide production. *Clin Exp Pharmacol Physiol* 1990;17:849–859.
151. Nielson CP, Vestal RE. Effects of adenosine on polymorphonuclear leucocyte function, cyclic 3':5' adenosine monophosphate and intracellular calcium. *Br J Pharmacol* 1989;97:882–888.
152. Fonteh AN, Winkler JD, Torphy TJ, Heravi J, Undem BJ, Chilton FH. Influence of adenosine 3', 5'-monophosphate on platelet activating factor biosynthesis in the human neutrophil. *J Immunol* 1993;151:1–12.
153. Boogaerts MA, Malbrain S, Meeus P, Van Houe L, Verhoef GEG. *In vitro* modulation of normal and disease human neutrophil function by pentoxifylline. *Blut* 1990;61:60–65.
154. Sheetz MP, Wang WP, Kreutzer DL. Polyphosphoinositides as regulators of membrane skeletal stability. In: *White cell mechanics: basic science and clinical aspects.* New York: Alan R. Liss, 1984;87–94.
155. Kay AB. Inflammatory cells in chronic asthma. *Agents Actions* 1989;28:147–161.
156. Plaut M, Pierce JH, Watson CJ, Hamley-Hyde J, Nordan RP, Paul WE. Mast cell lines produce lymphokines in response to cross-linkage of FcERI or to calcium ionophores. *Nature* 1989;339:64–67.
157. Galli SJ, Gordan JR, Wersbil BK. Cytokine production by mast cells and basophils. *Curr Opinion Immunol* 1991;3:865–873.
158. Tung RS, Lichtenstein LM. Cyclic AMP agonist inhibition increases at low levels of histamine release from human basophils. *J Pharmacol Exp Ther* 1981;218:642–646.
159. MacGlashan DW, Schleimer RP, Peters SP, et al. Comparative studies of human basophils and mast cells. *Fed Proc* 1983;43:2504–2509.
160. Undem BJ, Buckner CK. Mechanisms of β-adrenergic-induced inhibition of immunologic mediator release. In: Hollinger MA, ed. *Current topics in pulmonary pharmacology and toxicology,* vol 1. New York: Elsevier, 1985:57–88.
161. Peachell PT, Lichtenstein LM, Schleimer RP. Inhibition by adenosine of histamine and leukotriene release from human basophils. *Biochem Pharmacol* 1989;38:1717–1725.
162. Peachell PT, MacGlashan DW, Lichtenstein LM, Schleimer RP. Regulation of human basophil and lung mast cell function by cyclic adenosine monophosphate. *J Immunol* 1988;140:571–579.
163. Undem BJ, Peachell PT, Lichtenstein LM. Isoproterenol-induced inhibition of immunoglobulin E-mediated release of histamine and arachidonic acid metabolites from the human lung mast cell. *J Pharmacol Exp Ther* 1988;247:209–217.
164. Undem BJ, Torphy TJ, Goldman D, Chilton FH. Inhibition by adenosine 3':5'-monophosphate of eicosanoid and platelet-activating factor biosynthesis in the mouse PT-18 mast cell. *J Biol Chem* 1990;265:6750–6758.
165. Fuller RW. Macrophages. *Br Med Bull* 1992;48:65–71.
166. Snyderman R, Smith CD, Verghese MW. Model for leukocyte regulation by chemoattractant receptors: roles of a guanine nucleotide regulatory protein and polyphosphoinositide metabolism. *J Leukocyte Biol* 1986;40:785–800.
167. Fuller RW, O'Malley G, Baker AJ, MacDermot J. Human alveolar macrophage activation: inhibition by forskolin but not β-adrenoceptor stimulation or phosphodiesterase inhibition. *Pulmon Pharmacol* 1988;1:101–106.

168. Wilk P. Vasoactive intestinal peptide inhibits the respiratory burst in human monocytes by a cyclic AMP-mediated mechanism. *Regul Pept* 1989;25:187–197.
169. Turner NC, Wood LJ, Burns FM, Gueremy T, Souness JE. The effect of cyclic AMP and cyclic GMP phosphodiesterase inhibitors of the superoxide burst of guinea-pig peritoneal macrophages. *Br J Pharmacol* 1993;876–883.
170. Baker AJ, Fuller RW. Effect of cyclic adenosine monophosphate, 5'-(N-ethylcarbox-yamido)-adenosine and methylxanthines on the release of thromboxane and lyposomal enzymes from human alveolar macrophages and peripheral blood monocytes *in vitro*. *Eur J Pharmacol* 1992;211:157–161.
171. Dent G, Giembycz MA, Rabe KF, Barnes PJ, Magnussen H. Inhibition of human alveolar macrophage respiratory burst by theophylline: association with phosphodiesterase inhibition. *Br J Pharmacol* 1992;107:55P.
172. Elliott KRF, Leonard EJ. Interactions of formylmethionyl-leucyl-phenylalanine, adenosine, and phosphodiesterase inhibitors in human monocytes. *FEBS Lett* 1989;254:94–98.
173. Renz H, Gong J-H, Schmidt A, Naim M, Gemsa D. Release of tumour necrosis factor-α from macrophages. Enhancement and suppression are dose-dependently regulated by prostaglandin E_2 and cyclic nucleotides. *J Immunol* 1988;141:2388–2393.
174. Strieter RM, Remick DA, Ward PA, et al. Cellular and molecular regulation of tumour necrosis factor-alpha production by pentoxifylline. *Biochem Biophys Res Commun* 1988;155:1230–1236.
175. Feiren MWJA, van dem Bemd G-JCM, Ben-Efrain S, Bonta IL. Prostaglandin E_2 inhibits the release of tumour necrosis factor-α, rather than interleukin 1β, from human macrophages. *Immunol Lett* 1991;31:85–90.
176. Endres S, Fulle H-J, Sinha B, et al. Cyclic nucleotides differentially regulate the synthesis of tumor necrosis factor-a and interleukin-1β by human mononuclear cells. *Immunology* 1991;72:56–60.
177. Serkkola E, Hurme M, Palkama T. Prolonged elevation of intracellular cyclic AMP activates interleukin-1 production in human peripheral blood monocytes. *Scand J Immunol* 1992;35:203–208.
178. Corrigan CJ, Kay AB. Role of T-lymphocytes and lymphokines. *Br Med Bull* 1992;48:72–84.
179. Robinson DS, Hamid Q, Ying S, et al. Predominant T_{H2}-like bronchoalveolar T-lymphocyte population in atopic asthma. *N Engl J Med* 1992;326:298–304.
180. Hadden JW. Transmembrane signals in the activation of T lymphocytes by mitogenic antigens. *Immunol Today* 1988;9:235–239.
181. Altman A, Coggenhall KM, Mustelin T. Molecular events mediating T cell activation. *Adv Immunol* 1990;48:227–360.
182. Tamir A, Isakov N. Increased intracellular cyclic AMP levels block PKC-mediated T cell activation by inhibition of c-*jun* transcription. *Immunol Lett* 1991;27:95–100.
183. Alava MA, DeBell KE, Conti A, Hoffman T, Bonvini E. Increased intracellular cyclic AMP inhibits inositol phospholipid hydrolysis induced by pertubation of the T cell receptor/CD3 complex but not by G-protein stimulation. *Biochem J* 1992;284:189–199.
184. Maghazachi AA. Cholera toxin inhibits interleukin-2-induced, but enhances pertussis toxin-induced T-cell proliferation: regulation by cyclic nucleotides. *Immunology* 1992;75:103–107.
185. Plaut M, Marone G, Gillespie E. The role of cyclic AMP in modulating cytotoxic T lymphocytes. II. Sequential changes during culture in responsiveness of cytotoxic lymphocytes to cyclic AMP-active agents. *J Immunol* 1983;131:2945–2952.
186. Gajewski TF, Schell SR, Fitch FW. Evidence implicating utilization of different T cell receptor-associated signaling pathways by T_H1 and T_H2 clones. *J Immunol* 1990;144:4110–4120.
187. Snijdewint FGM, Kalinski P, Bos JD, Kapsenberg ML. The cytokine production profile of human T cell clones can selectively be affected by prostaglandin E_2. *Eur J Allergy Clin Immunol* 1992;12:220.
188. Lahat N, No E, Horenstein L, Colin AA. Effect of theophylline on the proportion and function of T-suppressor cells in asthmatic children. *Allergy* 1985;40:453–457.
189. Guillou PJ, Kerr MB, Ramsden CW, Giles GR. Studies of T-cell subset changes in patients receiving aminophylline as an adjunct to conventional immunosuppression for renal transplantation. In: Turner-Waiwick M, Levy J, eds. *New perspectives in theophylline therapy*. London: Royal Society of Medicine, 1984;157–164.

190. Patke CL, Orson FM, Shearer WT. Cyclic AMP-mediated modulation of immunoglobulin production in B cells by prostaglandin E_1. *Cell Immunol* 1991;137:36–45.
191. Vasquez A, Auffredou MT, Galanaud P, Leca G. Modulation of IL-2 and IL-4-dependent human B cell proliferation by cyclic AMP. *J Immunol* 1991;146:4222–4227.
192. Page CP. Platelet-activating factor. In: Barnes PJ, Rodger IW, Thomson NC, eds. *Asthma: basic mechanisms and clinical management.* London: Academic Press, 1988;283–304.
193. Capron A, Auriault C, Cesbron J-Y, Pancré V. In: Kaliner MA, Barnes PJ, Persson CGA, eds. *Platelets in asthma. Asthma its pathology and treatment.* New York: Marcel Dekker, 1991;231–246.
194. Fredén K, Olsson L-B, Vilén L, Kutti J. Peripheral platelet count in response to salbutamol before and after adrenergic beta-receptor blockade. *Acta Haematol* 1978; 60:310–315.
195. Weller MPI, Wright DJM. Inhibition by laevo-propranolol and naloxone of salbutamol-induced depression of white cell and platelet counts in mice. *Br J Pharmacol* 1981;73:298–299.
196. Vilén L, Kutti J, Fredén K, Lundborg P, Cronberg S. The peripheral platelet count and ADP-induced platelet aggregation in response to metoprolol and propranolol as studied in young healthy male volunteers. *Scand J Haematol* 1983;31:440–446.
197. Salzman EW. Cyclic AMP and platelet function. *N Engl J Med* 1972;286:358–363.
198. Perrson CGA, Svensjö E. Vascular responses and their suppression: drugs interfering with venular permeability. In: Bonta IL, Bray MA, Parnham MJ, eds. *Handbook of inflammation, vol 5: The pharmacology of inflammation.* Amsterdam: Elsevier, 1985:61–81.
199. Perrson CGA. Role of plasma exudation in asthmatic airways. *Lancet* 1986;1126–1129.
200. Chung KF, Rogers DF, Barnes PJ, Evans TW. The role of increased airway microvascular permeability and plasma exudation in asthma. *Eur Resp J* 1990;3:329–337.
201. Rogers DF, Evans TW. Plasma exudation and oedema in asthma. *Br Med Bull* 1992;48:120–134.
202. Renkonen R, Mattila P, Häyry P, Ustinov J. Interleukin 1-induced lymphocyte binding to endothelial cells: role of cAMP as a second messenger. *Eur J Immunol* 1990; 20:1563–1567.
203. Bouillon M, Fortieo MA, Boulianne R, Audette M. Biphasic effect of cAMP-elevating agents on ICAM-1 expression stimulated by retinoic acid and interferon γ. *Int J Cancer* 1992;50:281–288.
204. Langeler EG, van Hinsbergh VWM. Norepinephrine and iloprost improve barrier function of human endothelial cell monolayers: role of cAMP. *Am J Physiol* 1991; 260:C1052–C1059.
205. Suttorp N, Welsch T, Weber V, Richter U, Schudt C. Activation of cAMP-dependent protein kinase blocks hydrogen peroxide-induced enhanced endothelial permeability in vitro. *Am Rev Respir Dis* 1991;143:A572.
206. Rampart M, Williams TJ. Polymorphonuclear leukocyte-dependent plasma leakage in the rabbit skin is enhanced or inhibited by prostacyclin depending on the route of administration. *Am J Pathol* 1986;124:66–73.
207. Boschetto P, Roberts NM, Rogers DF, Barnes PJ. Effect of antiasthma drugs on microvascular leakage in guinea pig airways. *Am Rev Respir Dis* 1989;139:416–421.
208. Advenier C, Qian Y, Koune L, Molimard M, Candenas M-L, Naline E. Formoterol and salbutamol inhibit bradykinin- and histamine-induced airway microvascular leakage in guinea-pig. *Br J Pharmacol* 1992;105:792–798.
209. Raeburn D, Karlsson J-A. Comparison of the effects of isozyme-selective phosphodiesterase inhibitors and theophylline on PAF-induced plasma leakage in the guinea-pig airways in vivo. *Am Rev Respir Dis* 1992;145:A612.
210. Souness JE, Carter CM, Diocee BK, Hassall GA, Wood LJ, Turner NC. Characterization of guinea-pig eosinophil phosphodiesterase activity. Assessment of its involvement in regulating superoxide generation. *Biochem Pharmacol* 1991;42:937–965.
211. Giembycz MA. Could isoenzyme-selective phosphodiesterase inhibitors render bronchodilator therapy redundant in the treatment of bronchial asthma? *Biochem Pharmacol* 1992;43:2041–2051.
212. Schudt C, Winder S, Forderkunz S, Hatzelmann A, Ullrich V. Influence of selective phosphodiesterase inhibitors on human neutrophil functions and levels of cAMP and Ca_i. *Naunyn Schmiedebergs Arch Pharmacol* 1991;344:682–690.

213. Nielson CP, Vestal RE, Sturm RJ, Heaslip R. Effects of selective phosphodiesterase inhibitors on the polymorphonuclear leukocyte respiratory burst. *J Allergy Clin Immunol* 1990;86:801–808.
214. Wright CD, Kuipers PJ, Kobylarz-Singer D, Devall LJ, Klinkefus BA, Weishaar RE. Differential inhibition of human neutrophil functions. Role of cyclic AMP-specific, cyclic GMP-insensitive phosphodiesterase. *Biochem Pharmacol* 1990;40:699–707.
215. Engerson T, Legendre JL, Jones HP. Calmodulin-dependency of human neutrophil phosphodiesterase. *Inflammation* 1986;10:31–35.
216. Grady PG, Thomas LL. Characterization of cyclic-nucleotide phosphodiesterase activities in resting and *N*-formylmethionylleucylphenylalanine-stimulated human neutrophils. *Biochim Biophys Acta* 1986;885:282–293.
217. Peachell PT, Undem BJ, Schleimer RP, MacGlashan DW Jr, Lichtenstein LM, Torphy TJ. Preliminary identification and role of phosphodiesterase isozymes in human basophils. *J Immunol* 1992;148:2503–2510.
218. Torphy TJ, Livi GP, Balcarek JM, White JR, Undem BJ. Therapeutic potential of isozyme-selective phosphodiesterase inhibitors in the treatment of asthma. *Adv Second Messenger Phosphoprotein Res* 1992;25:289–305.
219. Bergstrand H, Lundqvist B, Schurmann A. Rat mast cell high affinity cyclic nucleotide phosphodiesterases: separation and inhibitory effects of two anti-allergic agents. *Mol Pharmacol* 1978;14:848–855.
220. Thompson WJ, Ross CP, Pledger WJ, Strada SJ. Cyclic adenosine 3′,5′-monophosphate phosphodiesterase. Distinct forms in human lymphocytes and monocytes. *J Biol Chem* 1976;251:4922–4929.
221. Thompson WJ, Ross CP, Strada SJ, Hersh EM, Lavis VR. Comparative analyses of cyclic adenosine 3′,5′-monophosphate phosphodiesterases of human peripheral blood monocytes and cultured P388D cells. *Cancer Res* 1980;40:1955–1960.
222. White JR, Torphy TJ, Christensen SB, Lee JA, Mong S. Purification and characterization of the rolipram-sensitive low K_m phosphodiesterase from human monocytes. *FASEB J* 1990;4:A1987.
223. Okonogi K, Gettys TW, Uhing RJ, Tarry WC, Adams DO, Prpic V. Inhibition of prostaglandin E$_2$-stimulated cAMP accumulation by lipopolysaccharide in murine peritoneal macrophages. *J Biol Chem* 1991;266:10305–10312.
224. Takemoto DJ, Wee W-NP, Kaplan SA, Appelman MM. Cyclic AMP phosphodiesterase in human lymphocytes and lymphoblasts. *J Cyclic Nucleotide Res* 1978;4:123–132.
225. Robicsek SA, Krzanowski JJ, Szentivanyi A, Polson JB. High pressure liquid chromatography of cyclic nucleotide phosphodiesterase from purified human T-lymphocytes. *Biochem Biophys Res Commun* 1989;163:554–560.
226. Robicsek SA, Blanchard DK, Djeu JY, Kryanowski JJ, Szentivanyi A, Polson JB. Multiple high-affinity cyclic AMP-phosphodiesterases in human T-lymphocytes. *Biochem Pharmacol* 1991;42:869–877.
227. Simpson AWM, Reeves ML, Rink TJ. Effects of SK&F 94120, an inhibitor of cyclic nucleotide phosphodiesterase type III, on human platelets. *Biochem Pharmacol* 1988;37:2315–2320.
228. MacPhee CH, Harrison SA, Beavo JA. Immunological identification of the major low-K_m cAMP phosphodiesterase: probable target for anti-thrombotic agents. *Proc Natl Acad Sci USA* 1986;83:6660–6663.
229. Souness JE, Diocee BK, Martin W, Moodie SA. Pig aortic endothelial-cell cyclic nucleotide phosphodiesterases. Use of phosphodiesterase inhibitors to evaluate their roles in regulating cyclic nucleotide levels in intact cells. *Biochem J* 1990;266:127–132.
230. Lugnier C, Schini VB. Characterization of cyclic nucleotide phosphodiesterases from cultivated bovine aortic endothelial cells. *Biochem Pharmacol* 1990;39:75–84.
231. Arch JRS, Laycock SM, Smith H, Spicer BA. Effects of type IV phosphodiesterase inhibitors on Sephadex-induced eosinophilia and hyperresponsiveness. In: Tarayre JP, Vargaftig BB, Carilla E, eds. *New concepts in asthma*. London: MacMillan, 1993.
232. Kings MA, Chapman I, Kristerson A, Sanjar S, Morley J. Human recombinant lymphokines and cytokines induce pulmonary eosinophilia in the guinea pig which is inhibited by ketotifen and AH21-132. *Int Arch Allergy Appl Immunol* 1990;91:354–361.

233. Sturm RJ, Osborne MC, Heaslip RJ. The effect of phosphodiesterase inhibitors on pulmonary inflammatory cell influx in ovalbumin sensitized guinea pigs. *J Cell Biochem* 1990;14C:337.
234. Underwood DC, Osborn RR, Novak LB. Inhibition of antigen-induced bronchoconstriction and eosinophil infiltration in the guinea-pig by the cyclic AMP-specific phosphodiesterase inhibitor, rolipram. *J Pharmacol Exp Ther* 1993;266:306–313.
235. Busse WW, Anderson CL. The granulocyte response to the phosphodiesterase inhibitor RO 20-1724 in asthma. *J Allergy Clin Immunol* 1981;67:70–74.
236. Frossard N, Landry Y, Pauli G, Ruckstuhl M. Effects of cyclic AMP- and cyclic GMP-phosphodiesterase inhibitors on immunological release of histamine and on lung contraction. *Br J Pharmacol* 1981;73:933–938.
237. Averill LE, Kammer GM. Inhibition of interleukin 2 production is mediated by a cyclic adenosine monophosphate (cAMP)-dependent pathway. *Clin Res* 1985;33:839A.
238. Cooper KD, Kang K, Chan K, Hanifin JM. Phosphodiesterase inhibition by Ro 20-1724 reduces hyper-1gE synthesis by atopic dermatitis cells in vitro. *J Invest Dermatol* 1985;84:477–482.
239. Muggli R, Tschopp TB, Mittelholzer E, Baumgartner HR. 7-Bromo-1,5-dihydro-3,6-dimethylimidazo [2,1-b] quinazolin-2 (3H)-one (Ro 15-2041), a potent antithrombotic agent that selectively inhibits platelet cyclic AMP-phosphodiesterase. *J Pharmacol Exp Ther* 1985;235:212–219.
240. Seiler S, Arnold AJ, Grove RI, Fifer CA, Keely SL Jr, Stanton HC. Effects of anagrelide on platelet cAMP levels, cAMP-dependent protein kinase and thrombin-induced Ca^{++} fluxes. *J Pharmacol Exp Ther* 1987;243:767–773.
241. Radomski MW, Palmer RM, Moncada S. The role of nitric oxide and cGMP in platelet adhesion to vascular endothelium. *Biochem Biohphys Res Commun* 1987;148:1482–1489.
242. Radomski MW, Palmer RMJ, Moncada S. The anti-aggregating properties of vascular endothelium: interactions between prostacyclin and nitric oxide. *Br J Pharmacol* 1987;92:639–649.
243. Mollace V, Salvemini D, Anggard E, Vane J. Nitric oxide from vascular smooth muscle cells: regulation of platelet reactivity and smooth muscle cell guanylate cyclase. *Br J Pharmacol* 1991;104:633–638.
244. Miot F, Erneux C, Wells JN, Dumont JE. The effects of alkylated xanthines on cyclic AMP accumulation in dog thyroid slices exposed to carbamylcholine. *Mol Pharmacol* 1984;25:261–266.
245. Erneux C, van Sande J, Miot F, Cochaux P, Decoster C, Dumont JE. A mechanism in the control of intracellular cAMP level: the activation of a calmodulin-sensitive phosphodiesterase by a rise of intracellular free calcium. *Mol Cell Endocrinol* 1985;43:123–134.
246. Meeker RB, Harden TK. Muscarinic cholinergic receptor-mediated control of cyclic AMP metabolism: agonist-induced changes in nucleotide synthesis and degradation. *Mol Pharmacol* 1983;23:384–392.
247. Tanner LI, Harden TK, Wells JN, Martin MW. Identification of the phosphodiesterase regulated by muscarinic cholinergic receptors of 1321N1 human astrocytoma cells. *Mol Pharmacol* 1986;29:455–460.
248. Miller-Hance WC, Miller JR, Wells JN, Stull JT, Kamm KE. Biochemical events associated with activation of smooth muscle contraction. *J Biol Chem* 1988;263:13979–13982.
249. Saitoh Y, Hardman JG, Wells JN. Differences in the association of calmodulin with cyclic nucleotide phosphodiesterase in relaxed and contracted arterial strips. *Biochemistry* 1985;24:1613–1618.
250. MacFarland RT, Zelus BD, Beavo JA. High concentration of a cGMP-stimulated phosphodiesterase mediates ANP-induced decreases in cAMP and steroidogenesis in adrenal glomerulosa cells. *J Biol Chem* 1991;266:136–142.
251. Whalin ME, Scammell JG, Strada SJ, Thompson WJ. Phosphodiesterase II, the cGMP-activatable cyclic nucleotide phosphodiesterase, regulates cyclic AMP metabolism in PC12 cells. *Mol Pharmacol* 1991;39:711–717.
252. Houslay MD, Wallace AV, Marchmont RJ, Martin BR, Heyworth CM. Insulin controls intracellular cyclic AMP concentrations in hepatocytes by activating specific cyclic

AMP phosphodiesterases: phosphorylation of the peripheral plasma membrane enzyme. *Adv Cyclic Nucleotide Res* 1984;16:159–176.

253. Pyne NJ, Cooper ME, Houslay MD. The insulin- and glucagon-stimulated dense-vesicle high affinity cyclic AMP phosphodiesterase from rat liver. Purification, characterization and inhibitor sensitivity. *Biochem J* 1987;242:33–42.

254. Grant PG, Mannarino AF, Colman RW. cAMP-mediated phosphorylation of the low-K_m cAMP phosphodiesterase markedly stimulates its catalytic activity. *Proc Natl Acad Sci USA* 1988;85:9071–9075.

255. Levin RI, Weksler BB, Jaffe EA. The interaction of sodium nitroprusside with human endothelial cells and platelets: nitroprusside and prostacyclin synergistically inhibit platelet function. *Circulation* 1982;66:1299–1307.

256. Shimokawa H, Flavahan NA, Lorenz RR, Vanhoutte PM. Prostacyclin releases endothelium-derived relaxing factor and potentiates its action in coronary arteries of the pig. *Br J Pharmacol* 1988;95:1197–1203.

257. Maurice DH, Haslam RJ. Molecular basis of the synergistic inhibition of platelet function by nitrovasodilators and activators of adenylate cyclase: inhibition of cyclic AMP breakdown by cyclic GMP. *Mol Pharmacol* 1990;37:671–681.

258. Maurice DH, Crankshaw D, Haslam RJ. Synergistic actions of nitrovasodilators and isoprenaline on rat aortic smooth muscle. *Eur J Pharmacol* 1991;192:235–242.

259. Lidbury PS, Antunes E, De Nucci G, Vane JR. Interactions of iloprost and sodium nitroprusside on vascular smooth muscle and platelet aggregation. *Br J Pharmacol* 1989;98:1275–1280.

260. Schwartz JP, Passonneau JV. Cyclic AMP-mediated induction of the cyclic AMP phosphodiesterase of C-6 glioma cells. *Proc Natl Acad Sci USA* 1974;71:3844–3848.

261. Prasad K, Kumar S. Cyclic 3',5'-AMP phosphodiesterase activity during cyclic AMP-induced differentiation of neuroblastoma cells in culture. *Proc Soc Exp Bio Med* 1973;142:406–409.

262. Ross PS, Manganiello VC, Vaughan M. Regulation of cyclic nucleotide phosphodiesterase in cultured hepatoma cells by dexamethasone and N^6,O^2-dibutyryl adneosine 3':5'-monophosphate. *J Biol Chem* 1977;252:1448–1452.

263. Bourne HR, Tomkins GM, Dion S. Regulation of phosphodiesterase synthesis: requirement for cyclic adenosine monophosphate dependent protein kinase. *Science* 1973;191:952–954.

264. Torphy TJ, Zhou H-L, Cieslinski LB. Stimulation of β-adrenoceptors in a human monocyte cell line (U937) up-regulates phosphodiesterase activity. *J Pharmacol Exp Ther* 1992;263:1195–1205.

265. Manganiello V, Vaughan M. Prostaglandin E_1 effects on adenosine 3':5'-cyclic monophosphate concentration and phosphodiesterase activity in fibroblasts. *Proc Natl Acad Sci USA* 1972;69:269–273.

266. Verhoeven G, Cailleau J, de Moor P. Hormonal control of phosphodiesterase activity in cultured rat Sertoli cells. *Moll Cell Endocrinol* 1981;24:41–47.

267. Torphy TJ, Barnette MS, Cieslinski LB, Zhou H-L. Identification and regulation of phosphodiesterase isozymes in U937 cells. *Am Rev Respir Dis* 1992;45:A283.

268. Swinnen JV, Joseph DR, Conti M. The mRNA encoding a high affinity cAMP phosphodiesterase is regulated by hormones and cAMP. *Proc Natl Acad Sci USA* 1989;86:8197–8201.

269. Swinnen JV, Tsikalas KE, Conti M. Properties and hormonal regulation of two structurally related cAMP phosphodiesterases from rat Sertoli cells. *J Biol Chem* 1991;266:18370–18377.

270. Grewe SR, Chan SC, Hanifin JM. Elevated leukocyte cyclic AMP-phosphodiesterase in atopic disease: a possible mechanism for cyclic AMP-agonist hyporesponsiveness. *J Allergy Clin Immunol* 1982;70:452–457.

271. Holden CA, Chan SC, Hanifin JM. Monocyte localization of elevated cAMP phosphodiesterase activity in atopic dermatitis. *J Invest Dermatol* 1986;87:372–376.

272. Parker CW, Smith JW. Alterations in cyclic adenosine monophosphate metabolism in human bronchial asthma. I. Leukocyte responsiveness to β-adrenergic agents. *J Clin Invest* 1973;52:48–59.

273. Busse WW. Decreased granulocyte response to isoproterenol in asthma during upper respiratory tract infections. *Am Rev Respir Dis* 1973;115:783–789.

274. Butler JM, Chan SC, Stevens S, Hanifen JM. Increased leukocyte histamine release with elevated cyclic AMP-phosphodiesterase activity in atopic dermatitis. *J Allergy Clin Immunol* 1983;71:490–497.
275. Chan SC, Grewe SR, Stevens SR, Hanifin JM. Functional desensitization due to stimulation of cyclic AMP-phosphodiesterase in human mononuclear leukocytes. *J Cyclic Nucleotide Res* 1982;8:211–224.
276. Holden CA, Chan SC, Norris S, Hanifin JM. Histamine induced elevation of cyclic AMP phosphodiesterase activity in human monocytes. *Agents Actions* 1987;22:36–42.
277. Hanifin JM. Pharmacological abnormalities in atopic dermatitis. *Allergy* 1989;44:S41–S46.
278. Barnes PJ. Endogenous catecholamines and asthma. *J Allergy Clin Immunol* 1986;77:791–795.
279. Leeman M, Lejeune P, Melot C, Naeije R. Reduction in pulmonary hypertension and in airway resistances by enoximone (MDL 17,043) in decompensated COPD. *Chest* 1987;91:662–666.
280. Ukena D, Rentz K, Reiber C, Engelstätter R, Sybrecht GW. Bronchodilator effect of a phosphodiesterase type III/IV selective inhibitor, zardaverine, in patients with chronic obstructive airways disease (OAD). *Am Rev Respir Dis* 1992;145:A757.
281. Israel E, Mathur PN, Tashkin D, Drazen JM. LY 186655 prevents bronchospasm in asthma of moderate severity. *Chest* 1988;94:71S.
282. Rudd RM, Gellert AR, Studdy PR, Geddes DM. Inhibition of exercise-induced asthma by an orally absorbed mast cell stabilizer (M&B 22,948). *Br J Dis Chest* 1983;77:78–86.
283. Reiser J, Yeang Y, Warner JO. The effect of zaprinast (M&B 22,948) an orally absorbed mast cell stabilizer on exercise-induced asthma in children. *Br J Dis Chest* 1986;80:157–163.
284. Wood MA, Hess ML. Review: long-term oral therapy of congestive heart failure with phosphodiesterase inhibitors. *Am J Med Sci* 1989;297:105–113.
285. Naccarelli GV, Goldstein RA. Electrophysiology of phosphodiesterase inhibitors. *Am J Cardiol* 1989;63:35–40A.
286. Horowski R, Sastre-Y-Hernandez M. Clinical effects of the neurotropic selective cAMP phosphodiesterase inhibitor rolipram in depressed patients: global evaluation of the preliminary reports. *Curr Ther Res* 1985;38:23–29.
287. Sturgess I, Searle GF. The acute effect of the phosphodiesterase inhibitor rolipram on plasma osmolality. *J Clin Pharmacol* 1990;29:369–370.
288. Lincoln TM. Cyclic GMP and mechanisms of vasodilation. *Pharmacol Ther* 1989;41:479–502.
289. Souness JE, Brazdil R, Diocee BK, Jordan R. Role of selective cyclic GMP phosphodiesterase inhibition in the myorelaxant actions of M&B 22,948, MY-5445, vinpocetine and 1-methyl-3-isobutyl-8-(methylamine)xanthine. *Br J Pharmacol* 1989;98:725–735.

Drugs and the Lung,
edited by C.P. Page and W.J. Metzger.
Raven Press, Ltd., New York © 1994

12

The Pharmacology of Bradykinin in Human Airways

Stephen G. Farmer

*Department of Pulmonary Pharmacology, Zeneca Pharmaceuticals Group,
Wilmington, Delaware 19897-2300*

Bradykinin (BK) is a potent inflammatory nonapeptide whose production in the body elicits numerous physiological responses (1–7). Kinins are generated from precursor proteins, the kininogens, by the kallikreins and other serine proteases in tissues and plasma. Many studies in experimental animals as well as a few in humans implicate BK, kallidin (Lys-BK, KD), and their hydroxyproline derivatives, [Hyp³]-BK and [Hyp⁴]-KD, in inflammatory diseases of the upper and lower airways (1,8–11). This chapter focuses on the effects of kinins in human airways, addresses the evidence for a role for these nocuous mediators in human pulmonary disease, and discusses the available data on effects of BK receptor antagonists in man.

KININ RECEPTORS

In the airways kinins, acting on specific, cell-surface receptors, may produce responses, including the following: neurogenic inflammation, via stimulation of sensory nerve fibers; arteriolar dilation, venoconstriction, and plasma protein extravasation, leading to mucosal edema, congestion, and swelling; airway smooth muscle contraction, causing bronchoconstriction; and release of many inflammatory mediators such as tachykinins, cytokines, and metabolites of arachidonic acid (1,3,5–7,9–14) (Fig. 1).

Kinin receptors are currently classified as B_1 and B_2 subtypes, based upon the relative potencies of various agonists and antagonists (for recent reviews, see refs. 5 and 7). In general, B_2 receptors exhibit much higher affinity for BK and KD than for their respective carboxypeptidase N products, desArg⁹-BK or desArg¹⁰-KD, whereas B_1 receptors are more sensitive to the desArginine metabolites.

B_1 Receptors have been characterized largely in rabbit vascular smooth muscle (15–18), although they have also been demonstrated in some other

449

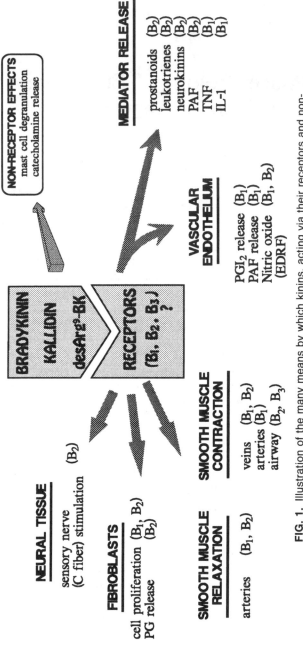

FIG. 1. Illustration of the many means by which kinins, acting via their receptors and non-specific actions, may stimulate mediator release and cellular responses in the different cells and tissues or the airways. The receptor subtypes listed as being responsible for physiological responses have been generalized from the literature. The receptor(s) mediating some effects frequently depends upon the species and cell type under investigation. (Adapted with permission from ref. 9.)

(human) cell types in tissue culture (19,20). To date, however, there is insufficient evidence supporting B_1-receptor expression in human airway tissues, and this subtype will not be further considered here. The pharmacology of B_1 receptors has recently been reviewed (5,13).

Most effects of BK are mediated by B_2 receptors, although there are increasing reports of heterogeneity among this subtype, in addition to the reputed existence of B_3 receptors (21,22). The evidence for heterogeneity among B_2 receptors, as well as other BK receptor subtypes, is discussed in detail elsewhere (3,7).

B_2 RECEPTOR ANTAGONISTS

Substitution with D-phenylalanine for L-proline in position 7 of the BK sequence renders [DPhe^7]-BK (NPC 361), the first known antagonist of B_2 receptors (23). Over the years, numerous analogues, based on NPC 361, have been described, and their structure-activity relationships and pharmacological actions are described elsewhere (3,24–26).

[DPhe^7]-substituted analogues of BK have had a significant influence on kinin pharmacology for almost 10 years, notwithstanding their relatively weak affinity for B_2 receptors (5,24–27). Furthermore, these peptides often elicit agonist-like responses that complicate, or render impossible, interpretation of experimental results.

More recently discovered B_2 receptor antagonists contain modified amino acids in positions 7 and 8 of bradykinin's primary sequence (28–32). Two such drugs are DArg-[Hyp^3,Thi^5,DTic^7,Oic^8]-BK (HOE 140) and DArg-[Hyp^3,Thi^5,DTic^7,Tic^8]-BK (NPC 16731), which are considerably more potent (and metabolically stable) B_2-receptor antagonists than any analogues of NPC 361 *in vitro* (28–30,33,34) and *in vivo* (31,34–36).

BK-RECEPTOR ANTAGONISTS IN ANIMAL MODELS OF ASTHMA

As of this writing (September, 1992) there are no data available on effects of BK antagonists in asthmatic patients, although pharmaceutical companies are certainly conducting clinical trials in this regard. There are, however, a few reports on effects of these drugs in experimental models of airway inflammation and hyperresponsiveness in animals. These studies have evidenced a potentially important role for BK in allergic asthma and, as such, are outlined below.

Sheep

In sheep with a natural hypersensitivity to *Ascaris suum* antigen, inhalation of an aqueous extract of the nematode elicits acute anaphylactic bronchospasm that is associated, approximately 2h later, with an increase in airway responsiveness to carbachol-induced bronchoconstriction (37,38). In addition, eosinophils and neutrophils infiltrate the airways (39,40). Pretreatment of allergic sheep with a B_2 receptor antagonist, DArg-[Hyp^3,DPhe^7]-BK (NPC 567), reduced or abolished antigen-induced airway hyperresponsiveness (40). Moreover, the BK antagonist reduced the airway inflammation that occurred after antigen inhalation (40).

That NPC 567, at a dose that inhibits bronchoconstrictor responses to exogenous BK (41), had no effect on the immediate response to antigen indicates that endogenous kinins are not involved in antigen-induced obstruction. Nevertheless, the ability of NPC 567 to abrogate antigen-induced airway hyperresponsiveness in sheep provides strong evidence for a role of BK in this phenomenon. Since NPC 567 was effective only when administered prior to allergen exposure, rather than postantigen, the authors suggested that BK is released during airway anaphylaxis, and that this mediator may have a function in modulating the inflammatory response (40).

Another study implicates kinins as important mediators in this animal model. In 30% to 50% of allergic sheep anaphylactic bronchoconstriction is followed, 6 to 8 h later, by late onset bronchial obstruction (37). Administration of aerosol NPC 567 inhibits completely the onset of late airway obstruction (42). Furthermore, inhalation of *A. suum* antigen also causes increased bronchoalveolar lavage (BAL) fluid levels of kinins and tosyl-L-arginine methyl ester esterase (TAME esterase) activity (an index of kininogenase activity), as well as prostaglandins, thromboxane, peptidoleukotrienes, and leukotriene B_4. The efficacy of NPC 567 to attenuate the late phase airway response was accompanied with reduced levels of the BAL inflammatory mediators noted (42). Further, the BK antagonist reduced the severity of antigen-induced airway infiltration by granulocytes.

Conversely, the delayed airway hyperresponsiveness that usually occurs at 24 h postantigen was unaffected by NPC 567 (42). Like other [DPhe^7]-BK analogue antagonists, NPC 567 is a peptide and, therefore, metabolically labile. In an effort to overcome the instability of NPC 567 *in vivo,* the drug was administered prior to and during antigen inhalation, as well as 4, 8, and 24 h postantigen. Under these circumstances, NPC 567 not only blocked late onset airway obstruction but also airway hyperresponsiveness occurring at 24 h (42). Thus, generation of airway kinins in an animal model of allergic asthma appears to stimulate the synthesis and release of several metabolic products of arachidonic acid, which, in turn, may contribute to the genesis of airway inflammation, hyperresponsiveness, and late onset responses.

Guinea Pigs

Sensitized guinea pigs repeatedly exposed to antigen for several weeks exhibit airway hyperresponsiveness to intravenous acetylcholine (ACh) and airway infiltration by eosinophils (43). Furthermore, there have been reports that antigen challenge causes increased circulating levels of kinins in this species, and that exposure of perfused lungs from sensitized guinea pigs to antigen results in kallikrein production *in vitro* (44,45). Therefore, it was of interest to investigate the effects of B_2-receptor antagonists on antigen-induced airway hyperresponsiveness in these animals. Inhalation of NPC 567 or NPC 16731 prior to and during each antigen challenge of sensitized guinea pigs inhibited both airway hyperresponsiveness and eosinophil influx (36). Furthermore, during the course of these studies we noted that NPC 16731 abrogated antigen-induced cyanosis and retarded significantly the onset of dyspnea, doubling the time taken for animals to exhibit respiratory distress (36). As with the sheep studies, the ability of BK receptor antagonists to inhibit antigen-induced airway hyperresponsiveness, in addition to eosinophilia, indicates an important role for endogenous kinins. Moreover, the decreased eosinophil infiltration, in animals administered the BK antagonists suggests that BK has a significant function in maintaining allergic inflammation of the airways.

AIRWAY EFFECTS OF BRADYKININ IN MAN

Nasopharyngeal Effects

The observation by Herxheimer and Stresemann (46) that inhalation of "0.5% bradykinin aerosol was very active in asthmatic patients, but not in normal subjects," was the first of many studies that observed BK to be a potent bronchoconstrictor agent in asthmatics, and yet was essentially inactive as an airway spasmogen in nonasthmatic subjects (47–50).

Although, at the doses employed, BK is not a bronchoconstrictor, in nonasthmatics it causes irritation of the upper airway passages. Thus, a common response of nonasthmatic subjects to inhaled BK is cough (49–52), possibly due to stimulation of pharyngeal sensory nerve endings. Similarly, there are reports of BK causing a "prickling sensation in the upper airways" (47), pharyngeal irritation (50), and retrosternal discomfort (49). Interestingly, in one study, irritation was elicited not only by BK, but also by KD and desArg⁹-BK (50), perhaps indicative of nonspecific (i.e., nonreceptor-mediated) effects of the peptides.

Comparatively more studies have been carried out on the effects of BK on nasopharyngeal function than on pulmonary actions of kinins. There are two major explanations for this. First, inhaled kinins elicit relatively little, if any, response in the lungs of nonasthmatics. Second, there is evidence that kinins are pivotal mediators in the pathophysiology of upper airway diseases such as rhinovirus infection (the common cold), influenza, and allergic rhinitis (1,8,11).

For example, intranasal challenge of nonallergic individuals with a solution containing BK mimics the symptoms of the common cold, apparently by a direct action and independently of histamine release (53). Thus, nasal instillation of BK potently caused nasal obstruction, rhinorrhea, increased concentrations of TAME esterase and albumin in nasal secretions (indicating elevated microvascular permeability), and a protracted sore throat in nonallergic and atopic individuals alike (53). (This "normal" author has experienced BK inhalation while rashly getting too close to a nebulizer in the laboratory, and can attest to coughing for several minutes and having a sore throat for 2 or 3 h.) Similar data were recently published by Doyle et al. (52), who found that BK increased nasal resistance, increased secretions, and caused cough, nasal and sinus pressure, and throat pain. In contrast to the results of Proud's group (53), the latter study noted that histamine was more potent in causing nasal obstruction than BK (52). This difference in relative potencies may have been due to the different methods of drug administration; in the Doyle study, BK and histamine were delivered via inhalation of nebulized mists (52), whereas in the Proud study they were instilled into the nostril from a syringe (53).

Several groups have investigated the possible role of eicosanoids in the nasal effects of kinins in man. Premedication of healthy human subjects with aspirin (650 mg) 2 h prior to intranasal challenge with BK was without effect upon subjective symptoms, such as congestion, rhinorrhea, sore throat and sneezing, increased secretion of albumin and TAME esterase activity in nasal lavage fluid (54). The dose of aspirin employed had been previously demonstrated to inhibit prostaglandin D_2 (PGD_2) production induced by allergen challenge. In a similar study, Baraniuk et al. (55) reported that although ibuprofen, a more potent cyclooxygenase inhibitor, altered neither BK-induced sneezing and nasopharyngeal pain nor the total protein content in nasal lavages, this drug potentiated BK-induced glycoconjugate secretion. They also noted that ibuprofen caused a marked augmentation in basal glycoconjugate secretion, although sensitivity to BK-induced glycoconjugate secretion was significantly increased in addition to the effects on basal release (55). This is a surprising observation since these investigators previously demonstrated that ibuprofen reduced BK-induced glycoconjugate release from human nasal mucosal cells *in vitro* (56). Moreover, many effects of BK are mediated by cyclooxygenase products of arachidonic acid metabolism and, as such, are suppressed by cyclooxygenase inhibitors (7,10). Overall, however, evidence to date suggests that the nasopharyngeal effects of BK in man are not mediated indirectly by prostaglandins.

Similarly, studies have confirmed that human nasal responses to kinins do not involve mast cell–derived mediators. Thus, Brunnée and colleagues (57) demonstrated that BK had no effect on nasal lavage levels of histamine, PGD_2, and leukotriene (LT) C_4, although the same dose caused irritation, pain, and congestion, as well as increased lavage concentrations of albumin

(57). Interestingly, this study also found that BK had a significantly greater effect in allergic subjects than in nonallergic subjects. In a preliminary report, the potent histamine H_1 receptor antagonist terfenadine (120 mg) has recently been demonstrated to be without significant effect on pain, rhinorrhea, and increased nasal resistance in response to intranasal challenge with BK (58). BK-induced nasal responses, therefore, probably do not involve endogenous histamine.

Furthermore, although BK is a potent stimulant of C-fiber nerve endings (59–62), which may lead to reflex activation of cholinergic pathways (49,59,63), local application of ipratropium bromide, an antimuscarinic drug, had no effect upon nasal responses of normal subjects or allergic rhinitics BK or KD (58,64).

Geppetti and co-investigators (65) confirmed the lack of effect of ipratropium on nasal symptoms induced by KD, in addition to demonstrating that desensitization to capsaicin, a C-fiber neurotoxin, did not influence the nasal actions of KD. This observation may suggest that the nasal effects of kinins in man are not mediated by stimulation of capsaicin-sensitive sensory nerve endings. In a related study, nasopharyngeal effects of kinins and capsaicin were compared. Rajakulasingam and colleagues (66) reported that intranasal BK induced discomfort or pain as well as increasing nasal airway resistance and stimulating protein secretion. In contrast, whereas capsaicin (at a considerably higher dose than employed by Geppetti et al.) caused marked and in some cases "unbearable" pain, the neurotoxin was without effect upon nasal resistance or microvascular leakage (66). Unfortunately, the effects of this high dose of capsaicin upon responses to BK were not determined. Nevertheless, the data suggested that the actions of kinins and capsaicin, in the human nose, are not identical. These investigators proposed that the ability of BK to cause pain is neuronal, while the peptide's effects on resistance and secretion reflect a direct action on the nasal vasculature (66).

Human Nasopharyngeal Kinin Receptors and Effects of Bradykinin Antagonists

The nasal effects of kinins in man appear not to be mediated by B_1 receptors, as several studies have shown that challenge with the B_1-receptor agonist desArg^9-BK elicits no subjective or measured responses (54,64,65). However, whether human nasal responses to kinins are mediated by B_2 receptors remains to be determined. Studies with a B_2-receptor antagonist have been frustrated by the apparent ineffectiveness of intranasal NPC 567 in man.

As discussed above, several studies have implicated the involvement of endogenous kinins in the symptoms of the common cold. This prompted the clinical testing of a B_2-receptor antagonist in rhinovirus-induced colds (67).

In this study, healthy volunteers were challenged with rhinovirus type 2 and rhinovirus strain EL. Individuals who developed symptomatic colds within 36 and 84 h of inoculation were administered intranasal NPC 567 (500 μg in 200 μl vehicle) or vehicle alone, six times per day for a maximum period of 5 days. Symptoms such as nasal congestion, rhinorrhea, sore throat, and cough were assessed subjectively on each day of the trial. In short, the mean clinical symptom scores, as well as total nasal secretion weights, were identical on day 1 in both the placebo and drug-treated groups (67). Furthermore, on day 6 postinoculation the mean nasal secretion was greater in those individuals who were administered NPC 567 than in the placebo group. In addition, several people noted an irritant effect of the kinin antagonist.

Thus, no evidence that NPC 567 has a beneficial effect in the common cold was produced in the study by Higgins and colleagues (67). These data, however, do not rule out a role of kinins in the symptoms of rhinovirus infection, as NPC 567 was recently demonstrated to be ineffective against the nasal effects of BK itself in man (68). Pongracic and coinvestigators (68) utilized an intranasal dose of 500 μg NPC 567, 5 min prior to challenge with 20 μg BK. BK-induced responses, subjective symptoms, nasal albumin secretion, and TAME esterase activity were unaffected by NPC 567. Because of the possibility that NPC 567 may be degraded by nasal peptidases prior to kinin application, these investigators conducted an additional study wherein NPC 567 was coadministered with BK. Under these circumstances, however, no effect of the antagonist was evident (68).

Thus, although Higgins et al. (67) found no apparent effect of NPC 567 in the common cold, Pongracic and colleagues (68) demonstrated clearly that, with the experimental protocols used, NPC 567 is ineffective as an antagonist of BK-induced nasal responses in man. There are several potential reasons underlying these observation. First, mucosal inflammation may limit the access of this relatively large, polar molecule, following its topical application, to nasal kinin receptors. Second, as it is a peptide NPC 567 may be subject to degradation by peptidases present in the inflamed nasal mucosa. In addition, NPC 567 has a relatively low affinity for B_2 receptors (5,7) such that it may not have been present in sufficiently high quantities to overcome endogenous BK. The latter two explanations are unlikely as NPC 567 was ineffective against BK even when coadministered with the agonist (68). Moreover, Pongracic et al. noted that, even at a 100-fold excess of antagonist compared to BK, no inhibitory effects were apparent.

There are other potential interpretations of the lack of effect of the BK antagonist. Thus, kinins may not be of major importance in producing the symptoms of the common cold, although there is abundant evidence to the contrary (1,11). Alternatively, there are reports that, in guinea pigs and sheep, responses of the trachea to BK may not be mediated by B_1 or B_2 receptors (21,33,69–71). If BK has a role in the symptoms of rhinovirus infection, and if these effects are mediated by B_3 receptors, one might predict that a B_2-selective antagonist, even a weak one like NPC 567, would have little clinical effect. Studies of the effects of more recently discovered and considerably more potent BK receptor antagonists such as NPC 16731 (33) or HOE 140 (28,31), discussed above, will prove useful. These agents should contribute significantly to our understanding of human nasopharyngeal kinin receptors and may provide novel therapies for upper airway diseases.

Pharmacology of Bradykinin-Induced Bronchoconstriction in Asthma

As discussed earlier, it has been recognized for 30 years that BK is a very potent bronchoconstrictor in asthmatic patients (46,48,72,73). Thus, in asthmatics, but not in nonasthmatic subjects, inhalation of BK or KD aerosols results in cough, wheezing, and bronchoconstriction (49,50,74–76).

Also noted above, the inhibitory effect of muscarinic receptor antagonists on BK-induced bronchoconstriction in man has been demonstrated with atropine (74) and ipratropium bromide (49). Thus, BK-induced bronchoconstriction in humans is probably mediated via vagal reflex.

That BK effects in human airways may be largely neuronal is supported by the fact that the kinin also causes cough (49,50,76). Further evidence for a role of neuronal mechanisms may be provided by the observation that disodium cromoglycate and nedocromil sodium provide significant protection against BK-induced bronchoconstriction and cough (49,76). There are several reports that indicate the effects of these drugs, at least in part, are due to their inhibition of sensory nerve function (77–81). As in the guinea pig, BK-induced bronchoconstriction, ensuing from its inhalation, is not affected by prior treatment of humans with cyclooxygenase inhibitors (49,82), suggesting that prostaglandins are not involved. However, contrary to observations in the guinea pig (83–85), the airway effects of BK in asthmatics are not affected by the angiotensin-converting enzyme (ACE) inhibitors captopril or ramipril (49,75). BK-induced bronchoconstriction in asthmatic subjects does not involve histamine, acting via H_1 receptors, as terfenadine has no effect (82).

Evidence for a role for kinins in the pathogenesis of asthma is provided by observations that elevated kinin levels were detected in plasma of asthmatic patients (86,87), and correlations between kinin levels and symptom severity were evident (86). Bronchoalveolar kinin-generating activity and levels of immunoreactive kinins increase, following allergen challenge, in allergic asthmatics (87,88). Analysis of the bronchoalveolar lavage fluid showed the predominant kinin to be kallidin. Further, the major kininogenase activity was compatible with tissue kallikreins. Thus, Christiansen and coworkers (87) speculated that the presence of tissue and plasma kallikrein activities in the asthmatic airways could, via kinin generation, participate in the cascade of events leading to asthma.

Intravenous BK was also reported to be a bronchodilator in asthmatic subjects, and Newball et al. (89) suggested that this effect resulted from the higher intrinsic bronchial tone in these patients. It is puzzling that in most studies in man BK is a bronchoconstrictor, whereas bronchodilation was evident in this study. An important difference in this study may lie in the fact that Newball and coworkers administered BK intravenously, whereas aerosolized kinin was inhaled in the other studies (46,47,49,50,74,76). It is possible that intravenous BK may not have ready access to airway luminal C fibers, stimulation of which may mediate bronchoconstriction in man. Moreover, catecholamines released from the adrenal medulla may have mediated the bronchodilation following intravenous BK. It is noteworthy that airway effects of BK in guinea pigs and their pharmacological manipulation are dependent upon the route of administration (90).

HUMAN AIRWAY KININ RECEPTORS

Similar to nasal responses, BK-induced bronchospasm is not mediated by B_1 receptors since a B_1-receptor agonist, desArg^9-BK, is without effect on pulmonary resistance (50,91). Although BK and KD are potent bronchoconstrictor substance in asthmatics, with BK being about three times more potent (50), the involvement of B_2 receptors or perhaps another BK receptor subtype will not be established until studies with antagonists of this receptor subtype have been conducted in humans. The results of these studies are eagerly awaited by several pharmaceutical companies currently searching for nonpeptide BK receptor antagonists.

Fuller and colleagues (49) first reported that, whereas repeated challenges with inhaled histamine in asthmatics were reproducible, tachyphylaxis to the bronchoconstrictor activity of BK was evident. Thus, although BK was approximately 20-fold more potent (PD_{35}, 0.07 µmol) than histamine upon initial administration, a second challenge with BK 60 min later yielded a PD_{35} value of 0.38 µmol. Interestingly, challenge with BK also reduced airway responsiveness to subsequent inhalation of histamine (49). The involvement of prostaglandins in this heterologous tachyphylaxis was negated since prior administration of aspirin neither altered responsiveness to BK nor inhibited tachyphylaxis. The authors speculated that congestion due to mucosal edema following the initial BK challenge may have limited delivery of subsequent doses of inhaled bronchoconstrictors (49). It is not known whether histamine or, indeed, another bronchoconstrictor induces tachyphylaxis to subsequently administered BK.

A more recent report confirmed the loss of airway responsiveness to BK following repeated challenge of asthmatics with the peptide, but, in contrast to above, inhaled BK did not inhibit histamine-induced bronchoconstriction (92). Polosa and colleagues (92) also verified that inhibition of cyclooxygenase with flurbiprofen neither affected BK-induced bronchospasm nor altered the airway tachyphylaxis.

In an interesting preliminary study, the same investigators found that, although desArg^9-BK failed to elicit bronchoconstriction in asthmatics, the B_1-receptor agonist reduced airway responsiveness to BK by a similar degree to that induced by prior inhalation of BK or KD (91). Since desArg^9-BK is essentially inactive, as an agonist or antagonist, at B_2 receptors at least in animal tissues (see refs. 5,7, and 12), it is difficult to invoke this receptor subtype in the cross-tachyphylaxis observed. Indeed, the B_1-receptor agonist does not displace the binding of [^{3}H]-BK in animal airway tissues (21,70). As noted earlier, desArg^9-BK was reported to cause cough and pharyngeal irritation in some subjects (50). This may indicate a nonspecific action on airway sensory nerve endings. If this is the case, then the ability of the B_1-receptor agonist to induce tachyphylaxis to BK may reflect a desensitization of C fibers that is unrelated to kinin receptors.

CONCLUSION

While it is unlikely that the clinical manifestations of asthma and its underlying pathophysiology are due to a single endogenous mediator, it is reasonable that BK may play a critical role (Fig. 2). Thus, BK has many effects in the airways consistent with a role in the pathogenesis of asthma. It is a potent airway spasmogen that also stimulates the release, from a variety of different cells, of many of the mediators commonly implicated with the disease: prostaglandins, peptidoleukotrienes, platelet-activating factor (PAF), and other inflammatory (neuro)peptides such as substance P and neurokinin A (Fig. 1). All of these substances cause bronchoconstriction, increase airway secretion, and decrease airway caliber.

Furthermore, several of the mediators that BK is capable of releasing— LTB$_4$, PAF, and substance P—are potent chemoattractants that may mediate infiltration by leukocytes, thereby augmenting the airway inflammatory response. BK is a potent vasodilator and increases microvascular permeability to macromolecules, its effects being mediated directly as well as indirectly by sensory neuropeptides and prostaglandins. Thus, kinins may be important in increasing airway blood flow and edema; these characteristics, too, can increase airway resistance (Fig. 2).

The bronchoconstrictor effector per se of BK may not be important in the asthmatic airways. Antigen-induced bronchoconstriction in guinea pigs and sheep is unaltered by a BK receptor antagonist. Rather, data suggest that kinins may be involved in airway hyperreactivity and inflammation and in the late onset response subsequent to antigen challenge in allergic animals. A characteristic feature of asthma is the nonspecific airway hyperreactivity, which manifests itself as excessive sensitivity of the airways to many stimuli

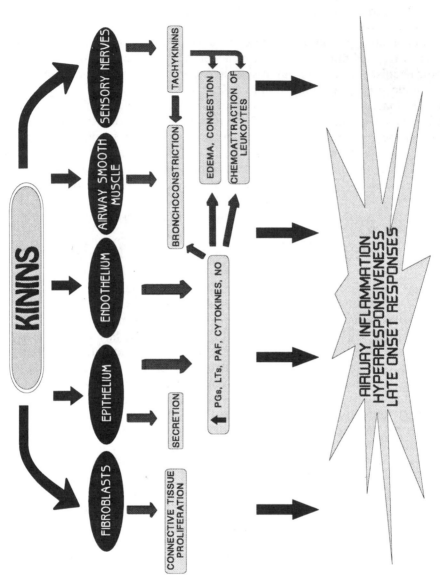

FIG. 2. Kinins, acting on many cell types (see Fig. 1), may have a central role in the onset and maintenance of the chronic inflammation and hyperresponsiveness of the asthmatic airways. (From ref. 9, with permission.)

(93–96). Late onset asthmatic responses, which are often not susceptible to bronchodilators and probably result from airway inflammation, are a characteristic feature of the disease (97–99). Kinin levels increase in the intraluminal airways of allergic animals and asthmatics following allergen challenge, and BK, accordingly, may contribute to airway hyperresponsiveness and late responses.

The data available with BK B_2-receptor antagonists in animals provide convincing testimony for a fundamental role for kinins in airway hyperresponsiveness and inflammation (36,40,42). However, data obtained in animal studies do not always reflect circumstances in humans. Only with clinical studies will the potential usefulness of BK antagonists in diseases of the upper and lower airways and the putative role of kinins in airway disease become apparent.

REFERENCES

1. Proud D, Kaplan AP. Kinin formation: mechanisms and role in inflammatory disorders. *Annu Rev Immunol* 1988;6:49–84.
2. Margolius HS. Tissue kallikreins and kinins: regulation and roles in hypertensive and diabetic diseases. *Annu Rev Pharmacol Toxicol* 1989;29:343–364.
3. Bathon JM, Proud D. Bradykinin antagonists. *Annu Rev Pharmacol Toxicol* 1991; 31:129–162.
4. DeLa Cadena RA, Colman RW. Structure and function of human kininogens. *Trends Pharmacol Sci* 1991;12:272–275.
5. Farmer SG, Burch RM. The pharmacology of bradykinin receptors. In: Burch RM, ed. *Bradykinin antagonists: basic and clinical research.* New York: Marcel Dekker, 1991; 1–31.
6. Bhoola KD, Figueroa CD, Worthy K. Bioregulation of kinins: kallikreins, kininogens, and kininases. *Pharmacol Rev* 1992;44:1–80.
7. Farmer SG, Burch RM. Biochemical and molecular pharmacology of kinin receptors. *Annu Rev Pharmacol Toxicol* 1992;32:511–536.
8. Baraniuk JN. Neural control of human nasal secretion. *Pulmon Pharmacol* 1991;4:20–31.
9. Farmer SG. Role of kinins in airway diseases. *Immunopharmacology* 1991;22:1–20.
10. Farmer SG. Airway pharmacology of bradykinin. In: Burch RM, ed. *Bradykinin antagonists: basic and clinical research.* New York: Marcel Dekker, 1991;213–236.
11. Pongracic JA, Churchill L, Proud D. Kinins in rhinitis. In: Burch RM, ed. *Bradykinin antagonists: basic and clinical research.* New York: Marcel Dekker, 1991;237–259.
12. Farmer SG, Burch RM. Airway bradykinin receptors. *Ann NY Acad Sci* 1991;629:237–249.
13. Marceau F, Regoli D. Kinin receptors of the B_1 type and their antagonists. In: Burch RM, ed. *Bradykinin antagonists: basic and clinical research.* New York: Marcel Dekker, 1991;33–49.
14. Steranka LR, Burch RM. Bradykinin antagonists in pain and inflammation. In: Burch RM, ed. *Bradykinin antagonists: basic and clinical research.* New York: Marcel Dekker, 1991;191–211.
15. Regoli D, Marceau F, Barabé J. *De novo* formation of vascular receptor for bradykinin. *Can J Physiol Pharmacol* 1978;56:674–677.
16. Regoli D, Marceau F, Lavigne J. Induction of B_1 receptors for kinins in the rabbit by a bacterial lipopolysaccharide. *Eur J Pharmacol* 1981;71:105–115.
17. Bouthillier J, DeBlois D, Marceau F. Studies on the induction of pharmacological responses to des-Arg⁹-bradykinin *in vitro* and *in vivo. Br J Pharmacol* 1987;92:257–264.

18. DeBlois D, Bouthillier J, Marceau F. Effect of glucocorticoids, monokines and growth factors on the spontaneously developing responses of the rabbit isolated aorta to des Arg^9 bradykinin. *Br J Pharmacol* 1988;93:969–977.
19. Straus DS, Pang KJ. Effects of bradykinin on DNA synthesis in resting NIL8 hamster cells and human fibroblasts. *Exp Cell Res* 1984;151:87–95.
20. Lerner UH, Modéer T. Bradykinin B$_1$ and B$_2$ receptor agonists synergistically potentiate interleukin-1-induced prostaglandin biosynthesis in human gingival fibroblasts. *Inflammation* 1991;15:427–436.
21. Farmer SG, Burch RM, Meeker SN, Wilkins DE. Evidence for a pulmonary bradykinin B$_3$ receptor. *Mol Pharmacol* 1989;36:1–8.
22. Field JL, Hall JM, Morton IKM. Bradykinin receptors in the guinea-pig taenia caeci are similar to proposed BK$_3$ receptors in the guinea-pig trachea, and are blocked by HOE 140. *Br J Pharmacol* 1992;105:293–296.
23. Vavrek RJ, Stewart JM. Competitive antagonists of bradykinin. *Peptides* 1985;6:161–164.
24. Steranka LR, Farmer SG, Burch RM. Antagonists of B$_2$ bradykinin receptors. *FASEB J* 1989;3:2019–2025.
25. Burch RM, Farmer SG, Steranka LR. Bradykinin receptor antagonists. *Med Res Rev* 1990;10:237–269.
26. Stewart JM, Vavrek RJ. Chemistry of peptide B$_2$ bradykinin antagonists. In: Burch RM, ed. *Bradykinin antagonists: basic and clinical research.* New York: Marcel Dekker, 1991;51–96.
27. Stewart JM, Vavrek RJ. Bradykinin competitive antagonists for classical kinin receptors. In: Greenbaum LM, Margolius HS, eds. *Kinins IV. Advances in experimental medicine and biology,* vol 198A. New York: Plenum Press, 1986;537–542.
28. Hock FJ, Wirth K, Albus U, et al. Hoe 140 a new potent and long acting bradykinin-antagonist: *in vitro* studies. *Br J Pharmacol* 1991;102:769–773.
29. Kyle DJ, Martin JA, Farmer SG, Burch RM. Design and conformational analysis of several highly potent bradykinin receptor antagonists. *J Med Chem* 1991;34:1230–1233.
30. Kyle DJ, Martin JA, Burch RM, et al. Probing the bradykinin receptor: mapping and geometric topography using ethers of hydroxyproline in novel peptides. *J Med Chem* 1991;34:2649–2653.
31. Wirth K, Hock FJ, Albus U, et al. Hoe 140 a new potent and long acting bradykinin-antagonist: *in vivo* studies. *Br J Pharmacol* 1991;102:774–777.
32. Burch RM, Kyle DJ. Recent developments in the understanding of bradykinin receptors. *Life Sci* 1992;50:829–838.
33. Farmer SG, Burch RM, Kyle DJ, Martin JA, Meeker SN, Togo J. DArg[Hyp^3-Thi^5-DTic^7-Tic^8]-bradykinin, a potent antagonist of smooth muscle BK$_2$ receptors and BK$_3$ receptors. *Br J Pharmacol* 1991;102:785–787.
34. Lembeck F, Griesbacher T, Eckhardt M, Henke S, Breipohl G, Knolle J. New, long-acting, potent bradykinin antagonists. *Br J Pharmacol* 1991;102:297–304.
35. Bao G, Qadri F, Stauss B, Stauss H, Gohlke P, Unger T. HOE 140, a new highly potent and long-acting bradykinin antagonist in conscious rats. *Eur J Pharmacol* 1991;200:179–182.
36. Farmer SG, Wilkins DE, Meeker S, Seeds EAM, Page CP. Effects of bradykinin receptor antagonists on antigen-induced respiratory distress, airway hyperresponsiveness and eosinophilia in guinea-pigs. *Br J Pharmacol* 1992; 107:653–659.
37. Abraham WM. Pharmacology of allergen-induced early and late airway responses and antigen-induced hyperresponsiveness in allergic sheep. *Pulmon Pharmacol* 1989;2:33–40.
38. Abraham WM. Bradykinin antagonists in a sheep model of allergic asthma. In: Burch RM, ed. *Bradykinin antagonists: basic and clinical research.* New York: Marcel Dekker, 1991;261–276.
39. Solér M, Sielczak MW, Abraham WM. A PAF antagonist blocks antigen-induced airway hyperresponsiveness and inflammation in sheep. *J Appl Physiol* 1989;67:406–413.
40. Solér M, Sielczak M, Abraham WM. A bradykinin antagonist blocks antigen-induced airway hyperresponsiveness and inflammation in sheep. *Pulmon Pharmacol* 1990;3:9–15.

41. Abraham WM, Ahmed A, Cortes A, et al. Airway effects of inhaled bradykinin, substance P and neurokinin A in sheep. *J Allergy Clin Immunol* 1991;87:557–564.
42. Abraham WM, Burch RM, Farmer SG, Ahmed A, Cortes A. A bradykinin antagonist modifies allergen-induced mediator release and late bronchial responses in sheep. *Am Rev Respir Dis* 1991;143:787–796.
43. Ishida K, Kelly LJ, Thompson RJ, Beattie LL, Schellenberg RR. Repeated antigen challenge induces airway hyperresponsiveness with tissue eosinophilia in guinea pigs. *J Appl Physiol* 1989;67:1133–1139.
44. Brocklehurst WE, Lahiri SC. The production of bradykinin during anaphylaxis. *J Physiol* 1962;160:15–16P.
45. Jonasson O, Becker EL. Release of kallikrein from guinea-pig lung during anaphylaxis. *J Exp Med* 1966;123:509–522.
46. Herxheimer H, Stresemann E. The effect of bradykinin aerosol in guinea-pigs and in man. *J Physiol* 1961;158:38P.
47. Varonier HS, Panzani R. The effect of inhalations of bradykinin on healthy and atopic (asthmatic) children. *Int Arch Allergy* 1968;34:293–296.
48. Lecomte J, Petit JM, Mélon J, Troquet J, Marcelle R. Propriétés bronchoconstrictrices de la bradykinine chez l'homme asthmatique. *Arch Int Pharmacodyn Ther* 1962;137:232–235.
49. Fuller RW, Dixon CMS, Cuss FMC, Barnes PJ. Bradykinin-induced bronchoconstriction in humans: mode of action. *Am Rev Respir Dis* 1987;135:176–180.
50. Polosa R, Holgate ST. Comparative airway responses to inhaled bradykinin, kallidin, and [des-Arg^9]bradykinin in normal and asthmatic subjects. *Am Rev Respir Dis* 1990;142:1367–1371.
51. Choudry NB, Fuller RW, Pride NB. Sensitivity of the human cough reflex: effect of inflammatory mediators prostaglandin E$_2$, bradykinin and histamine. *Am Rev Respir Dis* 1989;140:137–141.
52. Doyle WJ, Boehm S, Skoner DP. Physiologic responses to intranasal dose-response challenges with histamine, methacholine, bradykinin, and prostaglandin in adult volunteers with and without nasal allergy. *J Allergy Clin Immunol* 1990;86:924–935.
53. Proud D, Reynolds CJ, Lacapra S, Kagey-Sobotka A, Lichtenstein LM, Naclerio RM. Nasal provocation with bradykinin induces symptoms of rhinitis and a sore throat. *Am Rev Respir Dis* 1988;137:613–616.
54. Churchill L, Pongracic JA, Reynolds CJ, Naclerio RM, Proud D. Pharmacology of nasal provocation with bradykinin: studies of tachyphylaxis, cyclooxygenase inhibition, α-adrenergic stimulation, and receptor subtype. *Int Arch Allergy Appl Immunol* 1991;95:322–331.
55. Baraniuk JN, Silver PB, Kaliner MA, Barnes PJ. Ibuprofen augments bradykinin-induced glycoconjugate secretion by human nasal mucosa in vivo. *J Allergy Clin Immunol* 1992;89:1032–1039.
56. Baraniuk JN, Lundgren JD, Mizoguchi H, et al. Bradykinin and respiratory mucous membranes. Analysis of bradykinin binding site distribution and secretory responses *in vitro* and *in vivo*. *Am Rev Respir Dis* 1990;141:706–714.
57. Brunnée T, Nigam S, Kunkel G, Baumgarten CR. Nasal challenge studies with bradykinin: influence upon mediator generation. *Clin Exp Allergy* 1991;21:425–431.
58. Rajakulasingam K, Polosa R, Lau LCK, Church MK, Holgate ST, Howarth PH. Influence of terfenadine alone and in combination with ipratropium bromide on bradykinin induced nasal symptoms and plasma protein leakage. *J Allergy Clin Immunol* 1992;89:206.
59. Kaufman MP, Coleridge HM, Coleridge JCG, Baker DG. Bradykinin stimulates afferent vagal C-fibers in intrapulmonary airways of dogs. *J Appl Physiol* 1980;48:511–517.
60. Lundberg JM, Saria A. Capsaicin-induced desensitization of airway mucosa to cigarette-smoke, mechanical and chemical irritants. *Nature* 1983;302:251–253.
61. Saria A, Martling C-R, Yan Z, Theodorsson-Norheim E, Gamse R, Lundberg JM. Release of multiple tachykinins from capsaicin-sensitive sensory nerves in the lung by bradykinin, histamine, dimethylphenyl piperazinium, and vagal nerve stimulation. *Am Rev Respir Dis* 1988;137:1330–1335.
62. Geppetti P, Tramontana M, Santicioli P, Del Bianco E, Giuliani S, Maggi CA. Bradyki-

nin-induced release of calcitonin gene-related peptide in guinea-pig atria: mechanism of action and calcium requirements. *Neuroscience* 1990;3:687–692.
63. Roberts AM, Kaufman MP, Baker DG, Brown JK, Coleridge HM, Coleridge JCG. Reflex tracheal contraction induced by stimulation of bronchial C-fibers in dogs. *J Appl Physiol* 1981;51:485–493.
64. Rajakulasingam K, Polosa R, Holgate ST, Howarth PH. Comparative nasal effects of bradykinin, kallidin and [Des-Arg⁹]-bradykinin in atopic rhinitic and normal volunteers. *J Physiol* 1991;437:577–587.
65. Geppetti P, Fusco BM, Alessandri M, et al. Kallidin applied to the human nasal mucosa produces algesic response not blocked by capsaicin desensitization. *Regul Pept* 1991; 33:321–329.
66. Rajakulasingam K, Polosa R, Lau LCK, Church MK, Holgate ST, Howarth PH. Nasal effects of bradykinin and capsaicin: influence on plasma protein leakage and role of sensory neurons. *J Appl Physiol* 1992;72:1418–1424.
67. Higgins PG, Barrow GI, Tyrrell DAJ. A study of the efficacy of the bradykinin antagonist, NPC 567, in rhinovirus infections in human volunteers. *Antiviral Res* 1990;14:339–344.
68. Pongracic JA, Naclerio RM, Reynolds CJ, Proud D. A competitive kinin receptor antagonist, [D-Arg⁰,Hyp³,DPhe⁷]-bradykinin, does not affect the response to nasal provocation with bradykinin. *Br J Clin Pharmacol* 1991;31:287–294.
69. Farmer SG, Ensor JE, Burch RM. Evidence that cultured airway smooth muscle cells contain bradykinin B₂ and B₃ receptors. *Am J Respir Cell Mol Biol* 1991;4:273–277.
70. Mak JWC, Barnes PJ. Autoradiographic visualization of bradykinin receptors in human and guinea pig lung. *Eur J Pharmacol* 1991;194:37–43.
71. Perkins MN, Burgess GM, Campbell EA, et al. HOE140: a novel bradykinin analogue that is a potent antagonist at both B₂ and B₃ receptors *in vitro*. *Br J Pharmacol* 1991;102:171P.
72. Girard JP, Moret P. Action de la sérotonine et de la bradykinine en aérosols chez les asthmatiques. *Helv Med Acta* 1963;30:520–526.
73. Collier HOJ. Kinins and ventilation of the lungs. In: Erdös EG, ed. *Handbook of experimental pharmacology,* vol 25. Berlin, Heidelberg, New York: Springer-Verlag, 1970;409–420.
74. Simonsson BG, Skoogh B-E, Bergh NP, Andersson R, Svedmyr N. *In vivo* and *in vitro* effect of bradykinin on bronchial motor tone in normal subjects and patients with airways obstruction. *Respiration* 1973;30:378–388.
75. Dixon CMS, Fuller RW, Barnes PJ. The effect of an angiotensin converting enzyme inhibitor, ramipril, on bronchial responses to inhaled histamine and bradykinin in asthmatic subjects. *Br J Clin Pharmacol* 1987;23:91–93.
76. Dixon CMS, Barnes PJ. Bradykinin-induced bronchoconstriction: inhibition by nedocromil sodium and sodium cromoglycate. *Br J Clin Pharmacol* 1989;27:831–836.
77. Jackson DM. The effect of nedocromil sodium, sodium cromoglycate and codeine phosphate on citric acid induced cough in dogs. *Br J Pharmacol* 1988;93:609–612.
78. Eady RP, Jackson DM. Effect of nedocromil sodium on SO₂-induced airway hyperresponsiveness and citric acid-induced cough in dogs. *Int Arch Allergy Appl Immunol* 1989;88:240–243.
79. Dixon CMS, Ind PW. Inhaled sodium metabisulphite induced bronchoconstriction: inhibition by nedocromil sodium and sodium cromoglycate. *Br J Clin Pharmacol* 1990;30:371–376.
80. Wright W, Zhang YG, Salome CM, Woolcock AJ. Effect of inhaled preservatives on asthmatic subjects. I. Sodium metabisulfite. *Am Rev Respir Dis* 1990;141:1400–1404.
81. Mansour E, Ahmed A, Cortes A, Caplan J, Burch RM, Abraham WM. Mechanisms of metabisulfite-induced bronchoconstriction. Evidence for bradykinin B₂ receptor stimulation. *J Appl Physiol* 1992;72:1831–1837.
82. Polosa R, Phillips GD, Lai CKW, Holgate ST. Contribution of histamine and prostanoids to bronchoconstriction provoked by inhaled bradykinin. *Allergy* 1990;45:174–182.
83. Greenberg R, Osman GH, O'Keefe EH, Antonaccio MJ. The effects of captopril (SQ 14,225) on bradykinin-induced bronchoconstriction in the anesthetized guinea pig. *Eur J Pharmacol* 1979;57:287–294.

84. Karlsson J-A, Zackrisson C, Forsberg K. Effect of prolonged inhibition of angiotensin converting enzyme on MK-447. Studies on the irritant induced cough and bronchoconstriction in guinea-pigs. *Am Rev Respir Dis* 1988;137(suppl):508.
85. Ichinose M, Barnes PJ. The effect of peptidase inhibitors on bradykinin-induced bronchoconstriction in guinea-pigs *in vivo*. *Br J Pharmacol* 1990;101:77–80.
86. Abe K, Watanabe N, Kumagai N, Mouri T, Seki T, Yoshinaga K. Circulating plasma kinin in patients with bronchial asthma. *Experientia* 1967;23:626–627.
87. Christiansen SC, Proud D, Cochrane CG. Detection of tissue kallikrein in the bronchoalveolar lavage fluid of asthmatic subjects. *J Clin Invest* 1987;79:188–197.
88. Christiansen SC, Proud D, Sarnoff RB, Juergens U, Cochrane CG, Zuraw BL. Elevation of tissue kallikrein and kinin in the airways of asthmatic subjects after endobronchial allergen challenge. *Am Rev Respir Dis* 1992;145:900–905.
89. Newball HH, Keiser HR, Pisano JJ. Bradykinin and human airways. *Respir Physiol* 1975;24:139–146.
90. Ichinose M, Belvisi MG, Barnes PJ. Bradykinin-induced bronchoconstriction in guinea pig in vivo: role of neural mechanisms. *J Pharmacol Exp Ther* 1990;253:594–599.
91. Polosa R, Rajakulasingam K, Holgate ST. Cross-tachyphylaxis studies with inhaled kinins in asthma: evidence for partial antagonism induced by inhaled [desArg⁹]-BK. *J Allergy Clin Immunol* 1991;87:251.
92. Polosa R, Lai CKW, Robinson C, Holgate ST. The influence of cyclooxygenase inhibition on the loss of bronchoconstriction response to repeated bradykinin challenge in asthma. *Eur Respir J* 1990;3:914–921.
93. Boushey HA, Holtzman MJ, Sheller JR, Nadel JA. State of the art: bronchial hyperreactivity. *Am Rev Respir Dis* 1980;121:389–413.
94. Snashall PD, Pawels R. Introduction: definitions and historical perspective. In: Nadel JA, Pauwels R, Snashall PD, eds. *Bronchial hyperresponsiveness*. London: Blackwell Scientific, 1987;1–4.
95. Laitinen LA, Heino M, Laitinen A. Airway hyperresponsiveness, epithelial disruption, and epithelial inflammation. In: Farmer SG, Hay DWP, eds. *The airway epithelium. Physiology, pathophysiology, and pharmacology*. New York: Marcel Dekker, 1991;187–211.
96. Pueringer RJ, Hunninghake GW. Inflammation and airway reactivity in asthma. *Am J Med* 1992;92(suppl 6A):32S–38S.
97. Morley J, Page CP, Sanjar S. Pharmacology of the late response to allergen and its relevance to asthma prophylaxis. *Int Arch Allergy Appl Immunol* 1985;77:73–78.
98. O'Byrne PM, Dolovich J, Hargreave FE. Late asthmatic responses. *Am Rev Respir Dis* 1987;136:740–751.
99. Frew AJ, Corrigan CJ, Maestrelli P, et al. T lymphocytes in allergen-induced late-phase reactions and asthma. *Int Arch Allergy Appl Immunol* 1989;88:63–67.

Drugs and the Lung,
edited by C.P. Page and W.J. Metzger.
Raven Press, Ltd., New York © 1994

13

PAF Antagonists as Asthma Therapeutics

Dean A. Handley and *Franklin Cerasoli, Jr.

*Department of Atherosclerosis and Vascular Diseases, Preclinical Research
Department, Sandoz Research Institute, Sandoz Pharmaceuticals
Corporation, East Hanover, New Jersey 07936; and *Preclinical Development,
Ariad Pharmaceuticals, Inc., Cambridge, Massachusetts 02139*

HISTORICAL DEVELOPMENT

For a mediator of inflammation, platelet-activating factor (PAF) has led an enchanted life and has enjoyed a meteoric rise in attention since its discovery two decades ago (1). In terms of pathological properties, PAF subordinates the combined attributes of leukotrienes, thromboxanes, and prostaglandins, and accordingly has been embraced by both academia and industry alike. Academic researchers viewed PAF as an entirely new area of endeavor, somehow coexisting without their knowledge but markedly influencing experimental results. Industrial researchers likewise sprang into action, for PAF antagonists offered a potential new area of specific therapeutics to diseases that were poorly restrained by conventional anti-inflammatory drugs.

Structural identification of PAF by a triad of different groups in 1979 catapulted it into the forefront of biomedical research, notwithstanding the confusion that comes when one molecule is variously called (depending upon the allegiance of the researcher) acetyl glyceryl ether phosphorylcholine (AGEPC) (2), its original founding name of Paf-acether (3), and an antihypertensive polar renal-medullary lipid (APRL) (4). Studies in PAF were enhanced by the fact that there is little molecular heterogeneity, as the two dominant forms of PAF (C_{16} and C_{18}) vary only by potency. There seems to be one type of receptor and no real differences in terms of species specificity, such that PAF antagonists that were developed against the human platelet receptor antagonize PAF-mediated responses in mice through (hu)man. However, elucidating the etiology of PAF in disease has been hampered by difficulties in measuring endogenous production of PAF, as it may remain cell or tissue bound after formation. Quantitative extraction and chromatographic techniques must be applied to detect PAF in plasma, urine, saliva, or pleural fluids. PAF is short lived in the plasma ($T_{1/2}$ of 40 sec) and the degradation product (lyso-PAF) is the same as the substrate used in its formation, clouding estimations regarding extent of endogenous production (5).

It was soon realized that PAF did more than activate platelets, although it is still the most potent low molecular weight activator of platelets identified to date. PAF activates most cells of the immune and inflammatory system, such as neutrophils, monocytes, eosinophils, basophils, lymphocytes, endothelial cells, macrophages, and mast cells. Cellular responses to PAF are reported to include generation of inflammatory mediators, superoxide production, chemotaxis, aggregation, proliferation, exocytosis, adhesion, degranulation, shape change, and surface charge alterations (6). Furthermore, immune and inflammatory stimuli induce the production of PAF from mast cells (7,8), pleural cells (9), polymorphonuclear leukocytes (10), eosinophils (11), platelets (12), macrophages (13,14), glomerular mesangial cells (15), lymphocytes (16), cultured endothelial cells (17,18), and basophils (19,20).

PAF is produced by the retina (21), kidney (4,22), liver (23), and the lung (24). Organ dysfunction induced by PAF includes pulmonary artery hypertension, coagulopathies, cardiac and renal dysfunction, pulmonary (25) and circulatory (26) anaphylaxis, pulmonary edema (27,28), and death (29). For these reasons, PAF is felt to participate in the initiation or progression of ischemic bowel necrosis (30), colitis (31), myocardial ischemia (32), cold urticaria (33), adult respiratory distress syndrome (34), pancreatitis (35,36), ulcers (37), arthritis (38), asthma (39,40), cardiovascular diseases (41,42), glomerulonephritis (43), cerebrovascular ischemia, acute transplant rejection (45,46), immune anaphylaxis (47), shock (44,48,49), and even atherosclerosis (50,51). These diverse diseases, in terms of PAF generation, can be grouped into those mediated by immune complexes (45,52–56), endotoxin (30,57–61), or organ ischemia (62–64), as each is known to induce endogenous release of PAF.

In spite of this impressive list of PAF-mediated pathological involvement, the initial clinical indications and indeed trials, have been limited to studies of PAF antagonists solely in the area of asthma. Asthma is now recognized as an inflammatory disease characterized by symptomatic bronchoconstriction (reversible airway obstruction) and airway hyperreactivity, defined as an increased sensitivity, vulnerability, or exaggerated responsiveness of the upper airways to a variety of allergic and nonallergic stimuli (65). Airway hyperreactivity is considered a hallmark clinical feature of asthma and is thought to reflect underlying inflammation associated with increased mucus production, pulmonary eosinophilia, airway edema, epithelial desquamation, and mediator release.

PAF is a powerful inflammatory mediator that exhibits a striking ability to produce many of the symptoms of asthma, including bronchoconstriction, decreased lung compliance, airway edema, and eosinophil recruitment (66–

71). Most important is the unique ability of PAF to induce sustained airway hyperreactivity, reported in guinea pigs (72–77), rabbits (78), dogs (79), and sheep (67). These results strongly suggest a role for PAF in asthma (39,80–84) and a therapeutic potential for PAF antagonists (48,85–87).

The concept that PAF may contribute to asthma pathology may be more appropriately resolved through clinical trails with potent, bioavailable PAF antagonists (81,88). The ability of PAF antagonists to selectively inhibit pulmonary responses induced by PAF (79,89–92) as well as those of allergen (92–94) continues to highlight the importance of this mediator, as well as drugs that may attenuate or abrogate its effects. From synthetic and natural sources, a variety of PAF antagonists (structurally similar and dissimilar to PAF) have been produced. We will address the preclinical and clinical studies that substantiate the role of PAF in asthma and identify the therapeutic strengths and weaknesses of PAF antagonists as anti-asthma drugs.

DEVELOPMENTAL PAF ANTAGONISTS

A number of PAF antagonists have been developed, some structurally related to PAF and others quite dissimilar from PAF. None has been approved for clinical use, although many are considered specific, long-lasting, new, potent, and "novel" by their founders, such as BN 50739 (95), CV 6209 (96), WEB 2086 (97–100), SDZ 64-419 (101), E5990 (61), E6123 (102), SR 27417 (103), TCV-309 (104) and RP 59227 (105–107). The following subsections discuss the work of several pharmaceutical companies in this area of research.

Alter S.A.

PCA 4248 [2-(phenylthio) ethyl-5-methoxycarbonyl 2,4,6 triethyl 1,4-dihydropyridine-3-carboxylate] is reported to inhibit PAF, immune complex, and endotoxin reactions in mice and rats (108).

Boehringer Ingelheim KG

Initial studies showed that triazolobenzodiazepines possessed PAF receptor antagonist activity *in vitro* (109) and it was soon verified that other anti-anxiety drugs such as etizolam (110), brotizolam (111,112), alprazolam (111–113), and triazolam (111–113) exhibited PAF antagonist activity. PAF receptor activity could be dissociated from the CNS activity (111,112) and the first significant compound in this series was the thieno-triazolodiazepine compound WEB 2086 (Apafant) (Fig. 1A). WEB 2086 was shown to be a potent PAF-receptor antagonist *in vitro* and has been compared to L-652,731

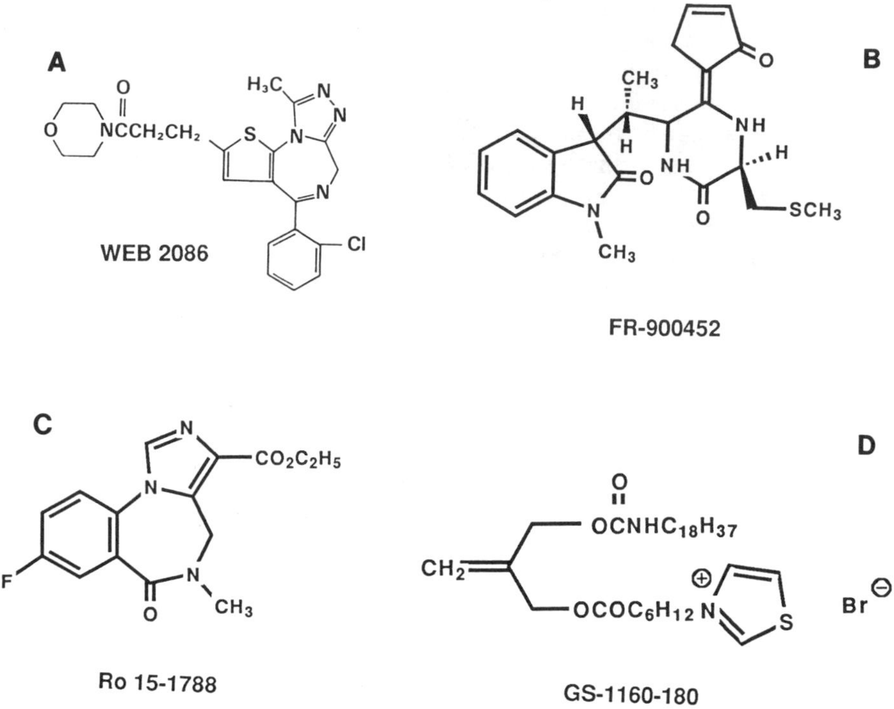

FIG. 1. A: WEB 2086: 3-[4-(2-chlorophenyl)-9-methyl -6H-thieno [3,2-f] [1,2,4] triazolo [4,3-a] [1,4] diazepin -2-yl]-1-(4-morpholinyl) -1-propanone. **B:** FR-900452: 1-methyl-3-(1-(5-methylthiomethyl-6-oxy-3-(2-oxy 3- cyclopenten -1- ylidene) -2- piperazinyl) ethyl) -2- indolinone. **C:** Ro 15-1788: (ethyl 8-fluoro 5-methyl-5,6-dihydro -6-oxo-4H- imidazo [1,5- a] [1,4] benzodiazepine-3-carboxylate). **D:** GS-1160-180: 3-[6-[[2- methylene -3-[[octadecylamino) carbonyl]-oxy] propoxy] carbonyl] hexyl] thiazolium bromide.

(114) and BN52021, where it is over 50-fold more potent (91). Newer compounds in this series include WEB 2170 (115) and WEB 2347 (116).

Eisai Co., Ltd.

E 5990, an 1-ethyl-2-[N-(2-methoxy) benzoyl-N-[(2R)2-methoxy 3-(4-octadecylcarbamoyloxy) piperidinocarbonyl oxypropyloxy] carbonyl] aminomethyl pyridinium chloride, has been shown to act as competitive receptor antagonist and inhibit vascular responses to PAF and endotoxin (61). Recently E6123,(S)-(+)6-(2-chloro-phenyl) 3-cyclopropanecarbonyl 8-11-dimethyl 2,3,4,5 tetrahydro 8H-pyrido [4′,3:4,5] thieno [3,2-f] [1,2,4] triazolo [4,3-a] [1,4] diazepine, has been shown to demonstrate exceptional oral potency in a number of PAF or antigen-mediated *in vivo* responses (102).

Fujisawa Pharmaceutical Co.

FR-900452 is a cyclo pentenopiperazinylindolinone (Fig. 1B) that was isolated from the fermentation broth from *Streptomyces phaeofaciens* (117), which acts as a specific PAF receptor antagonist (117,118).

Hoffmann-La Roche & Co., Ltd.

Ro 15-1788 (Fig. 1C), ethyl 8-fluoro 5-methyl-5,6-dihydro-6-oxo-4H-imidazo [1,5-a] [1,4] benzodiazepine-3-carboxylate, exhibits modest activity in the PAF-induced platelet aggregation assay (111) and hemorrhagic shock (119). Ro 19-3704 (3-(4((R)-2-((methoxycarbonyl) oxy-3-(octadecylcarbamoyl) oxy) propoxy) butyl) thiazolium iodide) is reported to inhibit PAF-induced platelet aggregation and a several pulmonary responses in the guinea pig (120).

Leo Pharmaceutical Products, Ltd.

GS-1160-180, a methylene octadecylamino carbonyl hexyl thiazolium bromide (Fig. 1D) PAF receptor antagonist, *in vivo* inhibits PAF-induced bronchoconstriction in the guinea pig and hypotension in the rat (121).

Merck Sharp & Dohme Research Labs

The first compound reported from this company was kadsurenone (Fig. 2A), an extract isolated from the Chinese herbal plant Piper futokadsura (122). *In vitro*, kadsurenone acts as competitive receptor antagonist (123, 124) and exhibits a 20 to 1 difference in the *in vitro* activity between the two tested enantiomers (123).

L-652,731 (124a), a trimethoxyphenyl tetrahydrofuran (Fig. 2B), is a very potent receptor antagonist that is orally active in several species (49,124–126). The most recent compound from the tetrahydrofuran series is L-659,989 (Fig. 2C), in which the chiral enantiomers exhibit a 27-fold potency difference *in vitro* (127).

Ono Pharmaceutical Co., Ltd.

Ono-6240 is a competitive receptor antagonist (124) and a structural analog of PAF (Fig. 2D), which has been shown to inhibit PAF-induced hypotension and vascular permeability effects (128).

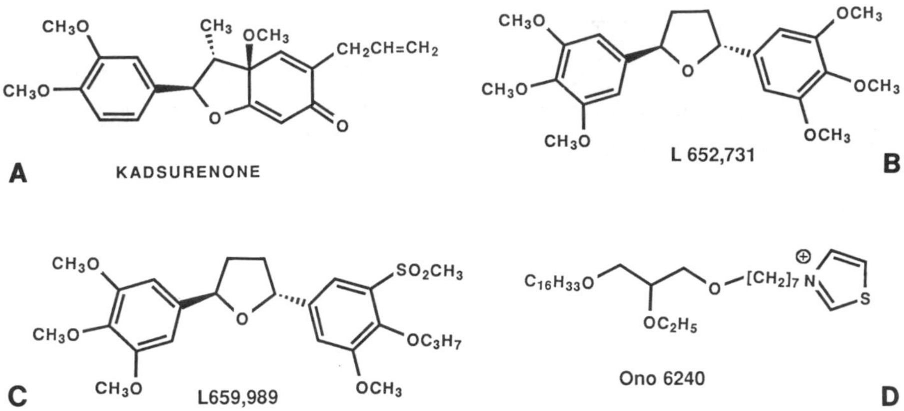

FIG. 2. A: Kadsurenone: [2-(3,4-dimethoxyphenyl) -2b,3-dihydro-3a, methoxy-3B-methyl-5-(allyl)-6-2H- oxobenzofuran. **B:** L-652,731: trans 2,5- bis (3,4,5- trimethoxyphenyl) tetrahydrofuran. **C:** L-659,989: trans -2-(3- methoxy-5-methylsufonyl 4-propoxyphenyl)5- (3,4,5-trimethoxyphenyl) tetrahydrofuran. **D:** Ono-6240: 1-O-hexadecyl-(2R,2S)-O-ethyl 3-O-(7-thiazolio-heptyl) glycerol chloride.

Rhône-Poulenc Sante

A distinct chemical series has been developed by this company, of which 48740 RP has been most extensively studied (Fig. 3A). 52770 RP (129; Fig. 3B) and 59227 RP (105) have recently been introduced and appear to possess much greater potency by parenteral or oral administration. In the *in vitro* rabbit aggregation assay, the enantiomers of 52770 show a 670-fold difference (130), and the 59227 enantiomers exhibit a 250-fold difference (106). The most recent of this series, 59227 RP, exhibits potent anti-PAF actions *in vivo* (107).

Sandoz Research Institute

The earliest PAF antagonist was SDZ 63-072 (Fig. 3C), which is comparable to CV-3988 but has a thiazolium group on carbon 3 and a tetrahydrofuran ring on carbon 2. This compound antagonized PAF-induced platelet aggregation (131), PAF-induced prostaglandin E_2 (PGE_2) synthesis by cultured glomerular mesangial cells (132), and systemic effects of PAF, endotoxin, and immune complexes in rats (133) and primates (134). The *d*- and *l*-enantiomers show similar inhibition of PAF-induced human platelet aggregation and receptor binding (131), indicating a lack of enantioselectivity.

SDZ 63-119 is a nonphosphorus thiazolium PAF receptor antagonist (Fig. 3D) that inhibits PAF-induced aggregation (131). As for SDZ 63-072, the en-

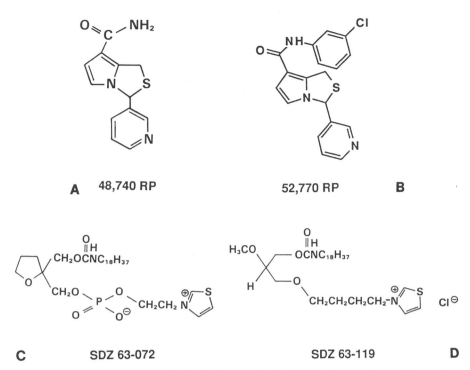

A 48,740 RP   52,770 RP **B**

C SDZ 63-072   SDZ 63-119 **D**

FIG. 3. **A:** 48740-RP: 3-(3- pyridyl)- 1H,3H- pyrrolo [1,2-c] tiazole -7-carboxamide, hydrochloride. **B:** 52770-RP: *N*-(3-chlorophenyl)- 3-(3-pyridinyl) 1H,3H- pyrrolo [1,2-c] thiazole -7-carboxamide. **C:** SDZ 63-072: (R,S)-3-[2-[(2- octadecylaminocarbonyloxy methyl tetrahydro -2-furanylmethoxy) hydroxyphosphinyl oxy] ethyl] thiazolium hydroxide inner salt 4-oxide. **D:** SDZ 63- 119: (R,S)-3- [4-[(3-oxtadecyl aminocarbonyloxy 2-methoxy) propoxybutyl] thiazolium bromide.

antiomers are equipotent *in vitro* as inhibitors of PAF-induced human platelet aggregation and receptor binding (131).

In SDZ 63-441, the glycerol fragment has been replaced with a cis 2,5 bis hydromethyltetrahydrofuran unit and the thiazolium group with a quinolinium (Fig. 4A). SDZ 63-441 inhibits PAF-induced platelet aggregation (135), vascular responses in rats, dogs, and primates (136), and is reported to be more potent than CV-3988 (137). SDZ 63-675 is an analog of 63-441, in which the hydrogens at carbons 2 and 5 have been replaced with methyl groups (Fig. 4B). SDZ 63-675 is slightly more potent than SDZ 63-441, and inhibits PAF-induced responses in rat, guinea pigs, dogs, and primates (138,139). The (+) form of SDZ 63-675 is fourfold more potent than the (−) form as an inhibitor of PAF-induced hemoconcentration in the guinea pig and in the Cebus primate (140). SDZ 63-675 has been shown to attenuate an number of responses in animals, as recently reviewed (141).

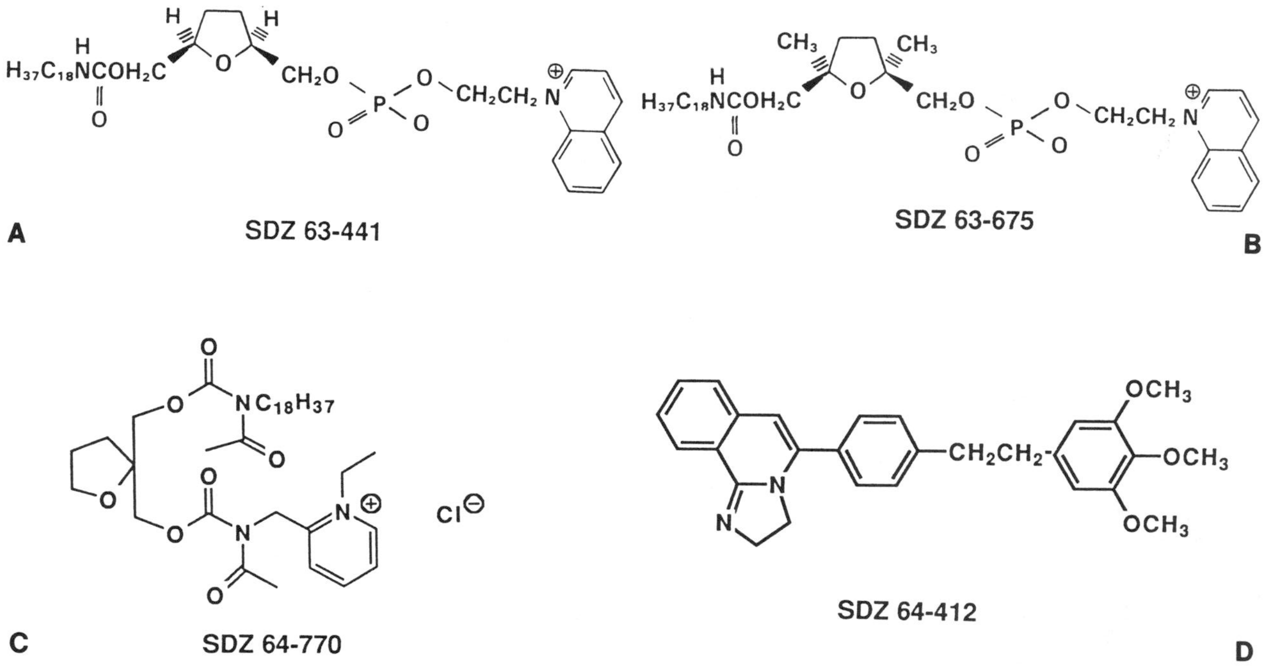

FIG. 4. A: SDZ 63-441: cis (±) -1-[2-[hydroxy[[tetrahydro -5- [(octadecylaminocarbonyl) oxy] methyl] furyl-2-yl] methoxy phosphinyloxy] ethyl] quinolinium hydroxide, inner salt. **B:** SDZ 63-675: cis (±) -1-[2-[hydroxy[[tetrahydro -2,5-dimethyl- 5-[(octadecyl aminocarbonyl) ocy] methyl]furan -2- yl] methoxy phosphinyloxy] ethyl] quinolinium hydroxide, inner salt. **C:** SDZ 64-770: 2-[acetyl [[tetrahydro-2- [[[[[acetyl] (octadecyl) amino]-carbonyl]oxy]methyl] furan -2-yl] methoxycarbonyl] aminomethyl]- -ethylpyridinium chloride. **D:** SDZ 64-412: 5-[4 (3',4',5' -trimethoxy phenylethyl) phenyl]-2,3-dihydro-imidazo [2,1-a] isoquinoline hydrochlo-ride.

The newer generation of antagonists exhibit potent inhibition of all major systemic responses to PAF in many species, such as demonstrated with SDZ 64-419 (101) and SDZ 64-770 (Fig. 4C). SDZ 64-770 shares several features of WEB 2086, where that phosphothiazolium group has been replaced with an *N*-acetyl carbamate pyridinium moiety. The resulting changes conferred exceptional potency and long duration of activity *in vivo*. SDZ 64-770 showed dose-dependent inhibition of PAF-induced bronchoconstriction and hemoconcentration in the guinea pig, with ED_{50} values of 5μg/kg for both responses (Fig. 5A). When administered at tenfold the ED_{50} value, 50% inhibition was observed at 1 h, denoting extended *in vivo* activity (Fig. 5B). SDZ 64-770 exhibited dose-dependence against PAF-induced hypotension in the rat (Fig. 5C), hemoconcentration and hypotension in the dog (Fig. 5D), and hemoconcentration in the cebus primate (Fig. 5E). Such broad inhibitory effects against different responses to PAF, involving different cell/tissue sites in different species, indicate an absence of receptor heterogeneity or species specificity. Furthermore, SDZ 64-770 showed potent dose-dependent reversal of endotoxin-induced hypotension in the rat (Fig. 6A), with potency that exceeded the activity of L 652,731 or WEB 2086 in the same model (Fig. 6B). SDZ 64-412 (Fig. 4D) is a 5-aryl imidazo [2,1-a] isoquinoline salt and is one of the most potent PAF receptor antagonists developed to date, with an IC_{50} of 60 nM (142) that exhibits again broad inhibitory effects against PAF- or endotoxin-mediated responses (142).

Sanofi Researche

The first of a new series of PAF antagonists, SR 27417 (*N*-(2 dimethylaminoethyl)-*N*-(3-pyridinylmethyl) [2,4,6-triisopropyl phenyl) thiazol-2-yl] amine) furmarate, inhibits PAF-, endotoxin-, or antigen-mediated responses in mice (103).

Schering-Plough Research

Sch 37370, 1-acetyl-4(8-chloro-5,6-dihydro 11H-benzo[5,6] cyclohepta [1,2-b] pyridine 11-ylidine) piperidine, is a dual antagonist of PAF and histamine that inhibits platelet responses to PAF and *in vivo* responses in the guinea pig (143).

Sumitomo Pharmaceuticals Co., Ltd.

SM-10661 is a water-soluble thiazolidine PAF antagonist (Fig. 7A) that has recently been reported to exhibit moderate *in vivo* activity (144).

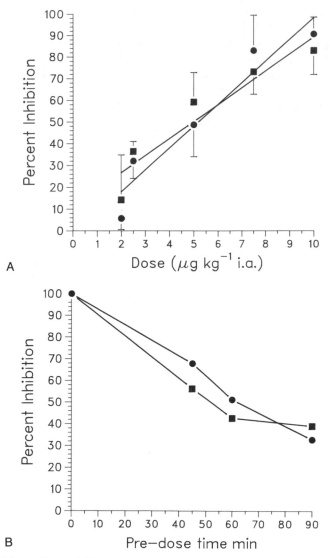

FIG. 5. Inhibitory effects of SDZ 64-770 against PAF-mediated responses. Shown are mean values (1 ± s.e.m.) from five to seven animals per dose. **A:** SDZ 64-770 was prepared in isotonic saline and given by i.a. injection at the indicated doses 1 min before a 150 ng/kg i.v. dose of synthetic C_{18} PAF, prepared in tris-Tyrode's buffer containing 1% BSA (protocol according to ref. 135). Dose-response profiles were generated in the guinea pig for inhibition of hemoconcentration (●) and bronchoconstriction (■), where the ED_{50} values for both parameters was 5 µg/kg. **B:** Guinea pigs were given SDZ 64-770 at 0.05 mg/kg (tenfold the ED_{50} value) and tested at the indicated times later with 150 ng/kg PAF i.v. (protocol according to ref. 101). About 50% inhibition of PAF-induced hemoconcentration (●) and bronchoconstriction (■) was observed 1 h following injection of SDZ 64-770.

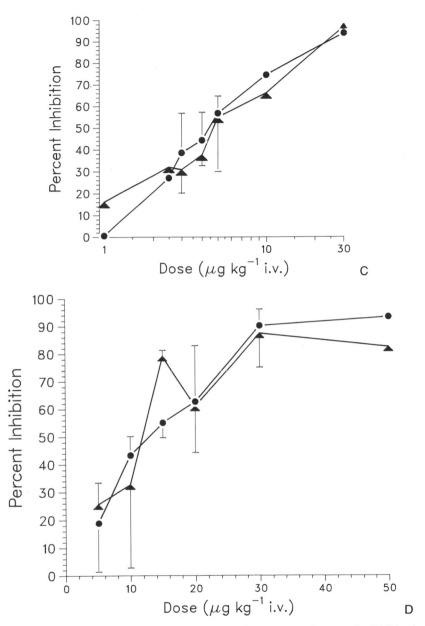

FIG. 5. *Continued.* **C:** Dose-dependent inhibition by SDZ 64-770 of 100 ng/kg PAF i.v. induced hypotension (●) and duration of the hypotensive response (▲) in the rat (protocol according to 135), where the ED_{50} values were 5 μg/kg for both responses. **D:** Dose-dependent inhibition by SDZ 64-770 of 1.5 μg/kg PAF i.v. induced hemoconcentration (●) and hypotension (▲) in the dog (protocol according to 135), where the ED_{50} values were 12 μg/kg for both responses.

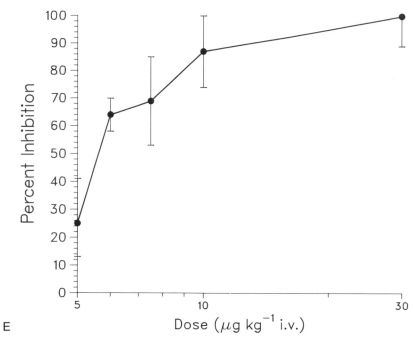

FIG. 5. *Continued.* **E:** Dose-dependent inhibition by SDZ 64-770 of 3.5 μg/kg PAF i.v. in-duced hemoconcentration in the primate (Cebus apella, protocol according to ref. 135), where the ED_{50} value is 6 μg/kg.

Takeda Chemical Co., Ltd.

The first synthetic PAF receptor antagonist reported in the literature was CV-3988 (Fig. 7B), a structural analog of PAF in which the quaternary moiety on carbon 3 has been replaced with a thiazolium, the ether linkage on carbon 1 replaced by a octadecyl carbamate group, and methyl ether on carbon 2 instead of an acetoxy. CV-3988 inhibits PAF-induced aggregation (145) and binding of PAF on human platelets (146) and liver membranes (124). CV-3988 has been used as a literature standard for comparison with other PAF receptor antagonists, such as Ono-6240 (147,148), L-652,731 (113,147), kadsurenone (147,149), Ginkgolide B (147–149), alprazolam (113), and triazolam (113).

CV-6209 (Fig. 7C) has an ethyl pyridinium group on carbon 3 and the phosphate group has been replaced by an *N*-acetyl carbamate linkage. *In vitro,* the enantiomers of CV-6209 at carbon 2 of the glycerol exhibit equal potency (96). The most recent compound of this series is TCV-309, 3-bromo-5 [*N*-phenyl-*N*-[2[[2-(1,2,3,4-tetrahydro 2-isoquinoly carbonyloxy) ethyl] carbomyl] ethyl]carbomyl] 1-propylpyridinium nitrate, which exhibits po-tent inhibition of several PAF- and endotoxin-mediated responses (104).

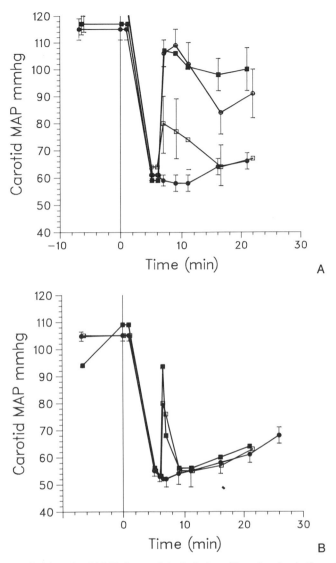

FIG. 6. A: Reversal of 1 mg/kg 0111B$_4$ i.v. endotoxin-induced hypotension in the rat (protocol according to ref. 133) by SDZ 64-770 at doses of 1 (□), 10 (○), or 100 (■) (μg/kg i.v.). Shown are mean values (1 ± s.e.m.) from three to seven animals per dose. Virtually complete reversal is seen with 100 μg/kg i.a. dose, in comparison to controls injected with saline (●). **B:** Similar evaluation for the PAF antagonists L 652,731 (■) and WEB 2086 (□) showing a small, temporary reversal of endotoxin-induced hypotension in comparison to controls injected with saline (●).

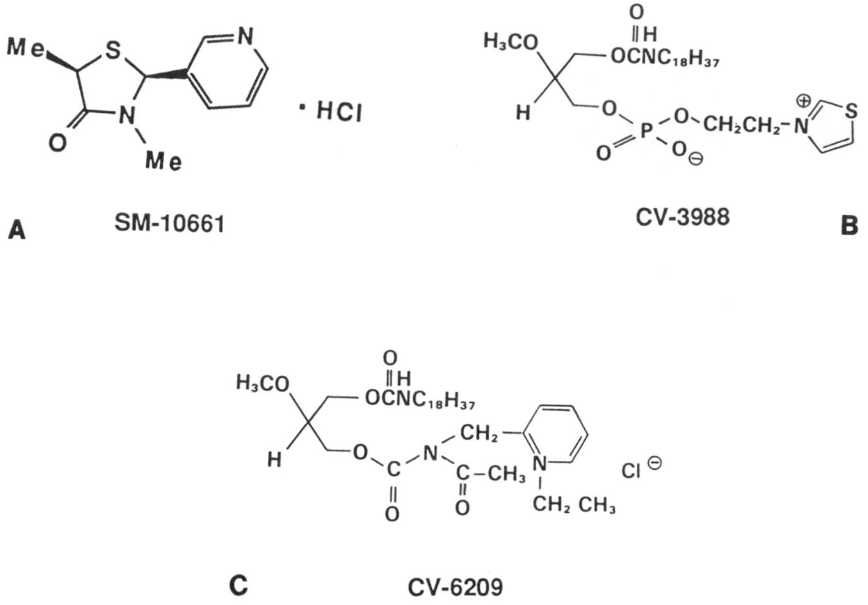

FIG. 7. A: SM-10661: (±) -2,5-cis -2- (3-pyridyl) -3,5-dimethyl-thiazolidin-4-one hydrochloride. **B:** CV-3988: (R,S)-2- methoxy -3-(octadecyl carbamoyloxy) propyl -2-(3-thazolio) ethyl phosphate. **C:** CV-6209: (R,S) -2-[N-2-acetyl -(N-2-methoxy -3- octadecyl carbonyl oxypropoxycarbonyl) aminoethyl]-1-ethylpyridinium chloride.

Yamanouchi Pharmaceutical Company

YM461, 1-(3-phenylpropyl) 4-[2-(3-pyridyl) thiazolidin 4 ylcarbonyl] piperazine fumarate, exhibits potent and long-lasting oral activity in the sheep model of allergen-induced responses (150).

Yoshitomi Pharmaceutical Industries, Ltd.

Etizolam, 6-(o-chlorophenyl) 8-ethyl-1-methyl 4H-s-triazolo [3,4-c] thieno [2,3-e] [1,4] diazepine, is an anti-anxiety drug that inhibits PAF-induced reactions in guinea pigs and mice (110).

PRECLINICAL EFFECTS OF PAF RELEVANT TO ASTHMA

Acute Bronchoconstriction

PAF is one of the most powerful bronchoconstrictor agents identified to date, over 20,000-fold more potent than histamine (115,151,152). This property and exceptional potency suggested a role for PAF as a mediator in allergen-induced acute bronchospasm. The bronchoconstrictor effects of PAF are platelet-dependent when PAF is given parenterally (34,72,78,153,154), but appear to be platelet-independent when PAF is given by aerosol or intratracheal administration (155,156). Vascular permeability effects of PAF are platelet-independent (153), significantly more potent than leukotrienes (157), and vary only by potency with different routes of administration (158). The guinea pig is the preferred animal for evaluation of PAF-induced bronchoconstriction (5), although the rat (159), cat (160), rabbit (78), sheep (28,34,67), and primates (161–165) have been evaluated. Species that possess platelets that are unresponsive to PAF, including rats (166,167) and Cebus primates, do not exhibit bronchoconstriction when challenged with PAF unless large doses of PAF are used (168).

Most PAF antagonists have been shown to inhibit PAF-induced bronchoconstriction (usually in the guinea pig), including CV-3988 (160,160), CV-6209 (49), L-652,731 (169), L-659,989 (127), Ono 6240 (128), 48740 RP (170,171), SDZ 63-119 (172), SDZ 63-072 (162,172), SDZ 63-441 (135), SDZ 63-675 (138,139), SDZ 64-412 (142), Sch 37370 (143), Sm-10661 (144), WEB 2086 (97,173,174), and WEB 2347 (116). Only Ro 15-1788 (orally or parenterally) reportedly failed to inhibit PAF-induced bronchoconstriction (111). As PAF exhibits a four log-fold stereoselective difference in platelet binding (147) and bronchoconstriction potency (127), it is reasonable to expect stereoselectivity in terms of antagonist activity. The *d*- and *l*-enantiomers of SDZ 63-119 (172,175), SDZ 63-072 (172), and SDZ 63-441 (49) are equipotent against PAF-induced bronchoconstriction in the guinea pig. However, the (+) form of SDZ 63-675 is fourfold more potent than the (−) form as an inhibitor of PAF-induced hemoconcentration in the guinea pig and in the Cebus primate (140).

In the case of allergen-induced bronchoconstriction, it is known that in the guinea pig the acute response is driven by release histamine (154). Accordingly, PAF antagonists such as CV-3988 (169), WEB 2086 (102,176), and SDZ 64-412 (177) did not inhibit acute allergen-induced bronchospasm in sensitized guinea pigs. The notable exception was E6123, which exhibited potent and dose-dependent inhibitory effects (102). SDZ 63-441 was not effective in inhibiting acute antigen-induced bronchoconstriction in the dog (178) or primate (163,179). WEB 2086 is able to inhibit bronchoconstriction induced in the guinea pig from passive or active anaphylaxis (102,180) and antigen-induced eosinophil infiltration triggered by PAF or antigen (181). However, other investigators have reported WEB 2086 as ineffective against active anaphylaxis *in vivo* (97) or antigen-induced airway vascular leakage (182). Ro 19-3704 is reported to inhibit allergen-induced bronchoconstriction in passively sensitized guinea pigs when the allergen is administered intravenously but not by aerosol (120). PAF antagonists seem to exhibit limited effectiveness in allergen-induced bronchoconstriction (139,149,183,184), suggesting that PAF may not have a prominent role in acute bronchospasm. Similarly, asthma drugs known to attenuate allegen-induced bronchoconstriction exhibit limited inhibition of PAF-induced effects (185). The inability of PAF antagonists to prevent symptomatic bronchospasm should not influence their usefulness or perceived benefit in asthma therapy, for other effective and widespread asthma therapies such as cromolyn and steroids similarly lack bronchodilation properties but are effective prophylactic agents.

Airways Eosinophilia

Several studies have identified a clear correlation between eosinophils and asthma. Eosinophils are a major cellular participant in the inflammatory response to allergen and are implicated as an effector cell in asthma pathology. It is reported that asthmatics exhibit pulmonary (186,187) and blood (188) eosinophilia and that bronchoalveolar lavage (BAL) eosinophils counts correlate with airway hyperreactivity (189,190).

Several studies have attempted to elucidate the role of eosinophil-derived products with bronchial inflammation and airway hyperreactivity. Not only do eosinophils synthesize PAF in response to immunoglobulin G (IgG)-dependent (191) and chemotactic peptides (11), but they respond to PAF in terms of potent chemotactic activation (192–195). Eosinophils exhibit high affinity receptors to PAF (100). Accordingly, PAF can induce pulmonary recruitment of eosinophils into the lungs of guinea pigs (181) and baboons (196). The reactions to PAF mimic the development of pulmonary eosinophilia following allergen challenge (181,197,198). PAF antagonists such as WEB 2086 (199), L-652-731 (199), and SRI 63-441 (199) inhibit PAF-induced eosinophil chemotaxis *in vitro*. PAF antagonists block PAF-induced pulmonary eosinophil recruitment (181,200), but in response to antigen-induced pulmonary eosinophilia, inhibitory (181,201) as well as noninhibitory (107,177,202) effects are reported. However, the role of the eosinophil in asthma pathology is not firmly established, as PAF antagonists such as SDZ 64-412 inhibit airway hyperreactivity without affecting airway eosinophilia (177), while other prophylactic antiasthma drugs inhibit eosinophilia but fail to modify airway hyperreactivity (200).

PAF antagonists such as WEB 2086 inhibit PAF-induced bronchial permeability (98) and the development of PAF-induced pulmonary eosinophilia, as shown for SDZ 64-412 (142,200).

Late Phase Responses

The late asthmatic response (LAR) develops 2 to 6 h after allergen challenge and is observed in about 50% of atopic asthmatics. LAR usually follows an acute asthmatic response, although isolated LAR—in the absence of early asthmatic response (EAR)—is seen in a subset of patients. Clinically, LAR may exhibit severe and protracted airway obstruction, which is refractory to most agents used for acute symptom relief. LAR is associated with subsequent increases in airway hyperreactivity (203). A number of animal models of LAR have been developed, including the rat (204), monkey (205), sheep (150,206), rabbit (203,207), and guinea pig (208–211), all of which exhibit airway hyperreactivity and eosinophil infiltration. These models are difficult to reproduce, as animals either are selected for natural IgE-allergen sensitivity or immunized to specific antigen by a neonatal immunization protocol.

A limited number of studies have demonstrated that LAR can be inhibited by pretreatment of guinea pigs with nedocromil sodium (210,211). The PAF antagonist YM461 shows potent inhibition of allergen-induced LAR in sheep (150). Lyso PAF is significantly elevated in human plasma 6 h after antigen challenge (212) and has been suggested to play a role in late-onset reactions following allergen inhalation (82).

Airway Hyperreactivity

Prolonged airway hyperreactivity and attendant airway inflammation are well established clinical characteristics of human asthma. A number of studies established that PAF could elicit sustained and nonspecific airway hyperreactivity in a variety of species, including guinea pigs (72–77), rabbits (78), dogs (79), sheep (67), and primates (213). As seen for other PAF-mediated effects, PAF-induced airway hyperreactivity is inhibited by the PAF antagonists SDZ 63-441 (214), CV-3988 (76), BN 52021 (76), WEB 2086 (76), and RP 59227 (61).

Animal models of allergen-induced airway hyperreactivity have involved passive sensitization using reagenic antibodies developed in donor animals (97,102,215), natural sensitivity (150), active sensitization to induce an IgE response to antigen by either repeated aerosol exposure (97,202,216–218) or immunization (102,176,177,210,219–223). In terms of abating allergen-induced hyperreactivity, the effects of PAF antagonists have been variable. WEB 2086 has been found to be ineffective (176) and effective (224), while E6123 showed potent inhibition of allergen-induced airway hyperreactivity (102), as did SDZ 64-412 (177,202) and YM461 (150). Other PAF antagonists such as BN 52021 showed modest effects at large doses (430,355). Thus, PAF antagonists do not exhibit a consistent inhibitory effect on allergen-mediated airway hyperreactivity in response to allergen.

CLINICAL EFFECTS OF PLATELET-ACTIVATING FACTOR RELEVANT TO ASTHMA

Recent identification of endogenously released platelet-associated mediators in asthmatics suggests that PAF may be an important mediator in asthma. A first piece of evidence demonstrated that inhaled allergen challenge of asthmatics results in elevated serum levels of platelet factor 4 (225). Asthmatics also have platelet products in their BAL fluid (226). PAF itself is present in the sputum (227) and BAL fluid (228) of asthmatics. Furthermore, baseline plasma PAF in asthmatics positively correlates with the severity of airway hyperreactivity that these patients express (229). PAF and lyso-PAF are present in BAL fluid from atopic subjects (some asthmatics) 20 h after segmental airway challenge with antigen (230). PAF is also elevated in the plasma of atopic asthmatic patients after allergen-induced bronchoconstriction, but not after methacholine-induced bronchoconstriction (229). The findings of endogenous platelet-associated mediators (including PAF) in asthmatics led to the hypothesis that PAF may play an important role in asthma. These findings also led to more sophisticated asthma-directed experimentation with PAF and PAF antagonists, in both animals and, more importantly, humans.

Acute Bronchoconstriction

Several clinical studies demonstrate that PAF is a potent bronchoconstricting agent. This raises the possibility that PAF may play a key role as a mediator of the reversible, acute bronchoconstriction observed in asthmatics. First evidence of PAF-induced bronchoconstriction in humans was provided by Cuss et al. (231). In this study PAF induced a dose-dependent bronchoconstriction, as evidenced by a decrease in expiratory flow at 30% of vital capacity (Vp_{30}), in normal humans. This bronchoconstriction onset was within 1 min of inhalation and did not completely reverse until approximately 8 h later. PAF-induced bronchoconstriction was confirmed by another independent study (232), where PAF, inhaled by both normal humans and mild asthmatics, produced a dose-dependent decrease in specific airway conductance (SG_{aw}). Vp_{30} is only minimally decreased in the asthmatics and is unaffected in the normal subjects. Forced expiratory volume in 1 sec (FEV_1) in asthmatics and normal subjects is almost unaffected. These data, in part, provide some suggestion that PAF may elicit airflow obstruction in the central airways to a greater extent than in the small, peripheral airways (232); however, this suggestion remains to be proven in light of the methodology in other studies (233,234). These studies demonstrate that PAF is capable of producing the acute bronchoconstriction associated with typical asthmatic responses.

The dose dependency of PAF-induced bronchoconstriction has been only recently observed due to rapid tachyphylaxis to repeated PAF inhalations (see below) (88). In this study, normal subjects were given single cumulative, increasing doses of inhaled PAF separated by 2 weeks between each dose. Only in this fashion is the dose dependency of PAF observed and not confounded by PAF's tachyphylactic effects observed by multiple dose challenges used in other studies (231,232). PAF-induced bronchoconstriction may be mediated through the release of lipoxygenase products (74,235) or histamine (236).

Asthmatics appear to be more sensitive to PAF than to other nonspecific spasmogens (e.g., methacholine). One study demonstrates that the provocative concentration that yields a 35% decrease in specific airway conductance ($PC_{35}SG_{aw}$) for PAF is 0.19 mmol/L (nebulizer concentration) in asthmatics and 0.88 mmol/L for normal subjects. Therefore, asthmatics are four to five times more sensitive to inhaled PAF than the normal subjects (232). This finding is also observed in asthmatic children where inhaled PAF induces six out of seven children to bronchoconstrict but only induces one out of seven normal children to bronchoconstrict (92). This increased sensitivity of asthmatics to PAF may be dependent on the recently observed finding that asthmatics express low serum activity of PAF acetylhydrolase, the enzyme responsible for PAF metabolism (237). This deficiency may result in increased PAF availability for the generation and expression of deleterious effects.

Although asthmatics may be more sensitive to PAF, both normal subjects and asthmatics rapidly become tachyphylactic to repeated PAF inhalations (231,232). Possible explanations for tachyphylaxis (232) include reduced sensitivity of the PAF receptors, increased metabolism of PAF, enhanced release of endogenous bronchodilatory mediators (238), and decreased PAF receptor density (239). Tachyphylaxis often makes bronchoconstriction, due to repeated ascending dosing with inhaled PAF, difficult to interpret since repetitive inhalations of PAF may result in no further airflow obstruction.

Late Phase Bronchoconstriction

Late phase bronchoconstriction is a characteristic found in many asthmatics. It is believed to be mediated, in part, by PAF (82) since lyso-PAF is elevated in the plasma of asthmatics 6 h following allergen challenge (212). However, late phase bronchoconstriction is often difficult to model in animal and clinical experimentation. In clinical experiments, PAF is not yet demonstrated to possess the ability to induce late phase bronchoconstriction. To date, only one experiment has had adequate design to assess the possible PAF-induced late phase bronchoconstriction. Lai et al. (88) assessed FEV_1 and Vp_{30} for up to 7 h after inhaled PAF challenges in atopic and nonatopic nonasthmatic human volunteers. Subsequently, each subject was observed for 14 days. Very high doses of PAF (400 μg) failed to induce late phase bronchoconstriction. It is possible that PAF may cause late phase bronchoconstriction between 7 and 24 h; however, this is not tested for in the above experiment or in any other experiment. Therefore, the data generated at present suggest that PAF is incapable of producing late phase bronchoconstriction.

Airway Hyperreactivity

Airway hyperreactivity is now recognized to be the underlying defect of asthmatics and stems from chronic airway inflammation. However, the specific events that relate airway inflammation to airway hyperreactivity remain unclear. PAF certainly is a potential link between the two; however, the role of PAF in airway hyperreactivity remains unclear.

The ability of PAF to induce airway hyperreactivity was first demonstrated by Cuss et al. (231). In this study approximately 60 μg aerosolized PAF was administered to normal volunteers, over 1 h. Airway reactivity to aerosolized methacholine was assessed for up to 14 days after the PAF challenge and the provocative methacholine concentration that resulted in a 40% decrease (PC_{40}) in Vp_{30} was documented. This study demonstrates that airway hyperreactivity, assessed as a twofold reduction in PC_{40}, is maximal 3 days after PAF administration. Varying degrees of airway hyperreactivity are evident for at least 7 days after PAF inhalation. The degree of airway hyperreactivity in this experiment is modest compared to that typically observed in asthmatics. However, the data demonstrate that PAF could be the *single* inflammatory mediator that induces prolonged airway hyperreactivity in normal human volunteers.

Other investigations expand the finding of PAF-induced airway hyperreactivity in normal subjects. PAF-induced airway hyperreactivity, in normal subjects, is confirmed by the initial investigators in subsequent experiments (240). This finding is also corroborated by independent investigations in which PAF produces a decrease in the methacholine $PC_{35}SG_{aw}$ from 26 to 11.3 mmol/L (232). In contrast to these three reports supporting PAF-induced airway hyperreactivity in normal subjects, several investigations (by two independent laboratories) do not support such findings (88,241,242). When 30 μg of aerosolized PAF was administered to normal human volunteers, airway hyperreactivity was not observed for the 6-day study period (241). This discrepancy is believed to be due to the low doses of PAF utilized in the study (241); however, as little as 23 μg of inhaled PAF induces airway hyperreactivity (232). Furthermore, another study demonstrates that larger PAF doses (100 to 400 μg) are unable to induce airway hyperreactivity in normal individuals (88). In this study, all doses of PAF do not elicit airway hyperreactivity at any time over 2 weeks; however, they produce tachyphylaxis over the first 2 to 3 days after PAF inhalation to the methacholine challenge used to assess airway reactivity. This tachyphylaxis is not demonstrated previously and remains unexplained. These data demonstrate that PAF has equivocal effects on the development of airway hyperreactivity in normal humans. The simple explanation that low doses of PAF do not cause airway hyperreactivity cannot account for the discrepancy in data obtained from normal humans. An alternative explanation may incorporate (especially at high PAF doses) tachyphylaxis linked to the mechanism that mediates PAF-induced airway hyperreactivity (88).

Although PAF's ability to induce airway hyperreactivity in normal subjects is evident but controversial, PAF lacks the ability to induce sustained airway hyperreactivity in asthmatics. This is demonstrated in several investigations (86,232,242). Rubin et al. (232) exposed six mild asthmatic subjects to aerosolized PAF. These subjects had substantial airway hyperreactivity demonstrated by an average of five fold less baseline methacholine $PC_{35}SG_{aw}$ than normal volunteers. Up to 45 min after PAF inhalation, methacholine challenges were repeated. The average $PC_{35}SG_{aw}$ was similar to baseline in each case. These data demonstrate that unlike the normal volunteers used in this study, the asthmatics do not develop *further* airway hyperreactivity after PAF inhalation. Subsequent studies corroborate the above finding. In mild asthmatics, aerosolized PAF administration elicits no airway hyperreactivity for up to 7 days (86). Recently, slight increases in airway hyperreactivity in asthmatics are suggested to occur 2 h after PAF inhalation (242); however, the airway hyperreactivity is transient—unlike that reported for normal volunteers. The reason for PAF's inability to produce sustained airway hyperreactivity in asthmatics is speculative and may be related to underlying tachyphylaxis due to increased basal levels of endogenous PAF. Alternatively, the degree of airway hyperreactivity in asthmatics, at the period of the study, may be maximal and may not be further enhanced by any mediator, including PAF.

Pulmonary-Directed Inflammatory Responses

Only now is asthma recognized as a chronic inflammatory disease of the airways despite the long-time recognition of airway inflammation and granulocyte infiltration. The role of eosinophils is believed to be of prime importance since most atopic asthmatics have some degree of blood eosinophilia. Asthmatics, on whom BAL has been performed, also have eosinophils in the lavagate (190). Furthermore, there is evidence of eosinophil activation in asthma since the eosinophils collected from this patient group are proportionately more hypodense than those collected from normal humans, suggesting eosinophil activation *in vivo* (243).

The relationship between PAF and eosinophils is very tight. Human eosinophils possess a high-affinity PAF receptor (234) and exhibit chemotaxis in response to PAF (192). PAF also induces the shift in eosinophil density, from normodense to hypodense, that is associated with eosinophil activation (245). PAF induces toxic oxygen radical release (246,247) and eosinophil degranulation, resulting in the release of eosinophil peroxidase (248). Activated eosinophils, and the mediators released from them, are demonstrated to be deleterious to human airway epithelium *in vitro* (249). These data suggest that PAF may induce blood and airway eosinophilia as well as eosinophil activation. Activated eosinophils may release several mediators that are capable of altering epithelial cell integrity and this in turn may lead to impaired airway regulation and airway hyperreactivity that is frequently observed in asthmatics (250–254).

In clinical studies, the role of PAF in airway eosinophilia and eosinophil activation is less clear. PAF's ability to induce airway eosinophilia in man is still undefined—unlike its role in the skin of atopic individuals where PAF, administered i.d., produces a rapid and remarkable eosinophilia (255). However, inhalation of PAF produces changes in circulating neutrophils (5,241,256) and airspace neutrophilia (5), rather than eosinophilia, without changes in circulating platelets (5,256). Upon inhalation of PAF, blood neutrophil counts rapidly decrease to 30% to 50% of baseline counts within 5 min (5,257). It is believed that the neutrophils sequester in the pulmonary circulation (5). Sequestration is confirmed by the use of ^{111}In-labeled neutrophils (257). Neutrophil sequestration in the pulmonary vasculature is followed by a rebound neutrophilia that occurs within 15 min after the PAF inhalation, suggesting demargination of a large neutrophil pool from the pulmonary circulation (5,256). Real-time measurement of ^{111}In-labeled neutrophils demonstrates that released neutrophils, previously sequestered in the pulmonary circulation, account for only a small portion of the blood neutrophil recovery and are not associated with the rebound (257). The rebound is apparently due to PAF-induced release of neutrophils from bone marrow. An increase in both leukocyte count and neutrophil differential, thereby greatly increasing the numbers of neutrophils, is observed in bronchoalveolar lavage fluid 4 h after PAF inhalation (5). Interestingly, the presence of this large number of airspace neutrophils is positively correlated with PAF-induced acute bronchoconstriction, but is negatively correlated with airway hyperreactivity (5). This is contrary to the large numbers of eosinophils in BAL fluid obtained from atopic asthmatics, and the coincident deficits in lung function.

Although inhaled PAF appears to induce pulmonary neutrophilia, rather than eosinophilia, it may still affect eosinophil (and other leukocytes) function *in vivo*. Eosinophils, obtained from the blood of asthmatic children, produce greater O_2^- release than neutrophils obtained from the same patient or eosinophils and neutrophils obtained from the blood of normal healthy volunteers (258). The control eosinophils can be made to release greater amounts of O_2^- by preincubation with PAF; however, such preincubation does not affect the increased levels of O_2 release already observed from the asthmatic eosinophils (258). This may be indirect evidence that PAF produces eosinophil priming *in vivo* (258), demonstrated by possible tachyphylaxis to PAF *in vitro*.

Basal levels of intracellular inositol triphosphate (IP$_3$) and Ca^{2+} in platelets from asthmatics are greater than in platelets from normal individuals (256). After PAF inhalation, intracellular IP$_3$ and Ca^{2+} levels increase in platelets from both asthmatics and normal volunteers; however, the platelets are refractory specifically to *in vitro* PAF stimulation (256). These data suggest that while the role of platelets in asthma is currently debated, PAF, whether endogenous in asthmatics or inhaled in both asthmatics and normal volunteers, appears to have specific effects on platelets and eosinophils, including *in vivo* priming and tachyphylaxis. These findings further suggest that endogenous PAF may play a role in the pulmonary inflammation observed in asthmatics, although that role remains undefined.

PLATELET-ACTIVATING FACTOR ANTAGONISTS IN MAN

The suggestion that PAF plays a major role in the pathophysiology of asthma leads to the aspiration of the therapeutic use of PAF antagonists in asthma. Many compounds are designed and synthesized to specifically antagonize the PAF receptor. PAF antagonists are well documented to inhibit atopic and PAF-induced dermal reactions in man (175,259–261). Several different PAF antagonists are efficacious in various animal models that mimic portions of the pathology associated with asthma (see above). However, the role of PAF antagonists in asthma is relatively undefined. At present, only a few clinical studies investigate their usage.

PAF Antagonists and Acute Bronchoconstriction

By far the best evidence that PAF antagonists work against human asthma symptoms is demonstrated by PAF-induced bronchoconstriction. Oral administration of the ginkgolide mixture BN 52063 (120 mg) to healthy volunteers, 2 h prior to five sequential inhalations of PAF (24 μg), produced a 10% to 15% reduction in the PAF-induced Vp_{30} decrease (233). This reduction was observed after each PAF inhalation and the amount of the reduction progressively increased. However, these results may be confounded by the well-documented tachyphylaxis associated with repeated PAF inhalations. A more active ginkgolide PAF antagonist, BN 52021, when inhaled, completely abolished inhaled PAF-induced (but not methacholine-induced) bronchoconstriction (92).

Similar data are observed with the triazolobenzodiazepine, WEB 2086 (90), which when administered orally (40 mg) 1.5 h prior to an inhaled PAF challenge, produces a complete inhibition of the twofold increase in R_{aw} (airway resistance) associated with PAF inhalation in this study. Preliminary evidence suggests that a third oral PAF antagonist, UK 74505 (25 and 100 mg), also completely inhibits inhaled PAF-induced (30 μg) bronchoconstriction in man (262). While PAF inhalation in man is an appropriate test for PAF antagonist efficacy studies in man, the real issues are (a) whether PAF *is* an important mediator in asthma and (b) whether PAF antagonists are able to produce therapeutic effects in asthma. The data generated with the ginkgolides and WEB 2086 suggest that if PAF were an important mediator of the acute bronchoconstriction response in asthma then the presence of a PAF antagonist should alleviate this symptom.

Clinical studies are beginning to focus on testing the efficacy of PAF antagonists in asthmatics and in response to various "clinically relevant" airway challenges. Orally administered BN 52063 (40 mg t.i.d.) significantly inhibits immediate bronchoconstriction induced by inhaled allergen in seven out of eight asthmatic subjects (93). These subjects are also rendered approximately sixfold less sensitive to the allergen challenge after this dosing regimen (93). A similar finding is observed with pretreatment of inhaled BN 52021, which prevents allergen-induced bronchoconstriction in three out of seven asthmatic children and decreases their airway sensitivity to allergen (92). BN 52063 also produces partial protection from exercise-induced asthma (183). Such findings suggest that PAF antagonists can inhibit allergen-induced bronchoconstriction in asthmatics.

These data are, in part, contradicted by more recent studies demonstrating that PAF antagonists are ineffective against allergen-induced acute bronchoconstriction. One such contradictory study demonstrates that WEB 2086, previously demonstrated to be effective against antigen-induced bronchoconstriction, is ineffective (263). Atopic asthmatics who received 100 mg oral WEB 2086 (t.i.d.) for 7 days prior to allergen challenge were not protected from allergen-induced acute bronchoconstriction (263). In an independent study, the formulation for WEB 2086 (WEB 2086 BS) was changed and aerosol administration was utilized to better target the PAF-mediated effects in the airways of asthmatics (264). Asthmatic patients received (250 μg) WEB 2086 BS q.i.d. for 7 days prior to antigen challenge. Upon challenge, acute bronchoconstriction was unchanged from placebo, despite inhibition of platelet aggregation, measured *ex vivo* (264). Another PAF antagonist, MKS 287 (500 mg, oral) administered to atopic asthmatics 1 h prior to allergen challenge, fails to inhibit the resultant acute bronchoconstriction (265). Therefore, the ability of PAF antagonists to inhibit PAF-induced bronchoconstriction in man is significant, suggesting that PAF antagonists may be an effective therapy for acute bronchoconstriction if PAF were a mediator of this symptom. However, the ability of PAF antagonists to inhibit allergen-induced bronchoconstriction remains equivocal.

PAF Antagonists and Late Phase Bronchoconstriction

Although specific PAF antagonists inhibit allergen-induced late phase bronchoconstriction in preclinical models, such as sheep (150), very little data are available regarding the effects of PAF antagonists on late phase bronchoconstriction in man. However, three independent preliminary reports, in man, suggest that PAF antagonists are ineffective against allergen-induced late phase bronchoconstriction. A single dose of MKS 287 (500 mg) administered 1 h prior to allergen challenge of asthmatic subjects is unable to inhibit the decrease in FEV_1 that occurred up to 7 h after challenge (265). Similarly, WEB 2086 (100 mg, oral, t.i.d. for 7 days) does not prevent the 21% fall in FEV_1 measured 3 to 7 h after allergen challenge of asthmatic patients (263). Furthermore, the changed formulation of WEB 2086 that accommodates aerosolization (WEB 2086 BS; 250 μg, inhaled, q.i.d. for 7 days) also is without effect on the late 25% decrease in FEV_1 observed in allergen-challenged asthmatics (264). These data demonstrate that PAF antagonists are unlikely to be effective, by either the oral or aerosol route, against the late phase bronchoconstriction demonstrated in many asthmatics.

PAF Antagonists and Airway Hyperreactivity

Similar to the case of late phase bronchoconstriction, few reports exist describing the efficacy of PAF antagonists against the underlying defect in asthma, airway hyperreactivity. One early report raised expectations that PAF antagonists may provide therapeutic benefit for this condition (93). In this study, oral t.i.d. treatment (40 mg) with BN 52063 marginally reduced airway hyperreactivity (approximately a 12% increase in acetylcholine PD_{100}), assessed 6 h after allergen challenge of asthmatics (93). More recently, preliminary evidence suggests that other PAF antagonists possess little efficacy against airway hyperreactivity. MKS 287 (500 mg, orally administered 1 h prior to antigen challenge) did not produce a rightward shift in the histamine $PC_{20}FEV_1$ after antigen challenge (265). Oral WEB 2086 (100 mg t.i.d. over 7 days) produces no change in the pre- versus post-antigen histamine PC_{20} (263). However, the inhaled WEB 2086 formulation (WEB 2086 BS; 250 μg q.i.d. for 7 days) produces a twofold increase in the methacholine PC_{20} from 0.11 mg/ml before the allergen challenge to 0.26 mg/ml after the allergen challenge. Despite this apparent decrease is airway hyperreactivity afforded by WEB 2086 BS, the decrease in statistically insignificant and considered small (264). To date, the efficacy of PAF antagonists against airway hyperreactivity remains unproven.

Pulmonary-Directed Inflammatory Responses

The ability of PAF antagonists to alter either PAF-induced pulmonary inflammation or the pulmonary inflammation associated with asthma is not well defined. For example, in addition to its inhibition of PAF-induced bronchoconstriction, WEB 2086 (oral, 40 mg) completely inhibits platelet aggregation, measured *ex vivo* (90). UK 74505, at oral doses up to 100 mg, also completely inhibits the PAF-induced neutropenia as well as acute bronchoconstriction (262). In contrast, BN 52063 (oral, 120 mg) administered to normal volunteers, 2 h before inhaled PAF challenge, fails to inhibit the

PAF-induced neutropenia (233). In contrast, inhaled BN 52021 inhibits the PAF-induced eosinopenia and neutropenia in normal volunteers; however, this effect was not observed with asthmatics (92). The lack of agreement between these studies questions the ability of PAF antagonists to inhibit the inflammation associated with PAF. This action of a PAF antagonist is especially important if it is to be used for modifying the asthma disease process, since chronic pulmonary inflammation is a recognized hallmark feature of asthma and is expected to be the major contributor to the disease process. Furthermore, few studies question the relevance of PAF antagonists in (a) the reversal of established pulmonary inflammation in asthmatics and (b) allergen-induced inflammatory responses in asthmatics. Until these issues are addressed the efficacy of PAF antagonists in asthma-related pulmonary inflammation remains to be proven.

CONCLUSIONS AND FUTURE DIRECTIONS

PAF is implicated as an important, if not pivotal, mediator in asthma. In preclinical studies, PAF produces the typical symptoms of asthma, including bronchoconstriction, decreased lung compliance, airway edema, and eosinophil recruitment. It is the only *single* mediator that possesses the ability to produce *sustained* airway hyperreactivity. This single finding is the most important observation that links PAF to asthma and is the reason for the great interest in PAF. Furthermore, antagonism of endogenous PAF release in preclinical animal models further implies there is a role for PAF as well as the therapeutic potential of PAF antagonists.

Although preclinical studies nearly always link PAF to asthmatic symptoms and demonstrate the promise of PAF antagonism in asthma therapy, clinical studies are less promising. Inhaled PAF produces bronchoconstriction in man that can often be blocked by PAF antagonists. However, the ability of PAF to produce other asthma symptoms in man, including pulmonary eosinophilia, late phase bronchoconstriction, and airway hyperreactivity, is equivocal. The ability of potent and specific PAF antagonists to inhibit these PAF-induced symptoms, when they are observed, is equally equivocal. Finally, the ability of PAF antagonists to inhibit these symptoms in asthmatics is still unclear. Some investigations speculate the promise of the therapeutic use of PAF antagonists in asthma while others speculate the demise.

What is required to settle the issues surrounding PAF and PAF antagonists in asthma? The most significant requirement is the definition of the role of PAF in asthmatics, specifically the role in each of the asthma symptoms— bronchoconstriction, pulmonary inflammation, late phase bronchoconstriction, and airway hyperreactivity. A continuation (with much perseverance) of the current investigations that utilize specific, potent, and bioavailable PAF antagonists is warranted. A clear picture of the role, nuances, and idiosyncrasies of PAF in asthmatic subjects must be elucidated through well-planned and controlled experimentation. Only with such a clear picture can the role of PAF in asthma be described and the therapeutic potential of PAF antagonists be elucidated.

REFERENCES

1. Benveniste J, Henson PM, Cochrane GC. Leukocyte dependent histamine release from rabbit platelets: the role of IgE-basophils and platelet activating factor. *J Exp Med* 1972;136:1356–1368.
2. Demopolus CA, Pinckard RN, Hanahan DJ. Platelet activating factor. Evidence for 1-O-alkyl 2-acetyl sn-glyceryl 3-phosphorylcholine as the active component (a new class of lipid chemical mediators). *J Biol Chem* 1979;254:9355–9358.
3. Benveniste J, Tence M, Varenne P, Bidault J, Boullet C, Polonsky J. Semi-synthese et structure proposee du facteur activant les plaquettes (P.A.F.): PAF-acether, un alkyl ether analogue de la lysophatidylcholine. *CR Acad Sci Paris* 1979;289D:1037–1041.
4. Blank ML, Synder F, Byers LW, Brooks B, Muirhead EE. Antihypertensive activity of an aklyl ether analog of phosphatidylcholine. *Biochem Biophys Res Commun* 1979;90:1194–1200.
5. Handley DA. Quantitation of in vitro and in vivo biological effects of platelet activating factor. In: Chang JY, Lewis AJ, eds. *Pharmacological methods in the control of inflammation.* New York: Alan R. Liss, 1989;23–58.
6. Pinckard R, Ludwig JC, McManus L. Platelet activating factors. In: Gallin JI, Goldstein IM, Snyderman R, eds. *Inflammation: basic principles and clinical correlates.* New York: Raven Press, 1986;1–39.
7. Schleimer RP, MacGlashan DW, Peters S, Pinckard N, Adkinson N, Lichtenstein LW. Characterization of inflammatory mediator release from purified human lung mast cells. *Am Rev Respir Dis* 1986;133:614–617.
8. Joly F, Bessou G, Benveniste J, Ninio E. Ketotifen inhibits Paf-acether biosynthesis and β-hexosaminidase release in mouse mast cells stimulate with antigen. *Eur J Pharmacol* 1987;144:133–139.
9. Hayashi M, Kimura J, Yamaki K, et al. Detection of platelet activating factor in exudates of rats with phorbol myristate acetate induced pleurisy. *Thromb Res* 1987;48:299–310.
10. Sisson JH, Prescott SM, McIntyre TM, Zimmerman GA. Production of platelet activating factor by stimulated polymorphonuclear leukocytes. *J Immunol* 1987;138:3918–3926.
11. Lee T, Lenihan D, Malone B, Roddy L, Wasserman S. Increased biosynthesis of platelet activating factor in activated human eosinophils. *J Biol Chem* 1984;259:5526–5530.
12. Chignard M, Le Couedic JP, Vargaftig BB, Benveniste J. Platelet activating factor (PAF-acether) secretion from platelets: effect of aggregating agents. *Br J Haematol* 1980;46:455–464.
13. Rylander R, Beijer L. Inhalation of endotoxin stimulates alevolar macrophage production of platelet activating factor. *Am Rev Respir Dis* 1987;135:83–86.
14. Albert DH, Snyder F. Biosynthesis of 1-alkyl 2-acetyl sn-glycero-3-phosphocholine by rat alevolar macrophages. *J Biol Chem* 1983;258:97–102.
15. Wang J, Kester M, Dunn M. The effects of endotoxin on platelet activating factor synthesis in cultured rat glomerular mesangial cells. *Biochim Biophys Acta* 1988;969:217–224.
16. Malavasi F, Tetta C, Funaro A, et al. Fc receptor triggering induced expression of surface activation antigens and release of platelet activating factor in large granulocytes. *Proc Natl Acad Sci USA* 1986;83:2443–2447.
17. Whately R, Zimmerman G, McIntyre T, Prescott S. Endothelium from diverse vascular sources synthesizes platelet activating factor. *Arteriosclerosis* 1988;8:321–331.

18. McIntyre T, Zimmerman G, Prescott S. Leukotrienes C_4 and D_4 stimulate human endothelial cells to synthesize platelet activating factor and bind neutrophils. *Proc Natl Acad Sci USA* 1986;83:2204–2208.

19. Betz S, Lotner GZ, Henson PM. Production and release of platelet activating factor (PAF): dissociation from degranulation and superoxide production in the human neutrophil. *J Immunol* 1980;125:2749–2763.

20. Hanahan DJ, Demopoulos CA, Liehr J, Pinckard RN. Identification of a platelet activating factor isolated from rabbit basophils as acetylglycerly ether phosphorylcholine. *J Biol Chem* 1980;255:5514–5516.

21. Bussolino F, Gremo F, Tetta C, Pescarmona G, Camussi G. Production platelet activating factor by chick retina. *J Biol Chem* 1986;261:16502–16508.

22. Zanglis A, Lianos EA. Platelet activating factor biosynthesis and degradation in the rat glomeruli. *J Lab Clin Med* 1987;110:330–337.

23. Renooij W, Snyder F. Biosynthesis of 1-alkyl 2-acetyl sn-glycero-3-phosphocholine (platelet activating factor and a hypotensive lipid) by cholinephosphotransferase in various rat tissues. *Biochim Biophys Acta* 1981;663:545–556.

24. Fitzgerald MF, Moncada S, Parente L. The anaphylactic release of platelet activating factor from perfused guinea pig lungs. *Br J Pharmacol* 1986;88:149–153.

25. Lellouch-Tubiana A, Lefort J, Pfister A, Vargaftig BB. Interactions between granulocytes and platelets with the guinea pigs lung passive anaphylactic shock. *Int Arch Allergy Appl Immunol* 1987;83:198–205.

26. Doebber TW, Wu MS, Biftu T. Platelet activating factor (PAF) mediation of rat anaphylactic responses to soluble immune complexes. Studies with a PAF receptor antagonist 1-752,731. *J Immunol* 1986;136:4659–4668.

27. Mojarad M, Hamasaki Y, Said SI. Platelet activating factor increases pulmonary microvascular permeability and induced pulmonary edema. *Bull Eur Physiopathol Respir* 1983;19:253–256.

28. Burhop KE, Van Der Zee H, Bizios R, Kaplan JE, Malik AB. Pulmonary vascular response to platelet activating factor in awake sheep and the role of cyclooxygenase metabolites. *Am Rev Respir Dis* 1986;134:548–554.

29. Myers A, Ramey E, Ramwell P. Glucocorticoid protection against PAF-acether toxicity in mice. *Br J Pharmacol* 1983;79:595–598.

30. Hsueh W, Gonazalez-Crussi F, Arroyave J. Platelet activating factor: an endogenous mediator of bowel necrosis endotoxemia. *FASEB J* 1987;1:403–406.

31. Wallace JL. Release of platelet activating factor (PAF) and accelerated healing induced by a PAF antagonist in an animal model of chronic colitis. *Can J Physiol Pharmacol* 1988;66:422–435.

32. Stahl GL, Terashita ZI, Lefer AM. Role of platelet activating factor on propagation of cardiac damage during myocardial ischemia. *J Pharmacol Exp Ther* 1986;244:898–904.

33. Grandel K, Farr R, Wanderer A, Eisenstadt T, Wasserman S. Association of platelet activating factor with primary acquired cold urticaria. *N Engl J Med* 1985;313:405–409.

34. Christman BW, Lefferts PL, King GA, Snapper JR. Role of circulating platelets and granulocytes in platelet activating factor (PAF)-induced pulmonary dysfunction in awake sheep. *J Appl Physiol* 1988;64:2033–2041.

35. Zhou W, Chao W, Levine BA, Olsen MS. Evidence for platelet activating factor as a late phase mediator of chronic pancreatitis in the rat. *Am J Pathol* 1990;137:1501–1508.

36. Emanuelli G, Montrucchio G, Gaia E, Dughera L, Corvetti G, Gubetta L. Experimental acute pancreatitis induced by platelet activating factor in rabbits. *Am J Pathol* 1989;134:315–325.

37. Rosam A, Wallace J, Whittle B. Potent ulcerogenic actions of platelet activating factor on the stomach. *Nature* 1986;319:54–56.

38. Pettipher ER, Higgs GA, Henderson B. PAF-acether in chronic arthritis. *Agents Actions* 1987;21:98–103.

39. Barnes PJ, Chung KF. PAF closely mimics pathology of asthma. *Trends Pharmacol Sci* 1987;8:285–287.

40. Page CP, Morley J. Evidence favouring PAF rather than leukotrienes in the pathogenesis of asthma. *Pharmacol Res Commun* 1986;18:217–237.

41. Jackson C, Schumacher W, Kunkel S, Driscoll E, Lucchesi B. Platelet activating factor

and the release of a platelet-derived coronary artery vasodilator stustance in the canine. *Circ Res* 1986;58:218–229.

42. Robertson DA, Wang DY, Lee CO, Levi R. Negative inotropic effect of platelet activating factor: association with a decrease in intracellular sodium activity. *J Pharmacol Exp Ther* 1988;245:124–128.

43. Perico N, Delaini F, Tagliaferri M, Abbate M, Cucchi M, Bertani T, Remuzzi G. Effect of platelet activating factor and its specific receptor antagonist on glomerular permeability to proteins in isolated perfused rat kidney. *Lab Invest* 1988;58:163–171.

44. Satoh K, Imaizumi T, Kawamura Y, et al. Activity of platelet activating factor (PAF) acetylhydrolase in plasma from patients with cerebrovascular disease. *Prostaglandins* 1988;35:685.

45. Makowka L, Chapman F, Cramer D, Qian S, Sun H, Starzel TE. Platelet activating factor and hyperacute rejection. *Transplantation* 1990;50:359–365.

46. Makowka L, Miller C, Chapchap P, et al. Prolongation of pig-to-dog renal xenograft survival by modification of the infammatory mediator response. *Ann Surg* 1987; 206:482–495.

47. Halonen M, Palmer J, Lohman I, McManus L, Pinckard R. Respiratory and circulatory alterations induced by acetyl glyceryl ether phosphorylcholine, a mediator of IgE anaphylaxis in the rabbit. *Am Rev Respir Dis* 1980;122:915–924.

48. Handley DA. New developments for clinical applications for PAF antagonists. *J Clin Exp Med* 1987;143:415–418.

49. Handley DA. Development and therapeutic indications of PAF receptor antagonists. *Drugs Future* 1988;13:137–152.

50. Handley DA, Lee M, Saunders RN. Extravasation and aortic changes accompaning acute and subacute intraperitoneal administration of PAF. In: Benveniste J, Arnout B, eds. *Platelet activating factor*. Amsterdam: Elsivier, 1983;243–250.

51. Handley DA, Saunders RN. Platelet activating factor and inflammation in atherosclerosis: targets for drug development. *Drug Devel Res* 1986;7:361–375.

52. Inarrea P, Gomez-Cambronero J, Pascual J, del Carmen Ponte M, Hernando L, Sanchez-Crespo M. Synthesis of PAF acether and blood volume changes in Gram negative sepsis. *Immunopharmacology* 1985;9:45–52.

53. Saunders R, Handley DA. PAF and immunopathological responses. In: Handley D, Saunders R, Houlihan W, Tomesch J, eds. *Platelet activating factor in immune complex and endotoxin mediated diseases*. New York: Marcel Dekker, 1990;223–244.

54. Camussi G, Neilsen N, Tetta C, Saunders RN, Milgrom F. Release of platelet activating factor from rabbit heart perfused in vitro by sera with transplantation alloantibodies. *Transplantation* 1987;44:113–118.

55. Hellewell PG. The contribution of platelet activating factor to immune complex mediated inflammation. In: Handley D, Saunders R, Houlihan W, Tomesch J, eds. *Platelet activating factor in immune complex and endotoxin mediated diseases*. New York: Marcel Dekker, 1990;367–386.

56. Ito S, Camussi G, Tetta C, Milgrom F, Andres G. Hyperacute renal allograft rejection in the rabbit. *Lab Invest* 1984;51:148–161.

57. Chang SW, Feddersen CO, Henson PM. Voelkel NF. Platelet activating factor mediates hemodynamic changes and lung injury in endotoxin treated rats. *J Clin Invest* 1987;79:1498–1509.

58. Doebber T, Wu MS, Robbins JC, Choy BM, Chang MN, Shen TY. Platelet activating factor (PAF) involvement in endotoxin-induced hypotension in rats. Studies with PAF receptor dadsurenone. *Biochem Biophys Res Commun* 1985;127:799–808.

59. Whittle B, Boughton-Smith N, Hutcheson I, Esplugues JV, Wallace JL. Increased intestinal formation of Paf in endotoxin induced damage in the rat. *Br J Pharmacol* 1987;92:3–4.

60. Handley DA. Platelet activating factor as a mediator of endotoxin mediated diseases. In: Handley D, Saunders R, Houlihan W, Tomesch J, eds. *Platelet activating factor in immune complex and endotoxin mediated diseases*. New York: Marcel Dekker, 1990;451–495.

61. Nagaoka J, Harada K, Kimura A, et al. Inhibitory effects of the novel platelet activating factor receptor antagonist, E 5990, an 1-ethyl-2-[N-(2-methoxy) benzoyl-N-[(2R) 2-methoxy 3-(4-octadecylcarbamoyloxy) piperidinocarbonyl oxypropyloxy] carbonyl] aminomethyl pyridinium chloride. *Drug Res* 1991;41:719–724.

62. Lepran I, Lefer AM. Ischemia aggravating effects of platelet activating factor in acute myocardial ischemia. *Basic Res Cardiol* 1985;80:135–141.
63. Stahl GL, Terachita Z, Lefer AM. Role of platelet activating factor in propagation of cardiac damage during myocardial ischemia. *J Pharmacol Exp Ther* 1988;244:898–904.
64. Montrucchio G, Alloatti G, Mariano F, et al. Role of platelet activating factor in the reperfusion injury of rabbit ischemic heart. *Am J Pathol* 1990;137:71–81.
65. O'Byrne PM. Allergen-induced airway hyperresponsiveness. *J Allergy Clin Immunol* 1988;81:119–127.
66. Barnes PJ. Platelet activating factor and asthma. *J Allergy Clin Immunol* 1988;81:152–160.
67. Christman BW, Lefferts PL, Snapper JR. Effect of platelet activating factor on aerosol histamine responsiveness in awake sheep. *Am Rev Respir Dis* 1987;135:1267–1270.
68. Evans TW, Chung KF, Rogers DF, Barnes PJ. Effect of platelet activating factor on airway permeability: possible mechanisms. *J Appl Physiol* 1987;63:479–484.
69. Page CP. The role of platelet activating factor in allergic respiratory diseases. *Br J Clin Pharmacol* 1990;30:99S–106S.
70. Rogers DF, Alton EW, Aursudkij B, Boschetto P, Dewar A, Barnes PJ. Effect of platelet activating factor on formation and composition of airway fluid in the guinea-pig trachea. *J Physiol* 1990;431:643–658.
71. Colditz IG, Topper EK. The effect of systemic treatment with platelet activating factor on the migration of eosinophils to the lung, pleural and peritoneal cavities in the guinea pig. *Int Arch Allergy Appl Immunol* 1991;95:94–96.
72. Lewis AJ, Dervinis A, Chang J. The effects of antiallergic and bronchodilator drugs on platelet activating factor (PAF-acether) bronchospasm and platelet aggregation. *Agents Actions* 1984;15:636–642.
73. Anderson G, Fennessy M. Effects of REV 5901, a 5-lipoxygenase inhibitor and leukotriene antagonist, on pulmonary responses to platelet activating factor in the guinea pig. *Br J Pharmacol* 1988;94:1115–1122.
74. Anderson GP, White HL, Fennessy MR. Increased airways responsiveness to histamine induced by platelet activating factor in the guinea pig: possible role of lipoxygenase metabolites. *Agents Actions* 1988;24:1–7.
75. Morley J, Mazzoni L, Sanjar S, Schaueblin E. Pharmacology of airway hyperreactivity in animals. In: Holme G, Morley J, eds. *PAF and asthma.* New York: Academic Press, 1990;291–311.
76. Dixon EJA, Wilsoncroft P, Roberston DN, Page CP. The effect of Paf antagonists on bronchial hyperresponsiveness induced by Paf, propranolol or indomethacin. *Br J Pharmacol* 1989;97:717–722.
77. Criscuoli M, Subissi A, Daffonchio L, Omini C. LG 30435, a new bronchodilator/antiallergic agent, inhibits PAF-acether induced platelet aggregation and bronchoconstriction. *Agents Actions* 1986;19:246–250.
78. Coyle AJ, Spina D, Page CP. PAF-induced bronchial hyperresponsiveness in the rabbit: contribution of platelets and airway smooth muscle. *Br J Pharmacol* 1990;101:31–38.
79. Chung KF, Aizawa H, Leikauf GD, Ueki IF, Evans TW, Nadel JA. Airway hyperresponsiveness induced by platelet activating factor: role for thromboxane generation. *J Pharmacol Exp Ther* 1986;236:580–584.
80. Morley J. Platelet activating factor and asthma. *Agents Actions* 1986;19:100–108.
81. Townley RG, Hopp RJ, Agrawal DK, Bewtra AK. Platelet activating factor and airway reactivity. *J Allergy Clin Immunol* 1989;83:997–1010.
82. Page CP, Guerriero D, Sanjar S, Morley J. Platelet activating factor (Paf-acether) may account for late onset reactions to allergen inhalation. *Agents Actions* 1985;16:30–32.
83. Page CP, Tomiak RHH, Sanjar S, Morley J. Suppression of Paf-acether responses: an anti-inflammatory effect of anti-asthma drugs. *Agents Actions* 1985;16:33–35.
84. Page CP. The role of platelet activating factor in asthma. *J Allergy Clin Invest* 1988;81:144–151.
85. Saunders RN, Handley DA. Platelet activating factor antagonists. *Annu Rev Pharmacol Toxicol* 1987;27:237–255.
86. Chung KF, Barnes PJ. Effects of platelet activating factor on airway calibre, airway responsiveness, and circulating cells in asthmatic subjects. *Thorax* 1989;44:108–115.

87. Chung KF, Barnes PJ. PAF antagonists. Their potential therapeutic role in asthma. *Drugs* 1988;35:93–103.
88. Lai CKW, Jenkins JR, Polosa R, Holgate ST. Inhaled PAF fails to induce airway hyperresponsiveness to methacholine in normal subjects. *J Appl Physiol* 1990;68:919–926.
89. Adamus WS, Heuer H, Meade CJ. PAF-induced platelet aggregation ex vivo as a method for monitoring pharmacological activity in healthy volunteers. *Methods Find Exp Clin Pharmacol* 1989;11:415–420.
90. Adamus WS, Heuer HO, Meade CJ, Schilling JC. Inhibitory effects of the new PAF acether antagonist WEB 2886 on pharmacological changes induced by PAF inhalation in human beings. *Clin Pharmacol Ther* 1990;47:456–462.
91. Chung KF, Dent G, McCusker M, Guinot PH, Page CP, Barnes PJ. Effect of a ginkgolide mixture (BN 52063) in antagonising skin and platelet responses to platelet activating factor in man. *Lancet* 1987;1:248–251.
92. Hsieh KH. Effects of PAF antagonist, BN 52021, on PAF-, methacholine-, and allergen-induced bronchoconstriction in asthmatic children. *Chest* 1991;99:877–882.
93. Guinot P, Brambilla C, Duchier J, Braquet P, Bonvoisin B, Cournot A. Effect of BN 52063, a specific PAF-acether antagonist, on bronchial provocation test to allergens in asthmatic patients. A preliminary study. *Prostaglandins* 1987;34:723–731.
94. Roberts NM, Page CP, Chung KF, Barnes PJ. Effect of a PAF antagonist, BN 52063, on antigen-induced, acute, and late-onset cutaneous responses in atopic subjects. *J Allergy Clin Immunol* 1988;82:236–241.
95. Rabinovici R, Yue T, Farhat M, Smith EF, Esser KM, Slivjak M, Feuerstein G. Platelet activating factor (PAF) and tumor necrosis factor-α (TNFα) interactions in endotoxemic shock: studies with BN 50739, a novel PAF antagonist. *J Pharmacol Exp Ther* 1990;255:256–263.
96. Takatani M, Yoshioka Y, Tasaka A, Terashita ZI, Imura Y, Nishikawa K, Tsuhima S. Platelet activating factors antagonists: synthesis and structure activity studies of a novel PAF antagonist modified in the phosphorylcholine moiety. *J Med Chem* 1989;32:56–64.
97. Pretolani M, Lefort J, Malanchere E, Vargaftig BB. Interference by the novel PAF-acether antagonist WEB 2086 with the bronchopulmonary responses to PAF-acether and to active and passive anaphylactic shock in guinea pigs. *Eur J Pharmacol* 1987;140:311–321.
98. Casals-Stenzel J, Franke J, Friedrich T, Lichey J. Bronchial and vascular effects of Paf in the rat isolated lung are completely blocked by WEB 2086, a novel specific Paf antagonist. *Br J Pharmacol* 1987;91:799–802.
99. Casals-Stenzel J. Effects of WEB 2086, a novel antagonist to platelet activating factor in active and passive anaphylaxis. *Immunopharmacology* 1987;13:117–124.
100. Ukena D, Krogel C, Yukawa T, Sybrecht G, Barnes PJ. PAF-receptors on eosinophils: identification with a novel ligand, [³H] WEB 2086. *Biochem Pharmacol* 1989;38:1702–1705.
101. Houlihan WJ, Cheon SH, Handley DA, Larson DA. Synthesis and pharmacology of a novel class of long-lasting PAF antagonists. *J Lipid Mediators* 1991;3:91–99.
102. Sakuma Y, Muramoto K, Harada K, Katayama S, Tsunoda H, Katayama K. Inhibitory effects of a novel PAF antagonist E6123 on anaphylactic responses in passively and actively sensitized guinea pigs and passively sensitized mice. *Prostaglandins* 1991; 42:541–555.
103. Herbert JM, Lespy L, Maffrand JP. Protective effect of SR 27417, a novel PAF antagonist, on lethal anaphylactic and endotoxin-induced shock in mice. *Eur J Pharmacol* 1991;205:271–276.
104. Terashita Z, Kawamura M, Takatani M, Tsushima S, Imura Y, Nishikawa K. Beneficial effects of TCV-309, a novel potent and selective platelet activating factor antagonist in endotoxin and anaphylactic shock in rodents. *J Pharmacol Exp Ther* 1992;260:748–755.
105. Robaut C, Mondot S, Floch A, Tahraoue L, Cavero I. Pharmacological profile of a novel, potent and specific PAF receptor antagonist, the 59227 RP. *Prostaglandins* 1988;35:838.
106. Mondot S, Cavero I. Cardiovascular profile of 59227 RP, a novel potent and specific PAF receptor antagonist. *Prostaglandins* 1988;35:827.

107. Underwood SL, Lewis SA, Raeburn D. RP 59227, a novel PAF receptor antagonist: effects in guinea pig models of airway hyperreactivity. *Eur J Pharmacol* 1992;210:97–102.
108. Fernandez-Gallardo S, Ortega M, Priego J, et al. Pharmacological actions of PCA 4248, a new platelet activating factor receptor antagonist: In vivo studies. *J Pharmacol Exp Ther* 1990;255:34–39.
109. Kornecki E, Ehrlich Y, Lenox R. Platelet activating factor induced aggregation of human platelets specifically inhibited by triazolobenzodiazepines. *Science* 1984;226:1954–1957.
110. Terasawa M, Mikashima H, Tahara T, Maruyama Y. Antagonistic activity of etizolam on platelet activating factor in vivo experiments. *Jpn J Pharmacol* 1987;44:381–386.
111. Casals-Stenzel J, Weber KH. Triazolodiazepines: dissociation of their Paf (platelet activating factor) antagonistic and CNS activity. *Br J Pharmacol* 1987;90:139–146.
112. Casals-Stenzel J. Triazolodiazepines are potent antagonists of platelet activating factor (PAF) in vitro and in vivo. *Arch Pharmacol* 1987;335:351–355.
113. Cox CP. Effects of CV-3988, an antagonist of platelet activating factor (PAF), on washed rabbit platelets. *Thromb Res* 1986;41:211–222.
114. Stewart A, Dusting G. Characterization of receptor for platelet activating factor on platelets, polymorphonuclear leukocytes and macrophages. *Br J Pharmacol* 1988;94:1225–1233.
115. Heuer HO. Inhibition of active anaphylaxis in mice and guinea pigs by the new hetrazepinoic PAF antagonist bepafant (WEB 2170). *Eur J Pharmacol* 1991;199:157–163.
116. Heuer HO. WEB 2347: pharmacology of a new very potent and long acting hetrazepinic PAF antagonist and its action in repeatedly sensitized guinea pigs. *J Lipid Mediators* 1991;4:39–44.
117. Okamoto M, Yoshida K, Nishikawa N, et al. FR-900452, a specific antagonist of platelet activating factor (PAF) produced by *Streptomyces phaeofaciens*. *J Antibiot* 1986;39:198–204.
118. Okamoto M, Yoshida K, Nishikawa M, Kohsaka M, Aoki H. Platelet activating factor (PAF) involvement in endotoxin induced thrombocytopenia in rabbits: studies with FR-900452, a specific inhibitor of PAF. *Thromb Res* 1986;42:661–671.
119. Bitterman H, Lefer D, Lefer A. Beneficial actions of RO 15-1788, a benzodiazepine receptor antagonist, in hemorrhagic shock. *Methods Find Exp Clin Pharmacol* 1987;9:341–347.
120. Lagente V, Desquand S, Hadvary P, et al. Interference of Paf antagonist Ro 19-3704 with Paf and antigen-induced bronchoconstriction in the guinea pig. *Br J Pharmacol* 1988;94:27–36.
121. Grue-Sorensen G, Nielsen I, Neilsen C. Derivatives of 2-methylene propane 1,3-diol as a new class of antagonists of platelet activating factor. *J Med Chem* 1988;31:1174–1178.
122. Shen TY, Hwang S, Chang M, Doebber T, Lam M, Wu M, Wang X, Han G, Li R. Characterization of a platelet activating factor receptor antagonist isolated from haifenteng (Piper futokadsura): specific inhibition of in vitro and in vivo platelet activating factor induced effects. *Proc Natl Acad Sci USA* 1985;82:672–676.
123. Ponipom M, Bugianesi R, Brokker S, Yue B, Hwang S, Shen T. Structure activity relationships of kadsurenone analogues. *J Med Chem* 1987;30:136–142.
124. Hwang SB. Specific receptor sites for platelet activating factor on rat liver plasma membranes. *Arch Biochem Biophys* 1987;257:339–344.
124a. Smallbone B, Taylor NE, McDonald JW. Effects of L652,731, a platelet activating factor (PAF) receptor antagonist, on PAF- and complement induced pulmonary hypertension in sheep. *J Pharmacol Exp Ther* 1987;242:1035–1040.
125. Doebber T, Wu M. Platelet activating factor induced cellular and pathophysiological responses in the cardiovascular system. *Drug Devel Res* 1988;12:151–161.
126. Hwang S, Lam M, Biftu T, Beattie T, Shen T. Trans 2,5 bis-(3,4,5-trimethoxyphenyl) tetrahydrofuran. *J Biol Chem* 1985;260:15639–15645.
127. Hwang SB, Lam M, Alberts A, Bugianesi R, Chabala J, Ponpipom M. Biochemical and pharmacological characterization of L-659,989: an extremely potent, selective and competitive receptor antagonist to platelet activating factor. *J Pharmacol Exp Ther* 1988;246:534–541.

128. Miyamoto T, Ohno H, Yano T, Okada T, Hamanaka N, Kawasaki A. Ono-6240: a new potent antagonist of platelet activating factor. In: Hayaishi O, Yamamoto S, eds. *Adv Prostaglandin Thromboxane Leukotriene Res* 1985;15:719–720.

129. Marquis O, Robaut C, Cavero I. [³H] 52770 RP, a platelet activating factor receptor antagonist, and tritiated platelet activating factor label a common specific binding site in human polymorphonuclear leukocytes. *J Pharmacol Exp Ther* 1988;244:709–715.

130. Robaut C, Durand G, James C, Lave D, Sedivy P, Floch A, Mondot S, Pacot D, Cavero I, Le Fur G. PAF binding sites. Characterization by [³H] 52770, a pyrrolo [1,2c] thiazole derivative, in rabbit platelets. *Biochem Pharmacol* 1987;36:3221–3229.

131. Winslow C, Anderson R, D'Aries F, Frisch G, DeLillo A, Lee M, Saunders RN. Toward understanding the mechanism of action of platelet activating factor antagonists. In: Winslow CM, Lee ML, eds. *New horizons in platelet activating factor research.* New York: John Wiley, 1987;153–164.

132. Neuwrith R, Singhal P, Satriano J, Braquet P, Schlondorff D. Effect of platelet activating factor antagonists on cultured rat mesangial cells. *J Pharmacol Exp Ther* 1987;243:409–414.

133. Handley DA, Van Valen RG, Melden MK, Flury S, Lee ML, Saunders RN. Inhibition and reversal of endotoxin-, aggregated IgG- and PAF-induced hypotension in the rat by SRI 63-072, a PAF receptor antagonist. *Immunopharmacology* 1986;12:11–17.

134. Handley DA, Van Valen RG, Saunders RN. Vascular responses of platelet-activating factor in the cebus apella primate and inhibitory profiles of PAF antagonists SRI 63-072 and SRI 63-119. *Immunopharmacology* 1986;11:175–182.

135. Handley DA, Tomesch JC, Saunders RN. Inhibition of PAF induced responses in the rat, guinea pig, dog and primate by the receptor antagonist SRI 63-441. *Thromb Haemost* 1986;56:40–44.

136. Handley DA, Van Valen RG, Tomesch JC, Melden MK, Jaffe JA, Ballard F, Saunders RN. Biological properties of the receptor antagonist SRI 63-441 in the PAF and endotoxin models of hypotension in the rat and dog. *Immunopharmacology* 1987;13:125–132.

137. Robertson DA, Genovese A, Levi R. Negative inotropic effect of platelet activating factor on human myocardium: a pharmacological study. *J Pharmacol Exp Ther* 1987;243:834–839.

138. Handley DA, Van Valen RG, Winslow CM, Tomesch JC, Saunders RN. In vitro and in vivo pharmacological effects of the PAF receptor antagonist SRI 63-675. *Thromb Haemost* 1987;57:187–190.

139. Ma Y, Dunham E. Antagonism of the vasodilator effects of a platelet activating factor precursor in anesthetized spontaneously hypertensive rats. *Eur J Pharmacol* 1988;145:153–162.

140. Handley D. Preclinical and clinical pharmacology of platelet activating factor receptor antagonists. *Med Res Rev* 1990;10:351–370.

141. Olson NC. SRI 63-675: a platelet activating factor receptor antagonist. *Cardiovasc Drug Rev* 1992;10:54–70.

142. Handley DA, Van Valen RG, Melden MK, Houlihan WJ, Saunders RN. Biological effects of the orally active PAF receptor antagonist SDZ 64-412. *J Pharmacol Exp Ther* 1988;247:617–628.

143. Billah MM, Chapman RW, Egan RW, Gilchrest H, Piwinski J, Sherwood J, Siegel M, West RE, Kreutner W. Sch 37370: a potent, orally active, dual antagonist of platelet activating factor. *J Pharmacol Exp Ther* 1990;252:1090–1096.

144. Komuro Y, Imanishi N, Uchida M, Morooka S. Biological effect of orally active platelet activating factor receptor antagonist SM-10661. *Mol Pharmacol* 1991;38:378–384.

145. Terashita ZI, Tsushima S, Yoshioka Y, Nomura H, Inada Y, Nishikawa K. CV-3988-a specific antagonist of platelet activating factor (PAF). *Life Sci* 1983;32:1975–1982.

146. Terashita Z, Imura Y, Nishikawa K. Inhibition by CV-3988 of the binding of [³H]-platelet activating factor (PAF) to the platelet. *Biochem Pharmacol* 1985;34:1491–1499.

147. Hwang SB, Lam M. Species difference in the specific receptor of platelet activating factor. *Biochem Pharmacol* 1986;35:4511–4518.

148. Terashita Z, Imura Y, Takatani M, Tsushima S, Nishikawa K. CV-6209: a highly potent platelet activating factor antagonist in vitro and in vivo. *J Pharmacol Exp Ther* 1987;242:263–268.

149. Nunez D, Chignard M, Korth R, Le Couedic J, Norel X, Spinnewyn B, Braquet P, Benveniste J. Specific inhibition of PAF-acether induced platelet activation by BN 52021 and comparison with the PAF acether inhibitors kadsurenone and CV-3988. *Eur J Pharmacol* 1986;123:197–205.
150. Tomioka K, Garrido R, Ahmed A, Stevenson JS, Abraham WM. YM 461, PAF antagonist, blocks antigen-induced late airway responses and airway hyperresponsiveness in allergic sheep. *Eur J Pharmacol* 1989;170:209–215.
151. Patterson R, Harris KE. The activity of aerosolized and intracutaneous synthetic platelet activating factor (AGEPC) in rhesus monkeys with IgE mediated airway responses and normal monkeys. *J Lab Clin Med* 1983;102:933–938.
152. Vilain B, Lagente V, Touvay C, et al. Pharmacological control of the in vivo passive anaphylactic shock by the PAF-acether antagonist compound BN 52021. *Pharmacol Res Commun* 1986;18:119–125.
153. Handley DA, Lee ML, Saunders RN. Evidence for a direct effect on vascular permeability of platelet activating factor induced hemoconcentration in the guinea pig. *Thromb Haemost* 1985;54:756–759.
154. Vargaftig BB, Lefort J, Chicnard M, Benveniste J. Platelet activating factor induced platelet-dependent bronchoconstriction unrelated to the formation of prostaglandin derivatives. *Eur J Pharmacol* 1980;65:185–192.
155. Desquand S, Touvay C, Randon J, et al. Interference of BN 52021 (Ginkgolide B) with bronchopulmonary effects of PAF-acether in the guinea pig. *Eur J Pharmacol* 1986; 127:83–95.
156. Vargaftig BB, Lefort J, Rotilio D. Route-dependent interactions between PAF-acether and guinea pig bronchopulmonary smooth muscle: relevance of cyclooxygenase mechanisms. In: Benveniste J, Arnoux B, eds. *Platelet activating factor. INSERM Symposium.* Amsterdam; Elsevier, 1983;307–313.
157. Handley DA, Farley C, Deacon RW, Saunders RN. Evidence for distinct systemic extravasation effects of platelet activating factor, leukotrienes B_4, C_4, D_4 and histamine in the guinea pig. *Prostaglandins Leukotrienes Med* 1986;21:269–277.
158. Handley DA, Van Valen RG, Melden MK, Saunders RN. Evaluation of dose and route effects of platelet activating factor-induced extravasation in the guinea pig. *Thromb Haemost* 1984;52:34–36.
159. Misawa M, Takata T. Effects of platelet activating factor on rat airways. *Jpn J Pharmacol* 1988;48:7–13.
160. Underwood DC, Kadowitz PJ. Analysis of bronchoconstrictor responses to platelet activating factor in the cat. *J Appl Physiol* 1989;67:377–382.
161. Patterson R, Bernstein PR, Harris KE, Krell PD. Airway responses to sequential challenges with platelet activating factor and leukotriene D_4 in rhesus monkey. *J Lab Clin Med* 1984;104:340–345.
162. Patterson R, Harris KE, Lee ML, Houlihan WJ. Inhibition of rhesus monkey airway and cutaneous responses to platelet activating factor (PAF) (AGEPC) with the anti-PAF agent SRI 63-072. *Int Arch Allergy Appl Immunol* 1986;81:265–272.
163. Patterson R, Harris KE, Bernstein PR, Krell RD, Handley DA, Saunders RN. Effects of combined receptor antagonists of leukotriene D_4 (LTD_4) and platelet activating factor (PAF) on rhesus airway responses to LTD_4, PAF and antigen. *Int Arch Allergy Appl Immunol* 1989;88:462–470.
164. Denjean A, Arnoux B, Benveniste J, Lockhart A, Masse R. Bronchoconstriction induced by intratracheal administration of platelet activating factor (PAF-acether) in baboons. *Agents Actions* 1981;11:567–568.
165. Denjean A, Arnoux B, Masse R, Lockart A, Benveniste J. Acute effects of intratracheal administration of platelet activating factor in baboons. *J Appl Physiol* 1983; 55:799–804.
166. Inarrea P, Gomez-Cambronero J, Nieto M, Sanchez Crespo M. Characteristics of the binding of platelet activating factor to platelets to different animal species. *Eur J Pharmacol* 1984;105:309–315.
167. Namm DH, Tadepalli AS, High JA. Species specificity of the platelet response to 1-O-alkyl-2-acetyl sn glycero-3-phosphocholine. *Thromb Res* 1982;25:341–350.
168. Dahlback M, Bergstrand H, Sorenby L. Bronchial anaphylaxis in actively sensitized Spraque Dawley rats: studies of mediators involved. *Acta Pharmacol Toxicol* 1984; 55:6–17.

169. Danko G, Sherwood JE, Grissom B, Kreutner W, Chapman RW. Effect of the PAF antagonists, CV-3988 and L-652,731 on the pulmonary and hematological responses to guinea pig anaphylaxis. *Pharmacol Res Commun* 1988;20:785–798.
170. Lefort J, Sedivy P, Desquand S, Randon J, Coeffier E, Floch A, Benveniste J, Vargaftig BB. Pharmacological profile of 48740 R.P., a PAF acether antagonist. *Eur J Pharmacol* 1988;150:257–268.
171. Coeffier E, Borrel MC, Lefort J, et al. Effects of PAF-acether and structural analogues on platelet activating factor activation and bronchoconstriction in guinea pigs. *Eur J Pharmacol* 1986;131:179–188.
172. Handley DA, Anderson RC, Saunders RN. Inhibition by SRI 63-072 and SRI 63-119 of PAF acether and immune complex effects in the guinea pig. *Eur J Pharmacol* 1987;141:409–416.
173. Casals-Stenzel J, Muacevic G, Weber KH. Pharmacological actions of WEB 2086, a new specific antagonist of platelet activating factor. *J Pharmacol Exp Ther* 1987; 241:974–981.
174. Lohman IC, Halonen M. Effects of the PAF antagonist WEB 2086 on PAF-induced physiological alterations and on IgE anaphylaxis in the rabbit. *Am Rev Respir Dis* 1990;142:390–397.
175. Guinot Ph, Braquet P, Duchier J, Cournot A. Effects of BN 52066 on PAF-acether induced weal and flare in man. *Agents Actions* 1987;21:229–234.
176. Desquand S, Lefort J, Dumarey C, Vargaftig BB. The booster injection of antigen during active sensitization of guinea pig modifies the anti-anapylactic activity of the PAF antagonist WEB 2086. *Br J Pharmacol* 1990;100:217–222.
177. Havill AM, Van Valen RG, Handley DA. Prevention of non-specific airway hyperreactivity after allergen challenge in guinea pigs by the PAF receptor antagonist SDZ 64-412. *Br J Pharmacol* 1990;99:396–400.
178. Senzel H, Hummer B, Hahn H. Effect of the PAF antagonist SRi 63-441 on the allergic response in wake dogs with natural asthma. *Agents Actions* 1987;21:253–260.
179. Patterson R, Harris KE, Handley DA, Saunders RN. Evaluation of the effect of a platelet activating factor (PAF) receptor antagonist on platelet activating factor and ascaris antigen-induced airway responses in rhesus monkeys. *J Lab Clin Med* 1987;110:606–611.
180. O'Donnell SR, Erjefalt I, Persson GA. Early and late tracheobronchial plasma exudation by platelet activating factor administered to the airway mucosal surface in guinea pigs: effects of WEB 2086 and enprofylline. *J Pharmacol Exp Ther* 1990;254: 65–70.
181. Lellouch-Tubiana A, Lefort J, Simon MT, Pfister A, Vargaftig BB. Eosinophil recruitment into guinea pig lungs after PAF-acether and allergen administration. *Am Rev Respir Dis* 1988;137:948–954.
182. Evans T, Dent G, Rogers D, Aursudkij B, Chung KF, Barnes P. Effect of a Paf antagonist, WEB 2086, on airway microvascular leakage in the guinea pig and platelet aggregation in man. *Br J Pharmacol* 1988;94:164–168.
183. Wilkens JH, Wilkens H, Uffmann J, Bovers J, Fabel H, Frolich JC. Effects of the PAF antagonist (BN 52063) on bronchoconstriction and platelet activation during exercise induced asthma. *Br J Clin Pharmacol* 1990;29:85–91.
184. Handley DA, Lee M, Farley C, Deacon R, Melden M, Van Valen RG, Winslow CM, Saunders R. Biological characterization of cyclimmonium PAF antagonists. In: Handley DA, Houlihan W, Saunders R, Tomesch J, eds. *Platelet activating factor in endotoxin and immune complex mediated diseases*. New York: Marcel Dekker, 1990;157–175.
185. Alving K, Matran R, Lundberg JM. Effect of nedocromil sodium on allergen-, PAF-, histamine- and bradykinin-induced airways vasodilation and pulmonary obstruction in the pig. *Br J Pharmacol* 1991;104:452–458.
186. Frigas E, Gleich GJ. The eosinophil and the pathophysiology of asthma. *J Allergy Clin Immunol* 1986;77:527–537.
187. Horn BR, Robin ED, Theodore J, Van Kessel A. Total eosinophil counts in the management of bronchial asthma. *N Engl J Med* 1975;292:1152–1155.
188. Durham SR, Kay AB. Eosinophils, bronchial hyperreactivity and late phase asthmatic reactions. *Clin Allergy* 1985;15:411–418.
189. Brusasco V, Crimi E, Gianiorio P, Lantero S, Rossi GA. Allergen-induced increase in

airway responsiveness and inflammation in mild asthma. *J Appl Physiol* 1990;69:2209–2214.

190. Wardlaw A. Eosinophils and mast cells in bronchoalveolar lavage in subjects with mild asthma. Relationship to bronchial hyperreactivity. *Am Rev Respir Dis* 1988;137:62–73.

191. Cromwell O, Wardlaw AJ, Champion A, Moqbel R, Osei D, Kay AB. IgG-dependent generation of platelet activating factor by normal and low density human eosinophils. *J Immunol* 1990;145:3862–3868.

192. Wardlaw AJ, Moqbel R, Cromwell O, Kay AB. Platelet activating factor. A potent chemotactic and chemokinetic factor for human eosinophils. *J Clin Invest* 1986; 78:1701–1706.

193. Tamura N, Agrawal DK, Suliaman FQ, Townley RG. Effects of platelet activating factor on the chemotaxis of normodense eosinophils from normal subjects. *Biochem Biophys Res Commun* 1987;142:638–644.

194. Sigal CE, Valone FH, Holtzman MJ, Goetzl EJ. Preferential human eosinophil chemotactic activity of platelet activating factor (PAF) 1-O-hexadecyl 2-acetyl sn-glyceryl-3-phosphocholine (AGEPC). *J Clin Immunol* 1987;7:179–184.

195. Kroegel C, Yakawa T, Westwick J, Barnes PJ. Evidence for two distinct platelet activating factor receptors on eosinophils: dissociation between PAF-induced intracellular calcium mobilization and superoxides anion generation in eosinophils. *Biochem Biophys Res Commun* 1989;162:511–521.

196. Arnoux A, Denjean A, Page CP, Nolibe D, Morley J, Benveniste J. Accumulation of platelets and eosinophils in baboon lung after Paf-acether challenge. *Am Rev Respir Dis* 1988;137:855–860.

197. Sanjar S, Aoki S, Kristersson A, Smith D, Morley J. Antigen challenge induces pulmonary eosinophil accumulation and airway hyperreactivity in sensitized guinea pigs: the effect of anti-asthma drugs. *Br J Pharmacol* 1990;99:679–686.

198. Dunn CJ, Elliot GA, Oostveen JA, Richards IM. Development of a prolonged eosinophil-rich inflammatory leukocyte infiltration in the guinea pig asthmatic response to ovalalbumin inhalation. *Am Rev Respir Dis* 1988;137:541–547.

199. Hakansson L, Venge P. Inhibition of neutrophil and eosinophil chemotactic responses to PAF by the PAF antagonists WEB 2086, L-652-731, and SRI 63-441. *J Leukoc Biol* 1990;47:449–456.

200. Sanjar S, Aoki S, Boubekeur K, Chapman I, Smith D, Kings M, Morley J. Eosinophil accumulation in pulmonary airways of guinea pigs induced by exposure to an aerosol of platelet activating factor: effect of anti-asthma drugs. *Br J Pharmacol* 1990;99:267–272.

201. Coyle AJ, Urwin S, Page CP, Touvay C, Villian B, Braquet P. The effect of the selective PAF antagonist BN 52021 on PAF- and antigen-induced bronchial hyperreactivity and eosinophil accumulation. *Eur J Pharmacol* 1988;148:51–58.

202. Ishida K, Thompson R, Beattie LL, Wiggs B, Schellenberg RR. Inhibition of antigen-induced airway hyperresponsiveness, but not acute hypoxia nor airway eosinophilia, by an antagonist of platelet-activating factor. *J Immunol* 1990;144:3907–3911.

203. Larson GL, Wilson MC, Clark RAF, Behrens BL. The inflammatory reaction in the airways in an animals model of the late asthmatic response. *Fed Proc* 1987;46:105–112.

204. Eidelman DH, Bellofiore S, Martin JG. Late airway responses to antigen challenge in sensitized inbred rats. *Am Rev Respir Dis* 1988;137:1033–1037.

205. Hamel R, McFarlane CS, Ford-Hutchinson AW. Late pulmonary responses induced by Ascaris allergen in conscious squirrel monkeys. *J Appl Physiol* 1986;61:2081–2087.

206. Abraham M, Delehunt JC, Yerger L, Marchette B. Characterization of a late phase pulmonary response after antigen challenge in allergic sheep. *Am Rev Respir Dis* 1983;128:839–844.

207. Murphy KR, Wilson MC, Irvin CG, et al. The requirement for polymorphonuclear leukocytes in the late asthmatic response and heightened airways reactivity in an animal model. *Am Rev Respir Dis* 1986;134:62–68.

208. Iijima H, Ishii M, Yamauchi K, et al. Bronchoalevolar lavage and histologic characterization of late asthmatic response in guinea pigs. *Am Rev Respir Dis* 1987;136:922–929.

209. Hutson PA, Church MK, Clay TP, Miller P, Holgate ST. Early and late-phase bronchoconstriction after allergen challenge of nonanesthetized guinea pigs. *Am Rev Respir Dis* 1988;137:548–557.

210. Church MK, Hutson PA, Holgate ST. Effect of nedocromil sodium on early and late phase responses to allergen challenge in the guinea pig. *Drugs* 1989;37:101–108.
211. Hutson PA, Holgate ST, Church MK. Inhibition by nedocromil sodium of early and late phase bronchoconstriction and airway cellular infiltration provoked by ovalalbumin inhalation in conscious sensitized guinea pigs. *Br J Pharmacol* 1988;94:6–8.
212. Nakamura T, Morita Y, Kuriyama M, Ishihara K, Ito K, Miyamoto T. Platelet activating factor in late asthmatic response. *Int Arch Allergy Appl Immunol* 1987;82:57–61.
213. Wegner CD, Clarke CC, Torcellini CA, Letts LG, Gundel RH. Effects of single and multiple inhalations of platelet activating factor on airway cell compositions and responsiveness in monkeys. *Clin Exp Allergy* 1992;22:51–57.
214. Anderson GP, Fennessy MR. Lipozygenase metabolites mediate increased airway responsiveness to histamine after acute platelet activating factor exposure in the guinea pig. *Agents Actions* 1988;24:8–19.
215. Lagente V, Touvay C, Randon J, et al. Inference of PAF-acether antagonist BN 52021 with passive anaphylaxis in the guinea pig. *Prostaglandins* 1987;33:265–274.
216. Ishida K, Kelly L, Thompson R, Beattie L, Schellenberg RR. Repeated antigen challenge induces airway hyperresponsiveness with eosinophilia in guinea pigs. *J Appl Physiol* 1989;67:1133–1139.
217. Shindoh J, Sugiyama S, Takagi K, Satake T, Ozawa T. Recovery time course of airway hyperresponsiveness to acetylcholine after ovalbumin challenge in guinea pigs. *Chest* 1991;99:1274–1279.
218. Schellenberg RR, Ishida K, Thompson RJ. Nedcromil sodium inhibits airway hyperresponsiveness and eosinophilic infiltration induced by repeated antigen challenge in guinea pigs. *Br J Pharmacol* 1991;103:1842–1846.
219. Becker AB, Hershkovich J, Simons E, Simons K, Lilley M, Depron M. Development of chronic airway hyperresponsiveness in ragweed-sensitized dogs. *J Appl Physiol* 1989;66:2691–2697.
220. Alving K, Matran R, Fornhem C, Lundberg JM. Late phase bronchial and vascular responses to allergen in actively sensitized guinea pigs. *Acta Physiol Scand* 1991;143:137–138.
221. Coyle AJ, Page CP, Atkinson L, Sjoerdsma K, Touvay C, Metzger WJ. Modification of allergen-induced airway obstruction and airway hyperresponsiveness in an rabbit allergic model by the selective platelet-activating factor antagonist, BN 52021. *J Allergy Clin Immunol* 1989;84:960–967.
222. Chung KF, Aizawa H, Becker AB, Frick O, Gold WM, Nadel JA. Inhibition of antigen-induced airway hyperresponsiveness by a thromboxane synthetase inhibitor (OKY-046) in allergic dogs. *Am Rev Respir Dis* 1986;134:258–261.
223. Handley DA, DeLeo J, Havill AM. Induction by aerosol allergen of sustained and nonspecific IgE-mediated airway hyperreactivity in the guinea pig. *Agents Actions* 1992;37:201–203.
224. Solèr M, Sielczak MW, Abraham WM. A PAF antagonist blocks antigen-induced airway hyperresponsiveness and inflammation in sheep. *J Appl Physiol* 1989;67:406–413.
225. Knauer KA, Lichtenstein LM, Adkinson N Jr, Fish JE. Platelet activation during antigen-induced airway reactions in asthmatic subjects. *N Engl J Med* 1981;304:1404–1407.
226. Metzger WJ, Hunninghake GW, Richerson HB. Late asthmatic responses: inquiry into mechanisms and significance. *Clin Rev Allergy* 1985;3:45–165.
227. Grandel KE, Wardlow ML, Fare RS. Platelet activating factor in sputum of patients with asthma and COPD. *Fed Proc* 1985;44:184.
228. Horii T, Okazaki H, Kino M, Kobayashi Y, Satouchi K, Saito K. Platelet-activating factor detected in bronchoalveolar lavage fluid from an asthmatic. *Lipids* 1991;26:1292–1296.
229. Chan-Yeung M, Lam S, Chan H, Tsem KS, Salari H. The release of platelet-activating factor into plasma during allergen-induced bronchoconstriction. *J Allergy Clin Immunol* 1991;87:667–673.
230. Averill FJ, Hubbard WC, Liu MC. Detection of platelet activating factor (PAF) and lyso-PAF in bronchoalveolar lavage fluids from allergic subjects following antigen challenge. *Am Rev Respir Dis* 1991;143:A811.

231. Cuss FM, Dixon CMS, Barnes PJ. Effects of inhaled platelet activating factor on pulmonary function and bronchial responsiveness in man. *Lancet* 1986;2:189–192.
232. Rubin A-HE, Smith LJ, Patterson R. The bronchoconstrictor properties of platelet activating factor in humans. *Am Rev Respir Dis* 1987;136:1145–1151.
233. Roberts NM, McCusker M, Chung KF, Barnes PJ. Effects of PAF antagonist, BN52063, on PAF-induced bronchoconstriction in normal subjects. *Br J Clin Pharmacol* 1988;26:65–72.
234. Wardlaw AJ, Chung KF, Moqbel R, MacDonald AJ, et al. Effects of inhaled PAF in humans on circulating and bronchoalveolar lavage fluid neutrophils: relationship to bronchoconstriction and changes in airway responsiveness. *Am Rev Respir Dis* 1990;141:386–392.
235. Spencer DA, Evans JM, Green SE, Piper PJ, Costello JF. Participation of the cysteinyl leukotrienes in the acute bronchoconstrictor response to inhaled platelet activating factor in man. *Thorax* 1991;46:441–445.
236. Smith LJ, Rubin AE, Patterson R. Mechanism of platelet-activating factor-induced bronchoconstriction in humans. *Am Rev Respir Dis* 1988;137:1015–1019.
237. Miwa M, Miyake T, Yamanaka T, et al. Characterization of platelet-activating factor (PAF) acetylhydrolase: correlation between deficiency of serum PAF acetylhydrolase and respiratory symptoms in asthmatic children. *J Clin Invest* 1988;82:1983–1991.
238. Hamasaki Y, Mojarad M, Saga T, Tai H-H, Said S. Platelet-activating factor raises airway and vascular pressures and induces edema in lungs perfused with platelet-free solution. *Am Rev Respir Dis* 1984;129:742–746.
239. Camussi G, Montrucchio G, Antro C, Tetta C, Bussolino F, Emanuelli G. *In vitro* spasmogenic effect on rabbit lung tissue of 1-0-octadecyl-2-acetyl-sn-glyceryl-3-phosphorylcholine (platelet-activating factor): specific desensitization after *in vivo* infusion. *Agents Actions* 1983;3:507–509.
240. Chung KF, Minette P, McCusker M, Barnes PJ. Ketotifen inhibits the cutaneous but not the airway responses to platelet-activating factor in man. *J Allergy Clin Immunol* 1989;81:1192–1198.
241. Hopp RJ, Bewtra AK, Nabe M, Agrawal DK, Townley RG. Effects of PAF-acether inhalation on nonspecific bronchial reactivity and adrenergic response in normal and asthmatic subjects. *Chest* 1990;98:936–941.
242. Hopp RJ, Bewtra AK, Agrawal DK, Townley RG. Effects of platelet activating factor inhalation on non-specific bronchial reactivity in man. *Chest* 1989;96:1070–1072.
243. Klopproge E, de Leeuw AJ, DeMonchy JGR, Kauffman HE. Hypodense eosinophilic granulocytes in normal individuals and patients with asthma: generation of hypodense cell populations in vitro. *J Allergy Clin Immunol* 1989;393–400.
244. Ukena G, Dent C, Chanez P, Barnes PJ, Sybrecht GW. Characterization of platelet activating factor (PAF)-receptors in neutrophilic and eosinophilic granulocytes. *Pneumologie* 1990;44:531–532.
245. Yukawa T, Kroegel C, Evans P, Fukuda T, Chung KF, Barnes PJ. Density heterogeneity of eosinophil leukocytes: induction of hypodense eosinophils by platelet-activating factor. *Immunology* 1989;68:140–143.
246. Capron M, Benveniste J, Braquet P, Capron A. Role of PAF-acether in IgE dependent activation of eosinophils. In: Braquet P, ed. *New trends in lipid mediator research. The role of PAF in immune disorders*, vol 2. Basel: Karger, 1989;10–17.
247. Zoratti EM, Sedgwick JB, Vrtis RR, Busse WW. The effects of platelet-activating factor on the generation of superoxide anion in human eosinophils and neutrophils. *J Allergy Clin Immunol* 1991;88:749–758.
248. Kroegel C, Yukawa T, Dent S, Chanez P, Chung KF, Barnes PJ. Platelet activating factor induces eosinophil peroxidase release from purified human eosinophils. *Immunology* 1988;64:559–562.
249. Ayars GH, Altman LC, Gleich GJ, Loegering DA, Baker CB. Eosinophil and eosinophil-granule mediated pneumocyte injury. *J Allergy Clin Immunol* 1985;76:595–604.
250. Cerasoli F Jr, Gilfillan A, Selig WM. Eosinophils, mast cells, and basophils: cellular mechanisms contributing to lung microvascular injury. In: Johnson A, Ferro TJ, eds. *Lung vascular injury: molecular and cellular responses*. New York: Marcel Dekker, 1992;263–307.

251. Cerasoli F Jr, Tocker J, Selig WM. Airway eosinophils from actively sensitized guinea pigs exhibit enhanced superoxide anion release in response to antigen challenge. *Am J Resp Cell Mol Biol* 1991;4:355–363.

252. Selig WM, Tocker J, Cerasoli F Jr. Eosinophil exacerbate antigen-induced edema formation in the perfused guinea pig lung. *FASEB J* 1991;5:A1243.

253. Kay AB. Asthma and inflammation. *J Allergy Clin Immunol* 1991;87:893–910.

254. Chung KF, Barnes PJ. Role for platelet-activating factor in asthma. *Lipids* 1991; 26:1277–1279.

255. Henocq E, Vargafig BB. Skin eosinophilia in atopic patients. *J Allergy Clin Immunol* 1988;81:691–696.

256. Block LH, Imhof E, Emmons LR, Roth M, Perruchoud AP. PAF-dependent phosphatidyl inositol turnover in platelets: differences between asthmatics and normal individuals. *Respiration* 1990;57:372–378.

257. Tam FWK, Clague J, Dixon CMS, Stuttle AWJ, et al. Inhaled platelet-activating factor causes pulmonary neutrophil sequestration in normal humans. *Am Rev Respir Dis* 1992;146:1003–1008.

258. Schauer U, Leinhaas C, Jager R, Rieger CH. Enhanced superoxide generation by eosinophils from asthmatic children. *Int Arch Allergy Appl Immunol* 1991;96:317–321.

259. Guinot P, Braquet P, Duchier J, Cournot A. Inhibition of PAF-acether induced wheal and flare reaction in man by a specific PAF antagonist. *Prostaglandins* 1986;32:160–163.

260. Markey AC, Barker JNWN, Archer CB, Guinot P, Lee TK, McDonald DM. Platelet activating factor-induced clinical and histopathologic responses in atopic skin and their modification by platelet activating factor antagonist BN52063. *J Am Acad Dermatol* 1990;23:263–268.

261. Hayes JP, Ridge SM, Griffith S, Barnes PJ, Chung KF. Inhibition of cutaneous and platelet responses to platelet-activating factor by oral WEB 2086 in man. *J Allergy Clin Immunol* 1991;88:83–88.

262. O'Conner BJ, Ridge SM, Chen-Worsdell YM, Uden S, Chung KF. Complete inhibition of airway and neutrophil responses to inhaled platelet activating factor (PAF) by an oral PAF antagonist, UK 74505. *Am Rev Respir Dis* 1991;143:A156.

263. Freitag A, Watson RM, Mastos G, Eastwood C, O'Byrne PM. The effects of treatment with an oral platelet activating factor antagonist (WEB 2086) on allergen induced asthmatic responses in human subjects. *Am Rev Respir Dis* 1991;143:A157.

264. Wilkens H, Wilkens JH, Bosse S, et al. Effects of an inhaled PAF-antagonist (WEB 2086 BS) on allergen-induced early and late asthmatic responses and increased bronchial responsiveness to methacholine. *Am Rev Respir Dis* 1991;143:A812.

265. Bel EH, De Smet M, Rossing TH, Timmers MC, Dijkman JH, Sterk PJ. The effect of a specific oral PAF antagonist, MK-287, on antigen-induced early and late asthmatic reactions in man. *Am Rev Respir Dis* 1991;143:A811.

Drugs and the Lung,
edited by C.P. Page and W.J. Metzger.
Raven Press, Ltd., New York © 1994

14

Tachykinin Receptor Antagonists

Carlo Alberto Maggi and *Stefano Manzini

Department of Pharmacology, Menarini Pharmaceuticals, 50131 Florence, Italy
*Department of Pharmacology, Menarini Ricerche
Sud, 00040 Pomezia, Rome, Italy

The term *neurogenic inflammation* labels a series of inflammatory events that follows the activation of a discrete subset of primary afferent neurons characterized by (a) polymodal nociceptive modalities of excitation, (b) a dual sensory and efferent function, and (c) a peculiar and unique sensitivity to the excitatory and desensitizing actions of capsaicin (1–3). A local release of sensory neuropeptides from the peripheral endings (the excited terminal or other endings activated through axon reflexes) of these capsaicin-sensitive primary afferent neurons is mandatory for the genesis of this type of neurogenic inflammatory response. Among sensory neuropeptides, tachykinins (TKs), stored in and released from capsaicin-sensitive nerves, play a central role in neurogenic inflammation (4). In view of the powerful motor and inflammatory actions of peptides of this family (see below), their potential role as mediators of a variety of inflammatory diseases has been put forward.

In the last few years increasing experimental evidence has suggested that neurogenic inflammation could play a role in asthma (5,6). A major support of this hypothesis is given by experimental data concerning the distribution, release, and biological actions of TKs in the airways of several animal species and humans. This chapter reviews the most recent advancements in this field, with special reference to human tissues. The basis for the rational design of specific TKs receptor antagonists, hopefully useful in the therapy of respiratory diseases, is also discussed.

OCCURRENCE AND DISTRIBUTION OF
TACHYKININ-CONTAINING NERVES

In mammals two genes encode for the TK family of peptides. The preprotachykinin I gene encodes the sequence of substance P and neurokinin A, while the preprotachykinin II gene encodes the sequence for neurokinin B

(7–10). TK-containing capsaicin-sensitive sensory nerves have been shown to exist in the upper and lower respiratory tract of various animal species (11,12). The presence of substance P immunoreactive nerve fibers has been confirmed in the human lung with a distribution within and beneath the epithelium, near submucosal glands, adjacent to some ganglionic structures, around blood vessels and, to a lesser extent, in proximity of smooth muscle layers (13–17). A co-storage of substance P and neurokinin A, but not neurokinin B, in nerve fibers has been demonstrated in human lower airways (15). Autoradiographic studies have evidenced that TK-containing nerve fibers are accompanied by the expression of TK receptors in various airway tissues from guinea pigs (18) and humans (19).

A substantial increase in the number and length of substance P immunoreactive nerves has been found in bronchial specimens obtained from asthmatic subjects as compared to controls or to patients with nonasthmatic chronic airflow obstruction (20). Likewise an increase in NK-1 binding sites (the preferential receptor for substance P) in bronchial samples obtained from asthmatic subjects has also been shown (21).

RELEASE OF TACHYKININS

Exposure of perfused lung or bronchial rings to capsaicin produces a calcium-dependent release of TKs (22,23), and the magnitude of this effect was greater at a bronchial than at a tracheal level, suggesting regional differences in nerve density (and/or amount of releasable TKs) (24). Capsaicin-induced TK release underwent desensitization (24), thus confirming the specificity of its action.

A capsaicin-sensitive release of sensory neuropeptides could be evoked also by exposing airway tissues to a number of endogenously released and generated inflammatory substances such as bradykinin, histamine, nicotinic agonist (22,25), platelet-activating factor (PAF) (26,27), and some lipoxygenase metabolites (27–29). Saria et al. (22) found a sizeable release of TKs also after antidromic vagal nerve stimulation. TK recovery in the perfusing medium following capsaicin challenge is enhanced by inhibitors of neutral endopeptidases (23,30), but not by angiotensin-converting enzyme (ACE) inhibitors (30).

Up to now, no clear evidence for a capsaicin-induced release of TKs from human bronchial specimens has been reported.

BIOLOGICAL EFFECTS OF TACHYKININS

Bronchomotor Actions

TKs are among the most potent and effective endogenous bronchoconstrictor substances, both *in vitro* and *in vivo* (31,32). This has been confirmed in human lung with neurokinin A being about two orders of magnitude more potent than substance P (33–35). Recently neuropeptide K, an elongated form of neurokinin A, has been demonstrated to act as the most potent contractile TK in isolated human bronchi (36). However, a release of neuropeptide K from capsaicin-sensitive nerves has never been demonstrated in the peripheral nervous system. Both inhaled and infused substance P generates bronchoconstriction in human volunteers (37,38). Joos et al. (39) demonstrated a marked leftward shift in bronchoconstrictor dose-response curves upon neurokinin A inhalation in asthmatic as compared to healthy subjects.

In certain species, TKs induce bronchodilatation by stimulating receptors localized on epithelial structures, and a consequent stimulation of epithelium-derived relaxing factor(s) (probably prostanoids) release (40,41). For example, in the mouse bronchus, where no contractile response could be evoked by TKs or capsaicin, a clear indomethacin-sensitive relaxation of precontracted bronchi could be induced by NK-1 receptor agonists, capsaicin, or nerve stimulation (42). Therefore a lack or a reduction of TK-induced bronchodilatation following the characteristic epithelial damage of asthmatic airways (43) could explain the exaggerated bronchoconstrictor responses of asthmatic patients to TK administration.

Effect on Vascular Permeability

Functional and electron microscopic studies indicate the ability of TKs and capsaicin to increase vascular permeability in rat and guinea pig airways, probably by the opening of endothelial gaps at postcapillary venules level (44–46). So far, no evidence for a similar inflammatory effect of TKs in human lung has been obtained, although it is well known that substance P remarkably increases microvascular leakage in human skin (47,48). Recently, several groups have demonstrated that a selective, nonpeptide antagonist of the NK-1 receptor (CP 96,345) blunted the neurogenic-, substance P–, or cigarette smoke–induced increase in plasma exudation and edema in guinea pig airways (49–51).

TKs have pronounced effects also on vascular blood flow in the pulmonary circulation. Substance P, most likely through generation of nitric oxide (52,53), causes a marked increase in pulmonary blood flow (54–56). However, at least in the guinea pig pulmonary artery, evidence has been obtained that following antidromical nerve stimulation of capsaicin-sensitive nerves, calcitonin gene-related peptide more than substance P could be involved in the nonadrenergic-noncholinergic (NANC) vasodilation (57). Substance P–induced vasodilation can produce synergistic effects, with enhanced vascular permeability to further increase the plasma protein extravasation and the consequent production of edema (58).

Effect on Inflammatory Cells

TKs, at least *in vitro,* can modulate the function of several inflammatory cells, although the pathophysiological relevance of such actions is unclear. In fact, some of these actions (e.g., mast cell and eosinophil degranulation) are evident only at rather high TK concentrations and are probably unrelated to stimulation of specific TK receptors since they are mimicked by TK analogues lacking the C-terminal portion, a motif essential for binding to specific TK receptors (59–61). However, some examples of receptorial TK effect on inflammatory cells with potential relevance for lung pathophysiology have been obtained. Alveolar macrophages are particularly stimulated by low concentrations of TKs (especially selective agonists of the NK-2 receptor) (62) and this response seems to be amplified in antigen-sensitized and -boosted guinea pigs (63). Of relevance is the recent anatomical evidence suggesting a close proximity of sensory nerves and alveolar macrophages (64).

There is evidence for and against a TK receptor–mediated stimulating effect of TKs on human neutrophil functions (65–67). A priming effect more than a direct stimulating action could also be involved (68–70). A stimulation of neutrophil chemotaxis has been shown, and this action is due to the C-terminal portion of the TK sequence (71). McDonald (72) found a massive recruitment of neutrophils in rat trachea during neurogenic inflammation. The expression of an endothelial leukocyte adhesion molecule (ELAM-1) by microvascular endothelium following substance P exposure (73) could be of relevance in such migration.

The most recent theory of asthma pathophysiology assumes a key role for T lymphocytes in the inflammatory response (74). An important role of TKs as modulators of proliferative and physiological responses of lymphocytes was proposed as early as 1983 by Payan et al. (75) and later confirmed by other groups (76–78). Further evidence indicates a stimulation by TKs also of the immunoglobulin synthesis and secretion by human B lymphocytes (79,80). Whether or not TKs act on specific lymphocyte cell populations of relevance for the induction, maintenance, and severity of the allergic response in the lung of asthmatic subjects is, however, still a matter requiring further research.

Further studies related to the ability of TKs to stimulate the expression, synthesis, and/or secretion of key inflammatory factors by pulmonary tissues and/or cells, such as cytokines and adhesion molecules, will probably yield important discoveries in the next few years.

Effect on Secretion

Substance P is a potent stimulant of myoepithelial cells of the submucosal gland (81). This could be the major mechanism through which substance P increases mucus secretion, as demonstrated in several animal species (82). By using selective agonist and antagonists, the involvement of NK-1 receptors in TK-induced airway mucus secretion has been further defined (83–85).

Substance P and NANC vagal nerve stimulation excite the secretory function of goblet cells as well and it is interesting to note that the vapor phase of the smoke elicits a largely capsaicin-sensitive goblet cell discharge (86).

Rogers et al. (87) have confirmed the potent secretagogue properties of substance P in human bronchi. This response is amplified by neutral endopeptidases blockade and mimicked by capsaicin (88). A stimulation by TKs of mucous and serous cell secretion has been shown also in human nasal mucosa *in vitro* (89).

Effect of TK Depletion on Antigen-Induced Bronchial Anaphylaxis

If TKs are relevant for the pathogenesis of asthma, their depletion should exert a protective effect in experimental models mimicking asthmatic response to antigen challenge. Indeed, contradictory results have appeared in the literature, with evidence for (90,91) and against (92–94) this hypothesis. An important experimental difference between these studies was the treatment sequence of antigen sensitization and chronic capsaicin treatment for TK depletion. Protection was observed when capsaicin treatment was carried out after the antigen sensitization. Recent findings indicate that blockade of TK metabolism by neutral endopeptidase inhibitors produces a significant enhancement of the bronchomotor response to antigen challenge (95) and that capsaicin pretreatment antagonized the increase in bronchial hyperreactivity elicited by repeated antigen aerosol challenges in guinea pigs (96).

METABOLISM OF TACHYKININS

The capsaicin-sensitive sensory nerves are not able to reuptake the released neuropeptides; therefore, postjunctional metabolic system(s) are the most important terminating factor of TK biological effects (97). In the lung both neutral endopeptidase (NEP, EC 3.4.24.11) and angiotensin converting enzyme (ACE, EC 3.4.15.1) are potentially able to cleave TKs. Various experimental studies with NEP or ACE inhibitors clearly indicate that in the lung NEP is by far the most important enzymatic system for metabolization of released TKs (30,58,98).

NEP is localized on the epithelium and, at least in the guinea pig, at submucosal and smooth muscle level (99). Endopeptidase activity has been also demonstrated on the surface of inflammatory cells, such as neutrophils (100–102). Interestingly, various factors that can elicit or exacerbate pulmonary neurogenic inflammation (such as viral infection, cigarette smoke, oxidants, toluene diisocyanate, etc.) produce a dramatic reduction in NEP activity (103–106). By contrast, corticosteroid treatment augments the expression of this enzyme, thus potentially reducing the proinflammatory action of TKs (107).

Several studies indicate that NEP inhibitors, such as thiorphan or phosphoramidon, amplify the biological effects of TKs on the airways, such as bronchial smooth muscle contraction (23,98), increase in vascular permeability (108), glandular mucus secretion (109), and cough (110). Furthermore, NEP inhibition enhances the TK release detected after chemical stimulation of sensory nerves (23).

Honda et al. (111) confirmed this metabolism of TKs in human bronchial tissues. In fact, pretreatment of bronchial tissues with phosphoramidon, but not with the ACE inhibitor captopril, greatly potentiates the contraction elicited by substance P or by capsaicin.

TACHYKININS RECEPTORS

To date, there is evidence for the existence of three distinct TK receptors mediating the biological effects of these peptides in mammalian tissues (112). These receptors are termed NK-1, NK-2, and NK-3 and recognize the C-terminal sequence of TKs, i.e., Phe-X-Gly-Leu-Met NH2. Some effects of TKs, such as mast cell degranulation, which are not related to the common C-terminal sequence, are, by definition, not mediated by NK-1, NK-2, or NK-3 receptors. Mast cells degranulation is produced by substance P (SP); this effect requires high concentrations of the peptide and has been explained through a direct interaction of basic aminoacid residues in the N-terminal region of SP with G protein on the mast cell membrane (113).

Natural TKs possess a different affinity for NK-1, NK-2, and NK-3 receptors. In the airways of various species, including humans, only NK-1 and NK-2 receptors have been described thus far (31). SP and NKA are the most potent endogenous ligands for NK-1 and NK-2 receptors, respectively. However, at high concentrations, all natural TKs act as full agonists of each receptor type.

Both NK-1 and NK-2 receptors have been isolated and cloned, also from human pulmonary tissues (114–116). They all belong to the superfamily of rhodopsin-like G protein–coupled receptors with seven hydrophobic transmembrane spanning segments that form the ligand recognition site. Recently, evidence has been presented to indicate that both NK-1 (117,118) and NK-2 receptors (119,120) are heterogeneous. Evidence supporting this idea originated from studies performed with novel antagonists, of both peptide and nonpeptide nature, having high selectivity for, e.g., NK-1 over NK-2 or

NK-3 receptors. It appears that this heterogeneity is largely species dependent; thus, the pharmacological profile of the human NK-1 receptor is similar to that of the guinea pig or rabbit NK-1 receptor, but very different, in
terms of antagonists affinities, from that of the rat or mouse NK-1 receptor
(118). Preliminary evidence suggesting the existence of an *intraspecies* heterogeneity for the NK-2 receptor has been also presented (63,121), however,
which would indicate the existence of true receptor subtypes. Owing to the
rapid progress in this field, it is likely that this aspect of TK research will
change rapidly in the next few years, with important consequences on the
therapeutic applications of this class of compounds.

TACHYKININ RECEPTOR ANTAGONISTS

The first generation of TK antagonists (Table 1), developed at the beginning of the 1980s by insertion of D-Trp residues in the sequence of SP, allowed the establishment of the transmitter role of SP (see 122 for a review).
However, such antagonists (the prototype of which is Spantide) suffer from
a number of drawbacks, including low potency, partial agonist activity, limited ability to discriminate between NK-1 and NK-2 receptors, neurotoxicity
after intrathecal administration, local anesthetic activity, induction of mast

TABLE 1. *Development of tachykinin receptor antagonists*

First generation: unselective peptide tachykinin receptor antagonists
[D-Pro^2, D-Trp^{7,9}] substance P
Spantide I: [D-Arg^1, D-Trp^{7,9}, Leu^{11}] substance P
Second generation: selective peptide tachykinin receptor antagonists
NK-1 selective
   L 668,169: cyclo (Gln- D-Trp- (NMe) Phe - (R)Gly [ANC-2] -Leu- Met)$_2$
   Spantide II: [D-NicLys^1, Pal^3,D-Cl$_2$Phe^5,Asn^6-, D-Trp^{7,9},Nle^{11}] substance P
   GR 82,334: [D-Pro^9 [spiro-γ-lactam] Leu^{10},Trp^{11}]physalaemin (1–11)
   FR 113,680: Ac-Thr-D-Trp(CHO)-Phe-NMeBzl
   FK888: (3-(N-Me)indolil)-CO-Hyp-2 Nal-NMeBzl
NK-2 selective
   L 659,877: cyclo (Gln-Trp-Phe-Gly-Leu-Met)
   MEN 10,207: [Tyr^5, D-Trp^{6,8,9},Arg^{10}] NKA (4–10)
   MEN 10,376: [Tyr^5, D-Trp^{6,8,9},Lys^{10}] NKA (4–10)
   R 396: Ac-Leu-Asp-Gln-Trp-Phe-GlyNH$_2$
   MDL 29,913: cyclo [Leu-Ψ (CH$_2$NCH$_3$)-Leu-Gln-Trp-Phe-Gly]
Third generation: selective nonpeptide tachykinin receptor antagonists
NK-1 selective
   CP 96,345: [(2S, 3S) -cis-2- (diphenylmethyl)-*N*-[(2-methoxyphenyl)-methyl]-1-
   azabicyclo[2,2,2] octan-3-amine]
   RP 67,580: {(3aR, 7aR) 7,7- diphenyl-2- [imino-2-(2 methoxyphenyl) ethyl]
   perhydroisoindol-4-one}
NK-2 selective
   SR 48,968: (S)-*N*-methyl- *N* [4- (4-acetylamino-4-phenylpiperidino) -2- (3,4
   dichlorophenyl) butyl] benzamide

---

cell degranulation, and ability to antagonize peptides unrelated to the TK family (123).

In the past few years, a second generation of peptide TK antagonists has been developed (Table 1); these new tools have the advantage of a greater potency and marked selectivity for only one of the three TK receptors. The improved profile also includes, at least for some examples, specificity in blocking TK action as compared to unrelated peptides (e.g., bombesin), lack of local anesthetic and mast cell–degranulating properties, and lower or absent neurotoxicity after intrathecal administration. Examples of these new compounds are L 668,169, Spantide II, GR 71,251, GR 82,334, and FK888 for the NK-1 receptor; L 659,877, MEN 10,207, MEN 10,376, MDL 29,913, and R 396 for the NK-2 receptor. Some of these molecules could be viewed as candidates for first clinical trials, but their peptide nature dictates important limits to their use as drugs.

The discovery of CP 96,345 (117), the first nonpeptide-potent and selective NK-1 receptor antagonist, represents the birth of a third generation of TK antagonists that will probably undergo further development and clinical evaluation in next few years. Examples of other nonpeptide antagonists are RP 67,580 (124) for the NK-1 receptor and SR 48,968 (125) for the NK-2 receptor (Table 1).

CONCLUSIONS

Available evidence indicates that multiple TK receptors are expressed on several target cells that are involved in the pathogenesis of asthma/bronchial hyperreactivity. In the current view about the pathophysiology of this syndrome, both motor and inflammatory components must be taken into account.

Thus, TK action on multiple targets in the airways and lungs must be considered to understand their possible role as mediators in airway disease. The type of TK receptors expressed on a given target may be different from one species to another and information about the type of TK receptors expressed on human target cells is of paramount importance for a rational drug development in this field. In view of the multiplicity of TK receptors in the airways, one could argue that a TK antagonist with high affinity for more than one of the three receptors known (as example an antagonist having similar affinity for NK-1 and NK-2 sites) might have a better therapeutic potential than an NK-1 or NK-2 receptor-selective antagonist. Until now, only one compound with such characteristics has been described, the peptide antagonist FK 224 (126). The affinity of this compound for NK-1 and NK-2 receptor is relatively low, however, and certainly much lower than that of natural TKs. On the other hand, extremely potent antagonists are available to selectively block NK-1 or NK-2 receptors. Such compounds could be viewed as potential novel classes of anti-inflammatory and antibronchospastic agents and some of them will be undoubtedly tested in humans in the next few years.

In conclusion, anatomical, biochemical, physiological, and pharmacological evidence indicates that TKs are important mediators of certain airway diseases. A place for TK antagonists in human therapy can be anticipated. The remarkable success obtained in recent years in the fast development of potent and selective NK-1 and NK-2 receptor antagonists allowed us to forecast their use as prototypes of a new class of anti-inflammatory, analgesic, and/or spasmolytic drugs in the future.

REFERENCES

1. Maggi CA, Meli A. The sensory-efferent function of capsaicin sensitive neurons. *Gen Pharmacol* 1988;19:1–43.
2. Holzer P. Local effector functions of capsaicin-sensitive sensory nerve endings: involvement of tachykinins, calcitonin gene-related peptide and other neuropeptides. *Neuroscience* 1988;24:739–768.
3. Holzer P. Capsaicin: cellular targets, mechanisms of action, and selectivity for thin sensory neurons. *Pharmacol Rev* 1991;4:143–201.
4. Maggi CA. The pharmacology of the efferent function of sensory nerves. *J Auton Pharmacol* 1991;11:173–208.
5. Barnes PJ. Asthma as an axon reflex. *Lancet* 1986;1:242–244.
6. Barnes PJ, Belvisi MG, Rogers DF. Modulation of neurogenic inflammation: novel approaches to inflammatory disease. *TIPS* 1990;11:185–189.
7. Nawa H, Hirose T, Takashima H, Inayama S, Nakanishi S. Nucleotide sequences of cloned cDNAs for two types of bovine substance P precursor. *Nature* 1983;306:32–36.
8. Nawa H, Kotani H, Nakanishi S. Tissue specific generation of two preprotachykinin mRNAs from one gene by alternative RNA splicing. *Nature* 1984;312:729–734.
9. Kotani H, Hoshimaru M, Nawa H, Nakanishi S. Structure and gene organization of bovine neuromedin K precursor. *Proc Natl Acad Sci USA* 1986;83:7074–7078.
10. Krause JE, Chirgwin JM, Carter MS, Xu ZS, Hershey AD. Three rat preprotachykinin mRNAs encode the neuropeptides substance P and neurokinin A. *Proc Natl Acad Sci USA* 1987;84:881–885.
11. Wharton J, Polak JM, Bloom SR, Will JA, Brown MR, Pearse AGE. Substance P-like immunoreactive nerves in mammalian lung. *Invest Cell Pathol* 1979;2:3–10.
12. Lundberg JM, Franco-Cereceda A, Hua X, Hokfelt T, Fischer JA. Coexistence of substance P and calcitonin gene-related peptide-like immunoreactivities in sensory nerves in relation to cardiovascular and bronchoconstrictor effects of capsaicin. *Eur J Pharmacol* 1985;108:315–319.
13. Polak JM, Bloom SR. Regulatory peptides and neuron specific enolase in the respiratory tract of man and other animals. *Exp Lung Res* 1982;3:313–328.
14. Lundberg JM, Hokfelt T, Martling CR, Saria A, Cuello C. Substance P immunoreactive sensory nerves in the lower respiratory tract of various mammals including man. *Cell Tissue Res* 1984;235:251–261.
15. Martling C-R, Theodorsson-Norheim E, Lundberg JM. Occurrence and effects of multiple tachykinins: substance P, neurokinin A and neuropeptide K in human lower airways. *Life Sci* 1987;40:1633–1643.
16. Baraniuk JN, Lundgren JD, Mullol J, Okayama M, Merida M, Kaliner M. Substance P and neurokinin A in human nasal mucosa. *Am J Respir Cell Mol Biol* 1991;4:228–236.
17. Komatsu T, Yamamoto M, Shimokata K, Nagura H. Distribution of substance P-immunoreactive and calcitonin gene-related peptide-immunoreactive nerves in normal human lungs. *Int Arch Allergy Appl Immunol* 1991;95:23–28.

18. Hoover DB, Hancock JC. Autoradiographic localization of SP binding sites in guinea-pig airways. *J Autonom Nerv System* 1987;19:171–174.
19. Castairs JR, Barnes PJ. Autoradiographic mapping of SP receptors in lung. *Eur J Pharmacol* 1986;127:295–296.
20. Ollerenshaw SL, Jarvis D, Sullivan CE, Woolcock AJ. Substance P immunoreactive nerves in airways from asthmatics and nonasthmatics. *Eur Respir J* 1991;4:673–682.
21. Peters MJ, Adcock IM, Gelder CM, et al. NK_1 receptor gene expression is increased in asthmatic lung and reduced by corticosteroids. *Am Rev Respir Dis* 1992;145:A835.
22. Saria A, Martling CR, Yan Z, Theodorsson-Norheim E, Gamse R, Lundberg JM. Release of multiple tachykinins from capsaicin-sensitive sensory nerves in the lung by bradykinin, histamine, dimethylphenyl piperazinium, and vagal nerve stimulation. *Am Rev Respir Dis* 1988;137:1330–1335.
23. Maggi CA, Patacchini R, Perretti F, et al. The effect of thiorphan and epithelium removal on contractions and tachykinin release produced by activation of capsaicin-sensitive afferents in the guinea-pig isolated bronchus. *Naunyn Schmiedebergs Arch Pharmacol* 1990;341:74–79.
24. Manzini S, Conti S, Maggi CA, et al. Regional differences in the motor and inflammatory responses to capsaicin in guinea pig airways. *Am Rev Respir Dis* 1989;140:936–941.
25. Takayanagi I, Moriya M, Kurata R, Koike K. Effects of ageing on nicotine-induced contraction and substance P-like materials release in guinea-pig bronchus. *Gen Pharmacol* 1991;22:783–785.
26. Rodrigue F, Hoff C, Touvay C, et al. Release of immunoreactive substance P and vasoactive intestinal peptide (VIP) from guinea-pig upper airways by platelet activating factor (PAF-acether). *Prostaglandins* 1987;34:A178.
27. Martins MA, Shore SA, Drazen JM. Release of tachykinins by histamine, methacholine, PAF, LTD_4, and substance P from guinea pig lungs. *Am J Physiol* 1991;261:L449–L455.
28. Manzini S, Meini S. Involvement of capsaicin-sensitive structures in the bronchomotor effects of arachidonic acid and melittin: a possible role for lipoxin A4. *Br J Pharmacol* 1991;103:1027–1032.
29. Meini S, Evangelista S, Geppetti P, Szallasi A, Blumberg PM, Manzini S. Pharmacologic and neurochemical evidence for the activation of capsaicin-sensitive sensory nerves by lipoxin A4 in guinea pig bronchus. *Am Rev Respir Dis* 1992;146:930–934.
30. Martins MA, Shore SA, Drazen JM. Capsaicin-induced release of tachykinins: effects of enzyme inhibitors. *J Appl Physiol* 1991;70:1950–1956.
31. Maggi CA. Tachykinin receptors in the airways and lung: what should we block? *Pharmacol Res* 1990;22:5.
32. Ballati L, Evangelista S, Maggi CA, Manzini S. Effects of selective tachykinin receptor antagonists on capsaicin- and tachykinin-induced bronchospasm in anaesthetized guinea-pigs. *Eur J Pharmacol* 1992;214:215–221.
33. Advenier C, Naline E, Drapeau G, Regoli D. Relative potencies of neurokinins in guinea-pig trachea and human bronchus. *Eur J Pharmacol* 1987;139:133–137.
34. Naline E, Devillier P, Drapeau G, et al. Characterization of neurokinin effects and receptor selectivity in human isolated bronchi. *Am Rev Respir Dis* 1989;140:679–686.
35. Frossard N, Barnes PJ. Effect of tachykinins in small human airways. *Neuropeptides* 1991;48:8–15.
36. Burcher E, Alouan LA, Johnson PR, Black JL. Neuropeptide gamma, the most potent contractile tachykinin in human isolated bronchus, acts via a "non-classical" NK2 receptor. *Neuropeptides* 1991;20:79–82.
37. Fuller RW, Conradson TB, Dixon CMS, Crossman DC, Barnes PJ. Sensory neuropeptide effects in human skin. *Br J Pharmacol* 1987;92:781–788.
38. Crimi N, Palermo F, Oliveri R, et al. Effect of nedocromil on bronchospasm induced by inhalation of substance P in asthmatic airways. *Clin Allergy* 1988;18:375–382.
39. Joos G, Pauwels R, Van der Straeten M. The effect of inhaled substance P and neurokinin A on the airways of normal and asthmatic subjects. *Thorax* 1987;42:779–783.
40. Fine JM, Gordon T, Sheppard D. Epithelium removal alters responsiveness of guinea pig trachea to substance P. *J Appl Physiol* 1989;66:232–237.

41. Frossard N, Rhoden KJ, Barnes PJ. Influence of epithelium on guinea pig airways responses to tachykinins: role of endopeptidases and cyclooxygenase. *J Pharmacol Exp Ther* 1989;248:292–298.
42. Manzini S. Bronchodilatation by tachykinins and capsaicin in the mouse main bronchus. *Br J Pharmacol* 1992;105:968–972.
43. Laitinen LA, Heino M, Laitinen A, Kava T, Haahtela T. Damage of the airway epithelium and bronchial respiratory tract in patients with asthma. *Am Rev Respir Dis* 1985;131:599–606.
44. McDonald DM, Mitchell RA, Gabella G, Haskell A. Neurogenic inflammation in the rat trachea. II. Identity and distribution of nerves mediating the increase in vascular permeability. *J Neurocytol* 1988;17:605–628.
45. Rogers DF, Belvisi MG, Aursudkij B, Evans TW, Barnes PJ. Effects and interactions of sensory neuropeptides on airway microvascular leakage in guinea-pigs. *Br J Pharmacol* 1988;95:1109–1116.
46. Abelli L, Maggi CA, Rovero P, et al. Effect of synthetic tachykinin analogues on airway microvascular leakage in rats and guinea-pigs: evidence for the involvement of NK-1 receptors. *J Auton Pharmacol* 1991;11:267–275.
47. Hagemark O, Hokfelt T, Pernow B. Flare and itch induced by substance P in human skin. *J Invest Dermatol* 1978;71:233–235.
48. Fuller RW, Maxwell DL, Dixon CMS. The effects of substance P on cardiovascular and respiratory function in human subjects. *J Appl Physiol* 1987;62:1473–1479.
49. Eglezos A, Giuliani S, Viti G, Maggi CA. Direct evidence that capsaicin-induced plasma protein extravasation is mediated through tachykinin NK-1 receptors. *Eur J Pharmacol* 1991;209:277–279.
50. Lei Y-H, Barnes PJ, Rogers DF. Inhibition of neurogenic plasma exudation in guinea-pig airways by CP-96,345, a new non peptide NK$_1$ receptor antagonist. *Br J Pharmacol* 1992;105:261–262.
51. Delay-Goyet P, Lundberg JM. Cigarette smoke-induced airway oedema is blocked by the NK1 antagonist, CP-96,345. *Eur J Pharmacol* 1991;203:157-158.
52. Whittle BJR, Lopez-Belmonte J, Rees DD. Modulation of the vasodepressor actions of acetylcholine bradykinin, substance P and endothelin in the rat by a specific inhibitor of nitric oxide formation. *Br J Pharmacol* 1989;98:646–652.
53. Persson MG, Hedqvist P, Gustafsson LE. Nerve-induced tachykinin mediated vasodilatation in skeletal muscle is dependent on nitric oxide formation. *Eur J Pharmacol* 1991;205:295–301.
54. Salonen RO, Webber SE, Widdicombe JG. Effects of neuropeptides and capsaicin on the canine tracheal vasculature in vivo. *Br J Pharmacol* 1988;95:1262–1270.
55. Matran R, Alving K, Martling CR, Lacroix JS, Lundberg JM. Effects of neuropeptides and capsaicin on tracheobronchial blood flow in the pig. *Acta Physiol Scand* 1989; 135:335–342.
56. Adnot S, Cigarini I, Herigault R, Harf A. Effects of substance P and calcitonin gene-related peptide on the pulmonary circulation. *J Appl Physiol* 1991;70:1707–1712.
57. Maggi CA, Patacchini R, Perrretti F, et al. Sensory nerves, vascular endothelium and neurogenic relaxation of the guinea-pig isolated pulmonary artery. *Naunyn Schmiedebergs Arch Pharmacol* 1990;342:78–84.
58. Lotvall JO, Skoogh B-E, Barnes PJ, Chung KF. Effects of aerosolised substance P on long resistance in guinea-pigs: a comparison between inhibition of neutral endopeptidase and angiotensin-converting enzyme. *Br J Pharmacol* 1990;100:69–72.
59. Repke H, Bienert M. Structural requirements for mast cell triggering by substance P-like peptides. *Agents Actions* 1988;23:207–210.
60. Repke H, Bienert M. Mast cell activation—a receptor-independent mode of substance P action? *FEBS Lett* 1987;221:236–240.
61. Kroegel C, Giembycz MA, Barnes PJ. Characterization of eosinophil cell activation by peptides. Differential effects of substance P, melittin, and FMET-Leu-Phe. *J Immunol* 1990;145:2581–2587.
62. Brunelleschi S, Vanni L, Ledda F, Giotti A, Maggi CA, Fantozzi R. Tachykinins activate guinea-pig alveolar macrophages: involvement of NK-2 and NK-1 receptors. *Br J Pharmacol* 1990;100:417–420.

63. Brunelleschi S. Tachykinin actions on alveolar macrophages. *Neuropeptides* 1992; 22:11.
64. Weihe E. Significance of neuropeptides at the neuroimmune connection in inflammatory pain. *Neuropeptides* 1992;22:69.
65. Wozniak A, Mclennan G, Betts WH, Murphy A, Scicchitano R. Activation of human neutrophils by substance P: effect on FMLP-stimulated oxidative and arachidonic acid metabolism and on antibody-dependent cell-mediated cytotoxicity. *Immunology* 1989; 68:359–364.
66. Wiedermann CJ, Wiedermann FJ, Apperl A, Kiselbach G, Konwalinka G, Braunsteiner H. In vitro human polymorphonuclear leukocyte chemokinesis and human monocyte chemotaxis are different activities of aminoterminal and carboxyterminal substance P. *Naunyn Schmiedebergs Arch Pharmacol* 1989;340:185–190.
67. Iwamoto I, Yamazaki H, Nakagawa N, Kimura A, Tomioka H, Yoshida S. Differential effects of two C-terminal peptides of substance P on human neutrophils. *Neuropeptides* 1990;16:103–107.
68. Perianin A, Snyderman R, Malfroy B. Substance P primes human neutrophil activation: a mechanism for neurological regulation of inflammation. *Biochem Biophys Res Commun* 1989;2:520–524.
69. Wiedermann CJ, Niedermuhlbichler M, Zilian U, Geissler D, Lindley I, Braunsteiner H. Priming of normal human neutrophils by tachykinins: tuftsin-like inhibition of in vitro chemotaxis stimulated by formylpeptide or interleukin-8. *Regul Pep* 1991;36:359–368.
70. Brunelleschi S, Tarli S, Giotti A, Fantozzi R. Priming effects of mammalian tachykinins on human neutrophils. *Life Sci* 1991;48:PL1–PL5.
71. Marasco WA, Showell HJ, Becker EL. Substance P binds to the formyl peptide chemoaxis receptor on the rabbit neutrophil. *Biochem Biophys Res Commun* 1981;99: 1065–1068.
72. McDonald DM. Neurogenic inflammation in the rat trachea. I. Changes in venules, leucocytes and epithelial cells. *J Neurocytol* 1988;17:583–603.
73. Matis WL, Lavker RM, Murphy GF. Substance P induces the expression of an endothelial-leukocyte adhesion molecule by microvascular endothelium. *J Invest Dermatol* 1990;94:492–495.
74. Corrigan CJ, Kay AB. T-lymphocytes. In: Barnes PJ, Rodger IW, Thomson NC, eds. *Asthma: basic mechanisms and clinical management.* London: Academic Press, 1992;125–141.
75. Payan DG, Brewster DR, Goetzl EJ. Specific stimulation of human T-lymphocytes by substance P. *J Immunol* 1983;131:1613–1615.
76. Payan DG, Brewster DR, Missirian-Bastian A, Goetzl EJ. Substance P recognition by a subset of human T-lymphocytes. *J Clin Invest* 1984;74:1532–1539.
77. Casini A, Geppetti P, Maggi CA, Surrenti C. Effects of calcitonin gene-related peptide (CGRP) neurokinin A and neurokinin A(4-10) on the mitogenic response of human peripheral blood mononuclear cells. *Naunyn Schmiedebergs Arch Pharmacol* 1989; 339:354–358.
78. McGillis JP, Mitsuhashi M, Payan DG. Immunomodulation by tachykinin neuropeptides. *Ann N Y Acad Sci* 1990;594:85–94.
79. Laurenzi MA, Persson MAA, Dalsgaard CJ, Ringden O. Stimulation of human B lymphocyte differentiation by the neuropeptides substance P and neurokinin A. *Scand J Immunol* 1989;30:695–701.
80. Pascual DW, Xu-Amano J, Kiyono H, McGhee JR, Bost KL. Substance P acts directly upon cloned B lymphoma cells to enhance IgA and IgM production. *J Immunol* 1991;146:2130–2136.
81. Coles SJ, Neil KH, Reid LM. Potent stimulation of glycoprotein secretion in canine trachea by substance P. *J Appl Physiol* 1984;57:1323–1327.
82. Barnes PJ, Baraniuk JN, Belvisi MG. Neuropeptides in the respiratory tract. Part I. *Am Rev Respir Dis* 1991;144:1187–1198.
83. Gentry SE. Tachykinin receptors mediating airway macromolecular secretion. *Life Sci* 1991;48:1609–1618.
84. Meini S, Manzini S, Barnes PJ, Rogers DF. Effect of selective tachykinin agonists on

mucus secretion and smooth muscle contraction in ferret airways. *Am Rev Respir Dis* 1992;145:A370.

85. Geppetti P, Bertrand C, Bacci E, Snider RM, Maggi CA, Nadel JA. The NK-1 receptor antagonist CP 96,345 blocks substance P-evoked mucus secretion from the ferret trachea in vitro. *Neuropeptides* 1992;22:25.

86. Kuo H-P, Rohde JAL, Barnes PJ, Rogers DF. Cigarette smoke induced goblet cell secretion: neural involvement in guinea pig trachea. *Eur Respir J* 1990;3:189.

87. Rogers DF, Aursudkij B, Barnes PJ. Effects of tachykinins on mucus secretion in human bronchi in vitro. *Eur J Pharmacol* 1989;174:283–286.

88. Rogers DF, Barnes PJ. Opioid inhibition of neurally mediated mucus secretion in human bronchi. *Lancet* 1989;1:930.

89. Mullol J, Rieves RD, Baraniuk JN, et al. The effects of neuropeptides on mucous glycoprotein secretion from human nasal mucosa in vitro. *Neuropeptides* 1992;21:231–238.

90. Saria A, Lundberg JM, Skofitsch G, Lembeck F. Vascular protein leakage in various tissues induced by substance P, capsaicin, bradykinin, serotonin, histamine and by antigen challenge. *Naunyn Schmiedebergs Arch Pharmacol* 1983;324:212–218.

91. Manzini S, Maggi CA, Geppetti P, Bacciarelli C. Capsaicin desensitization protects from antigen-induced bronchospasm in conscious guinea-pigs. *Eur J Pharmacol* 1987;138:307–308.

92. Ahlstedt S, Alving K, Hesselmar B, Olaisson E. Enhancement of the bronchial reactivity in immunized rats by neonatal treatment with capsaicin. *Int Arch Allergy Appl Immunol* 1986;80:262–266.

93. Lai YL. Endogenous tachykinins in antigen-induced acute bronchial responses of guinea pigs. *Exp Lung Res* 1991;17:1047–1060.

94. Ingenito EP, Pliss LB, Martins MA, Ingram RH. Effects of capsaicin on mechanical, cellular and mediator responses to antigen in sensitized guinea pigs. *Am Rev Respir Dis* 1991;143:572–577.

95. Kohrogi H, Yamaguchi T, Kawano O, Honda I, Ando M, Araki S. Inhibition of neutral endopeptidase potentiates bronchial contraction induced by immune response in guinea pigs *in vitro*. *Am Rev Respir Dis* 1991;144:636–641.

96. Matsuse T, Thomson RJ, Chen X-R, Salari H, Schellenberg RR. Capsaicin inhibits airway hyperresponsiveness but not lipoxygenase activity or eosinophilia after repeated aerosolized antigen in guinea pigs. *Am Rev Respir Dis* 1991;144:368–372.

97. Krause JE. On the physiological metabolism of substance P. In: Jordan CC, Oehme P, eds. *Substance P, metabolism and biological actions.* London and Philadelphia: Taylor and Francis, 1985;13–32.

98. Djokic TD, Nadel JA, Dusser DJ, Sekizawa K, Graf PD, Borson DB. Inhibitors of neutral endopeptidase potentiate electrically and capsaicin-induced noncholinergic contraction in guinea-pig bronchi. *J Pharmacol Exp Ther* 1989;248:7–11.

99. Dusser DJ, Jacoby DB, Djokic TD, Rubinstein I, Borson DB, Nadel JA. Virus induces airway hyperresponsiveness to tachykinins: role of neutral endopeptidase. *J Appl Physiol* 1989;67:1504–1511.

100. Erdos EG, Wagner B, Harbury CB, Painter RG, Skidgel RA, Fa X-G. Down-regulation and inactivation of neutral endopeptidase 24.11 (Enkephalinase) in human neutrophils. *J Biol Chem* 1989;264:14519–14523.

101. Skidgel RA, Jackman HL, Erdos EG. Metabolism of substance P and bradykinin by human neutrophils. *Biochem Pharmacol* 1991;41:1335–1344.

102. Shipp MA, Stefano GB, Switzer SN, Griffin JD, Reinherz EL. CD10 (CALLA)/neutral endopeptidase 24.11 modulates inflammatory peptide-induced changes in neutrophil morphology, migration and adhesion proteins and is itself regulated by neutrophil activation. *Blood* 1991;78:1834–1841.

103. Dusser DJ, Djokic TD, Borson DB, Nadel JA. Cigarette smoke induces bronchoconstrictor hyperresponsiveness to substance P and inactivates airway neutral endopeptidase in the guinea pig. *J Clin Invest* 1989;84:900–906.

104. Piedimonte G, Nadel JA, Umeno E, McDonald DM. Sendai virus infection potentiates neurogenic inflammation in the rat trachea. *J Appl Physiol* 1990;68:754–760.

105. Murlas CG, Murphy TP, Lang Z. HOCl causes airway substance P hyperresponsiveness and neutral endopeptidase hypoactivity. *Am J Physiol* 1990;258:L361–L368.
106. Sheppard D, Thompson JE, Scypinski L, Dusser D, Nadel JA, Borson DB. Toluene diisocyanate increases airway responsiveness to substance P and decreases airway enkephalinase. *J Clin Invest* 1988;81:1111–1115.
107. Piedimonte G, Macdonald IM, Nadel JA. Glucocorticoids inhibit neurogenic protein extravasation and prevent virus-potentiated extravasation in the rat trachea. *J Clin Invest* 1990;86:1409–1415.
108. Umeno E, Nadel JA, Huang H-T, McDonald DM. Inhibition of neutral endopeptidase potentiates neurogenic inflammation in the rat trachea. *J Appl Physiol* 1989;66:2647–2652.
109. Borson DB, Corrales R, Varsano S, et al. Enkephalinase inhibitors potentiate substance P-induced secretion of $^{35}SO_4$-marcomolecules from ferret trachea. *Exp Lung Res* 1987;12:21–36.
110. Kohrogi H, Graf PD, Sekizawa K, Borson DB, Nadel JA. Neutral endopeptidase inhibitors potentiate substance P- and capsaicin-induced cough in awake guinea pigs. *J Clin Invest* 1988;82:2063–2068.
111. Honda I, Kohrogi H, Yamaguchi T, Ando M, Araki S. Enkephalinase inhibitor potentiates substance P- and capsaicin-induced bronchial smooth muscle contractions in humans. *Am Rev Respir Dis* 1991;143:1416–1418.
112. Nakanishi S. Mammalian tachykinin receptors. *Annu Rev Neurosci* 1991;14:123–136.
113. Mousli M, Bueb JL, Bronner C, Rouot B, Landry Y. G protein activation: a receptor independent mode of action for cationic amphiphilic neuropeptides and venom peptides. *TIPS* 1990;11:358–362.
114. Gerard NP, Eddy RL, Shows TB, Gerard C. The human neurokinin A (substance K) receptor. *J Biol Chem* 1990;265:20455–20462.
115. Gerard NP, Garraway LA, Eddy RL, et al. Human substance P receptor (NK-1): organization of the gene, chromosome localization, and functional expression of cDNA clones. *Biochemistry* 1991;30:10640–10646.
116. Hopkins B, Powell SJ, Danks P, Briggs I, Graham A. Isolation and characterisation of the human lung NK-1 receptor cDNA. *Biochem Biophys Res Commun* 1991;180:1110–1117.
117. Snider RM, Constantine JW, Lowe III JA, et al. A potent nonpeptide antagonist of the substance P (NK-1) receptor. *Science* 1991;251:435–437.
118. Gitter BD, Waters DC, Bruns RF, Mason NR, Nixon JA, Howbert JJ. Species differences in affinities of nonpeptide antagonists for substance P receptors. *Eur J Pharmacol* 1991;197:237–238.
119. Maggi CA, Patacchini R, Giuliani S, et al. Competitive antagonists discriminate between NK-2 tachykinin receptor subtypes. *Br J Pharmacol* 1990;100:588–592.
120. Maggi CA, Patacchini R, Astolfi M, Rovero P, Giuliani S, Giachetti A. NK-2 receptor agonists and antagonists. *Ann N Y Acad Sci* 1991;632:184–191.
121. Nimmo AJ, Carstairs JR, Maggi CA, Morrison JFB. Evidence for the co-existence of multiple NK_2 tachykinin receptor subtypes in rat bladder. *Neuropeptides* 1992;22:48.
122. Maggi CA, Patacchini R, Rovero P, Giuliani S, Giachetti A. Tachykinin receptor antagonists and potential clinical applications at peripheral level. *Biochem Soc Trans* 1991;19:909–912.
123. Buck SH, Shatzer SA. Agonist and antagonist binding to tachykinin peptide NK-2 receptors. *Life Sci* 1988;42:2701–2708.
124. Garret C, Carruette A, Fardin V, et al. Pharmacological properties of a potent and selective nonpeptide substance P antagonist. *Proc Natl Acad Sci USA* 1991;88:10208–10211.
125. Emonds AX, Vilain P, Goulaouic P, et al. A potent and selective nonpeptide antagonist of the neurokinin A (NK-2) receptor. *Life Sci Pharmacol Lett* 1992;50:101–106.
126. Fujii T, Mural M, Morimoto H, Maeda Y. Effects of FK888 and FK224 on airway constriction and airway edema induced by either neurokinins or capsaicin. *Am Rev Respir Dis* 1992;145:A42.

Drugs and the Lung,
edited by C.P. Page and W.J. Metzger.
Raven Press, Ltd., New York © 1994

15

Drug Therapy for the Adult Respiratory Distress Syndrome

Jonathan D. Plitman and James R. Snapper

Department of Pulmonary and Critical Care Medicine,
Vanderbilt University School of Medicine,
Nashville, Tennessee 37232-2650

The adult respiratory distress syndrome (ARDS), first described by Ashbaugh and colleagues in 1967 (1), is an often-fulminant form of acute respiratory failure. It has a widely quoted (although crudely estimated) incidence of 150,000 cases per year in the United States (2) and is 50% to 70% fatal (2–5). Although it is felt to be the result of increased pulmonary microvascular permeability, ARDS is a true "syndrome" in that it is defined not by a specific pathogenesis but rather by an array of clinical criteria: hypoxemia, pulmonary edema in the absence of left heart failure, and stiff, noncompliant lungs (1,6). Experimental evidence suggests that the sequence of events leading to increased permeability involves an acute inflammatory cascade. Events capable of triggering this process are many, the most common being sepsis, aspiration, trauma, near-drowning, and multiple transfusions (7–9). Sepsis, the most prevalent and most lethal cause of ARDS (10), has been the subject of intense scrutiny in recent years, and merits separate mention. In sepsis (11), an infection (often gram-negative, not necessarily with discernible bacteremia) initiates the release of a barrage of endogenous mediators that can lead to inflammation, alteration of vascular tone, and organ dysfunction, including, in up to 25% of cases, ARDS. These events can culminate in systemic hypotension and, frequently, death. Experimental investigations concerning sepsis and ARDS intersect to a large degree, and we will deal with these entities somewhat interchangeably.

More than two decades of energetic research have not yielded effective drug therapy for ARDS. The obduracy of this problem reflects the multiple biochemical avenues along which the pathogenetic cascade can proceed and the brevity of the "window of opportunity" early in the syndrome during which drug therapies have their greatest chance of success. [Many therapies studied in animal models of ARDS seem to work best (or sometimes only)

521

when administered before the pulmonary insult—an opportunity rarely afforded us in clinical medicine.] This chapter examines the current evidence concerning potential ARDS pharmacotherapies, but we emphasize to the reader that the value of *all* of these therapies remains speculative. Optimal patient care in ARDS continues to consist of treatment of the underlying condition and of supportive measures such as appropriate fluid therapy (12), ventilator management (13,14), body positioning (15,16), and prevention of nosocomial infection.

The mechanisms presumed responsible for the pathogenesis of ARDS have been frequently reviewed (e.g., 17–21), and we will not do so at length. A model is presented, however, in Fig. 1. An initiating stimulus triggers an inflammatory cascade in which cells release mediators that can either further amplify the cascade, directly harm the lungs, or both. These mediators include eicosanoids, platelet-activating factor, cytokines, proteolytic enzymes, and oxygen radicals. The result of this process is increased endothelial and epithelial permeability, increased pulmonary vascular pressures, altered lung mechanics, and impaired alveolar surfactant function.

Proposed ARDS pharmacotherapies belong to the following categories:

1. Anti-endotoxin immunotherapy
2. Classic anti-inflammatory drugs
   a. Corticosteroids
   b. Cyclooxygenase inhibitors
3. Novel anti-inflammatory drugs
   a. Anticytokine antibodies and receptor antagonists
   b. Platelet-activating factor receptor antagonists
   c. Pentoxifylline
4. Exogenous lipid mediators (prostaglandins E_1 and E_2)
5. Antioxidants
6. Antiproteases
7. Surfactant replacement

We will discuss the agents in this order. In a volume focusing on novel management of asthma, the parallels between the presumed mechanisms and proposed treatments of asthma and of ARDS are obvious. Indeed, ARDS is associated with increased reversible resistance to airflow and airway hyperresponsiveness in animals and humans (22–25).

ANTI-ENDOTOXIN IMMUNOTHERAPY

Endotoxin is an extremely toxic lipopolysaccharide found in the cell walls of all gram-negative bacteria. Purified endotoxin can trigger the events characteristic of sepsis and ARDS (11,20; and numerous references below). Endotoxin is immunogenic (26,27), and passive immunotherapy directed

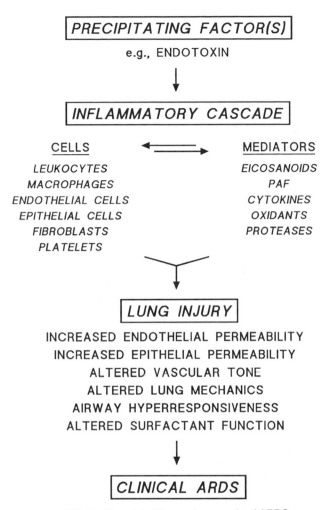

FIG. 1. A model of the pathogenesis of ARDS.

against it is thus a possibility. Endotoxin molecules consist of a non-toxic O side chain composed of repeating oligosaccharide units and of a toxic core region composed of lipid A and a number of sugars (28). Passive immunization against O side chains is protective against endotoxin in some animal models (e.g., 29–31), but anti-O immunity is felt to be of limited value in humans (26,32). O side chains, furthermore, are antigenically variable among different bacteria, while the structure of lipid A is highly conserved. Recent studies have thus focused on the use of anti-core antibodies.

The current phase of anti-endotoxin immunotherapy began in 1982. Ziegler et al. (33) showed, in a randomized, controlled trial, that mortality among patients with serious gram-negative infections was reduced by treatment with antiserum from healthy humans who had been immunized against the J5 mutant strain of *Escherichia coli* O111, a bacterium whose endotoxin lacks O chains but has an intact core region. The J5 antiserum was not felt to be of clinical utility, however, because of the problems of establishing a standardized supply and of potential disease transmission to recipients (34). Attempts were then made to identify and utilize the active principle of the antiserum. In a double-blind, randomized study by Calandra et al. (35), purified immunoglobulin G (IgG) from humans immunized against J5 *E. coli* had no effect on morbidity and mortality among patients with serious gram-negative infections. IgM anti-core, however, may be more protective against endotoxin than IgG (36). Two monoclonal IgM antibodies against J5 lipid A have been developed. These have been designated E5 (derived from mouse splenocytes) (37) and HA-1A (a human antibody) (34).

Both E5 and HA-1A have been the subject of large randomized, double-blind, controlled trials in patients with suspected gram-negative sepsis. In the E5 study of Greenman et al. (37), the antibody ($n = 242$) or saline ($n = 226$) was given intravenously twice at 24-h intervals in patients with suspected gram-negative sepsis. No overall decrease in 30-day mortality was detectable, although there was a statistically significant reduction in mortality among the 137 patients without shock (blood pressure <90 mm Hg) refractory to fluid resuscitation and pressors. In the HA-1A study, Ziegler et al. (34) gave a single intravenous dose of either the antibody ($n = 262$) or human albumin ($n = 281$). There was no overall difference in 28-day mortality. The subgroup with gram-negative bacteremia ($n = 200$) did have a significant decrease in mortality if treated with HA-1A; the decrease was more clearly demonstrable in those patients in shock (blood pressure <90 mm Hg or requiring pressors). It is difficult to reach a conclusion from these data; the test drugs only worked in a minority of subjects, and a different minority benefited in each study. From the specific standpoint of ARDS, pretreatment with the E5 antibody has been found to have minimal inhibitory effect on the ARDS-like pulmonary response to endotoxin in sheep (38). No effects of antibody treatment on the incidence or resolution of ARDS were noted in the human trials, although analysis of this issue was not a specific goal of these studies and the number of ARDS cases was relatively small.

Both the E5 and the HA-1A studies have been criticized on immunological grounds (39), and, in particular, the study design and data analysis of the HA-1A trial have been questioned (40). As of the writing of this review, the agents had not been approved by the Food and Drug Administration (FDA) for general use. Based on currently available information, they are of unclear benefit to the majority of sepsis patients and are of unknown usefulness in ARDS.

CORTICOSTEROIDS

The decades-long debate over the use of high-dose corticosteroids in sepsis and ARDS is quiescent at the moment, and there appears to be general agreement that the drugs are not useful in the acute management of these conditions. These data have been frequently reviewed (e.g., 41,42). We will summarize them and then touch on other aspects of corticosteroid therapy.

Corticosteroids are usually classified as anti-inflammatory drugs (43,44), although their precise mechanism of action is debated. Many studies show that these drugs decrease morbidity and mortality in various animal models of sepsis and lung injury if they are administered before or simultaneously with the experimental insult. This is true in bacteremia (45–47), endotoxemia (45,48,49), and acid aspiration (50). In 1976, Schumer (51) published a widely cited study in which high-dose corticosteroids significantly reduced mortality in septic patients. The study has been criticized, however, for a number of reasons (41,42,52). Part of the data collection was randomized and prospective (although not blinded) and part was retrospective. Not all patients received the same antibiotics and some patients received an extra dose of corticosteroids. Fluid resuscitation, furthermore, may not have been adequate.

Subsequently, a number of large, well-designed, randomized, controlled, prospective trials have reexamined high-dose corticosteroids. The first of these, by Sprung et al. (53), found no overall change in mortality of sepsis, although there was a trend toward reversal of shock with early corticosteroid therapy. The Veterans Administration Cooperative Study (54) and the study of Bone et al. (55) found no benefit in sepsis; in the latter study there was increased mortality among the septic patients with elevated creatinine who received corticosteroids. In neither of these studies did corticosteroids seem to reduce the risk of ARDS. The smaller study of Luce et al. (56), whose specific purpose was to examine the effect of corticosteroids on incidence of ARDS in sepsis, reached a similar conclusion. Finally, Bernard et al. (57) observed no improvement in either physiologic parameters or mortality in a trial of corticosteroids early in the course of established ARDS of various etiologies.

In general, therefore, high-dose corticosteroids are not useful as therapy for sepsis or early established ARDS, and should not be used. It is important to note, however, that such therapy may still be of value in a minority of ARDS variants. One example is the fat embolism syndrome (58). Several studies have shown that patients at risk for fat embolism due to long bone fractures have significantly less risk of respiratory failure if treated with corticosteroids (59–61). It should be emphasized that this is a prophylactic therapy. Patients with established ARDS, such as were included in the Bernard study (57), would be less likely to benefit. Corticosteroids are probably useful in respiratory failure due to *Pneumocystis carinii* pneumonia (62–64), which has features (65,66) reminiscent of ARDS.

Longer-term corticosteroid therapy has been considered later in the course of ARDS in an attempt to enhance lung healing. While some ARDS survivors improve rapidly, others undergo a more sluggish recovery associated with a scarring, fibroproliferative process that can progress to airspace obliteration or cyst formation (67–71). Two uncontrolled studies (72,73) have reported improvement after corticosteroid therapy in established ARDS with pulmonary fibrosis documented by open lung biopsy. The therapy was begun, on average, after 10 to 15 days of ARDS. Prospective, placebo-controlled studies would be required to substantiate the value of such therapy, but it would probably be difficult to document a survival benefit. The most common cause of death in established ARDS is not intractable respiratory failure *per se,* but rather ongoing sepsis and its sequelae (4). It is possible that corticosteroid therapy would hasten healing and shorten the hospital stay, but this potential benefit would need to be weighed carefully against the risk of corticosteroid complications. A related issue is whether such therapy might reduce the persistent abnormalities in pulmonary function, such as airflow obstruction, reduced vital capacity, and reduced diffusion capacity, to which some ARDS survivors are subject (74). While there are some correlations between physiological indices during ARDS and subsequent pulmonary function (74), the degree of fibrosis, inflammation, and airspace organization in ARDS open lung biopsies does not correlate with pulmonary function measured 1 year or more after ARDS (75).

CYCLOOXYGENASE INHIBITORS

Cyclooxygenase metabolites of arachidonic acid appear to be integral to the pathogenesis of sepsis-related ARDS. After administration of endotoxin, eicosanoids promptly and predictably appear in the plasma and lung lymph of animals (76–80). These products appear to be synthesized in the lung, as their concentration is greater in lung lymph than in plasma (80). Of primary interest are thromboxane A_2 (TxA_2), a vasoconstrictor and promoter of platelet aggregation, prostacyclin (PGI_2), a vasodilator and inhibitor of platelet aggregation, and prostaglandin E_2 (PGE_2), a vasodilator with numerous suppressive effects on inflammatory cells (20,81–83). Compelling data argue that TxA_2 is a key mediator of much of the pulmonary response to endotoxin in sheep; many aspects of this response are attenuated by cyclooxygenase inhibition (78,79,84) and by specific inhibitors of TxA_2 synthesis or thromboxane receptor blockers (85,86). One could infer potential therapeutic value of the elimination of TxA_2 in ARDS, and, in fact, a body of preliminary data (reviewed below) support the use of cyclooxygenase inhibitors in sepsis and ARDS.

Complicating issues must be acknowledged, however. Cyclooxygenase blockade also prevents the synthesis of metabolites that could potentially be beneficial in ARDS. These include PGE_2 (discussed with PGE_1, below) and prostacyclin, which reduce the pulmonary response to endotoxin in sheep (87,88). These benefits, of course, remain items of speculation, and vasodilator eicosanoids could also have deleterious effects. They may, for example, mediate a loss of hypoxic vasoconstriction in ARDS (77,89,90), which could worsen gas exchange. Infusions of prostacyclin into ARDS patients can impair ventilation-perfusion matching and increase shunt fraction (91), but this effect may simply be a pharmacological one illustrating the "typical" response of ARDS patients to exogenous vasodilators (see below). Also of concern is that TxA_2 and other cyclooxygenase products appear not to be responsible for the entire pulmonary endotoxin response, particularly the late changes in pulmonary microvascular permeability (78,79,84,92).

Treatment with the cyclooxygenase inhibitor ibuprofen is effective in a number of models of sepsis and lung injury when given before or with the experimental insult. For example, in addition to its effects in sheep, it reduces the pulmonary response to oleic acid and inhibits septic manifestations due to endotoxin in dogs (93,94), and reduces lung injury in bacteremic pigs (95). Of potentially greater importance are the observations of benefit when ibuprofen is administered *after* the initial insult, a protocol that more closely resembles a clinical situation. Gnidec et al. (96) administered ibuprofen after the onset of sepsis in a sheep model of bowel perforation and bacterial peritonitis. The drug attenuated the increase in pulmonary artery pressure and lung lymph flow, although lung lymph protein concentration was unaffected.

The currently available human data are also encouraging. Ibuprofen inhibits the fever and tachycardia caused by endotoxin in human volunteers (97). A recent double-blind, placebo-controlled trial of ibuprofen by Bernard et al. (98) in 30 sepsis patients showed that the drug decreased fever, tachycardia, and peak airway pressure while reducing the patients' previously elevated urinary excretion of degradation products of TxA_2 and prostacyclin. There was also a trend toward more rapid reversal of shock in the ibuprofen-treated patients. No significant toxicity, including nephrotoxicity, was noted.

A large multicenter trial of ibuprofen in sepsis is currently in progress. Other cyclooxygenase inhibitors may also prove useful, but one must exercise caution in generalizing among such agents. They often have dissimilarities of action that are potentially relevant to their value in sepsis and ARDS (99,100). Concerns about the suppression of potentially beneficial eicosanoids could be obviated by the use of specific TxA_2 synthesis or receptor blockers. All such drugs remain experimental at this time, and while under consideration in asthma (101,102), their use in ARDS has not been systematically studied.

ANTICYTOKINE ANTIBODIES AND RECEPTOR ANTAGONISTS

Cytokines are small proteins released by various inflammatory effector cells, primarily macrophages and monocytes, in response to insults such as infection. Their function and potential role in sepsis have been the subject of recent reviews (103,104). We will briefly summarize the salient background information. The cytokines of particular current interest in sepsis and ARDS are tumor necrosis factor-α (hereafter referred to as TNF), interleukin-1β (hereafter referred to as IL-1), and interleukin-6 (IL-6). Normally present in small quantities, these compounds are felt to have important roles in host defense. In higher amounts such as can appear during sepsis, however, they are highly toxic. TNF has effects that to a large extent resemble those of endotoxin: exogenous TNF infusion leads to a sepsis-like syndrome, ARDS-like lung injury, and death in a variety of animal models (105–110), and ibuprofen can attenuate this effect (111). Exogenous IL-1 shares many of the actions of TNF but appears less potent (107,112). TNF and IL-1 appear to act synergistically, however, and their combination is highly toxic (112,113). [Exogenous interleukin-2 also causes a sepsis-like state and increased microvascular permeability (114,115), but its role in sepsis is less established than that of TNF and IL-1 (103).]

Endogenous cytokines may be involved in sepsis and ARDS. Experimental exposure to endotoxin causes release of circulating TNF in animals (116,117) and humans (118). TNF release in animals is associated with the subsequent appearance of IL-1 and IL-6 (119,120). Circulating TNF tends to rise in human sepsis, although it is not detectable in many patients, and prognosis seems to worsen as TNF level rises (121–124). Whether elevated TNF in sepsis portends the development ARDS is debated (124,125), but serum and bronchoalveolar lavage (BAL) fluid levels of TNF have been found to be elevated acutely in half of ARDS patients (126). Increased serum IL-1 also implies a poor prognosis in sepsis (123). Increases in IL-1 have been found in BAL fluid from ARDS patients and those at risk for ARDS, although serum levels were not changed (127). Finally, in one study, circulating IL-6 was elevated in a majority of sepsis patients, although levels were not of prognostic value (128).

It thus is reasonable to think that reduction of cytokine levels might be beneficial in sepsis and ARDS. The approach that has been most widely studied is administration of antibodies against cytokines. There are theoretical factors that imply that such therapy may be more effective than anti-endotoxin immunotherapy. While anti-endotoxin therapy is, in principle, limited to gram-negative sepsis, TNF and IL-1 are released during the sepsis syndrome even in the absence of endotoxin (129). Also, there is lag time in the sequence of appearance of cytokines after endotoxin exposure. While the current data are rather variable, the time between endotoxin and peak levels of TNF appears to be 1 to 2 h (117,130), with IL-1 and IL-6 rising an hour or more thereafter (119,120). There thus might be, compared to anti-endotoxin therapy, additional time in the clinical setting for the preemptive administration of a therapeutic agent.

Beutler et al. (131) showed that pretreatment with polyclonal anti-TNF antibodies greatly prolongs survival of mice after exposure to endotoxin, and Tracey et al. (132) found that pretreatment with monoclonal anti-TNF antibodies completely protected baboons against the lethal effects of bacteremia. Similar results have been obtained by others in rabbits (130) and neutropenic rats (133). Anti-TNF antibodies also attenuate the release of IL-1 and IL-6 after bacteremia (119). In a subsequent baboon study, anti-TNF therapy greatly decreased mortality due to *E. coli* bacteremia when the antibody was given 30 min after the bacteria (134). Mice survived significantly longer after *E. coli* challenge when treated with an anti-TNF antibody up to 1.5 hours after the bacterial exposure (135). Interestingly, the monoclonal antibody use in the last-cited study was less effective versus other gram-negative bacilli tested. In two preliminary studies, murine monoclonal antibodies against TNF have been given to patients in septic shock (136,137). No significant adverse reactions were observed, and some patients experienced transient hemodynamic improvement.

Monoclonal anti-IL-6 antibodies seem to protect mice against lethal challenge with *E. coli* and with TNF (138). Research concerning anti-IL-1 therapy has centered on the IL-1 receptor antagonist (IL-1ra), a naturally occurring polypeptide. In rabbits, treatment with IL-1ra increases survival after endotoxin challenge (139) and reduces shock and granulocytic infiltration of the lungs after *E. coli* exposure (140).

Anticytokine therapy is thus a promising modality in the therapy of sepsis and ARDS. It will be important to study these treatments thoroughly in large trials, as more limitations and adverse effects may become apparent. For example, the systemic TNF response may be, to some extent, influenced by the route of endotoxin exposure. In rats, the blood TNF levels and the protective effect of anti-TNF antibodies were significantly less during gram-negative peritonitis than after intravenous infusion of endotoxin (141). Also, it is possible that "tonic exposure" to inflammatory cytokines is protective against subsequent septic or cytokine-mediated insult (117,142,143), and that anticytokine therapy may disrupt this (regulatory?) mechanism. Finally, as is true of many anti-inflammatory pharmacotherapies, anticytokine antibodies may, under certain circumstances, impair host defenses and exacerbate infection (144–146).

PLATELET-ACTIVATING FACTOR RECEPTOR ANTAGONISTS

Platelet-activating factor (PAF) is a lipid mediator derived from the membrane phospholipids of a variety of cells. It is an extremely potent inflammatory mediator, promoting platelet aggregation, activating granulocytes, altering vascular tone, and increasing vascular permeability and airway responsiveness (147–149). PAF is released *in vivo* in guinea pigs and rats after inhaled or intravenous endotoxin (150,151). In isolated perfused lungs, exogenous PAF causes increased vascular pressures and edema (152,153). Intravenous administration of PAF to sheep mimics the intravenous endotoxin model of lung injury, causing transient pulmonary vascular hypertension, egress of protein-rich fluid from the vasculature, reduced compliance, and increased resistance to airflow (154–156). PAF receptor antagonists reduce the adverse pulmonary effects of endotoxin in sheep (157,158), pigs (159), and various smaller animals (151,160,161). They also attenuate some of the manifestations of the pulmonary response to exogenous cytokines in isolated guinea pig lungs (162) and in the sheep (163). PAF receptor antagonists are actively under investigation as potential asthma drugs, but their role in human sepsis and ARDS remains to be studied. The positive results in a variety of animal models suggest that sepsis and ARDS are likely areas for future development of these drugs.

PENTOXIFYLLINE

Pentoxifylline is a xanthine derivative that is currently in use for its ability to improve perfusion in human peripheral vascular disease. Its mechanisms of action are not completely understood, but it is a phosphodiesterase (PDE) inhibitor and adenosine receptor antagonist (164,165). It has diverse anti-inflammatory actions. It reduces oxygen radical release, phagocytosis, and response to PAF by human peripheral leukocytes (166,167). It also inhibits platelet aggregation (168). It inhibits the release of TNF into the circulation of mice (169), rats (170), and humans (171) in response to intravenous exposure to endotoxin, although, in the human volunteers, it did not reduce the fever and flu-like illness that occurred after endotoxin infusion (171). It does, however, appear to reduce the ability of cytokines to activate granulocytes *in vitro* (172). Aminophylline, a more widely used xanthine-based PDE inhibitor with anti-inflammatory actions, has been observed to reduce lung edema in animal models of ARDS in part by reducing pulmonary vascular pressures (173,174). Pentoxifylline appears not to decrease pulmonary vascular pressures (175), but it also lacks aminophylline's tendency to lower systemic arterial blood pressure in sepsis (176).

A number of studies in animal models of sepsis and ARDS have shown that pentoxifylline has a beneficial effect. The drug prolongs survival after exposure to endotoxin in mice and rats (169,170), producing statistically significant increases in survival in the murine model when administered up to 4 h after the initial insult. In dogs, it reduces the development of increased lung permeability after protease injury (177). It also reduces pulmonary edema in a lung lavage model of ARDS in rabbits (175). In guinea pigs, pentoxifylline diminishes the granulocyte sequestration, increased vascular permeability and accumulation of oxidants in the lungs after gram-negative sepsis (176,178), and blocks the lung injury caused by intravenous TNF (179).

These data imply that pentoxifylline may be of value in human sepsis and ARDS, but this value is wholly speculative at present and remains to be studied. Of more general importance may be studies with selective and specific PDE inhibitors. For example, inhibitors of the calcium-independent, adenosine $3',5'$-cyclic monophosphate cAMP–specific PDE type 4 have diffuse anti-inflammatory actions and are under consideration as anti-asthma drugs (180). New classes of compounds such as PDE 4 inhibitors will be studied for their potential utility in sepsis and ARDS.

PROSTAGLANDINS E_1 and E_2

ARDS is associated with increased pulmonary arterial pressure (PAP) and pulmonary vascular resistance (PVR), which are probably the result of both active vasoconstriction and of the loss of microvasculature (18). Elevated pulmonary arterial pressure and PVR correlate with a poor prognosis (181,182), and vasodilator therapy thus has theoretical appeal. It is important to recognize, however, that pulmonary vasoconstriction may at times serve an adaptive purpose in ARDS by diverting blood away from the more damaged areas of lung (183). The loss of hypoxic vasoconstriction in ARDS (89,90) may contribute to the gas exchange abnormalities, and almitrine, a pulmonary vasoconstrictor agent, has been observed to increase arterial oxygen tension transiently in ARDS patients, at the expense of further elevation in pulmonary arterial pressure (184). The actions of exogenous pulmonary vasodilators on ARDS are complex (91,185; see below). Typically, as pulmonary arterial pressure and PVR fall, ventilation-perfusion matching deteriorates and arterial oxygen tension drops. There is often, however, a simultaneous rise in cardiac output, and net oxygen delivery either does not change or increases somewhat.

PGE_1 is a vasodilatory lipid mediator that has anti-inflammatory actions (82,186). In sheep given intravenous endotoxin, it reduces PAP and the rate of lung extravascular fluid accumulation (88). In dogs with oleic acid lung injury, PGE_1 improves gas exchange but does not alter hemodynamics (187). The vasodilator PGE_2 also has anti-inflammatory actions (83), including suppression of endotoxin-induced TNF production (188). The two agents share some suppressive actions on inflammatory cells, such as attenuation of release of leukotriene B_4, oxygen radicals, and cytotoxic enzymes from activated granulocytes (e.g., 189,190). PGE_2 also blunts the pulmonary response to endotoxin of the sheep (87). We will focus on PGE_1, which has been the subject of extensive human studies.

In patients with ARDS, PGE_1 lowers pulmonary arterial pressures and increases shunt fraction; arterial oxygen tension falls in most studies, but oxygen uptake and/or delivery are either preserved or increased due to increased cardiac output (191–193). A prospective trial by Holcroft et al. (194) of a 7-day intravenous infusion of PGE_1 in 41 surgical patients with ARDS demonstrated a significant survival benefit at 30 days, although the overall survival benefit at day 75 did not achieve statistical significance ($p < .08$). The patients' gas exchange generally improved, and they tolerated the therapy well, with the exception of mild hypotension. A subsequent prospective multicenter trial by Bone et al. (195) in 100 medical and surgical ARDS patients did not show any survival benefit from PGE_1 therapy. In fact, there was a statistically nonsignificant trend toward increased mortality among the treated patients at 30 days and 6 months. Side effects of PGE_1 were more serious, and included hypotension, fever, diarrhea, and supraventricular dysrhythmia. It is possible that this study contained sicker patients. In the Holcroft study, the subjects seemed to have less severe gas exchange abnormalities, and any patients with congestive heart failure were excluded. Another multicenter trial is currently in progress in which liposome-bound PGE_1 will be used. Pending such data, however, the use of the drug in ARDS is not recommended.

ANTIOXIDANTS

Highly reactive "free radical" metabolites of oxygen, which include hydrogen peroxide (H_2O_2), the hydroxyl radical (•OH), the superoxide anion (•O_2^-), and hypochlorous acid (HOCl), are among the potentially destructive substances released by activated inflammatory phagocytes (196,197). These substances are normally held in check in the lung by elaborate defense mechanisms that include antioxidant enzyme systems [superoxide dismutase (SOD), catalase, and the glutathione (GSH) redox cycle] and various smaller-molecular-weight soluble oxidant scavengers (e.g., vitamin E, β-carotene, vitamin C, uric acid, and free GSH) (198). It has been proposed, however, that in states of unusual inflammatory activity and oxidant stress, such as ARDS, these defenses may fail and expose lung tissues to oxidant damage (198,199). Increased amounts of H_2O_2 have been found in the expired breath of patients with ARDS (200,201). Oxidant-mediated damage has been demonstrated in endothelial cell cultures (202,203) and in explants of pulmonary parenchyma (204), as well as in isolated perfused lungs, where oxidant injury results in increased permeability edema reminiscent of ARDS (205,206). A number of pharmacologic strategies to enhance pulmonary antioxidant defenses are potentially applicable to ARDS (198). These include augmentation of stores of antioxidant enzymes (superoxide dismutase, catalase), augmentation of glutathione stores, and addition of small-molecular-weight free radical scavengers.

Supplementing antioxidant enzyme stores with exogenous SOD and/or catalase has so far produced mixed results in animal models of sepsis and ARDS. The inconsistent nature of these data may be due to the heterogeneous models and dosing schedules used, to the poor ability of native SOD and catalase to cross membranes, and to the potential for SOD, under certain circumstances, to create injurious amounts of H_2O_2 and •OH (198,207,208). Administration of native enzyme, alone or in a cocktail with other antioxidants, has, in various studies, appeared beneficial (209–212), ineffective (213–216), or deleterious (207). Delivering exogenous enzymes via liposomes to enhance transmembrane penetration appears to attenuate pulmonary oxygen toxicity (217,218), as does administration of enzyme stabilized by polyethylene glycol (219), which also appears to reduce septic lung injury in guinea pigs (220). A future consideration will be targeted augmentation of enzymes by transfective gene therapy (221).

Oxidant-induced lung injury is associated with depletion of GSH in lung tissue (222) and ARDS patients have reduced amounts of GSH in BAL fluid (223). N-acetylcysteine (NAC) has dual potential therapeutic mechanisms in oxidant injury: it may replenish GSH (224) and is a direct free radical scavenger (225). NAC has been shown to reduce significantly the lung injury due to endotoxemia in sheep and pigs (226,227) and hyperoxic injury in dogs (228). A pilot study in ARDS patients by Bernard et al. (229) showed that NAC did replenish GSH (measured as red blood cell GSH stores). With the exception of increased cardiac output, oxygen uptake, and oxygen delivery, however, there were no significant changes in the patients (gas exchange, thoracic compliance, chest radiograph appearance) (229). Further data in humans need to be collected on NAC [and potentially on related GSH congeners (230)].

Dimethylthiourea is a small-molecular-weight oxygen radical scavenger, primarily of •OH, that can prevent oxidant lung injury in rats (231,232). It has also been observed to inhibit pulmonary hypertension, increased lung permeability, hypoxemia, and lung edema due to endotoxin infusion in pigs (233). It is ineffective, however, in a similar model in sheep (234), and may be difficult to use clinically due to its limited scavenging capacity per molecule, necessitating high concentrations of the compound *in vivo* (198).

In summary, despite the large amount of data that have been collected on antioxidant manipulations in animal models of ARDS and ARDS itself, the value of these therapies remains unknown. More studies are required before we will be able to evaluate fully these theoretically appealing options.

ANTIPROTEASES

Enzymes such as the serine protease elastase and the metallopeptidases collagenase and gelatinase are important elements in the armamentarium of phagocytic inflammatory cells that can damage lung tissue, and thus may be involved in ARDS (199,235–237). Both McGuire et al. (238) and Lee et al. (239) found that a majority of ARDS patients had elevated levels of proteolytic activity in BAL fluid; this activity seems to consist predominantly of neutrophil elastase. Elevated levels of granulocyte collagenase have also been found in ARDS BAL fluid (240). Other studies, however, have not shown physiologically relevant elastase activity, probably due to inactivation of the enzyme by endogenous antiproteases (241–243). The issue remains unsettled, and the data may reflect heterogeneity among patients. The amount of available antiprotease activity in the lung is certain to vary from patient to patient, and to be complexly influenced by the rate of antiprotease inactivation by granulocytes (244–247), the individual's premorbid state (cigarette smoking?, preexisting lung disease?), and the rate of leakage of plasma protease inhibitor into the extravascular space versus the rate of protease release by activated leukocytes. Urinary desmosine excretion, an indicator of *in vivo* elastolysis, however, has been found to correlate with the degree of lung injury in ARDS (248). Similarly, elevated circulating plasma levels of elastase bound to α_1-antiprotease (α_1AP) correlate with an increased risk of ARDS in trauma patients (249).

Some preliminary animal data imply that exogenous antiproteases can block lung injury (e.g., 250,251) and antiprotease therapy in ARDS is an appropriate subject for further study. An important issue to be resolved is that of the optimum mode of antiprotease delivery. The lack of toxicity of exogenous α_1AP in humans has been shown (252), but α_1AP may poorly penetrate the compartmentalized microenvironment that inflammatory cells maintain between themselves and the targets of proteolysis (235). The use of small-molecular-weight serine protease inhibitors (251) or gene therapy (253–256) could prove preferable.

SURFACTANT REPLACEMENT

Pulmonary surfactant is a complex of phospholipids, neutral lipids, and proteins that is secreted into the alveoli by type II pneumocytes and whose primary function is to reduce alveolar surface tension (257). Experimental disruption of surfactant function in adult animals results in increased extravascular lung fluid (possibly due to increased hydrostatic driving force between the pulmonary microvasculature and the adjacent high-surface-tension alveoli) and reduced lung compliance (258–260). ARDS is associated with surfactant abnormalities. Petty et al. (261,262) recognized that the lung surfactant of ARDS patients had abnormal physical characteristics associated with abnormal lung pressure-volume behavior. Surfactant isolated from ARDS patients by BAL has an abnormally high surface tension (263,264). This seems to result, at least in part, from abnormal composition: ARDS surfactant apparently has a reduced lecithin/sphingomyelin ratio and reduced content of phosphatidylcholine and phosphatidylglycerol (263–265).

Surfactant is also inactivated by pulmonary edema fluid from various animal models of ARDS (266–268); soluble proteins, e.g., fibrin monomers, albumin, or hemoglobin, may be responsible (266,267,269). The oxidant and proteolytic factors released by human granulocytes also inactivate surfactant (270). Finally, decreased overall surfactant synthesis has been noted in a rat model of sepsis (271). There is little, if any, evidence that surfactant defects are an important factor in the genesis of ARDS. They may, however, help to perpetuate pulmonary edema (by imposing a hydrostatic burden that opposes the removal of alveolar fluid) and atelectasis. Reduced lung compliance may complicate patients' ventilator management and predispose them to barotraumatic complications.

Surfactant replacement therapy in the neonatal respiratory distress syndrome has been widely studied (257,272). The experience in ARDS is much less extensive. The effect of administration of exogenous surfactant has been studied in several animal models of ARDS. Rabbits with pulmonary edema after vagotomy, for example, have improved gas exchange and lung compliance after the administration of exogenous surfactant (267). Rabbits with hyperoxic lung injury have less pulmonary edema and better ventilation-perfusion matching when given exogenous surfactant (273). Analogous positive results have been obtained using other models: guinea pigs with pulmonary edema after lung lavage (274), mineral acid or bile acid aspiration in rabbits (275,276), and postviral ARDS in rats (277).

The published experience with surfactant replacement in humans with ARDS remains scant. Richman et al. (278) gave exogenous surfactant to three such patients. All three achieved modest improvement in gas exchange, although this was transient in two of the three. No changes in lung mechanics or radiographic abnormalities occurred. There were no complications. Larger trials are reportedly in progress, but, until such data become available, the routine use of exogenous surfactant in ARDS cannot be recommended.

CONCLUSION

A number of potential pharmacotherapies for sepsis and ARDS are logical within the limits of our understanding of the disorder. That their efficacy has yet to be demonstrated may reflect in part the difficult and time-consuming nature of data collection from patients in large trials and in part a multifactorial pathogenesis. We await the results of the ongoing clinical trials mentioned above. In the long run, combinations of complementary pharmacotherapies may be the key to greater success (84,279,280). For now, the primary task facing the clinician is to provide the ARDS patient with aggressive supportive care while minimizing the complications inherent in the aggressive management of the critically ill patient.

ACKNOWLEDGMENT

Supported by HL27274 and the Allen & Hanburys Respiratory Institute.

REFERENCES

1. Ashbaugh DG, Bigelow DB, Petty TL, Levine BE. Acute respiratory distress in adults. *Lancet* 1967;2:319–323.
2. Murray JF, and the staff of the Division of Lung Diseases, National Heart, Lung and Blood Institute. Mechanisms of acute respiratory failure. *Am Rev Respir Dis* 1977;115:1071–1078.
3. Fowler AA, Hamman RF, Zerbe GO, et al. Adult respiratory distress syndrome: prognosis after onset. *Am Rev Respir Dis* 1985;132:472–478.
4. Montgomery AB, Stager MA, Carrico CJ, Hudson LD. Causes of mortality in patients with the adult respiratory distress syndrome. *Am Rev Respir Dis* 1985;132:485–489.
5. Bartlett RH, Morris AH, Fairley HB, et al. A prospective study of acute hypoxic respiratory failure. *Chest* 1986;89:684–689.
6. Murray JF, Matthay MA, Luce JM, Flick MR. An expanded definition of the adult respiratory distress syndrome. *Am Rev Respir Dis* 1988;138:720–723.
7. Pepe PE, Potkin RT, Reus DH, et al. Clinical predictors of the adult respiratory distress syndrome. *Am J Surg* 1982;144:124–130.
8. Fowler AA, Hamman RF, Good JT, et al. Adult respiratory distress syndrome: risk with common predispositions. *Ann Intern Med* 1983;98:593–597.
9. Maunder RJ. Clinical prediction of the adult respiratory distress syndrome. *Clin Chest Med* 1985;6:413–426.
10. Fein AM, Lippmann M, Holtzman H, et al. The risk factors, incidence, and prognosis of ARDS following septicemia. *Chest* 1983;83:40–42.
11. Bone RC. The pathogenesis of sepsis. *Ann Intern Med* 1991;115:457–469.
12. Haupt MT, Kaufman BS, Carlson RW. Fluid resuscitation in patients with increased vascular permeability. *Crit Care Clin* 1992;8:341–353.
13. Hickling KG. Ventilatory management of ARDS: can it affect the outcome? *Intensive Care Med* 1990;16:219–226.
14. Hinson JR Jr, Marini JJ. Principles of mechanical ventilator use in respiratory failure. *Annu Rev Med* 1992;43:3411–361.
15. Langer M, Mascheroni D, Marcolin R, Gattinoni L. The prone position in ARDS patients: a clinical study. *Chest* 1988;94:103–107.
16. Schmitz TM. The semi-prone position in ARDS: five case studies. *Crit Care Nurse* 1991;11:22–33.
17. Brigham KL. Mechanisms of lung injury. *Clin Chest Med* 1982;3:9–24.
18. Newman JH. Sepsis and pulmonary edema. *Clin Chest Med* 1985;6:371–391.
19. Snapper JR. Lung mechanics in pulmonary edema. *Clin Chest Med* 1985;6:393–412.
20. Brigham KL, Meyrick B. Endotoxin and lung injury. *Am Rev Respir Dis* 1986;133:913–927.
21. Rinaldo JE, Christman JW. Mechanisms and mediators of the adult respiratory distress syndrome. *Clin Chest Med* 1990;11:621–632.
22. Hutchison AA, Hinson JM Jr, Brigham KL, Snapper JR. Effect of endotoxin on airway responsiveness to aerosol histamine in sheep. *J Appl Physiol* 1983;54:1463–1468.
23. Wright P, Ishihara Y, Bernard GR. Effects of nitroprusside on lung mechanics and hemodynamics after endotoxemia in awake sheep. *J Appl Physiol* 1988;64:2026–2032.
24. Simpson DL, Goodman M, Spector SL, Petty TL. Long-term follow-up and bronchial reactivity testing in survivors of the adult respiratory distress syndrome. *Am Rev Respir Dis* 1978;117:449–454.
25. Wright PE, Bernard GR. The role of airflow resistance in patients with the adult respiratory distress syndrome. *Am Rev Respir Dis* 1989;139:1169–1174.
26. McCabe WR. Gram-negative bacteremia. *Adv Intern Med* 1974;19:135–158.

27. Mattsby-Baltzer I, Alving CR. Antibodies to lipid A: occurrence in humans. *Rev Infect Dis* 1984;6:553–557.
28. Rietschel ET, Seydel U, Zähringer U, et al. Bacterial endotoxin: molecular relationships between structure and activity. *Infect Dis Clin North Am* 1991;5:753–779.
29. Markley K, Smallman E. Protection by vaccines against *Pseudomonas* infection after thermal injury. *J Bacteriol* 1968;96:867–874.
30. Kaijser B, Olling S. Experimental hematogenous pyelonephritis due to *Escherichia coli* in rabbits: the antibody response and its protective capacity. *J Infect Dis* 1973;128:41–49.
31. Baumgartner JD, Heumann D, Gerain J, et al. Association between protective efficacy of anti-lipopolysaccharide (LPS) antibodies and suppression of LPS-induced tumor necrosis factor α and interleukin 6: comparison of O side chain-specific antibodies with core LPS antibodies. *J Exp Med* 1990;171:889–896.
32. Zinner SH, McCabe WR. Effects of IgM and IgG antibody in patients with bacteremia due to gram-negative bacilli. *J Infect Dis* 1976;133:37–45.
33. Ziegler EJ, McCutchan JA, Fierer J, et al. Treatment of gram-negative bacteremia and shock with human antiserum to a mutant *Escherichia coli*. *N Engl J Med* 1982;307:1225–1230.
34. Ziegler EJ, Fisher CJ Jr, Sprung CL, et al. Treatment of gram-negative bacteremia and septic shock with HA-1A human monoclonal antibody against endotoxin: a randomized, double-blind, placebo-controlled trial. *N Engl J Med* 1991;324:429–436.
35. Calandra T, Glauser MP, Schellekens J, et al. Treatment of gram-negative septic shock with human IgG antibody to *Escherichia coli* J5: A prospective, double-blind, randomized trial. *J Infect Dis* 1988;158:312–319.
36. McCabe WR, DeMaria A Jr, Berberich H, Johns MA. Immunization with rough mutants of *Salmonella minnesota:* protective activity of IgM and IgG antibody to the R595 (Re chemotype) mutant. *J Infect Dis* 1988;158:291–300.
37. Greenman RL, Schein RMH, Martin MA, et al. A controlled clinical trial of E5 murine monoclonal IgM antibody to endotoxin in the treatment of gram-negative sepsis. *JAMA* 1991;266:1097–1102.
38. Wheeler AP, Hardie WD, Bernard G. Studies of an antiendotoxin antibody in preventing the physiologic changes of endotoxemia in awake sheep. *Am Rev Respir Dis* 1990;142:775–781.
39. Baumgartner J-D. Immunotherapy with antibodies to core lipopolysaccharide: a critical appraisal. *Infect Dis Clin North Am* 1991;5:915–927.
40. Warren HS, Danner RL, Munford RS. Anti-endotoxin monoclonal antibodies. *N Engl J Med* 1992;326:1153–1157.
41. Goldstein G, Luce JM. Pharmacologic treatment of the adult respiratory distress syndrome. *Clin Chest Med* 1990;11:773–787.
42. Sheagren JN. Corticosteroids for the treatment of septic shock. *Infect Dis Clin North Am* 1991;5:875–882.
43. Fauci AS, Dale DC, Balow JE. Glucocorticosteroid therapy: mechanisms of action and clinical considerations. *Ann Intern Med* 1976;84:304–315.
44. Van Hal PTW, Hoogsteden HC. Inflammatory mediators and glucocorticoids. In: Bray MA, Anderson WH, eds. *Mediators of pulmonary inflammation.* New York: Marcel Dekker, 1991;593–617.
45. Thomas CS Jr, Brockman SK. The role of adrenal corticosteroid therapy in *Escherichia coli* endotoxin shock. *Surg Gynecol Obstet* 1968;126:61–69.
46. Pitcairn M, Schuler J, Erve PR, et al. Glucocorticoid and antibiotic effect on experimental gram-negative bacteremic shock. *Arch Surg* 1975;110:1012–1015.
47. Modig J, Bord T. High-dose methylprednisolone in a porcine model of ARDS induced by endotoxemia. *Acta Chir Scand (Suppl)* 1985;526:94–103.
48. White GL, Archer LJ, Beller BK, et al. Increased survival with methylprednisolone therapy in canine endotoxin shock. *J Surg Res* 1978;25:357–364.
49. Brigham KL, Bowers RE, McKeen CR. Methylprednisolone prevention of increased lung vascular permeability following endotoxemia in sheep. *J Clin Invest* 1981;67:1103–1110.
50. Toung TJK, Bordos D, Benson DW, et al. Aspiration pneumonia: experimental evaluation of albumin and steroid therapy. *Ann Surg* 1976;183:179–184.

51. Schumer W. Steroids in the treatment of clinical septic shock. *Ann Surg* 1976;184:333–341.
52. Shine KI, Kuhn M, Young LS, Tillisch JH. Aspects of the management of shock. *Ann Intern Med* 1980;93:723–734.
53. Sprung CL, Caralis PV, Marcial EH, et al. The effects of high-dose corticosteroids in patients with septic shock: a prospective, controlled study. *N Engl J Med* 1984; 311:1137–1143.
54. Veterans Administration Systems Sepsis Cooperative Study Group. Effect of high-dose glucocorticoid therapy on mortality in patients with clinical signs of systemic sepsis. *N Engl J Med* 1987;317:659–665.
55. Bone RC, Fisher CJ, Clemmer TP, et al. A controlled clinical trial of high-dose methylprednisolone in the treatment of severe sepsis and septic shock. *N Engl J Med* 1987;317:653–658.
56. Luce JM, Montgomery AB, Marks JD, et al. Ineffectiveness of high-dose methylprednisolone in preventing parenchymal lung injury and improving mortality in patients with sepsis. *Am Rev Respir Dis* 1988;138:62–68.
57. Bernard GR, Luce JM, Sprung CL, et al. High-dose corticosteroids in patients with the adult respiratory distress syndrome. *N Engl J Med* 1987;317:1565–1570.
58. Levy D. The fat embolism syndrome: a review. *Clin Orthop* 1990;261:281–286.
59. Schonfeld SA, Ploysongsang Y, DiLisio R, et al. Fat embolism prophylaxis with corticosteroids: a prospective study in high-risk patients. *Ann Intern Med* 1983;99:438–443.
60. Lindeque BGP, Schoeman HS, Dommisse GF, et al. Fat embolism and the fat embolism syndrome: a double-blind therapeutic study. *J Bone Joint Surg* 1987;69B:128–131.
61. Kallenbach J, Lewis M, Zaltzman M, Feldman C, et al. "Low-dose" corticosteroid prophylaxis against fat embolism. *J Trauma* 1987;27:1173–1176.
62. Montaner JSG, Lawson LM, Levitt N, et al. Corticosteroids prevent early deterioration in patients with moderately severe *Pneumocystis carinii* pneumonia and the acquired immunodeficiency syndrome (AIDS). *Ann Intern Med* 1990;113:14–20.
63. Gagnon S, Boota AM, Fischl MA, et al. Corticosteroids as adjunctive therapy for severe *Pneumocystis carinii* pneumonia in the acquired immunodeficiency syndrome. A double-blind, placebo-controlled trial. *N Engl J Med* 1990;323:1444–1450.
64. Bozzette SA, Sattler FR, Chiu J, et al. A controlled trial of early adjunctive treatment with corticosteroids for *Pneumocystis carinii* pneumonia in the acquired immunodeficiency syndrome. California Collaborative Treatment Group. *N Engl J Med* 1990; 323:1451–1457.
65. Mason GR, Duane GB, Mena I, Effros RM. Accelerated solute clearance in *Pneumocystis carinii* pneumonia. *Am Rev Respir Dis* 1987;135:864–868.
66. O'Doherty MJ, Page CJ, Harrington C, Nunan T, et al. Haemophilia, AIDS and lung epithelial permeability. *Eur J Haematol* 1990;44:252–256.
67. Zapol WM, Trelstad RL, Coffey JW, et al. Pulmonary fibrosis in severe acute respiratory failure. *Am Rev Respir Dis* 1979;119:547–554.
68. Hogg JC. Morphologic features of the lung in the respiratory failure associated with hypovolemic and septic shock. *Prog Clin Biol Res* 1989;308:27–35.
69. Snyder LS, Hertz MI, Harmon KR, Bitterman PB. Failure of lung repair following acute lung injury: regulation of the fibroproliferative response (Part 1). *Chest* 1990; 98:733–738.
70. Snyder LS, Hertz MI, Harmon KR, Bitterman PB. Failure of lung repair following acute lung injury: regulation of the fibroproliferative response (Part 2). *Chest* 1990; 98:989–993.
71. Snyder LS, Hertz MI, Peterson MS, et al. Acute lung injury: pathogenesis of intraalveolar fibrosis. *J Clin Invest* 1991;88:663–673.
72. Ashbaugh DG, Maier RV. Idiopathic pulmonary fibrosis in adult respiratory distress syndrome: diagnosis and treatment. *Arch Surg* 1985;120:530–535.
73. Meduri GU, Belenchia JM, Estes RJ, et al. Fibroproliferative phase of ARDS; clinical findings and effects of corticosteroids. *Chest* 1991;100:943–952.
74. Elliott CG. Pulmonary sequelae in survivors of the adult respiratory syndrome. *Clin Chest Med* 1990;11:789–800.
75. Suchyta MR, Elliott CG, Colby T, Rasmusson BY, et al. Open lung biopsy does not

correlate with pulmonary function after the adult respiratory distress syndrome. *Chest* 1991;99:1232–1237.

76. Cook JA, Wise WC, Halushka PV. Elevated thromboxane levels in the rat during endotoxic shock: protective effects of imidazole, 13-azaprostanoic acid, or essential fatty acid deficiency. *J Clin Invest* 1980;65:227–230.

77. Hales CA, Sonne L, Peterson M, et al. Role of thromboxane and prostacyclin in pulmonary vasomotor changes after endotoxin in dogs. *J Clin Invest* 1981;68:497–505.

78. Ogletree ML, Brigham KL. Effects of cyclooxygenase inhibitors on pulmonary vascular responses to endotoxin in unanesthetized sheep. *Prostaglandins Leukot Med* 1982;8:489–502.

79. Snapper JR, Hutchison AA, Ogletree ML, Brigham KL. Effects of cyclooxygenase inhibitors on the alterations in lung mechanics caused by endotoxemia in the unanesthetized sheep. *J Clin Invest* 1983;72:63–76.

80. Ogletree ML, Begley CJ, King GA, Brigham KL. Influence of steroidal and nonsteroidal anti-inflammatory agents on the accumulation of arachidonic acid metabolites in plasma and lung lymph after endotoxemia in awake sheep: measurements of prostacyclin and thromboxane metabolites and 12-HETE. *Am Rev Respir Dis* 1986;133:55–61.

81. Dusting GJ, Moncada S, Vane JR. Prostacyclin: its biosynthesis, actions, and clinical potential. *Adv Prostaglandin Thromboxane Leukotriene Res* 1982;10:59–106.

82. Kunkel SL, Chensue SW. Prostaglandins and regulation of the immune response. *Adv Inflammation Res* 1984;7:93–109.

83. Oates JA. Prostaglandins and pulmonary pathophysiology. In: Brigham KL, Stahlman MT, eds. *Respiratory distress syndromes: molecules to man.* Nashville: Vanderbilt University Press, 1990;144–149.

84. Begley CJ, Ogletree ML, Meyrick BO, Brigham KL. Modification of pulmonary responses to endotoxemia in awake sheep by steroidal and nonsteroidal anti-inflammatory agents. *Am Rev Respir Dis* 1984;130:1140–1146.

85. Henry CL Jr, Ogletree ML, Brigham KL, Hammon JW Jr. Attenuation of the pulmonary vascular response to endotoxin by a thromboxane synthesis inhibitor (UK-38485) in unanesthetized sheep. *J Surg Res* 1991;50:77–81.

86. Kühl PG, Bolds JM, Loyd JE, et al. Thromboxane receptor-mediated bronchial and hemodynamic responses in ovine endotoxemia. *Am J Physiol* 1988;254:R310–R319.

87. Brigham KL, Serafin W, Zadoff A, et al. Prostaglandin E_2 attenuation of sheep lung responses to endotoxin. *J Appl Physiol* 1988;64:2568–2574.

88. Smith ME, Gunther R, Zaiss C, Demling RH. Prostaglandin infusion and endotoxin-induced lung injury. *Arch Surg* 1982;117:175–180.

89. Weir EK, Mlczoch J, Reeves JT, Grover RF. Endotoxin and prevention of hypoxic pulmonary vasoconstriction. *J Lab Clin Med* 1976;88:975–983.

90. Newman JH, McMurtry IF, Reeves JT. Blunted pulmonary pressor responses to hypoxia in blood perfused, ventilated lungs isolated from oxygen toxic rats: possible role of prostaglandins. *Prostaglandins* 1981;22:11–20.

91. Radermacher P, Santak B, Wüst HJ, et al. Prostacyclin for the treatment of pulmonary hypertension in the adult respiratory distress syndrome: effects on pulmonary capillary pressure and ventilation-perfusion distributions. *Anesthesiology* 1990;72:238–244.

92. Bowers RE, Ellis EF, Brigham KL, Oates JA. Effects of prostaglandin cyclic endoperoxides on the lung circulation of unanesthetized sheep. *J Clin Invest* 1979;63:131–137.

93. Fuhrman TM, Hollon MF, Reines HD, et al. Beneficial effects of ibuprofen in oleic acid induced lung injury. *J Surg Res* 1987;42:284–289.

94. Jacobs ER, Soulsby ME, Bone RC, et al. Ibuprofen in canine endotoxin shock. *J Clin Invest* 1982;70:536–541.

95. Byrne K, Carey PD, Sielaff TD, Jenkins JK, et al. Ibuprofen prevents deterioration in static transpulmonary compliance and transalveolar protein flux in septic porcine acute lung injury. *J Trauma* 1991;31:155–164.

96. Gnidec AG, Sibbald WJ, Cheung H, Metz CA. Ibuprofen reduces the progression of permeability edema in an animal model of hyperdynamic sepsis. *J Appl Physiol* 1988;65:1024–1032.

97. Revhaug A, Michie HR, Manson JM, et al. Inhibition of cyclo-oxygenase attenuates the metabolic response to endotoxin in humans. *Arch Surg* 1988;123:162–170.
98. Bernard GR, Reines HD, Halushka PV, et al. Prostacyclin and thromboxane A_2 formation is increased in human sepsis syndrome: effects of cyclooxygenase inhibition. *Am Rev Respir Dis* 1991;144:1095–1101.
99. Perlman MB, Johnson A, Malik AB. Ibuprofen prevents thrombin-induced lung vascular injury: mechanism of effect. *Am J Physiol* 1987;252:H605–H614.
100. Perianin A, Giroud J-P, Hakim J. Differential in vivo effects of indomethacin, ibuprofen, and flurbiprofen on oxygen-dependent killing activities of neutrophils elicited by acute nonimmune inflammation in the rat. *Inflammation* 1988;12:181–189.
101. Fujimura M, Nishioka S, Kumabashiri I, et al. Effects of aerosol administration of a thromboxane synthetase inhibitor (OKY-046) on bronchial responsiveness to acetylcholine in asthmatic subjects. *Chest* 1990;98:276–279.
102. Fujimura M, Sakamoto S, Matsuda T. Attenuating effect of a thromboxane synthetase inhibitor (OKY-046) on bronchial responsiveness to methacholine is specific to bronchial asthma. *Chest* 1990;98:656–660.
103. Christman JW, Wheeler AP, Bernard GR. Cytokines and sepsis: what are the therapeutic implications? *J Crit Care* 1991;6:172–182.
104. Dinarello CA. The proinflammatory cytokines interleukin-1 and tumor necrosis factor and treatment of the septic shock syndrome. *J Infect Dis* 1991;163:1177–1184.
105. Tracey KJ, Beutler B, Lowry SF, et al. Shock and tissue injury induced by recombinant human cachectin. *Science* 1986;234:470–474.
106. Remick DG, Kunkel RG, Larrick JW, Kunkel SL. Acute *in vivo* effects of human recombinant tumor necrosis factor. *Lab Invest* 1987;56:583–590.
107. Eichacker PQ, Hoffman WD, Farese A, et al. TNF but not IL-1 causes lethal lung injury and multiple organ dysfunction similar to human sepsis. *J Appl Physiol* 1991;71:1979–1989.
108. Stephens KE, Ishizaka A, Larrick JW, Raffin TA. Tumor necrosis factor causes increased pulmonary permeability and edema: comparison to septic acute lung injury. *Am Rev Respir Dis* 1988;137:1364–1370.
109. Johnson J, Meyrick B, Jesmok G, Brigham KL. Human recombinant tumor necrosis factor alpha infusion mimics endotoxemia in awake sheep. *J Appl Physiol* 1989;66:1448–1454.
110. Wheeler AP, Jesmok G, Brigham KL. Tumor necrosis factor's effects on lung mechanics, gas exchange, and airway reactivity in sheep. *J Appl Physiol* 1990;68:2542–2549.
111. Wheeler AP, Hardie WD, Bernard GR. The role of cyclooxygenase products in lung injury induced by tumor necrosis factor in sheep. *Am Rev Respir Dis* 1992;145:632–639.
112. Waage A, Espevik T. Interleukin 1 potentiates the lethal effect of tumor necrosis factor α/cachectin in mice. *J Exp Med* 1988;167:1987–1992.
113. Okusawa S, Gelfand JA, Ikejima T, et al. Interleukin-1 induces a shock-like state in rabbits. *J Clin Invest* 1988;81:1162–1172.
114. Ognibene FP, Rosenberg SA, Lotze M, et al. Interleukin-2 administration causes reversible hemodynamic changes and left ventricular dysfunction similar to those seen in septic shock. *Chest* 1988;94:750–754.
115. Lee RE, Lotze MT, Skibber JM, et al. Cardiorespiratory effects of immunotherapy with interleukin-2. *J Clin Oncol* 1989;7:7–20.
116. Beutler BA, Milsark IW, Cerami A. Cachectin/tumor necrosis factor: production, distribution, and metabolic fate in vivo. *J Immunol* 1985;135:3972–3977.
117. Waage A. Production and clearance of tumor necrosis factor in rats exposed to endotoxin and dexamethasone. *Clin Immunol Immunopathol* 1987;45:348–355.
118. Michie HR, Manogue KR, Spriggs DR, et al. Detection of circulating tumor necrosis factor after endotoxin administration. *N Engl J Med* 1988;318:1481–1486.
119. Fong Y, Tracey KJ, Moldawer LL, et al. Antibodies to cachectin/tumor necrosis factor reduce interleukin 1β and interleukin 6 appearance during lethal bacteremia. *J Exp Med* 1989;170:1627–1633.
120. Shalaby MR, Waage A, Aarden L, Espevik T. Endotoxin, tumor necrosis factor-α and interleukin 1 induce interleukin 6 production *in vivo*. *Clin Immunol Immunopathol* 1989;53:488–498.

121. Debets JMH, Kampmeijer R, van der Linden MPMH, et al. Plasma tumor necrosis factor and mortality in critically ill septic patients. *Crit Care Med* 1989;17:489–494.
122. Damas P, Reuter A, Gysen P, et al. Tumor necrosis factor and interleukin 1 serum levels during severe sepsis in humans. *Crit Care Med* 1989;17:975–978.
123. Calandra T, Baumgartner J-D, Grau GE, et al. Prognostic values of tumor necrosis factor/cachectin, interleukin-1, interferon-α, and interferon-γ in the serum of patients with septic shock. *J Infect Dis* 1990;161:982–987.
124. Marks JD, Marks CB, Luce JM, et al. Plasma tumor necrosis factor in patients with septic shock: mortality rate, incidence of adult respiratory distress syndrome, and effects of methylprednisolone administration. *Am Rev Respir Dis* 1990;141:94–97.
125. Roten R, Markert M, Feihl F, Schaller MD, et al. Plasma levels of tumor necrosis factor in the adult respiratory distress syndrome. *Am Rev Respir Dis* 1991;143:590–592.
126. Hyers TM, Tricomi SM, Dettenmeier PA, Fowler AA. Tumor necrosis factor levels in serum and bronchoalveolar lavage fluid of patients with the adult respiratory distress syndrome. *Am Rev Respir Dis* 1991;144:268–271.
127. Siler TM, Swierkosz JE, Hyers TM, et al. Immunoreactive interleukin-1 in bronchoalveolar lavage fluid of high-risk patients and patients with the adult respiratory distress syndrome. *Exp Lung Res* 1989;15:881–894.
128. Calandra T, Gerain J, Heumann D, et al. High circulating levels of interleukin-6 in patients with septic shock: evolution during sepsis, prognostic value, and interplay with other cytokines: the Swiss-Dutch J5 Immunoglobulin Study Group. *Am J Med* 1991;91:23–29.
129. Wakabayashi G, Gelfand JA, Jung WK, et al. *Staphylococcus epidermidis* induces complement activation, TNF, IL-1, a shock-like state and tissue injury in rabbits without endotoxemia: comparison to *Escherichia coli. J Clin Invest* 1991;87:1925–1935.
130. Mathison JC, Wolfson E, Ulevitch RJ. Participation of tumor necrosis factor in the mediation of gram negative bacterial lipopolysaccharide-induced injury in rabbits. *J Clin Invest* 1988;81:1925–1937.
131. Beutler B, Milsark IW, Cerami AC. Passive immunization against cachectin/tumor necrosis factor protects mice from lethal effect of endotoxin. *Science* 1985;229:869–871.
132. Tracey KJ, Fong Y, Hesse DG, et al. Anti-cachectin/TNF monoclonal antibodies prevent septic shock during lethal bacteraemia. *Nature* 1987;330:662–664.
133. Opal SM, Cross AS, Kelly NM, et al. Efficacy of a monoclonal antibody directed against tumor necrosis factor in protecting neutropenic rats from lethal infection with *Pseudomonas aeruginosa. J Infect Dis* 1990;161:1148–1152.
134. Hinshaw LB, Tekamp-Olson P, Chang ACK, et al. Survival of primates in LD_{100} septic shock following therapy with antibody to tumor necrosis factor (TNFα). *Circ Shock* 1990;30:279–292.
135. Silva AT, Bayston KF, Cohen J. Prophylactic and therapeutic effects of a monoclonal antibody to tumor necrosis factor-α in experimental gram-negative shock. *J Infect Dis* 1991;162:421–427.
136. Exley AR, Cohen J, Buurman W, et al. Monoclonal antibody to TNF in severe septic shock. *Lancet* 1990;335:1275–1277.
137. Vincent J-L, Bakker J, Marécaux G, et al. Administration of anti-TNF antibody improves left ventricular function in septic shock patients: results of a pilot study. *Chest* 1992;101:810–815.
138. Starnes HF Jr, Pearce MK, Tewari A, et al. Anti-IL-6 monoclonal antibodies protect against lethal *Escherichia coli* infection and lethal tumor necrosis factor-α challenge in mice. *J Immunol* 1990;145:4185–4191.
139. Ohlsson K, Björk P, Bergenfeldt M, et al. Interleukin-1 receptor antagonist reduces mortality from endotoxin shock. *Nature* 1990;348:550–552.
140. Wakabayashi G, Gelfand JA, Burke JF, et al. A specific receptor antagonist for interleukin 1 prevents *Escherichia coli*-induced shock in rabbits. *FASEB J* 1991;5:338–343.
141. Bagby GJ, Plessala KJ, Wilson LA, et al. Divergent efficacy of antibody to tumor necrosis factor-α in intravascular and peritonitis models of sepsis. *J Infect Dis* 1991;163:83–88.
142. Alexander HR, Sheppard BC, Jensen JC, et al. Treatment with recombinant human tumor necrosis factor-alpha protects rats against the lethality, hypotension, and hypothermia of gram-negative sepsis. *J Clin Invest* 1991;88:34–39.

143. Sheppard BC, Norton JA. Tumor necrosis factor and interleukin-1 protection against the lethal effects of tumor necrosis factor. *Surgery* 1991;109:698–705.
144. Nakane A, Minagawa T, Kato K. Endogenous tumor necrosis factor (cachectin) is essential to host resistance against *Listeria monocytogenes* infection. *Infect Immun* 1988;56:2563–2569.
145. Havell EA. Evidence that tumor necrosis factor has an important role in antibacterial resistance. *J Immunol* 1989;143:2894–2899.
146. Kindler V, Sappino A-P, Grau GE, et al. The inducing role of tumor necrosis factor in the development of bactericidal granulomas during BCG infection. *Cell* 1989;56:731–740.
147. Pinckard RN, McManus LM, Hanahan DJ. Chemistry and biology of acetyl glycerol ether phosphorylcholine (platelet-activating factor). *Adv Inflammation Res* 1982;4:147–180.
148. Schlondorff D, Neuwirth R. Platelet-activating factor and the kidney. *Am J Physiol* 1986;251:F1–F11.
149. Chung KF, Barnes PJ. Platelet-activating factor and asthma. In: Kaliner MA, Barnes PJ, Persson CGA, eds. *Asthma: its pathology and treatment*. New York: Marcel Dekker, 1991;267–300.
150. Rylander R, Beijer L. Inhalation of endotoxin stimulates alveolar macrophage production of platelet-activating factor. *Am Rev Respir Dis* 1987;135:83–86.
151. Chang S-W, Fedderson CO, Henson PM, Voelkel NF. Platelet-activating factor mediates hemodynamic changes and lung injury in endotoxin-treated rats. *J Clin Invest* 1987;79:1498–1509.
152. Heffner JE, Shoemaker SA, Canham EM, et al. Acetyl glyceryl ether phosphorylcholine-stimulated human platelets cause pulmonary hypertension and edema in isolated rabbit lungs: role of thromboxane A$_2$. *J Clin Invest* 1983;71:351–357.
153. Hamasaki Y, Mojarad M, Saga T, et al. Platelet-activating factor raises airway and vascular pressures and induces edema in lungs perfused with platelet-free solution. *Am Rev Respir Dis* 1984;129:742–746.
154. Burhop KE, van der Zee H, Bizios R, et al. Pulmonary vascular response to platelet-activating factor in awake sheep and the role of cyclooxygenase metabolites. *Am Rev Respir Dis* 1986;134:548–554.
155. Burhop KE, Garcia JGN, Selig WM, et al. Platelet-activating factor increases lung vascular permeability to protein. *J Appl Physiol* 1986;61:2210–2217.
156. Christman BW, Lefferts PL, King GA, Snapper JR. Role of circulating platelets and granulocytes in PAF-induced pulmonary dysfunction in awake sheep. *J Appl Physiol* 1988;64:2033–2041.
157. Sessler CN, Glauser FL, Davis D, Fowler AA III. Effects of platelet-activating factor antagonist SRI 63-441 on endotoxemia in sheep. *J Appl Physiol* 1988;65:2624–2631.
158. Christman BW, Lefferts PL, Blair IA, Snapper JR. Effect of platelet-activating factor receptor antagonism on endotoxin-induced lung dysfunction in awake sheep. *Am Rev Respir Dis* 1990;142:1272–1278.
159. Olson NC, Joyce PB, Fleisher LN. Role of platelet-activating factor and eicosanoids during endotoxin-induced lung injury in pigs. *Am J Physiol* 1990;258:H1674–H1686.
160. Rylander R, Beijer L, Lantz RC, et al. Modulation of pulmonary inflammation after endotoxin inhalation with a platelet-activating factor antagonist (48740 RP). *Int Arch Allergy Appl Immunol* 1988;86:303–307.
161. Lantz RC, Keller GE III, Burrell R. The role of platelet-activating factor in the pulmonary response to inhaled bacterial endotoxin. *Am Rev Respir Dis* 1991;144:167–172.
162. Hocking DC, Phillips PG, Ferro TJ, Johnson A. Mechanisms of pulmonary edema induced by tumor necrosis factor-α. *Circ Res* 1990;67:68–77.
163. Horvath CJ, Kaplan JE, Malik AB. Role of platelet-activating factor in mediating tumor necrosis factor alpha-induced pulmonary vasoconstriction and plasma-lymph protein transport. *Am Rev Respir Dis* 1991;144:1337–1341.
164. Ward A, Clissold SP. Pentoxifylline: a review of its pharmacodynamic and pharmacokinaetic properties, and its therapeutic efficacy. *Drugs* 1987;34:50–97.
165. Nicholson CD. Pharmacology of nootropics and metabolically active compounds in relation to their use in dementia. *Psychopharmacol* 1990;101:147–159.

166. Bessler H, Gilgal R, Djaldetti M, Zahavi I. Effect of pentoxifylline on the phagocytic activity, cAMP levels, and superoxide anion production by monocytes and polymorphonuclear cells. *J Leukocyte Biol* 1986;40:747–754.
167. Hammerschmidt DE, Kotasek D, McCarthy T, et al. Pentoxifylline inhibits granulocyte and platelet function, including granulocyte priming by platelet activating factor. *J Lab Clin Med* 1988;112:254–263.
168. Nenci GG, Gresele P, Agnelli G, Ballatori E. Effect of pentoxifylline on platelet aggregation. *Pharmatherapeutica* 1981;2:532–538.
169. Schade UF. Pentoxifylline increases survival in murine endotoxin shock and decreases formation of tumor necrosis factor. *Circ Shock* 1990;31:171–181.
170. Noel P, Nelson S, Bokulic R, et al. Pentoxifylline inhibits lipopolysaccharide-induced serum tumor necrosis factor and mortality. *Life Sci* 1990;47:1023–1029.
171. Zabel P, Wolter D, Schönharting M, Schade UF. Oxpentifylline in endotoxemia. *Lancet* 1989;2:1474–1477.
172. Sullivan GW, Carper HT, Novick WJ Jr, et al. Inhibition of the inflammatory action of interleukin-1 and tumor necrosis factor (alpha) on neutrophil function by pentoxifylline. *Infect Immun* 1988;56:1722–1729.
173. Foy T, Marion J, Brigham KL, Harris TR. Isoproterenol and aminophylline reduce lung capillary filtration during high permeability. *Am Rev Respir Dis* 1979;46:146–151.
174. Mizus I, Summer W, Farrukh I, et al. Isoproterenol or aminophylline attenuate pulmonary edema after acid lung injury. *Am Rev Respir Dis* 1985;131:256–259.
175. Seear MD, Hannam VL, Kaapa P, et al. Effect of pentoxifylline on hemodynamics, alveolar fluid reabsorption, and pulmonary edema in a model of acute lung injury. *Am Rev Respir Dis* 1990;142:1083–1087.
176. Harada H, Ishizaka A, Yonemaru M, et al. The effects of aminophylline and pentoxifylline on multiple organ damage after *Escherichia coli* sepsis. *Am Rev Respir Dis* 1989;140:974–980.
177. Rosenfeld BA, Toung TJK, Sendak MJ, et al. Pentoxifylline attenuates edema formation in proteolytic enzyme-induced lung injury. *Crit Care Med* 1990;18:1394–1397.
178. Ishizaka A, Wu Z, Stephens KE, et al. Attenuation of acute lung injury in septic guinea pigs by pentoxifylline. *Am Rev Respir Dis* 1988;138:376–382.
179. Lilly CM, Sandhu JS, Ishizaka A, et al. Pentoxifylline prevents tumor necrosis factor-induced lung injury. *Am Rev Respir Dis* 1989;139:1361–1368.
180. Torphy TJ, Undem BJ. Phosphodiesterase inhibitors: new opportunities for the treatment of asthma. *Thorax* 1991;46:512–523.
181. Zapol WM, Snider MT. Pulmonary hypertension in severe acute respiratory failure. *N Engl J Med* 1977;296:476–480.
182. Sibbald WJ, Paterson NAM, Holliday RL, et al. Pulmonary hypertension in sepsis: measurement by the pulmonary arterial diastolic-pulmonary wedge pressure gradient and the influence of passive and active factors. *Chest* 1978;73:583–591.
183. Harris TR, Bernard GR, Brigham KL, et al. Lung microvascular transport properties measured by multiple indicator dilution methods in patients with adult respiratory distress syndrome: a comparison between patients reversing respiratory failure and those failing to reverse. *Am Rev Respir Dis* 1990;141:272–280.
184. Reyes A, López-Messa JB, Alonso P. Almitrine in acute respiratory failure: effects on pulmonary gas exchange and circulation. *Chest* 1987;91:388–393.
185. Melot C, Naeije R, Mols P, et al. Pulmonary vascular tone improves pulmonary gas exchange in the adult respiratory distress syndrome. *Am Rev Respir Dis* 1987;136:1232–1236.
186. Zurier RB. Role of prostaglandins E in inflammation and immune responses. *Adv Prostaglandin Thromboxane Leukotriene Res* 1990;21:947–953.
187. Slotman GJ, Machiedo GW, Casey KF, Lyons MJ. Histologic and hemodynamic effects of prostacyclin and prostaglandin E_1 following oleic acid infusion. *Surgery* 1982;92:93–100.
188. Kunkel SL, Spengler M, May MA, et al. Prostaglandin E_2 regulates macrophage-derived tumor necrosis factor gene expression. *J Biol Chem* 1988;263:5380–5384.
189. Ham EA, Soderman DD, Zanetti ME, et al. Inhibition by prostaglandins of leukotriene B_4 release from activated neutrophils. *Proc Natl Acad Sci USA* 1983;80:4349–4353.

190. Hecker G, Ney P, Schrör K. Cytotoxic enzyme release and oxygen centered radical formation in human neutrophils are selectively inhibited by E-type prostaglandins but not by PGI$_2$. Naunym Schmiedebergs Arch Pharmacol 1990;341:308–315.
191. Shoemaker WC, Appel PL. Effects of prostaglandin E$_1$ in adult respiratory distress syndrome. Surgery 1986;99:275–283.
192. Radermacher P, Santak B, Becker H, Falke KJ. Prostaglandin E$_1$ and nitroglycerin reduce pulmonary capillary pressure but worsen ventilation-perfusion distributions in patients with adult respiratory distress syndrome. Anesthesiology 1989;70:601–606.
193. Mélot C, Lejeune P, Leeman M, et al. Prostaglandin E$_1$ in the adult respiratory distress syndrome: benefit for pulmonary hypertension and cost for pulmonary gas exchange. Am Rev Respir Dis 1989;139:106–110.
194. Holcroft JW, Vassar MJ, Weber CJ. Prostaglandin E$_1$ and survival in patients with the adult respiratory distress syndrome: a prospective trial. Ann Surg 1986;203:371–378.
195. Bone RC, Slotman G, Maunder R, et al. Randomized double-blind, multicenter study of prostaglandin E$_1$ in patients with the adult respiratory distress syndrome. Chest 1989;96:114–119.
196. Brigham KL. Role of free radicals in lung injury. Chest 1986;89:859–863.
197. Cross CE, Halliwell B, Borish ET, et al. Oxygen radicals and human disease. Ann Intern Med 1987;107:526–545.
198. Heffner JE, Repine JE. Pulmonary strategies of antioxidant defense. Am Rev Respir Dis 1989;140:531–554.
199. Weiss SJ. Tissue destruction by neutrophils. N Engl J Med 1989;320:365–376.
200. Sznajder JI, Fraiman A, Hall JB, et al. Increased hydrogen peroxide in the expired breath of patients with acute hypoxemic respiratory failure. Chest 1989;96:606–612.
201. Baldwin SR, Simon RH, Grum CM, et al. Oxidant activity in expired breath of patients with adult respiratory distress syndrome. Lancet 1986;1:11–14.
202. Harlan JM, Killen PD, Harker LA, et al. Neutrophil-mediated endothelial injury in vitro: mechanisms of cell detachment. J Clin Invest 1981;68:1394–1403.
203. Brigham KL, Meyrick B, Berry LC Jr, Repine JE. Antioxidants protect cultured bovine lung endothelial cells from injury by endotoxin. J Appl Physiol 1987;63:840–850.
204. Martin WJ II, Gadek JE, Hunninghake GW, Crystal RG. Oxidant injury of lung parenchymal cells. J Clin Invest 1981;68:1277–1288.
205. Shasby DM, Vanbenthuysen KM, Tate RM, et al. Granulocytes mediate acute edematous lung injury in rabbits and in isolated rabbit lungs perfused with phorbol myristate acetate: role of oxygen radicals. Am Rev Respir Dis 1982;125:443–447.
206. Tate RM, Vanbenthuysen KM, Shasby DM, et al. Oxygen-radical-mediated permeability edema and vasoconstriction in isolated perfused rabbit lungs. Am Rev Respir Dis 1982;126:802–806.
207. Traber DL, Adams T Jr, Sziebert L, et al. Potentiation of lung vascular response to endotoxin by superoxide dismutase. J Appl Physiol 1985;58:1005–1009.
208. Scott MD, Meshnick SR, Eaton JW. Superoxide dismutase-rich bacteria: paradoxical increase in oxidant activity. J Biol Chem 1987;262:3640–3645.
209. Perkowski SZ, Havill AM, Flynn JH, Gee MH. Role of intrapulmonary release of eicosanoids and superoxide anion as mediators of pulmonary dysfunction and endothelial injury in sheep with intermittent complement activation. Circ Res 1983;53:574–583.
210. Flick MR, Hoeffel JM, Staub NC. Superoxide dismutase with heparin prevents increased lung vascular permeability during air emboli in sheep. J Appl Physiol 1983;55:1284–1291.
211. Milligan SA, Hoeffel JM, Goldstein IM, Flick MR. Effect of catalase on endotoxin-induced acute lung injury in unanesthetized sheep. Am Rev Respir Dis 1988;137:420–428.
212. Schneider J, Friderichs E, Heintze K, Flohe L. Effects of recombinant human superoxide dismutase on increased lung vascular permeability and respiratory disorder in endotoxemic rats. Circ Shock 1990;30:97–106.
213. Warner BW, Hasselgren P-O, James JH, et al. Superoxide dismutase in rats with sepsis: effect on survival rate and amino acid transport. Arch Surg 1987;122:1142–1146.
214. Novotny MJ, Laughlin MH, Adams HR. Evidence for lack of importance of oxygen free radicals in Escherichia coli endotoxemia in dogs. Am J Physiol 1988;254:H954–H962.

215. Broner CW, Shenep JL, Stidham GL, et al. Effect of antioxidants in experimental *Escherichia coli* septicemia. *Circ Shock* 1989;29:77–92.
216. Redl H, Lieners C, Bahrami S, et al. SOD in rat models of shock and organ failure. *Adv Exp Med Biol* 1990;264:17–27.
217. Turrens JF, Crapo JD, Freeman BA. Protection against oxygen toxicity by intravenous injection of liposome entrapped catalase and superoxide dismutase. *J Clin Invest* 1984;73:879–885.
218. Padmanabhan RV, Gudapathy R, Liener IE, et al. Protection against pulmonary oxygen toxicity in rats by the intratracheal administration of liposome-encapsulated superoxide dismutase or catalase. *Am Rev Respir Dis* 1985;132:164–167.
219. White CW, Jackson JH, Abuchowski A, et al. Polyethylene glycol-attached antioxidant enzymes decrease pulmonary oxygen toxicity in rats. *J Appl Physiol* 1989;66:584–590.
220. Suzuki Y, Tanigaki T, Heimer D, et al. Polyethylene glycol-conjugated superoxide dismutase attenuates septic lung injury in guinea pigs. *Am Rev Respir Dis* 1992;145:388–393.
221. Elroy-Stein O, Bernstein Y, Croner Y. Overproduction of human Cu/Zn-superoxide dismutase in transfected cells: extenuation of paraquat-mediated cytotoxicity and enhancement of lipid peroxidation. *EMBO J* 1986;5:615–622.
222. Schraufstätter IU, Revak SD, Cochrane CG. Proteases and oxidants in experimental pulmonary inflammatory injury. *J Clin Invest* 1984;73:1175–1184.
223. Pacht ER, Timerman AP, Lykens MG, Merola AJ. Deficiency of alveolar fluid glutathione in patients with sepsis and the adult respiratory distress syndrome. *Chest* 1991;100:1397–1403.
224. Bernard GR. N-acetylcysteine in experimental and clinical acute lung injury. *Am J Med* 1991;91(suppl 3C):54S–59S.
225. Aruoma OI, Halliwell B, Hoey BM, Butler J. The antioxidant action of N-acetylcysteine: its reaction with hydrogen peroxide, hydroxyl radical, superoxide, and hypochlorous acid. *Free Radical Biol Med* 1989;6:593–597.
226. Bernard GR, Lucht WD, Niedermeyer ME, et al. Effect of N-acetylcysteine on the pulmonary response to endotoxin in the awake sheep and upon in vitro granulocyte function. *J Clin Invest* 1984;73:1772–1784.
227. Modig J, Sandin R. Haematological, physiological and survival data in a porcine model of adult respiratory distress syndrome induced by endotoxaemia. Effects of treatment with N-acetylcysteine. *Acta Chir Scand* 1988;154:169–177.
228. Wagner PD, Mathieu-Costello O, Bebout DE, et al. Protection against pulmonary O_2 toxicity by N-acetylcysteine. *Eur Respir J* 1989;2:116–126.
229. Bernard GR, Swindell BB, Meredith MJ, et al. Glutathione (GSH) repletion by N-acetylcysteine (NAC) in patients with the adult respiratory distress syndrome (ARDS). *Am Rev Respir Dis* 1989;139:A221.
230. Morris P, Wheeler AP, Berry L, et al. Glutathione ethyl ester attentuates LPS-mediated bovine pulmonary artery endothelial cell injury. *Am Rev Respir Dis* 1992;145:A571.
231. Fox RB, Harada RN, Tate RM, Repine JM. Prevention of thiourea-induced pulmonary edema by hydroxyl radical scavengers. *J Appl Physiol* 1983;55:1456–1459.
232. Fox RB. Prevention of granulocyte-mediated oxidant lung injury in rats by a hydroxyl radical scavenger, dimethylthiourea. *J Clin Invest* 1984;74:1456–1464.
233. Olson NC, Anderson DL, Grizzle MK. Dimethylthiourea attenuates endotoxin-induced acute respiratory failure in pigs. *J Appl Physiol* 1987;63:2426–2432.
234. Wong C, Fox R, Demling RH. Effect of hydroxyl radical scavenging on endotoxin-induced lung injury. *Surgery* 1985;97:300–307.
235. Campbell EJ, Senior RM, Welgus HG. Extracellular matrix injury during lung inflammation. *Chest* 1987;92:161–167.
236. Rinaldo JE. Role of antiprotease therapy in the adult respiratory distress syndrome. In: Brigham KL, Stahlman MT, eds. *Respiratory distress syndromes: molecules to man.* Nashville: Vanderbilt University Press, 1990;271–282.
237. Petty TL. Protease mechanisms in the pathogenesis of acute lung injury. *Ann NY Acad Sci* 1991;624:267–277.
238. McGuire WW, Spragg RG, Cohen AB, Cochrane CG. Studies on the pathogenesis of the adult respiratory distress syndrome. *J Clin Invest* 1982;69:543–553.

239. Lee CT, Fein AM, Lippmann M, et al. Elastolytic activity of pulmonary lavage fluid from patients with adult respiratory-distress syndrome. *N Engl J Med* 1981;304:192–196.
240. Christner P, Fein A, Goldberg S, et al. Collagenase in the lower respiratory tract of patients with adult respiratory distress syndrome. *Am Rev Respir Dis* 1985;131:690–695.
241. Idell S, Kucich U, Fein A, et al. Neutrophil elastase-releasing factors in bronchoalveolar lavage from patients with adult respiratory distress syndrome. *Am Rev Respir Dis* 1985;132:1098–1105.
242. Weiland JE, Davis WB, Holter JF, et al. Lung neutrophils in the adult respiratory distress syndrome: clinical and pathophysiological significance. *Am Rev Respir Dis* 1986;133:218–225.
243. Wewers MD, Herzyk DJ, Gadek JE. Alveolar fluid neutrophil elastase activity in the adult respiratory distress syndrome is complexed to alpha-2-macroglobulin. *J Clin Invest* 1988;82:1260–1267.
244. Carp H, Janoff A. In vitro suppression of serum elastase-inhibitory capacity by reactive oxygen species generated by phagocytosing polymorphonuclear leukocytes. *J Clin Invest* 1979;63:793–797.
245. Cochrane CG, Spragg R, Revak SD. Pathogenesis of the adult respiratory distress syndrome: evidence of oxidant activity in bronchoalveolar lavage fluid. *J Clin Invest* 1983;71:754–761.
246. Ossanna PJ, Test ST, Matheson NR, et al. Oxidative regulation of neutrophil elastase-alpha-1-proteinase inhibitor interactions. *J Clin Invest* 1986;77:1939–1951.
247. Desrochers PE, Weiss SJ. Proteolytic inactivation of alpha-1-proteinase inhibitor by a neutrophil metalloproteinase. *J Clin Invest* 1988;81:1646–1650.
248. Tenholder MF, Rajagopal KR, Phillips YY, et al. Urinary desmosine excretion as a marker of lung injury in the adult respiratory distress syndrome. *Chest* 1991;100:1385–1390.
249. Nuytinck JKS, Goris RJA, Redl H, et al. Posttraumatic complications and inflammatory mediators. *Arch Surg* 1986;121:886–890.
250. Niehaus GD, Kimura R, Traber LD, et al. Administration of a synthetic antiprotease reduces smoke-induced lung injury. *J Appl Physiol* 1990;69:694–699.
251. Kuratomi Y, Lefferts PL, Snapper JR. Effect of SC-39026 (putative neutrophil elastase inhibitor) on endotoxin-induced changes in lung lymph flow in awake sheep. *Am Rev Respir Dis* 1989;139(4):A301.
252. Wewers MD, Casolaro MA, Sellers SE, et al. Replacement therapy for alpha₁-antitrypsin deficiency associated with emphysema. *N Engl J Med* 1987;316:1055–1062.
253. Brigham KL, Meyrick B, Christman B, et al. *In vivo* transfection of murine lungs with a functioning prokaryotic gene using a liposome vehicle. *Am J Med Sci* 1989;298:278–281.
254. Rosenfeld MA, Siegfried W, Yoshimura K, et al. Adenovirus-mediated transfer of recombinant α1-antitrypsin gene to the lung epithelium in vivo. *Science* 1991;252:431–434.
255. Canonico AE, Conary JT, Meyrick BO, Brigham KL. In vivo expression of a CMV promoter driven α-1 antitrypsin (α1AT) gene after intravenous or airway administration of DNA/liposome complex. *Am Rev Respir Dis* 1992;145:A200.
256. Plitman JD, Canonico AE, Conary JT, et al. The effects of inhaled and intravenous DNA/liposomes on lung function and histology in the rabbit. *Am Rev Respir Dis* 1992;145:A588.
257. Jobe A, Ikegami M. Surfactant for the treatment of respiratory distress syndrome. *Am Rev Respir Dis* 1987;136:1256–1275.
258. Albert RK, Lakshminarayan S, Hildebrandt J, et al. Increased surface tension favors pulmonary edema formation in anesthetized dogs' lungs. *J Clin Invest* 1979;63:1015–1018.
259. Bredenberg CE, Paskanik AM, Nieman GF. High surface tension pulmonary edema. *J Surg Res* 1983;34:515–523.
260. Nieman GF, Bredenberg CE. High surface tension pulmonary edema induced by detergent aerosol. *J Appl Physiol* 1985;58:129–136.

261. Petty TL, Reiss OK, Paul GW, et al. Characteristics of pulmonary surfactant in adult respiratory distress syndrome associated with trauma and shock. *Am Rev Respir Dis* 1977;115:531–536.
262. Petty TL, Silvers GW, Paul GW, Stanford RE. Abnormalities in lung elastic properties and surfactant function in adult respiratory distress syndrome. *Chest* 1979;75:571–574.
263. Hallman M, Spragg R, Harrell JH, et al. Evidence of lung surfactant abnormality in respiratory failure: study of bronchoalveolar lavage phospholipids, surface activity, phospholipase activity, and plasma myoinositol. *J Clin Invest* 1982;70:673–683.
264. Gregory TJ, Longmore WJ, Moxley MA, et al. Surfactant chemical composition and biophysical activity in acute respiratory distress syndrome. *J Clin Invest* 1991;88:1976–1981.
265. Pison U, Seeger W, Buchhorn R, et al. Surfactant abnormalities in patients with respiratory failure after multiple trauma. *Am Rev Respir Dis* 1989;140:1033–1039.
266. Seeger W, Stöhr G, Wolf HRD, Neuhof H. Alteration of surfactant function due to protein leakage: special interaction with fibrin monomer. *J Appl Physiol* 1985;58:326–338.
267. Berry D, Ikegami M, Jobe A. Respiratory distress and surfactant inhibition following vagotomy in rabbits. *J Appl Physiol* 1986;61:1741–1748.
268. Kobayashi T, Nitta K, Ganzuka M, et al. Inactivation of exogenous surfactant by pulmonary edema fluid. *Pediatr Res* 1991;29:353–356.
269. Holm BA, Notter RH. Effects of hemoglobin and cell membrane lipids on pulmonary surfactant activity. *J Appl Physiol* 1987;63:1434–1442.
270. Ryan SF, Ghassabi Y, Liau DF. Effects of activated polymorphonuclear leukocytes upon pulmonary surfactant *in vitro*. *Am J Respir Cell Mol Biol* 1991;4:33–41.
271. Oldham KT, Guice KS, Stetson PS, Wolfe RR. Bacteremia-induced suppression of alveolar surfactant production. *J Surg Res* 1989;47:397–402.
272. Shapiro DL. Surfactant replacement therapy for respiratory distress syndrome. In: Brigham KL, Stahlman MT, eds. *Respiratory distress syndromes: molecules to man.* Nashville: Vanderbilt University Press, 1990;236–249.
273. Matalon S, Holm BA, Notter RH. Mitigation of pulmonary hyperoxic injury by administration of exogenous surfactant. *J Appl Physiol* 1987;62:756–761.
274. Berggren P, Lachmann B, Curstedt T, et al. Gas exchange and lung morphology after surfactant replacement in experimental adult respiratory distress syndrome induced by repeated lung lavage. *Acta Anaesthesiol Scand* 1986;30:321–328.
275. Kobayashi T, Ganzuka M, Taniguchi J, et al. Lung lavage and surfactant replacement for hydrochloric acid aspiration in rabbits. *Acta Anaesthesiol Scand* 1990;34:216–221.
276. Kaneko T, Sato T, Katsuya H, Miyauchi Y. Surfactant therapy for pulmonary edema due to intratracheally injected bile acid. *Crit Care Med* 1990;18:77–83.
277. van-Daal GJ, So KL, Gommers D, et al. Intratracheal surfactant administration restores gas exchange in experimental adult respiratory distress syndrome associated with viral pneumonia. *Anesth Analg* 1991;72:589–595.
278. Richman PS, Spragg RG, Merritt TA, et al. Administration of porcine-lung surfactant to humans with ARDS; initial experience. *Am Rev Respir Dis* 1987;135:A5.
279. Sielaff TD, Sugerman HJ, Tatum JL, Blochner CR. Successful treatment of adult respiratory distress syndrome by histamine and prostaglandin blockade in a porcine *Pseudomonas* model. *Surgery* 1987;102:350–357.
280. Opal SM, Cross AS, Sadoff JC, et al. Efficacy of antilipopolysaccharide and anti-tumor necrosis factor monoclonal antibodies in a neutropenic rat model of *Pseudomonas* sepsis. *J Clin Invest* 1991;88:885–890.

Drugs and the Lung,
edited by C.P. Page and W.J. Metzger.
Raven Press, Ltd., New York © 1994

16

Mechanisms of Airway Inflammation and Implications for Treatment of Asthma and Bronchitis

Michael J. Holtzman, Vickie R. Shannon, A. M. Masi, and Dwight C. Look

Division of Pulmonary and Critical Care Medicine, Department of Internal Medicine, Washington University School of Medicine, St. Louis, Missouri 63110

Evidence of airway inflammation in airway diseases such as asthma and bronchitis is well established by both clinical and experimental observation. Similarly, the use of anti-inflammatory drugs (especially glucocorticoids) is common (if not universal) practice in the treatment of asthma. The challenge that now confronts researchers and clinicians is twofold: defining the biochemical mechanisms responsible for airway inflammation and then determining the pharmacologic means to more effectively potentiate anti-inflammatory compounds and inhibit inflammatory ones. This chapter reviews some of the biochemical pathways (phospholipid–arachidonic acid metabolites, cell adhesion molecules, and cytokines) that modulate airway inflammation and some of the potential strategies for using this new information to improve airway function.

PHOSPHOLIPID–ARACHIDONIC ACID METABOLISM

Airway cells and tissues contain an intricate enzymatic network for phospholipid–fatty acid metabolism that leads to the formation of bioactive phospholipids such as platelet-activating factor (PAF) and to the oxygenation of fatty acids (especially arachidonic acid). At least two of the three enzymatic pathways capable of arachidonic acid oxygenation—cyclooxygenase [prostaglandin H (PGH) synthase] and lipoxygenase—are expressed at a high level in airway tissues. A third pathway—the cytochrome P-450 monooxygenase—may be expressed in the pulmonary airway (1), but experiments to date using isolated airway epithelial cells (in contrast to epidermal cells) have not provided evidence of eicosanoid formation solely by this mechanism (2). This section separately reviews (a) the phospholipase A_2 (PLA_2)

activity leading to the formation of unesterified arachidonic acid and lyso-phospholipid, (b) acetyltransferase activity responsible for converting lyso-phospholipid to PAF, (c) the PGH synthase/prostaglandin (PG) isomerase pathways that convert arachidonic acid to prostaglandins with physiologic and inflammatory activity, (d) the 15-lipoxygenase pathway capable of per-oxidatively damaging cell membranes, and (e) the 5-lipoxygenase pathway for generating leukotrienes with biologic activity. In each case, a proposal is made for modifying the expression or activity of these pathways in an at-tempt to improve function in the inflamed airway.

PLA$_2$ Activity and the Search for Selective Inhibitors

The action of phospholipases in the generation of biologically active lipids is essential, because the synthesis of eicosanoids generally requires that the substrate (arachidonic acid) be available in a nonesterified form and synthe-sis of PAF requires the concomitant generation of a lysophospholipid pre-cursor. Although the endogenous release of arachidonic acid could arise by hydrolytic cleavage from a number of cellular lipid pools (cholesterol esters, mono-, di-, and triacylglycerols, or phosphatides), it is the phosphatide frac-tion that constitutes the major source of precursor in most cell types.

At least three pathways exist for arachidonic acid release from cellular phospholipids: (a) PLA$_2$ activity directed at phosphatidylethanolamine, phosphatidylcholine, and/or phosphatidylinositol; (b) phospholipase C (PLC) plus diacylglycerol lipase directed at phosphatidylinositol and phosphatidyl-choline or PLC plus the sequential actions of a diacylglycerol kinase and a specific PLA$_2$; and (c) phospholipase D (PLD) acting on phosphatidylcholine generating free arachidonic acid by the subsequent action of a PLA$_2$. The precise quantitative importance of various phospholipases for arachidonate release is uncertain, but much of the evidence suggests that an arachidonyl-specific PLA$_2$ may be primarily responsible for substrate release leading to eicosanoid formation in some cells (3). Some members of this family of en-zymes exhibit variation with the state of cellular differentiation (4), coupling to cell surface receptors via pertussis toxin-sensitive G proteins (5), modu-lation by protein kinase C, epidermal growth factor, and cytokines (6), and calcium-dependent translocation from cytosol to membrane (7). The calcium dependency of phospholipase activity is the basis for using calcium-mobiliz-ing agents to stimulate arachidonate metabolism.

A cytosolic PLA$_2$ that fits the criteria for the type of enzyme responsible for arachidonate release has now been isolated, purified, and subjected to molecular cloning (8,9). The recombinant enzyme sequence has been used to generate cDNA probes and selective antibodies that suggest PLA$_2$ expres-sion may be increased by inflammatory cytokines such as interleukin-1α (IL-1α) and decreased by glucocorticoids (10). Additional studies of PLA$_2$ regulation may provide better definition of the molecular mechanisms that alter PLA_2 activity during airway inflammation. These studies will also have to account for possible heterogeneity of the PLA_2 family of enzymes and the complexity of their interaction with arachidonate-acceptor molecules. For example, genetically distinct isoforms of PLA_2 may be expressed and may have corresponding (stable) arachidonyl-enzyme intermediates (11). The arachidonic acid in intermediate form might then be specifically transferred to putative nucleophilic acceptors such as water (PLA_2 activity), lipids (transacylase activity), proteins in oxidative cascades (e.g., PGH synthases and lipoxygenases), or proteins that facilitate spatial translocation of arachidonic acid (i.e., extracellular release to a neighboring cell). If interaction of the arachidonyl-PLA_2 intermediate with an adjacent protein is isoform-specific, it may therefore be possible to achieve pharmacologic selectivity by drugs that are also isoform-specific.

Phospholipase Inhibitors

PLA_2 blockade would serve to decrease the formation of eicosanoids and other bioactive molecules such as lysophospholipids and PAF, but attempts to design specific and safe PLA_2 inhibitors have not yet been successful. One hypothesis for the anti-inflammatory activity of glucocorticoids has been that they inhibit phospholipase activity, and in some systems glucocorticoids appear to inhibit PLA_2 preferentially (12). This biologic effect of glucocorticoids may reflect their ability to increase the synthesis of lipocortins, but whether this mechanism represents the main activity of glucocorticoids is in doubt. Lipocortin sequence reveals consensus with other calcium- and phospholipid-binding proteins implying that lipocortins bind to phospholipids (rather than enzyme) as a basis for their inhibition of PLA_2 (13). The data cast doubt on the specificity of lipocortins as PLA_2 inhibitors because a variety of other homologous proteins exhibit the same activity. It appears more likely that glucocorticoids suppress PLA_2 synthesis by blocking mRNA synthesis and posttranscriptional expression (14). Glucocorticoids may also inhibit eicosanoid production by diminishing PGH synthase activity (see below). The availability of molecular probes to assay steady-state levels of the enzymes of arachidonate metabolism and the mRNAs encoding for them will provide an opportunity to directly assess which of these biochemical mechanisms is more important. An understanding of glucocorticoid effect might help elucidate why some cell types and some patients are relatively resistant to their pharmacologic effect (15,16).

PAF Biosynthesis and Inhibition

Platelet-activating factor (1-O-alkyl-2-acetyl-sn-glycero-3-phosphocholine) is a potent phospholipid mediator of inflammation and thrombosis. Cells involved in the inflammatory response (especially platelets, leukocytes, and endothelial cells) synthesis PAF only in response to specific stimuli, and in turn, the PAF may activate platelets and leukocytes. The PAF produced by endothelial cells is not secreted but remains bound to the surface, where it acts in concert with P-selectin to mediate the adhesion of neutrophils (17). Thus, the controlled local synthesis of PAF by endothelial cells is probably a normal early step in the inflammatory response and excessive PAF production could lead to an exaggerated local inflammatory response and resulting tissue damage. The capacity of PAF to selectively stimulate eosinophil chemotaxis (18) as well as its capacity to cause airway constriction and hypersensitivity in some studies (19) provided a further basis for its potential role as a mediator of asthmatic airway inflammation.

PAF Biosynthesis, Metabolism, and Regulation

There are two biosynthetic pathways for PAF: (a) de novo synthesis that is proposed to produce a small amount of PAF constitutively in tissues in which PAF may serve some basal physiologic role (20), and (b) a two-step remodeling pathway that is initiated by agonist binding and that is likely to be more active during inflammation (21,22). The first step involves hydrolysis of a long chain fatty acid from a precursor phospholipid via a PLA_2 to yield a lyso-PAF and free fatty acid (most frequently arachidonic acid); the second step consists of acetylation of lyso-PAF via a specific arachidonyl-CoA:lyso-PAF acetyltransferase. The acetyltransferase of endothelial cells is rapidly and transiently activated, and increases in its activity result in increased PAF biosynthesis and accumulation (23). The primary pathway for the cellular degradation of PAF is catalyzed by PAF-acetylhydrolase, which preferentially hydrolyzes the sn-2 acetyl group from PAF, resulting in the formation of biologically inactive lyso-PAF (24). Acetylhydrolase may exist either as an intracellular enzyme or as a lipoprotein-associated enzyme that exists in plasma (24). Both enzyme forms have identical substrate specificities, but differ in molecular weight, susceptibility to inhibitors and proteases, and antigenicity (25). The selective production of one form of PAF-acetylhydrolase over the other by certain cell types may be important in regulating the cellular accumulation of PAF. For instance, monocytes preferentially produce the intracellular form of the enzyme. Upon differentiation into macrophages, the plasma form of acetylhydrolase predominates. The selective production of the plasma enzyme by differentiated macrophages is associated with a marked decrease in PAF accumulation (26).

Cellular Sources of PAF

Since the discovery of PAF using rabbit basophils and platelets (27), the list of cells capable of synthesizing this compound (in humans) has expanded to include neutrophils, eosinophils, macrophages, and vascular endothelial cells (28). Some studies indicate that PAF may also be generated by human basophils and certain B- and T-cell lines (29). Activated mast cells and alveolar macrophages release PAF in response to specific allergens (30,31), suggesting that PAF formation may be important in the pathophysiology of atopic diseases.

Based on the possibilities that airway epithelial cells are a source of inflammatory mediators and that PAF may be a critical mediator for airway inflammation and hypersensitivity, we compared PAF production by airway epithelial and vascular endothelial cells using stable isotope dilution negative-ion chemical-ionization gas chromatography–mass spectrometry (GC-MS) (32). Both primary cultures of airway epithelial cells isolated from human and ovine tracheal mucosa and cultures of human umbilical vein endothelial cells generated measurable amounts of PAF under basal culture conditions and significantly increased amounts upon stimulation with a calcium ionophore. The findings suggest that both the de novo pathway for PAF biosynthesis via CDP-choline:alkyl-acetyl-glycerol cholinephosphotransferase activity, and the stimulatable pathway for biosynthesis via phospholipase A_2 and acetyltransferase activity may be active in these cell types. The 1-O-hexadecyl molecular species of PAF was much more abundant than the 1-O-octadecyl species in each of these cell populations. The levels of PAF produced either by tracheal epithelial or vascular endothelial cells are lower than for neutrophils on a per cell basis. However, metabolism of PAF to long-chain acylphosphatidylcholine molecular species may be rapid in lung epithelial cells (33) and rates of PAF biosynthesis may therefore be underestimated in this cell type. Preliminary results suggest that PAF is relatively inactive for modifying β_2-integrin–mediated adhesion to airway epithelial cells (unpublished observation, B. T. Keller, D. C. Look, M. J. Holtzman), but the capacity of epithelial cell-derived PAF for modifying other cell functions (e.g., selectin-mediated adhesion) still needs to be examined.

Platelet-Activating Factor Receptors and Receptor Antagonists

An unexpected finding was that PAF exerts its biologic effect by binding to specific PAF receptors. Receptor characteristics include stereospecific activation at subnanomolar agonist concentrations, specific tachyphylaxis, linkage to phosphoinositide hydrolysis, and increases in intracellular calcium. Similar sequences for the receptor have been deduced from guinea pig lung and human leukocyte cDNA libraries (34,35), but receptor heterogeneity among cell types is still a possibility. This receptor-binding property of PAF has led to the development of compounds with PAF-antagonistic properties, which include structurally related synthetic compounds (CV-3988 and Ro-193704), unrelated synthetic compounds (hetrazepines such as WEB-2086 and isoquinolines such as SDZ-64412), naturally occurring antagonists (kadsurenone and ginkgolides such as BN-52063), and nonspecific PAF inhibitors (reviewed in ref. 36). Although these compounds are extremely effective in blocking PAF- and antigen-induced bronchoconstriction and hypersensitivity in experimental models, their efficacy remains unproven for preventing or reversing airway inflammation due to asthma or bronchitis.

PGH Synthase/Isomerase Heterogeneity and Prostaglandins

Each of three enzymatic steps in the production of biologically active prostaglandins—PLA_2 release of arachidonic acid substrate, PGH synthase conversion of arachidonic acid to prostaglandin endoperoxides (PGG_2 and PGH_2), and PG isomerase/synthase conversion of PGH_2 to biologically active compounds (thromboxane, prostacyclin, and other prostaglandins)—appears to be actively regulated in human airway tissue (37). In turn, each of the prominent prostaglandin products (PGE_2, $PGF_{2\alpha}$, and PGD_2) is implicated in modulating human airway function. A physiologic, anti-inflammatory role for PGE_2 is evidenced by its capacity to promote epithelial growth and differentiation (38,39), facilitate ion transport and clearance (40–42), inhibit inflammatory cytokine and leukotriene production (43,44), inhibit T cell activation and function (45), decrease the capacity of epithelial cells to be infected (46), inhibit neutrophil adherence (47,48), and act as a bronchodilator (49). By seeming contrast, $PGF_{2\alpha}$ and PGD_2 may exert a proinflammatory effect by causing bronchoconstriction (50), mucous secretion (51), cough, and hyperreactivity (52). These functional profiles fit with the observation that PGE_2 levels are decreased whereas $PGF_{2\alpha}$ and PGD_2 are increased during airway inflammation and allergen challenge (53,54). The biochemical basis for controlling the relative amounts of the different prostaglandins is based on heterogeneity and differential regulation of specific prostaglandin-forming enzymes.

PGH Synthase Heterogeneity

PGH synthase (commonly called cyclooxygenase) catalyzes the conversion of arachidonic acid (and certain other polyunsaturated fatty acids) to prostaglandin endoperoxides. The cyclooxygenase activity of PGH synthase inserts two molecules of oxygen into arachidonic acid to yield prostaglandin G_2 (PGG_2) and a peroxidase activity of the enzyme reduces PGG_2 to PGH_2 (the 15-hydroxy analogue). Nonsteroidal anti-inflammatory drugs inhibit the cyclooxygenase but not the hydroperoxidase activity of the enzyme. In particular, aspirin selectively acetylates and irreversibly inactivates the enzyme, and this action is responsible for both therapeutic effects of the drug and idiosyncratic reactions to it. Identification of the aspirin-acetylation site and other structural features of PGH synthase have been facilitated by purification of the 70-kDa enzyme from bovine and ovine seminal vesicle and by molecular cloning of the corresponding 2.7 to 3.0 kb cDNA encoding for the complete protein from ovine seminal vesicle, murine fibroblast, and human platelet cDNA libraries (55–59) and a human genomic library (60).

The PGH synthase identified in these initial studies was designated PGH synthase-1 after studies from several laboratories detected an additional form of PGH synthase mRNA and protein designated PGH synthase-2 (61–66). Molecular cloning from chicken and murine fibroblast and human endothelial cDNA libraries indicate that PGH synthase-2 mRNA is larger (4.0–4.7 kb) and contains an open-reading frame encoding for a polypeptide that is homologous (59–61%) with PGH synthase-1. Each of the two types of recombinant polypeptides exhibit PGH synthase activity in assays of transfected cells (58,64,66,67), but the possibility that the two PGH synthase isoforms might be catalytically or pharmacologically distinct was not deduced from these studies.

Previous work from our laboratory also detected a PGH synthase mRNA (4.0 kb) that was expressed at higher levels in cultured (vs. freshly isolated) ovine tracheal epithelial cells (61). We subsequently observed that aspirin treatment of the cultured epithelial cells caused a dose-dependent increase in arachidonic acid conversion to 15-hydroxyeicosatetraenoic acid (15-HETE) production from arachidonic acid (68). The 15-HETE formed by aspirin-treated ovine tracheal epithelial cells was generated by a PGH synthase-dependent mechanism because the 15-HETE–forming activity was sensitive to selective inhibition by indomethacin and was quantitatively immunoprecipitated by anti-PGH synthase antiserum. Additional immunoprecipitation experiments indicated that anti-PGH synthase monoclonal antibodies raised against the aspirin-inhibited form of the enzyme (PGH synthase-1) did not recognize the aspirin-stimulated 15-HETE–forming PGH synthase. Thus, sequential immunoprecipitation of cultured epithelial cell material first with excess anti-PGH synthase-1 monoclonal antibody (mAb) followed by anti-PGH synthase antiserum indicated that two isoforms of PGH synthase (70 and 72 kDa) were expressed in airway epithelial cells. Our findings indicated that isozymes of PGH synthase exist that are pharmacologically distinct, but these studies did not yet provide structural evidence linking the PGH synthase-related mRNA and the pharmacologically distinct PGH synthase polypeptide in cultured airway epithelial cells and did not allow direct comparison to results obtained in other cell types. Subsequently, we have isolated and sequenced a full-length cDNA for ovine PGH synthase-2 from a tracheal epithelial cell cDNA library. Analysis of PGH synthase-2 from ovine tracheal epithelial cells indicates that it contains a unique sequence that is homologous with chicken, murine, and human PGH synthase-2 (69). Recent studies indicate that human airway epithelial cells express a homologous 4.5-kb PGH synthase-2 mRNA species and exhibit the same aspirin-evoked 15-HETE forming activity found in ovine cells as an index of PGH synthase-2 catalytic activity (unpublished observations, V. Zhang, A. M. Masi, H. Hussain, and M. J. Holtzman).

Regulation of Prostaglandin-Forming Activities

Eicosanoid production from prostaglandin-generating pathways may be regulated at several levels. In addition to phospholipase-regulated substrate availability, there may be direct regulation of PGH synthases and/or isomerases by transcriptional or posttranscriptional mechanisms. The availability of genomic sequence and suitable expression systems for PGH synthases will likely uncover a host of regulatory events, but, so far, interest in cellular control of prostaglandin production has focused on regulation by growth factors, cytokines, endotoxin, and glucocorticoids. For example, prostaglandin biosynthesis is stimulated by transforming growth factors (TGF-α and -β), epidermal growth factor (EGF), and platelet-derived growth factor (PDGF) (70,71). Inhibition of growth factor–induced prostaglandin formation by actinomycin D (72) suggested that growth factors enhance transcription of the PGH synthase gene. Alternatively, the lack of actinomycin D inhibition (despite increased PGH synthase mRNA levels) in some cell types (73) suggested enhanced mRNA stability as a basis for increased PGH synthase activity. The possibility that growth factor–stimulated prostaglandin formation is actually due in some cases to stimulation of phospholipase activity has also been shown (74) and may operate via a phospholipase-activating protein (75). As additional examples, IL-1 (76), IL-2 (77), interferon-γ (78), TNF-α (79), granulocyte macrophage–colony stimulating factor (GM-CSF) (80), endotoxin (81), sphingosine (82), and phorbol ester (83) have been shown to stimulate prostaglandin generation, which in some cases occurred via de novo synthesis of PGH synthase protein (84). The enhanced synthesis was often inhibitable by glucocorticoids (81,85).

These interesting (and sometimes contradictory) effects on prostaglandin formation were difficult to understand until PGH synthase-1 and PGH synthase-2 cDNAs were isolated. The availability of these molecular probes permitted the first direct studies of transcriptional regulation of the PGH synthase pathway and results soon indicated that PGH synthase regulation is more complicated than predicted for a single gene–single polypeptide system. One of the initial studies to report that induction of a second PGH synthase gene might be responsible for augmented prostaglandin synthesis was performed in ovine tracheal epithelial cells. Analysis of epithelial cell PGH synthase mRNA suggested that PGH synthase synthesis and activity in cultured epithelial cells is increased by augmented transcription of the 2.8-kb PGH synthase-1 gene and by increased transcription of a second 4.0-kb PGH synthase gene (PGH synthase-2) (61). Subsequent studies from other laboratories using transformed chicken and mouse fibroblasts and human vascular endothelial cells also detected an additional PGH synthase-2 mRNA (62–64,66). Evidence of selective regulation of PGH synthase-2 mRNA levels by stimulatory factors and by glucocorticoids has led to the proposal of a regulated PGH synthase-2 gene (implicated in inflammation and/or cell growth) and a constitutive PGH synthase-1 gene (for physiologic activities) (66,67,86).

In some cell types, there are distinct features that may contribute further to the overall hypothesis for PGH synthase-1 versus PGH synthase-2 function. For example, human tracheal epithelial cells convert arachidonic acid not only to PGE_2 (as ovine cells do), but also form significant amounts of $PGF_{2\alpha}$ and PGD_2 (37). It is possible that regulatory factors cause alterations in the relative amounts of PGE_2, $PGF_{2\alpha}$, and PGD_2 due to selective alterations in the levels of PGH synthase-1, PGH synthase-2, or prostaglandin isomerases. Studies are under way to sort out the mechanisms for possible alterations in prostaglandin-forming activities in order to further develop the hypothesis that PGH synthase-1/PGE isomerase activity leads to "physiologic" PGE_2 formation, whereas PGH synthase-2/PGF synthetase/PGD isomerase activity leads to "inflammatory" $PGF_{2\alpha}$ and PGD_2 formation.

Prostaglandin Function and New Uses of Inhibitors

Initial results suggest that the prostaglandin-forming activity of PGH synthase-2 (in contrast to its 15-HETE forming activity) may be inhibited by lower concentrations of aspirin and indomethacin than required for blocking prostaglandin formation by PGH synthase-1 (68). Aspirin irreversibly inhibits PGH synthase by acetylating a single serine residue so that enhancement of the nucleophilicity of the serine hydroxyl would increase its rate of acetylation. This could result from a conformational change of the protein that juxtaposes the serine residue and an electron-rich residue such as histidine. In any case, this finding may imply that prostaglandin formation by PGH synthase-2 can be selectively inhibited by low concentrations of nonsteroidal anti-inflammatory agents and may account for some of the variability in inhibitory concentrations of these agents among tissues (87). This differential sensitivity may also offer a therapeutic advantage, e.g., if the end point is selective inhibition of PGH synthase-2 in inflammatory cells. The high degree of sensitivity may also form the basis for the reactivity of some subjects to extremely low doses of aspirin (in aspirin-evoked syndromes of asthma and/or anaphylaxis). Preliminary reports also indicate that some inhibitors may offer additional selectivity for inhibiting PGH synthase-2 but not PGH synthase-1—a finding that further supports differences in catalytic mechanism between the two isoforms. Isoform-selective drugs may offer another mechanism for specific inhibition of inflammatory prostaglandins with preservation of physiologic prostaglandins.

15-Lipoxygenase and Cell Damage

Lipoxygenases catalyze the incorporation of one oxygen molecule into polyunsaturated fatty acids containing a 1,4-*cis,cis*-pentadiene structure to yield a 1-hydroperoxy-2,4-*trans,cis*-pentadiene product. The initial catalytic step is stereospecific removal of a hydrogen atom followed by antarafacial addition of molecular oxygen. Mammalian lipoxygenases also possess regiospecificity during interaction with substrate and on that basis have been designated as arachidonate 5-, 12-, or 15-lipoxygenase. The three distinct enzyme types insert oxygen at carbon 5, 12, or 15 of arachidonic acid, and the primary product is a 5*S*-, 12*S*-, or 15*S*-hydroperoxyeicosatetraenoic acid (5-, 12-, or 15-HPETE). The enzymes may also catalyze the formation of unstable epoxide intermediates that can be further metabolized to a variety of compounds, including leukotrienes (LTs) dihydroxy acids (diHETEs), epoxyhydroxy acids (hepoxilins), trihydroxy acids (lipoxins), aldehydes, and glutathione adducts.

Following the discovery of arachidonate 5-, 12-, and 15-lipoxygenases in leukocytes and platelets, a natural question was whether these enzymes were also expressed in nonhematopoietic cell types. Subsequent work has defined a highly active 15-lipoxygenase pathway in human airway epithelial cells (88–90), a related 12-lipoxygenase in bovine and rabbit tracheal epithelial cells (91–93), and 5-lipoxygenase activity in canine, ovine, and equine airway epithelial cell preparations (89,94–96). It is possible that the heterogeneity among species represents molecular divergence within a family of closely related enzymes. This hypothesis is most plausible with respect to 12- and 15-lipoxygenases in view of their highly similar enzymatic characteristics and primary structure (97,98).

Biology of the 15-lipoxygenase pathway takes on added interest because it is also the predominant pathway for arachidonic acid metabolism in whole lung tissue (99,100) and may be increased in asthmatic bronchial tissue (101). In addition, the major 15-lipoxygenase end product derived from arachidonic acid (15-HETE) is found in lavage fluid from asthmatic airways (102) and is released selectively by airway epithelial cells and eosinophils (103), two cell types that are implicated in the development of asthmatic airway inflammation.

The high level of 15-lipoxygenase activity in isolated human airway epithelial cells is distinctly unusual. The enzymatic activity is abundant in nasal and tracheal mucosal epithelial cells (88–90). Among other cell types, only eosinophils and reticulocytes exhibit comparable levels of activity (103). Comparison of the level of 15-lipoxygenase activity in airway epithelial cells to levels in cultured cells may be misleading, however, because 15-lipoxygenase activity appears to be lost under some culture conditions (104) and may be present in a cryptic form in other conditions (105). Immunohistochemical studies of the distribution of 15-lipoxygenase suggest that the enzyme may be expressed (at lower levels) in mucous cells, perineural cells, and vascular endothelial cells and myocytes of the upper airway and trachea of healthy humans (93,106). In contrast to airway tissue from normal subjects in which 15-lipoxygenase antigen is confined to the uppermost airways (nose and trachea) and is almost undetectable in bronchi, the bronchial tissue obtained from subjects with asthma or chronic bronchitis exhibits markedly positive immunostaining of mucosal epithelial cells with anti-15-lipoxygenase antibodies (107). The increased levels of 15-lipoxygenase antigen in bronchial epithelial cells of asthmatic and bronchitic subjects compared to the same cell population in normal subjects coupled with the previous findings of increased 15-lipoxygenase activity in asthmatic airways indicate that the epithelial 15-lipoxygenase is induced by airway inflammatory disease (107). In an analogous manner, the related 12-lipoxygenase is induced in the colonic epithelium in subjects with inflammatory bowel disease (108).

15-Lipoxygenase Function in the Airway

Evidence for proinflammatory and anti-inflammatory functions of 15-lipoxygenase products (especially 15-HETE) has been presented and recently reviewed (104). In addition, products of the 15-lipoxygenase pathway have effects on cell growth (109) and may participate in signal transduction events in neurons, endocrine cells, and perhaps mucus secreting cells (110–112). Taken together, however, there is little consensus for a biologic role of 15- (or related 12-) lipoxygenase products as mediators of airway function in humans, and the view that the products are often biologically inactive has been proposed (104,113).

An alternative role for the 15-lipoxygenase is its capacity to alter membrane composition. 15-Lipoxygenase products are incorporated into membrane phospholipids (114–117), and the enzyme actively utilizes intact phospholipid as a substrate *in vitro* and *in vivo* (118–122). Recent findings have established a link between 12-lipoxygenase and the regulation of cellular oxidation-reduction conditions (105). Cultured ovine tracheal epithelial cells may express a 12-lipoxygenase, but the enzyme may be bound to microsomal membranes (by a non–calcium-dependent mechanism) in a form that is inactive unless it is dissociated from the cytoplasm. In addition, the cytosolic inhibition of the microsomal-type 12-lipoxygenase is due at least in part to the selective sensitivity of the enzyme to cellular levels of GSH versus hydroperoxide. The pattern of sensitivity is distinct from the cytosolic 12-lipoxygenase or PGH synthase/isomerase pathways found in airway epithelial cells and may suggest that the microsomal-type 12-lipoxygenase is actively linked to the chain of enzymes that regulate cellular oxidation-reduction conditions. Activation of the airway epithelial 12-lipoxygenase by oxidant stress suggests that the enzyme may be responsible for peroxidation of membrane phospholipids (and consequent epithelial damage) during inflammation (105). These findings are analogous to the role of the enzyme in erythrocyte maturation. Reticulocyte mitochondrial membranes contain increased levels of the oxygenated derivatives of linoleic and arachidonic acids (121), and the formation of these products may destabilize membrane structure and predispose it to proteolysis during erythrocyte maturation.

Airway Epithelial Function and Arachidonic Acid Metabolism

Epithelial tissues (in skin, gut, and airway) bear the responsibility of maintaining and regulating the boundary between host and environment. This task includes protection against injury by controlling molecular access to the host and actively modulating immune and inflammatory responses to environmental agents (104). A unifying scheme for how these cellular functions are regulated at a molecular level by the products of phospholipid–arachidonic acid metabolism may be proposed that includes (a) PGH synthase-1/PGE isomerase as the physiologic pathway for PGE_2 required for normal epithelial barrier function, (b) PGH synthase-2/PGF synthase/PGD isomerase as the pathway for inflammatory prostanoids (in particular $PGF_{2\alpha}$ and PGD_2) and as such may be induced to higher levels of expression and activity by inflammation, and (c) 12- and related 15-lipoxygenases that contribute to the abnormal physiology and epithelial damage during inflammation and as such are also induced by inflammation and are activated by oxidant stress. Preservation (and improvement) in airway function therefore may rest on continuation of epithelial PGE_2 biosynthesis without induction of other PGH synthase- or lipoxygenase-catalyzed reactions.

5-Lipoxygenase and the Leukotrienes

Biosynthetic Pathways for the Leukotrienes

The arachidonate 5-lipoxygenase converts arachidonic acid to 5-HPETE and also catalyzes the formation of an unstable allylic epoxide (LTA_4) from 5-HPETE. LTA_4 may be hydrolyzed enzymatically to LTB_4 (by LTA hydrolase) or converted to LTC_4 upon addition of glutathione (by LTC synthase). Both LTB_4 and LTC_4 are exported from the cell by a carrier-mediated process (123), and both are also subject to further metabolism. LTB_4 is metabolized via cytochrome P-450 to 20-hydroxy-LTB_4 and then to 20-carboxy-LTB_4 in neutrophils, and specific ω-1 and ω-3 hydroxylation reactions have also been described (124). LTC_4 undergoes removal of glutamic acid by γ-glutamyl transpeptidase to yield LTD_4, and subsequent removal of glycine by a dipeptidase yields LTE_4.

The 5-lipoxygenase is specifically stimulated by calcium, and other enzymes in the cascade to leukotriene formation do not exhibit this requirement (125). In addition, the 5-lipoxygenase activity is enhanced by adenosine triphosphate (ATP) and to a lesser extent by other nucleotides and is sensitive to inhibition by peroxides (125). In contrast to the 12- and 15-lipoxygenases, the substrate specificity of the 5-lipoxygenase pathway is quite restricted. In contrast to the PGH synthase/isomerase pathway (where the first step is rate limiting), the rate limiting step in leukotriene biosynthesis occurs at the levels of the LTA hydrolase and LTC synthase (glutathione transferase).

Subcellular fractionation of 5-lipoxygenase activity indicates that the 5-lipoxygenase and LTA-hydrolase are soluble cytosolic enzymes. However, isolating the 5-lipoxygenase in the presence of excess calcium may increase its degree of membrane association, and this effect may mimic physiologic activation and translocation of the enzyme (126). Pharmacologic inhibitors of the translocation process may be useful in blocking leukotriene formation. In fact, at least three classes of such inhibitors have been identified and are used to isolate and clone a membrane activating protein necessary for leukotriene synthesis (127). Expression of this 5-lipoxygenase activating protein (FLAP) and the 5-lipoxygenase correlates closely with cellular leukotriene synthesis in some cells (128).

The 5-lipoxygenase has been purified and its full sequence determined by molecular cloning (129). Primary structural features have been reviewed (130). Expression of the 5-lipoxygenase cDNA in a baculovirus/insect cell system (131) and in osteosarcoma cells (132) and isolation of the complete 5-lipoxygenase gene from genomic DNA libraries (133) have now been accomplished. These advances are likely to lead to further insight into transcriptional and posttranscriptional mechanisms for lipoxygenase regulation. The 5-lipoxygenase gene appeared to be activated constitutively in mature cells of myeloid lineage, and this characteristic was consistent with the structure of the 5'-flanking region of the gene. However, it now appears that the gene may be inducible in B lymphocytes *in vitro* and *in vivo* (134,135).

The cDNA for LTA-hydrolase has also been isolated (136). The enzyme appears to be expressed in virtually all tissues and a variety of cell types, including those that lack 5-lipoxygenase activity (137). For example, LTA hydrolase but not 5-lipoxygenase is present in erythrocytes so that LTA_4 released from leukocytes can be converted to LTB_4 in the blood (138). Stimulation of LTB_4 production may also be potentiated by exercise-induced asthma (139). The mechanism of priming neutrophils for subsequent stimulation is uncertain, but a similar augmentation was observed for lipopolysaccharide treatment and was invoked as a mechanism for the pathogenesis of gram-negative sepsis (140). The possibility that 5-HETE and LTB_4 may in turn augment the release of additional inflammatory mediators has also been demonstrated (141).

Leukotriene Function

The leukotrienes derived from 5-HPETE have been implicated as critical mediators of inflammation, and their effects on the airways and on the microcirculation have been reviewed (142). LTB$_4$ is a potent chemoattractant and binds with high affinity in a stereospecific and saturable manner to receptors on the cell membrane of neutrophils (143). Leukotrienes C$_4$ and D$_4$, but to a lesser extent E$_4$, are potent inducers of contraction of airway, vascular, and intestinal smooth muscle by mechanisms dependent on calcium mobilization (144). The importance of the leukotrienes for pathophysiologic events has become even more convincing with the availability of specific inhibitors of the 5-lipoxygenase pathway. A variety of orally active 5-lipoxygenase inhibitors and LTD- and LTB-receptor antagonists have reached the stage of clinical testing, and some of the compounds appear to be effective in blocking bronchoconstriction (145). Results also suggest considerable heterogeneity in eicosanoid release and/or action depending on the inflammatory condition and on the individual.

Eicosanoids and Pharmacologic Approaches

The drive to establish treatment for over- or underproduction of eicosanoids has led to the development of useful agonist and antagonist drugs. The use of the eicosanoids themselves as drugs, e.g., PGE analogues as antiviral anti-inflammatory agents (146), is also under way, and the establishment of new roles for old drugs, e.g., theophylline's effects on leukotriene generation (147), is also an interesting side effect of research on arachidonic acid metabolism.

There are four critical components involved in the reaction for oxygenation of arachidonic acid: enzyme, two substrates (arachidonic acid and oxygen), and activator (e.g., lipid hydroperoxide). Any agent that interferes with the availability or function of any of these components will inhibit the generation of oxygenation products. Once the reaction is complete, pharmacologic inhibition can still be effective if cellular release of products or the subsequent binding to specific cellular receptors is prevented. The available strategies for phospholipid-arachidonate pharmacology are based on each of the biochemical steps involved in PAF and eicosanoid generation, release, and receptor binding (Fig. 1).

Substrate Availability

Arachidonic acid is a fatty acid of the n-6 type and is oxygenated rapidly under conditions in which the n-3 type (with the last double bond three carbons from the methyl end) is oxidized at an undetectable rate. This differ-

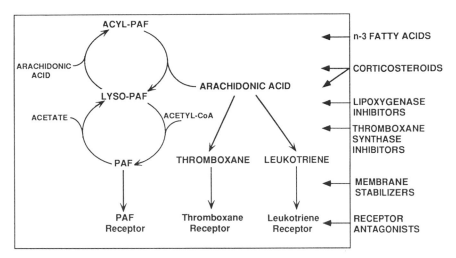

FIG. 1. Pharmacologic strategies for modulating phospholipid-arachidonic acid metabolism. Each of the biochemical steps involved in PAF/eicosanoid generation, release, and receptor binding are diagrammed inside the box, and some of the current approaches to inhibition of these steps are listed outside the box.

ence is the basis for the antagonism of n-6 eicosanoid formation by n-3 fatty acids such as eicosapentaenoic acid (EPA). EPA ingestion may lower normal stores of arachidonate, compete with arachidonate for oxygenation, and potentially alter substrate milieu to influence arachidonate uptake and releasability (148). Dietary supplementation with EPA can markedly attenuate the capacity of the leukocytes to generate leukotriene, and may also attenuate the late asthmatic response to allergen (149). So far, however, EPA treatment has resulted in little effect on the severity of asthma (149,150).

A second point of pharmacologic attack on the arachidonate cascade is aimed at inhibition of phospholipase and consequent diminution in substrate release. As noted above, a theory of anti-inflammatory activity of glucocorticoids is based on blocking mediator generation via suppression of PLA_2 (12), and so far, these agents have been the only practical means of PLA_2 inhibition for airway inflammation in humans. Significant advances in the use of these agents has been restricted to developing compounds that can be restricted to the lung and that yield higher potency and duration of action.

Product Biosynthesis and Binding

Similarity of the initial enzymatic reaction of cyclo- and lipooxygenation gives rise to the corollary that the pathways are susceptible to so-called dual inhibitors. Certain acetylenic fatty acids, such as eicosatetraynoic acid (ETYA) inhibit the enzymes by acting as suicide substrates, and others like nordihydroguaiaretic acid (NDGA) and phenidone or its pyrazoline analogues (e.g., BW755C) most likely act as free radical scavengers or antioxidants. The nonspecificity of these drugs render them only modestly useful for defining enzymatic mechanisms *in vitro,* and their toxicity make them unacceptable for human use. However, the strategy of an effective dual inhibitor for *in vivo* use remains attractive.

The most thorough understanding of a mechanism for selective oxidative inhibition is the one for PGH synthase inactivation by aspirin as noted above. In fact, one of the best examples of altered arachidonate metabolism affecting airway physiology is the link between PGH synthase inhibition and asthmatic bronchoconstriction (aspirin-evoked asthma). Proposed mechanisms include (a) loss of the influence of PGs on airway function, e.g., the loss of PGE bronchodilatory tone; (b) augmented production of other mediators (e.g., lipoxygenase products); and (c) an altered sensitivity to the effects of lipoxygenase products. Recent studies in support of these possibilities demonstrate that aspirin-sensitive asthmatics release higher levels of histamine and LTC_4 (but not lower levels of PGE_2) into nasal secretions after aspirin challenge (151) and that airway responsiveness to LTE_4 is increased compared to subjects without sensitivity or in the same subjects following desensitization (152). A unifying hypothesis is that endogenous PGE might be responsible for tonic inhibition of 5-lipoxygenase activity, and that a decrease of PGE would lead to leukotriene formation is susceptible individuals (so-called disinhibition). Efforts to test this hypothesis (and prevent aspirin-evoked syndromes) by treatment with PGE analogues have reported initial success.

Perhaps the most successful new drugs aimed at specifically decreasing airway inflammation are those capable of inhibiting the action of leukotrienes. A variety of orally active 5-lipoxygenase inhibitors have reached the stage of clinical testing (e.g., LY-170,680, A-64077, WY-50,295, Ro 24-5913) and have proven to be effective in blocking bronchoconstriction induced by cold, dry air (153). LT biosynthesis may also be blocked by drugs that have no effect on the 5-lipoxygenase itself but may prevent lipoxygenase-activation by blocking translocation of the enzyme from the cytosol to the membrane (see above). Whether this approach will offer an effective strategy is currently being tested *in vivo.* Specific LTD/E receptor antagonists (e.g., MK-571, SKF-104,353, and ICI-204,219) that inhibit antigen- and LT-induced bronchoconstriction have also been developed (154–156) and are more potent and selective than the first generation FPL-55712 or LY-171,883. One of these agents (MK-571) is effective in blocking bronchoconstriction induced by exercise (157) and shows clinical efficacy in mild asthma (158).

A focus of arachidonate-pharmacologic interaction has been the role of eicosanoids in both the early and late asthmatic response to allergen (159). During the early response, detection of thromboxane (Tx) release (160–162) and slight inhibition of bronchoconstriction by thromboxane receptor antagonists (e.g., GR32191) (163) suggest a small role for TxA_2 in the physiologic response. Release of histamine, PAF, and sulfidopeptide leukotrienes (presumably from mast cells) may contribute to the remainder of the early bronchoconstrictor response and therefore be inhibitable by drugs that prevent mediator release and/or relax smooth muscle such as cromolyn or β_2-adrenergic agonists (164). Identification of the mediators responsible for the late response are less certain but increases in LTC_4 (165) and inhibition by indomethacin (160) suggest a role for eicosanoids. Studies of LTD receptor antagonists or LTC synthesis inhibitors are under way. A selective LTB receptor antagonist has also been used to inhibit bronchopulmonary eosinophil influx during the late response in guinea pigs (166) but is untested in humans. The development of the late response appears dissociable from the attendant change in airway reactivity because indomethacin may have no effect on the late response but still inhibit the concomitant increase in reactivity in some patients (167). By contrast, other states of nonspecific airway hyperreactivity are unaffected by indomethacin (168). Taken together, the results suggest considerable heterogeneity in eicosanoid release and/or action depending on the inflammatory condition and on the individual.

CELL ADHESION MOLECULES

The influx of inflammatory cells (particularly eosinophils, neutrophils, and lymphocytes) into the airway is a central process in the development of late-phase reactions to allergen, bronchial hyperresponsiveness to inhaled agonists, and presumably to the clinical manifestations of asthma. The migration of leukocytes into the airway is dependent upon a series of cellular and molecular interactions that enable the resident airway cells to selectively recruit and command leukocytes in defense of the underlying tissues. By developing monoclonal antibodies against epitopes on the leukocyte surface and screening the hybridoma clones for blocking activity, investigators have discovered that a crucial step in the migration of these leukocytes is the coordinated expression and interaction of specific cell adhesion molecules on both the lung parenchymal cells and the migrating leukocytes (169–171). Thus, a new scheme for leukocyte recruitment has developed that revolves around the regulated expression of three distinct families of cell adhesion receptors, notably the cell adhesion molecule (CAM) members of the immunoglobulin supergene family, the integrins, and the selectins. In experimental models, the inhibition of cell adhesion molecule function also blocks inflammation and the alterations in biologic function that accompany the inflammatory response (172–176).

At least three interactions of cell adhesion molecules have been implicated in the development of airway inflammation. The best studied is the interaction between intercellular adhesion molecule-1 (ICAM-1) on endothelial and epithelial cells with the leukocyte β_2-integrins LFA-1 or Mac-1. ICAM-1 is up-regulated on vascular endothelial and airway epithelial cells and β_2-integrins are activated on leukocytes after cytokine or lipid mediator stimulation (177–182). ICAM-1 also serves as the receptor for the major group of human rhinoviruses (183,184). Immunohistochemical studies have demonstrated increased immunostaining for ICAM-1 in airway biopsy or brush specimens from asthmatic compared to normal subjects, and the level of immunostaining may correlate with disease severity (185,186). In two animal models of asthma (guinea pig and cynomolgus monkey), intravenous or inhaled treatment of the animals with a blocking monoclonal antibody directed against either ICAM-1 or β_2-integrins attenuated both leukocyte (particularly eosinophil) influx and airway hyperreactivity (173,180). In addition, treatment with both glucocorticoids and anti-ICAM-1 monoclonal antibodies were more effective than glucocorticoids alone in the model of chronic airway inflammation and hyperreactivity in cynomolgus monkeys (187). In the same model, an anti-Mac-1 blocking antibody did not inhibit eosinophil influx, but it did decrease eosinophil activation and airway hyperreactivity (188). The results suggest that leukocyte influx versus activation are regulated by distinct β_2-integrin–dependent mechanisms and that each is required for the development of airway hyperreactivity.

Two other molecular interactions have been implicated in the development of airway inflammation: endothelial-leukocyte adhesion molecule-1 (ELAM-1 or E-selectin) binding to its leukocyte sialyl–Lewis X carbohydrate ligand and vascular cell adhesion molecule-1 (VCAM-1) binding to the leukocyte β_1-integrin VLA-4. It appears that an initial event in leukocyte recruitment is adhesion to the vascular endothelium (mediated by selectin) followed by diapedesis through the vascular endothelium (regulated by ICAM-1) (189–191). ELAM-1 has also been shown to be expressed at a higher level in bronchial biopsies from asthmatic patients (186). In the cynomolgus monkey model of acute asthma, pretreatment of the animals with an anti-ELAM-1 monoclonal antibody blocked both neutrophil influx and late-phase airway obstruction after a single antigen challenge (192). Thus, it appears that anti-ELAM-1, anti-ICAM-1, and anti-Mac-1 monoclonal antibodies are able to selectively inhibit different aspects of the leukocytic infiltrate and the consequent physiologic response *in vivo* in nonhuman primate models of antigen-induced airway inflammation (180,188,192). Granulocyte influx into the airway following segmental antigen challenge in humans is also accompanied by activation of ELAM-1 and increases in Mac-1 (193), suggesting that these molecular mechanisms are actively utilized. The same investigators observed no increase in VLA-4 levels on recruited eosinophils, but this may be a reflection of the fact that integrin avidity (not level) is the important regulatory event in some systems (194,195). Eosinophil influx into the airway is common in asthmatic airway inflammation (196) and eosinophil adherence to vascular endothelium is dependent on VCAM-1/VLA-4 interaction (197–199). Results to date do not yet explain the selective recruitment of eosinophils into the airway after antigen challenge and serve to underscore the need for VCAM-1/VLA-4 blocking experiments performed *in vivo*.

Regulation of Cell Adhesion Molecules

Because leukocytes must (or at least often do) reach the airway lumen during inflammation, it is reasonable to propose that the epithelial cells lining the airway surface may express cell adhesion molecules analogous to those on the endothelial cells (181,194). A challenging question is just how the epithelial cells coordinate their expression of cell adhesion molecules with that in the underlying vascular plexus so that the leukocytes migrate through the tissues in an efficient, stimulus-specific manner. A recent clue to this process is the finding that vascular endothelial and airway epithelial cells have distinct but complementary profiles of cytokine-responsiveness in the transcriptional activation of the ICAM-1 gene (181). In vascular endothelial cells, the ICAM-1 gene responds to tumor necrosis factor-α (TNF-α) and interleukin-1β (IL-1β) much better than to interferon-γ (IFN-γ), whereas in airway epithelial cells, the gene responds much better to IFN-γ than to TNF-α or IL-1β. These profiles in ICAM-1 expression result in a parallel enhancement of endothelial-leukocyte adhesion by TNF-α or IL-1β stimulation and epithelial-leukocyte adhesion by IFN-γ treatment (200). The biologic basis for the difference in cytokine responsiveness is uncertain, but it is possible that the difference sets up the appropriate gradient of ICAM-1 expression for efficient localization of leukocytes. Thus, in the case of intracellular pathogens (such as respiratory viruses) entering from the airway luminal side, it may be advantageous to have the highest concentration of ICAM-1 near the lumen (where the pathologic process leads to IFN-γ production). In contrast, when there is invasion from the circulation (such as bacterial sepsis), it may be more utilitarian for leukocyte signaling to originate on the vascular luminal surface (where the pathology leads to TNFα or IL-1β formation). The coordination of leukocyte migration by the push and pull of endothelial and epithelial cell adhesion molecules will require further study but may allow strategies for blocking detrimental leukocyte migration (e.g., asthmatic inflammation) but not beneficial leukocyte migration (e.g., defense against infectious agents).

Differences in cytokine responsiveness between cell types offer an opportunity to decipher the genetic code of airway inflammation. Analysis of the 5'-flanking sequence of many of the cytokine-responsive genes indicates that their transcriptional control is regulated by sequence-specific DNA binding proteins (*trans*-acting factors) attaching to (or detaching from) *cis*-acting regulatory elements near the promoter region. In the case of ICAM-1 expression, this hypothesis is reinforced by studies of transformed epithelial cells indicating that the 5'-regulatory region of the ICAM-1 gene may contain one or more IFN-γ-stimulatable response elements and other cytokine response elements (201). Initial studies of primary culture cells indicate that specific genetic elements near the transcription start site are responsive to IFN-γ stimulation in airway epithelial but not in endothelial cells (202). Therefore, airway epithelial and vascular endothelial cells would be expected to generate different patterns of *trans*-acting factors in response to IFN-γ stimulation. A distinct set of nuclear proteins generated in epithelial cells might cause ICAM-1 gene activation after IFN-γ stimulation, whereas these proteins may be absent or modified in endothelial cells. Recent studies of the VCAM-1 gene indicate that two *cis*-acting elements bind distinct subsets of nuclear proteins (NF-κB type) and both sites are required for cytokine-responsiveness in endothelial cells but not in other cell types (203). Thus, the combination of specific DNA elements and factors that selectively bind to them may convey a tissue-specific or stimulus-specific response to cytokines.

Defining the *cis*-acting enhancing elements and the *trans*-acting binding factors that mediate the cytokine-induction of cell adhesion molecules will no doubt provide a clearer understanding of how airway cells utilize RNA transcription to respond to inflammatory stimuli and ultimately will provide information for the pathogenesis of inflammatory disease. In addition, this information may suggest strategies for treating inflammation by altering adhesion molecule expression at the cellular or molecular level. For example, cell adhesion molecule genes and in turn the gene products that control them are candidates for abnormal expression in inflammatory diseases. In fact, mutations of the β_2-integrins that follow an autosomal recessive mode of inheritance and lead to an aberrant inflammatory response have already been well defined (204). The characterization of transcriptional repressors and silencers (as well as cytokine-responsive enhancers) may offer the critical leads toward developing selective inhibitors of abnormal and/or normal cell adhesion molecule expression and ultimately airway inflammation. In particular, potentiation of repressor pathways and blockade of enhancer pathways for cell adhesion molecule expression represent new pharmacologic targets for specific anti-inflammatory therapy.

Strategies for Inhibition of Adhesion Molecules

Inhibition of cell adhesion molecule expression or function is an attractive target in the therapy of airway inflammatory diseases such as asthma (176). Current anti-inflammatory agents (such as glucocorticoids and sodium cromoglycate) may owe part of their efficacy to the attenuation of cell adhesion molecule function (205,206). However, agents that offer more selective blockade of cell adhesion molecules offers the potential for decreasing the side effects of therapy. Most studies to date have been limited to blocking cell adhesion molecule function in animal models of airway inflammation by administering monoclonal antibodies or synthetic peptides directed against cell adhesion molecules (173,180,187,188,192). These types of strategies have also been used to block rhinovirus attachment to epithelial cells in order to prevent infection *in vitro* (207,208).

Although blocking antibodies may be effective for acute therapy, they are usually ineffective for chronic therapy due to the immune system response to foreign protein and the consequent development of anti-idiotype antibodies. One solution to this problem has been to generate chimeric antibodies with human components (176). Another approach has been to engineer soluble forms of the adhesion molecules (usually the portion of the extracellular domain that is directly involved in protein–protein binding) or to manufacture small, synthetic peptide analogs or drugs that interfere with binding. Blockade of ICAM-1 function *in vitro* has been achieved using a 28 amino acid synthetic peptide modeled after a potential ICAM-1 binding domain (209).

Perhaps an even more selective route to inhibiting cell adhesion molecule function is to administer molecules that interfere with the regulation of cell adhesion molecules. Thus far, this approach has been utilized successfully *in vitro* by using (a) protein kinase C inhibitors to block a signal transduction mechanism for ICAM-1 up-regulation in cultured endothelial cells (210), (b) a microfilament disrupting agent to interfere with the interaction between ICAM-1 and the cytoskeleton of epithelial and lymphoid cells (thus interfering with the mobility of ICAM-1 on the cell surface) (211), and (c) antisense oligonucleotides to inhibit ICAM-1 gene expression in epithelial and endothelial cells (212). Taken together, the results to date suggest that anti-adhesive therapy may be effective as a sole treatment for airway inflammation or may render other anti-inflammatory drugs more effective. The latter effect may translate into a lower requirement for glucocorticoid treatment. Future studies will no doubt aim to determine the efficacy versus side effects for acute and chronic blockade of cell adhesion molecule function.

CYTOKINES

Two trends emerge from studies of cytokines and the role of these polypeptide mediators in the development of airway inflammation: (a) T lymphocytes (and mast cells) actively utilize a diverse set of cytokines to recruit and locally modulate the function of cells in the pulmonary airway; and (b) among the various types of cytokines capable of regulating immune function in the airway, the IL-4 family of cytokines (that includes IL-3, IL-4, IL-5, and GM-CSF) exhibit some of the most potent effects on critical features of asthmatic phenotype, i.e., the influx and activation of eosinophils and the enhanced production of IgE.

T-Cell Subsets and Airway Inflammation

The total number of lymphocytes are not consistently increased in the airways or peripheral blood of asthmatics, but the number of activated helper T cells (recognized by the CD4 surface marker and the IL-2 receptor, HLA-DR, and VLA-1 activation markers) are found in increased numbers in bronchoalveolar lavage, bronchial biopsy, and peripheral blood of asthmatic subjects (Table 1). The expression of all three activation markers on $CD4^+$ cells may correlate with the development of more severe asthma, while IL-2 receptor expression may decrease with improvement of asthma during treatment with glucocorticoids (213).

Definition of human T cell subsets in inflammation has begun by the construction of analogies to a simpler system worked out in the mouse (214). In the murine model, two antigen-activated helper T-cell subsets (T_H1 and T_H2) are each responsible for a different type of immune response: T_H1 cells produce IFN-γ, TNF-β, and IL-2, and appear to regulate delayed-type hyper-

TABLE 1. *Examples of cytokines that have been reported to be increased in biological specimens from asthmatic subjects*

Cytokine	Specimen	Cell source	Reference
IL-1β	BAL	AEC/monocyte	(Mattoli, 1991)
	BAL	nd	(Broide, 1992)
	BAL	Monocyte	(Marini, 1992)
	BAL	Alveolar Mac	(Borish, 1992)
IL-2	BAL	nd	(Robinson, 1992; Broide, 1992)
	BAL/blood	T-cell	(Walker, 1992)
IL-3	BAL	nd	(Robinson, 1992)
IL-4	BAL	T-cell	(Robinson, 1992)
	BAL/blood	T-cell	(Walker, 1992)
IL-5	BAL	T-cell	(Robinson, 1992, Marini, 1992)
	TBBx	nd	(Hamid, 1991)
	BAL/blood	T-cell	(Walker, 1992)
	BAL	Eosinophil/monocyte	(Broide, 1992)
IL-6	BAL	Alveolar Mac	(Gosset, 1991)
	BAL	nd	(Broide, 1992)
	TBBx	AEC	(Marini, 1992)
IL-8	TBBx	AEC	(Marini, 1992)
INF-γ	Blood	T-cell	(Corrigan, 1990)
TNF-α	BAL	Alveolar Mac	(Gosset, 1991)
	BAL	nd	(Broide, 1992)
GM-CSF	BAL	nd	(Robinson, 1992)
	Blood	nd	(Brown, 1991)
	TBBx	AEC	(Marini, 1992, Soloperto, 1991)
	BAL	T-cell	(Marini, 1992)
	BAL	T-cell, alveolar Mac	(Broide, 1991)
	BAL	Eosinophil/monocyte	(Broide, 1992)

BAL, bronchoalveolar lavage; TBBx, transbronchial biopsy; AEC, airway epithelial cell; Alveolar Mac, alveolar macrophage; nd, not determined.

sensitivity: TH2 cells release IL-4, IL-5, and IL-6, and are capable of stimulating humoral immunity mediated by B cells. For example, the TH2 cell may utilize IL-4 to promote B-cell synthesis of IgE in response to antigen. Both TH1 and TH2 cells synthesize GM-CSF, TNF-α and IL-3, and other cytokines may mediate interactions between T-cell subsets. For example, IL-10 produced by TH2 cells may help to regulate the immune response to an antigenic stimulus by inhibiting production of mediators from TH1 cells.

Characteristics of TH2 cell–mediated humoral immunity in mice may extend (at least in part) to the regulation of IgE biosynthesis in atopic or asthmatic human subjects. For example, a TH2-like pattern of cytokine production was found in bronchoalveolar lavage cells from subjects with mild atopic asthma using *in situ* hybridization (215). However, IL-2 levels were also increased in these subjects so that exclusive production of cytokines could not be definitively attributed to $CD4^+$ cells (215). A comparison of the pattern of T-cell activation and cytokine production between atopic and nonatopic asthmatic subjects has also yielded a pattern of immune response that is not as simple as the murine model (216); atopic subjects exhibited increases levels of activated $CD4^+$ T cells as well as IL-4 and IL-5 in blood and lavage samples, but nonatopic subjects had elevated levels of activated $CD4^+$ and $CD8^+$ cells and increased synthesis of IL-2 and IL-5 (216). Definition of atopic status and heterogeneity of asthmatic subsets has made these types of observations difficult to interpret. In addition, mast cells may also serve as a source for some of the same cytokines (217), and their contribution to the cytokine pool in IgE-activated reactions may be important.

IL-4 Family and Airway Function

There now appears to be enough functional, genetic, and structural similarities between IL-4, IL-5, GM-CSF, and IL-3 to designate this group as the IL-4 family of cytokines (218). Some of the shared characteristics of the family members include biologic activity, binding to the hematopoietin class of surface receptors, location on the long arm of chromosome 5, gene exon organization, and proposed three-dimensional structure. As noted above, biologic activities of the IL-4 family that are relevant to airway inflammation include regulation of eosinophil function and stimulation of IgE biosynthesis. IL-3, IL-5, and GM-CSF promote eosinophil differentiation, survival, chemotaxis, and activation (219–222). In a guinea pig model of airway inflammation induced by aerosolized ovalbumin, anti-IL-5 blocking antibodies can prevent eosinophil accumulation (223,224). In asthmatic subjects, anti-IL-5 antibodies can inhibit the T-cell–dependent survival of cultured peripheral blood eosinophils (225).

The discovery of IL-4 itself was based on its capacity to stimulate B-cell growth (226), but subsequent work has indicated that the substance has multiple effects via receptors expressed on diverse cell types. In particular, IL-

4 co-stimulates the proliferation of activated B and T cells; augments the cytotoxic activity of lymphocytes and monocytes; enhances the functional activity of myeloid cells; enhances adhesiveness of endothelial cells for T cells (by induction of VCAM-1); and enhances the production of specific immunoglobulin subclasses, most notably IgE (227). As is the case for other cytokines, IL-4 may also affect PGH synthase/isomerase and lipoxygenase activities (228,229), but the implications of these effects for immune regulation are uncertain. Elevated levels of IL-4 have been found in lavage and blood samples of allergic asthmatic subjects with increased IgE levels (216), but the effect of IL-4 blockade on the inflammatory response in these types of subjects still needs to be tested.

Strategies for Cytokine Inhibition

The development of reagents and drugs to specifically inhibit cytokine biosynthesis or action has just begun, so that only little information is available for effects on the immune response or on airway inflammation. Inhibition of multiple cytokines (IL-1, IL-2, IL-3, IL-5, GM-CSF, INF-γ, and TNF-α) on a variety of cell types (monocytes, macrophages, endothelial cells, and T lymphocytes) may be achieved by treatment with glucocorticoids (213,230–232). It appears that cyclosporin (which has been used extensively for promoting allograft survival) may be an agent that targets the T lymphocyte for its therapeutic effect, although mast cells and basophils may also be affected by the drug (233). Cyclosporin blocks T-cell activation by a process that includes inhibition of cytokine biosynthesis at the transcriptional level (234,235). Chronic treatment with cyclosporin achieved significant improvement in the airway function of glucocorticoid-dependent asthmatics (236). The molecular basis for this therapeutic effect is still uncertain, but the results provide a basis for the development of other (perhaps more specific) inhibitors of the cytokine-mediated immune response.

SUMMARY

This chapter encompassed only a fraction of the information obtained in recent studies of the biochemistry and physiology of airway inflammation. We have concentrated on some of the biochemical pathways (phospholipid–arachidonic acid metabolism, cell adhesion molecules, and cytokines) that have well-developed pharmacologic strategies, but other molecular targets (e.g., neuropeptides, proteases, major basic protein, endothelin, or nitric oxide synthase) may yield alternative strategies for inhibition of airway inflammation and improvement in airway function. Each of these biochemical cascades has been implicated as a source of "good" and "bad" activities with respective roles in physiologic and in pathophysiologic processes. The apparent paradoxes will ultimately be resolved by studies carried out *in vivo* using inhibitors that target specific molecular mechanisms.

ACKNOWLEDGMENTS

Some of the work cited in this chapter was supported by grants from the National Institutes of Health, the Monsanto–G. D. Searle–Washington University Research Agreement, and the Schering Career Investigator Award from the American Lung Association.

REFERENCES

1. Chichester CH, Philpot RM, Weir AJ, Buckpitt AR, Plopper CG. Characterization of the cytochrome P-450 monooxygenase system in nonciliated bronchiolar epithelial (Clara) cells isolated from mouse lung. *Am J Respir Cell Mol Biol* 1990;4:179–186.
2. Holtzman MJ, Turk J, Pentland A. A regiospecific monooxygenase with novel stereopreference in the major pathway for arachidonic acid oxygenation in isolated epidermal cells. *J Clin Invest* 1989;84:1446–1453.
3. Diez E, Mong S. Purification of a phospholipase A_2 from human monocytic leukemic U937 cells. Calcium-dependent activation and membrane association. *J Biol Chem* 1990;265:14654–14661.
4. Gao G, Serrero G. Phospholipase A_2 is a differentiation-dependent enzymatic activity for adipogenic cell line and adipocyte precursors in primary culture. *J Biol Chem* 1990;265:2431–2434.
5. Murayama T, Kajiyama Y, Nomura Y. Histamine-stimulated GTP-binding proteins-mediated phospholipase A_2 activation in rabbit platelets. *J Biol Chem* 1990;265:4290–4295.
6. Bonventre JV, Gronich JH, Nemenoff RA. Epidermal growth factor enhances glomerular mesangial cell soluble phospholipase A_2 activity. *J Biol Chem* 1990;265:4934–4938.
7. Channon JY, Leslie CC. A calcium-dependent mechanism for associating a soluble arachidonoyl-hydrolyzing phospholipase A_2 with membrane in the macrophage cell line RAW 264.7. *J Biol Chem* 1990;265:5409–5413.
8. Clark JD, Lin L-L, Kriz RW, et al. A novel arachidonic acid-selective cytosolic PLA_2 contains a Ca^{2+}-dependent translocation domain with homology to PKC and GAP. *Cell* 1991;65:1043–1051.
9. Wery JP, Schevitz RW, Clawson DK, et al. Structure of recombinant human rheumatoid arthritic synovial fluid phospholipase A_2 at 2.2 A resolution. *Nature* 1991;352:79–82.
10. Lin L-L, Lin AY, DeWitt DL. Interleukin-1α induces the accumulation of cytosolic phospholipase A_2 and the release of prostaglandin E_2 in human fibroblasts. *J Biol Chem* 1992;267:23451–23454.
11. Zupan LA, Steffens DL, Berry CA, Landt M, Gross RW. Cloning and expression of a human 14-3-3 protein mediating phospholipolysis. *J Biol Chem* 1992;267:8707–8710.
12. DeGeorge JJ, Ousley AH, McCarthy KD, Morell P, Lapetina EG. Glucocorticoids inhibit the liberation of arachidonate but not the rapid production of phospholipase C-dependent metabolites in acetylcholine-stimulated C62B glioma cells. *J Biol Chem* 1987;262:9979–9983.
13. Gassama-Diagne A, Fauvel J, Chap H. Calcium-independent phospholipases from guinea pig digestive tract as probes to study the mechanism of lipocortin. *J Biol Chem* 1990;265:4309–4314.
14. Nakano T, Ohara O, Teraoka H, Arita H. Glucocorticoids suppress group II phospholipase A_2 production by blocking mRNA synthesis and post-transcriptional expression. *J Biol Chem* 1990;265:12745–12748.
15. Cohan VL, Undem BJ, Fox CC, et al. Dexamethasone does not inhibit the release of

mediators from human mast cells residing in airway, intestine, or skin. *Am Rev Respir Dis* 1989;140:951–954.

16. Wilkinson JRW, Crea AEG, Clark JJH, Lee TH. Identification and characterization of a monocyte-derived neutrophil-activating factor in corticosteroid-resistant bronchial asthma. *J Clin Invest* 1989;84:1930–1941.

17. Lorant DE, Patel KD, McIntyre TM, et al. Coexpression of GMP-140 and PAF by endothelium stimulated by histamine or thrombin: a juxtacrine system for adhesion and activation of neutrophils. *J Cell Biol* 1991;115:223–224.

18. Wardlaw AJ, Moqbel R, Cromwell O, Kay AB. Platelet-activating factor: a potent chemotactic and chemokinetic factor for human eosinophils. *J Clin Invest* 1986;78:1701–1706.

19. Cuss FM, Dixon CMS, Barnes PJ. Effects of inhaled platelet activating factor on pulmonary function and bronchial responsiveness in man. *Lancet* 1986;2:189–192.

20. Lee T, Malone B, Snyder F. A new de novo pathway for the formation of 1-alkyl-2-acetyl-sn-glycerols, precursors of platelet activating factor. Biochemical characterization of 1-alkyl-2-lyso-sn-glycero-3-p:acetyl-CoA acetyltransferase in rat spleen. *J Biol Chem* 1986;261:5373–5377.

21. Snyder F. Platelet-activating factor and related acetylated lipids as potent biologically active cellular mediators. *Am J Physiol (Cell Physiol)* 1990;259:C697–C708.

22. Prescott SM, Zimmerman GA, McIntyre TM. Platelet-activating factor. *J Biol Chem* 1990;265:17381–17384.

23. Holland MR, Venable ME, Whatley RE, et al. Activation of the acetyl-coenzyme A: lysoplatelet-activating factor acetyltransferase regulates platelet-activating factor synthesis in human endothelial cells. *J Biol Chem* 1992;267:22883–22890.

24. Stafforini D, Prescott S, McIntyre T. Human plasma platelet-activating factor acetylhydrolase. *J Biol Chem* 1987;262:4223–4230.

25. Stafforini DM, Elstad ME, Zimmerman GA, McIntyre TM, Prescott SM. Human macrophages secret platelet-activating factor acetylhydrolase. *J Biol Chem* 1990;265:9682–9687.

26. Elstad MR, Stafforini DM, McIntyre TM, Prescott SM, Zimmerman GA. Platelet-activating factor acetylhydrolase increases during macrophage differentiation. A novel mechanism that regulates accumulation of platelet-activating factor. *J Biol Chem* 1989;264:8467–8470.

27. Benveniste J, Henson P, Cochrane C. Leukocyte dependent histamine release from rabbit platelets: the role of IgE, basophils, and a platelet-activating factor. *J Exp Med* 1972;136:1356–1377.

28. Whatley RE, Fennell DF, Kurrus JA, et al. Synthesis of platelet-activating factor by endothelial cells. *J Biol Chem* 1990;265:15550–15559.

29. Bussolino F, Fou R, Malavasi F, Ferrando M, Cammussi G. Release of platelet-activating factor (PAF)-like material from human lymphoid cell lines. *Exp Hematol* 1984;12:688–693.

30. Tonnel A, Joseph M, Gosset P, Fournier E, Capron A. Stimulation of alveolar macrophages in asthmatic patients after local provocation tests. *Lancet* 1983;1:1406.

31. Arnoux B, Jouvin-Marche E, Arnoux A, Benveniste J. Release of paf-acether from human blood monocytes. *Agents and Actions* 1982;12:713.

32. Holtzman MJ, Ferdman B, Bohrer A, Turk J. Synthesis of the 1-O-hexadecyl molecular species of platelet-activating factor by airway epithelial cells and vascular endothelial cells. *Biochem Biophys Res Commun* 1991;177:357–364.

33. Kumar R, King RJ, Martin HM, Hanahan DJ. Metabolism of platelet-activating factor (alkylacetylphosphocholine) by type-II epithelial cells and fibroblasts from rat lungs. *Biochim Biophys Acta* 1987;917:33–41.

34. Honda Z, Nakamura M, Miki I, et al. Cloning by functional expression of platelet-activating factor receptor from guinea-pig lung. *Nature* 1991;349:342–346.

35. Kunz D, Gerard NP, Gerard C. The human leukocyte platelet-activating factor receptor. cDNA cloning, cell surface expression, and construction of a novel epitope-bearing analog. *J Biol Chem* 1992;267:9101–9106.

36. Hosford D, Page CP, Barnes PJ, Braquet P. PAF-receptor antagonists. In: Barnes PJ, Page CP, Henson PM, ed. *Platelet activating factor and human disease.* Cambridge: Blackwell Scientific, 1989;83–116.

37. Holtzman MJ. Arachidonic acid metabolism in airway epithelial cells. *Annu Rev Physiol* 1992;54:303–329.
38. Pentland AP, Needleman P. Modulation of keratinocyte proliferation in vitro by endogenous prostaglandin synthesis. *J Clin Invest* 1986;77:246–251.
39. Konda Y, Nishisaki H, Nakano O, et al. Prostaglandin protects isolated guinea pig chief cells against ethanol injury via an increase in diacylglycerol. *J Clin Invest* 1990; 86:1897–1903.
40. Al-Bazzaz F, Yadava VP, Westenfelder C. Modification of Na and Cl transport in canine tracheal mucosa by prostaglandins. *Am J Physiol* 1981;240:F101–F105.
41. Gerrity TR, Cotromanes E, Garrard CS, Yeates DB, Lourenco RV. The effect of aspirin on lung mucociliary clearance. *N Engl J Med* 1983;308:139–141.
42. Widdicombe JH, Coleman DL, Finkbeiner WE, Tuet IK. Electrical properties of monolayers cultured from cells of human tracheal mucosa. *J Appl Physiol* 1985; 58:1729–1735.
43. Ferreri NR, Sarr T, Askenase PW, Ruddle NH. Molecular regulation of tumor necrosis factor-α and lymphotoxin production in T cells. *J Immunol* 1992;267:9443–9449.
44. Wightman PD, Dallob A. Regulation of phosphatidylinositol breakdown and leukotriene synthesis by endogenous prostaglandins in resident mouse peritoneal macrophages. *J Biol Chem* 1990;265:9176–9180.
45. Plaut M, Marone G, Gillespie E. The role of cyclic AMP in modulating cytotoxic T lymphocytes. *J Immunol* 1983;131:2945–2952.
46. Santoro MG, Benedetto A, Carruba G, Garaci E, Jaffe BM. Prostaglandin A compounds as antiviral agents. *Science* 1980;209:1032–1034.
47. Faden H, Hong JJ, Ogra PL. Interaction of polymorphonuclear leukocytes and viruses in humans: adherence of polymorphonuclear leukocytes to respiratory syncytial virus infected cells. *J Virol* 1984;52:16–23.
48. Chopra J, Webster RO. PGE$_1$ inhibits neutrophil adherence and neutrophil-mediated injury to cultured endothelial cells. *Am Rev Respir Dis* 1988;138:915–920.
49. Stuart-Smith K, Vanhoutte PM. Arachidonic acid evokes epithelium-dependent relaxations in canine airways. *J Appl Physiol* 1988;65:2170–2180.
50. Smith AP, Cuthbert MF, Dunlop LS. Effects of inhaled prostaglandins E1, E2, and F2a on the airway resistance of healthy and asthmatic man. *Clin Sci* 1975;48:421–430.
51. Marom Z, Shelhamer JH, Kaliner M. Effects of arachidonic acid, monohydroxyeicosatetraenoic acid and prostaglandins on the release of mucous glycoproteins from human airways in vitro. *J Clin Invest* 1981;67:1695–1702.
52. O'Byrne PM, Aizawa H, Bethel RA, et al. Prostaglandin F$_{2\alpha}$ increases responsiveness of pulmonary airways in dogs. *Prostaglandins* 1984;28:537–543.
53. Skoner DP, Page R, Asman B, Gillen L, Fireman P. Plasma elevations of histamine and a prostaglandin metabolite in acute asthma. *Am Rev Respir Dis* 1988;137:1009–1014.
54. Wenzel SE, Westcott JY, Smith HR, Larsen GL. Spectrum of prostanoid release after bronchoalveolar allergen challenge in atopic asthmatics and in control groups. *Am Rev Respir Dis* 1989;139:450–457.
55. Merlie JP, Fagan D, Mudd J, Needleman P. Isolation and characterization of the complementary DNA for sheep seminal vesicle prostaglandin endoperoxide synthase (cyclooxygenase). *J Biol Chem* 1988;263:3550–3553.
56. DeWitt DL, Smith WL. Primary structure of prostaglandin G/H synthase from sheep vesicular gland determined from the complementary DNA sequence. *Proc Natl Acad Sci USA* 1988;85:1412–1416.
57. Yokoyama C, Takai T, Tanabe T. Primary structure of sheep prostaglandin endoperoxide synthase deduced from cDNA sequence. *FEBS Lett* 1988;231:347–351.
58. DeWitt DL, El-Harith EA, Kraemer SA, et al. The aspirin and heme-binding sites of ovine and murine prostaglandin endoperoxide synthases. *J Biol Chem* 1990;265:5192–5198.
59. Funk CD, Funk LB, Kennedy ME, Pong AS, Fitzgerald GA. Human platelet/erythroleukemia cell prostaglandin G/H synthase: cDNA cloning, expression, and gene chromosomal assignment. *FASEB J* 1991;5:2304–2312.
60. Yokoyama C, Tanabe T. Cloning of the human gene encoding prostaglandin endoperoxide synthase and primary structure of the enzyme. *Biochem Biophys Res Commun* 1989;165:888–894.

61. Rosen GD, Birkenmeier T, Raz A, Holtzman MJ. Identification of a cyclooxygenase-related gene and its potential role in prostaglandin formation. *Biochem Biophys Res Commun* 1989;164:1358–1365.
62. Xie W, Chipman JG, Robertson DL, Erikson RL, Simmons DL. Expression of a mitogen-responsive gene encoding prostaglandin synthase is regulated by mRNA splicing. *Proc Natl Acad Sci USA* 1991;88:2692–2696.
63. Kujubu DA, Fletcher BS, Varnum BC, Lim RW, Herschman HR. TIS10, a phorbol ester tumor promoter-inducible mRNA from Swiss 3T3 cells, encodes a novel prostaglandin synthase/cyclooxygenase homologue. *J Biol Chem* 1991;266:12866–12872.
64. O'Banion MK, Sadowski HB, Winn V, Young DA. A serum- and glucocorticoid-regulated 4-kilobase mRNA encodes a cyclooxygenase-related protein. *J Biol Chem* 1991;266:23261–23267.
65. Sirois J, Richards JS. Purification and characterization of a novel, distinct isoform of prostaglandin endoperoxide synthase induced by human chorionic gonadotropin in granulosa cells of rat preovulatory follicles. *J Biol Chem* 1992;267:6382–6388.
66. Hla T, Neilson K. Human cyclooxygenase-2 cDNA. *Proc Natl Acad Sci USA* 1992;89:7384–7388.
67. Fletcher BS, Kujubu DA, Perrin DM, Herschman HR. Structure of the mitogen-inducible TIS10 gene and demonstration that the TIS10-encoded protein is a functional prostaglandin G/H synthase. *J Biol Chem* 1992;267:4338–4344.
68. Holtzman MJ, Turk J, Shornick LP. Identification of a pharmacologically-distinct prostaglandin H synthase in cultured epithelial cells. *J Biol Chem* 1992;267:21438–21445.
69. Zhang V, Hussain H, Wilson JD, Roswit WT, Holtzman MJ. Molecular cloning and expression of a pharmacologically-distinct, cytokine-regulated prostaglandin H synthase-2. Submitted.
70. Casey ML, Korte K, MacDonald PC. Epidermal growth factor stimulation of prostaglandin E_2 biosynthesis in amnion cells. *J Biol Chem* 1988;263:7846–7854.
71. Diaz A, Varga J, Jimenez SA. Transforming growth factor-β stimulation of lung fibroblast prostaglandin E_2 production. *J Biol Chem* 1989;264:11554–11557.
72. Yokota K, Kusaka M, Ohshima T, et al. Stimulation of prostaglandin E_2 synthesis in cloned osteoblastic cells of mouse (MC3T3-E1) by epidermal growth factor. *J Biol Chem* 1986;261:15410–15415.
73. Bailey JM, Makheja AN, Pash J, Verma M. Corticosteroids suppress cyclooxygenase messenger RNA levels and prostanoid synthesis in cultured vascular cells. *Biochem Biophys Res Commun* 1988;157:1159–1163.
74. Lin AH, Bienkowski MJ, Gorman RR. Regulation of prostaglandin H synthase mRNA levels and prostaglandin biosynthesis by platelet-derived growth factor. *J Biol Chem* 1989;264:17379–17383.
75. Clark MA, Conway TM, Shorr RGL, Crooke ST. Identification and isolation of a mammalian protein which is antigenically and functionally related to the phospholipase A_2 stimulatory peptide melittin. *J Biol Chem* 1987;262:4402–4406.
76. Baracos V, Rodemann P, Dinarello CA, Goldberg AL. Stimulation of muscle protein degradation and prostaglandin E_2 release by leukocytic pyrogen (interleukin-1). *N Engl J Med* 1983;308:553–558.
77. Frasier-Scott K, Hatzakis H, Seong D, Jones CM, Wu KK. Influence of natural and recombinant interleukin-2 on endothelial cell arachidonate metabolism. *J Clin Invest* 1988;82:1877–1883.
78. Eldor A, Fridman R, Vlodavsky I, et al. Interferon enhances prostacyclin production by cultured vascular endothelial cells. *J Clin Invest* 1984;73:251–257.
79. Elias JA. Tumor necrosis factor interacts with interleukin-1 and interferons to inhibit fibroblast proliferation via fibroblast prostaglandin-dependent and independent mechanisms. *Am Rev Respir Dis* 1988;138:652–658.
80. Silberstein DS, Owen WF, Gasson JC, et al. Enhancement of human eosinophil cytotoxicity and leukotriene synthesis by biosynthetic (recombinant) granulocyte-macrophage colony-stimulating factor. *J Immunol* 1986;137:3290–3294.
81. Masferrer JL, Zweifel BS, Seibert K, Needleman P. Selective regulation of cellular cyclooxygenase by dexamethasone and endotoxin in mice. *J Clin Invest* 1990;86:1375–1379.
82. Ballou LR, Chao CP, Holness MA, Barker SC, Raghow R. Interleukin-1-mediated

PGE$_2$ production and sphingomyelin metabolism. Evidence for the regulation of cyclooxygenase gene expression by sphingosine and ceramide. *J Biol Chem* 1992;267: 20044–20050.

83. Wu KK, Hatzakis H, Lo SS, et al. Stimulation of de novo synthesis of prostaglandin G/H synthase in human endothelial cells by phorbol ester. *J Biol Chem* 1988; 263:19043–19047.

84. Raz A, Wyche A, Siegel N, Needleman P. Regulation of fibroblast cyclooxygenase synthesis by interluekin-1. *J Biol Chem* 1988;263:3022–3028.

85. Fu J-Y, Masferrer JL, Seibert K, Raz A, Needleman P. The induction and suppression of prostaglandin H$_2$ synthase (cyclooxygenase) in human monocytes. *J Biol Chem* 1990;265:16737–16740.

86. O'Banion MK, Winn VD, Young DA. cDNA cloning and functional activity of a glucocorticoid-regulated inflammatory cyclooxygenase. *Proc Natl Acad Sci USA* 1992; 89:4888–4992.

87. Flower RJ. Drugs which inhibit prostaglandin biosynthesis. *Pharmacol Rev* 1974; 26:33–67.

88. Hunter JA, Finkbeiner WE, Nadel JA, Goetzl EJ, Holtzman MJ. Predominant generation of 15-lipoxygenase metabolites of arachidonic acid by epithelial cells from human trachea. *Proc Natl Acad Sci USA* 1985;82:4633–4637.

89. Holtzman MJ, Hansbrough JR, Rosen GD, Turk J. Uptake, release, and novel species-dependent oxygenation of arachidonic acid in human and animal airway epithelial cells. *Biochim Biophys Acta* 1988;963:401–413.

90. Henke D, Danilowicz RM, Curtis JF, Boucher RC, Eling TE. Metabolism of arachidonic acid by human nasal and bronchial epithelial cells. *Arch Biochem Biophys* 1988;267:426–436.

91. Hansbrough JR, Atlas AB, Turk J, Holtzman MJ. Arachidonate 12-lipoxygenase and cyclooxygenase: PGE isomerase are predominant pathways for oxygenation in bovine tracheal epithelial cells. *Am J Respir Cell Mol Biol* 1989;1:237–244.

92. Alpert SE, Kramer CM, Brashler JR, Bach MK. Generation of lipoxygenase metabolites of arachidonic acid by monolayer cultures of tracheal epitithelial cells and intact tracheal segments from rabbits. *Exp Lung Res* 1990;16:207–230.

93. Shannon VR, Crouch EC, Ueda N, et al. Related expression of arachidonate 12- and 15-lipoxygenases in animal and human lung tissue. *Am J Physiol (Lung Cell Mol Physiol)* 1991;261:L399–L405.

94. Holtzman MJ, Aizawa H, Nadel JA. Goetzl EJ. Selective generation of leukotriene B$_4$ by tracheal epithelial cells from dogs. *Biochem Biophys Res Commun* 1983;114:1071–1076.

95. Eling TE, Danilowicz RM, Henke DC, et al. Arachidonic acid metabolism by canine tracheal epithelial cells. *J Biol Chem* 1986;261:12841–12849.

96. Gray PR, Derksen FJ, Robinson NE, Slocombe RF, Peters-Golden ML. Epithelial strips: an alternative technique for examining arachidonate metabolism in equine tracheal epithelium. *Am J Respir Cell Mol Biol* 1992;6:29–36.

97. Hansbrough JR, Takahashi Y, Ueda N, Yamamoto S, Holtzman MJ. Identification of a novel arachidonate 12-lipoxygenase in bovine tracheal epithelial cells distinct from leukocyte and platelet forms of the enzyme. *J Biol Chem* 1990;265:1771–1776.

98. Yoshimoto T, Suzuki H, Yamamoto S, et al. Cloning and sequence analysis of the cDNA for arachidonate 12-lipoxygenase of porcine leukocytes. *Proc Natl Acad Sci USA* 1990;87:2142–2146.

99. Hamberg M, Hedqvist P, Radegran K. Identification of 15-hydroxy-5,8,11,13-eicosatetraenoic acid (15-HETE) as a major metabolite of arachidonic acid in human lung. *Acta Physiol Scand* 1980;110:219–221.

100. Dahlen S, Hansson G, Hedqvist P, et al. Allergen challenge of lung tissue from asthmatics elicits bronchial contraction that correlates with the release of leukotrienes C$_4$, D$_4$, and E$_4$. *Proc Natl Acad Sci USA* 1983;80:1712–1716.

101. Kumlin M, Hamberg M, Granstrom E, et al. 15(S)-Hydroxyeicostetraenoic acid is the major arachidonic acid metabolite in human bronchi: association with airway epithelium. *Arch Biochem Biophys* 1990;282:254–262.

102. Murray JJ, Tonnel AB, Brash AR, et al. Release of prostaglandin D$_2$ into human airways during acute antigen challenge. *N Engl J Med* 1986;315:800–804.

103. Holtzman MJ, Pentland A, Baenziger NL, Hansbrough JR. Heterogeneity of cellular

expression of arachidonate 15-lipoxygenase: implications for biological activity. *Biochim Biophys Acta* 1989;1003:204–208.

104. Holtzman MJ. Epithelial cell regulation of arachidonic acid oxygenation. In: Farmer SG, Hay DWP, ed. *The airway epithelium: physiology, pathophysiology, and pharmacology; lung biology in health and disease.* New York: Marcel Dekker, 1991;65–115.

105. Shornick LP, Holtzman MJ. A cryptic, microsomal-type arachidonate 12-lipoxygenase is tonically inactivated by oxidation-reduction conditions in cultured epithelial cells. *J Biol Chem* 1993;268:371–376.

106. Shannon VR, Hansbrough JR, Takahashi Y, et al. Biochemical and immunohistochemical evidence for selective expression of novel epithelial lipoxygenases. In: Samuelsson B, Paoletti R, Ramwell PW, Folco G, Granstom E, eds. *Adv Prostaglandin Thromboxane Leukotriene Res* 1990;37–40.

107. Shannon VR, Chanez P, Bousquet J, Holtzman MJ. Histochemical evidence for induction of arachidonate 15-lipoxygenase in airway disease. *Am Rev Respir Dis* 1993;147:1024–1028.

108. Shannon VR, Stenson WF, Holtzman MJ. Induction of epithelial arachidonate 12-lipoxygenase at active sites of inflammatory bowel disease. *Am J Physiol (Gastrointest Liver Physiol)* 1993;264:G104–G111.

109. Setty BNY, Graeber JE, Stuart MJ. The mitogenic effect of 15- and 12-hydroxyeicosatetraenoic acid on endothelial cells may be mediated by diacylglycerol kinase inhibition. *J Biol Chem* 1987;262:17613–17622.

110. Piomelli D, Volterra A, Dale N, et al. Lipoxygenase metabolites of arachidonic acid as second messengers for presynaptic inhibition of aplysia sensory cells. *Nature* 1987;328:38–43.

111. Shannon VR, Ramanadhan S, Turk J, Holtzman MJ. Selective expression of an arachidonate 12-lipoxygenase by pancreatic islet β-cells. *Am J Physiol (Endocrinol Metab)* 1992;263:E828–836.

112. Marom Z, Shelhamer JH, Sun F, Kaliner M. Human airway monohydroxyeicosatetraenoic acid generation and mucus release. *J Clin Invest* 1983;72:122–127.

113. Brash AR. Review of the possible roles of the platelet 12-lipoxygenase. *Circulation* 1985;72:702–707.

114. Stenson WF, Parker CW. Metabolism of arachidonic acid in ionophore-stimulated neutrophils. *J Clin Invest* 1979;64:1457–1465.

115. Funk CD, Powell WS. Release of prostaglandins and monohydroxy and trihydroxy metabolites of linoleic and arachidonic acids by adult and fetal aortae and ductus arteriosus. *J Biol Chem* 1985;260:7481–7488.

116. Brezinski ME, Serhan CN. Selective incorporation of (15S)-hydroxyeicosatetraenoic acid in phosphatidylinositol of human neutrophils: agonist-induced deacylation and transformation of stored hydroxyeicosanoids. *Proc Natl Acad Sci USA* 1990;87:6248–6252.

117. Legrand AB, Lawson JA, Meyrick BO, Blair IA, Oates JA. Substitution of 15-hydroxyeicostetraenoic acid in the phosphoinositide signaling pathway. *J Biol Chem* 1991;266:7570–7577.

118. Jung G, Yang DC, Nakao A. Oxygenation of phosphatidylcholine by human polymorphonuclear leukocyte 15-lipoxygenase. *Biochem Biophys Res Commun* 1985;130:559–566.

119. Brash AR, Ingram CD, Harris TM. Analysis of a specific oxygenation reaction of soybean lipoxygenase with fatty acids esterified in phospholipids. *Biochemistry* 1987;26:5465–5471.

120. Murray JJ, Brash AR. Rabbit reticulocyte lipoxygenase catalyzes specific 12(S) and 15(S) oxygenation of arachidonoyl-phosphatidylcholine. *Arch Biochem Biophys* 1988;265:514–523.

121. Kuhn H, Brash AR. Occurrence of lipoxygenase products in membranes of rabbit reticulocytes. *J Biol Chem* 1990;265:1454–1458.

122. Kuhn H, Belkner J, Wiesner R, Brash AR. Oxygenation of biological membranes by the pure reticulocyte lipoxygenase. *J Biol Chem* 1990;265:18351–18361.

123. Lam BK, Gagnon L, Austen KF, Soberman RJ. The mechanism of leukotriene B_4 export from human polymorphonuclear leukocytes. *J Biol Chem* 1990;265:13438–13441.

124. Powell WS, Gravelle F. Metabolism of arachidonic acid by peripheral elicited rat poly-morphonuclear leukocytes. *J Biol Chem* 1990;265:9131–9139.
125. Rouzer CA, Samuelsson B. On the nature of the 5-lipoxygenase reaction in human leukocytes: enzyme purification and requirement for multiple stimulatory factors. *Proc Natl Acad Sci USA* 1985;263:10135–10140.
126. Rouzer CA, Kargman S. Translocation of 5-lipoxygenase to the membrane in human leukocytes challenged with ionophore A23187. *J Biol Chem* 1988;263:10980–10988.
127. Dixon RAF, Diehl RE, Opas E, et al. Requirement of a 5-lipoxygenase-activating protein for leukotriene synthesis. *Nature* 1990;343:282–284.
128. Reid GK, Kargman S, Vickers PJ, et al. Correlation between expression of 5-lipoxygenase-activating protein, 5-lipoxygenase, and cellular leukotriene synthesis. *J Biol Chem* 1990;265:19818–19823.
129. Dixon RAF, Jones RE, Diehl RE, et al. Cloning of the cDNA for human 5-lipoxygenase. *Proc Natl Acad Sci USA* 1988;85:416–420.
130. Samuelsson B, Funk CD. Enzymes involved in the biosynthesis of leukotriene B_4. *J Biol Chem* 1989;264:19469–19472.
131. Funk CD, Gunne H, Steiner H, Izumi T, Samuelsson B. Native and mutant 5-lipoxygenase expression in a baculovirus/insect cell system *Proc Natl Acad Sci USA* 1989;86:2592–2596.
132. Rouzer CA, Rands E, Kargman S, et al. Characterization of cloned human leukocyte 5-lipoxygenase expressed in mammalian cells. *J Biol Chem* 1988;263:10135–10140.
133. Funk CD, Hoshiko S, Matsumoto T, Radmark O, Samuelsson B. Characterization of the human 5-lipoxygenase gene. *Proc Natl Acad Sci USA* 1989;86:2587–2591.
134. Jakobsson P-J, Steinhilber D, Odlander B, et al. On the expression and regulation of 5-lipoxygenase in human lymphocytes. *Proc Natl Acad Sci USA* 1992;89:3521–3525.
135. Shannon VR, Holtzman MJ. In situ evidence for 5-lipoxygenase induction in mantle-zone B-lymphocytes at active sites of inflammation. *J Cell Biochem* 1993; 17B:242.
136. Funk CD, Radmark O, Fu JY, et al. Molecular cloning and amino acid sequence of leukotriene A4 hydrolase. *Proc Natl Acad Sci USA* 1987;84:6677–6681.
137. Medina J, Odlander B, Funk CD, et al. B-lymphocytic cell line Raji expresses the leukotriene A_4 hydrolase gene but not the 5-lipoxygenase gene. *Biochem Biophys Res Commun* 1989;161:740–745.
138. McGee JE, Fitzpatrick FA. Erythrocyte-neutrophil interactions: formation of leuko-triene B_4 by transcellular biosynthesis. *Proc Natl Acad Sci USA* 1986;83:1349–1353.
139. Arm JP, Horton CE, House F, et al. Enhanced generation of leukotriene B_4 by neutro-phils stimulated by unopsonized zymosan and by calcium ionophore after exercise-induced asthma. *Am Rev Respir Dis* 1988;138:47–53.
140. Doerfler ME, Danner RL, Shelhamer JH, Parrillo JE. Bacterial lipopolysaccharides prime human neutrophils for enhanced production of leukotriene B_4. *J Clin Invest* 1989;83:970–977.
141. Tessner TG, O'Flaherty JT, Wykle RL. Stimulation of platelet-activating factor syn-thesis by a nonmetabolizable bioactive analog of platelet-activating factor and influ-ence of arachidonic acid metabolites. *J Biol Chem* 1989;264:4794–4799.
142. Lewis RA, Austen KF, Soberman RJ. Leukotrienes and other products of the 5-lipox-ygenase pathway. *N Engl J Med* 1990;323:645–655.
143. Goldman DW, Goetzl EJ. Specific binding of leukotriene B_4 to receptors on human polymorphonuclear leukocytes. *J Immunol* 1982;129:1600–1604.
144. Sjolander A, Gronroos E, Hammarstrom S, Andersson T. Leukotriene D_4 and E_4 in-duce transmembrane signaling in human epithelial cells. *J Biol Chem* 1990;265:20976–20981.
145. Holtzman MJ. Arachidonic acid metabolism: implications of biological chemistry for lung function and disease. *Am Rev Respir Dis* 1991;143:188–203.
146. Sinclair SB, Greig PD, Blendis LM, et al. Biochemical and clinical response of fulmi-nant viral hepatitis to administration of prostaglandin E. *J Clin Invest* 1989;84:1063–1069.
147. Nielson CP, Crowley JJ, Morgan ME, Vestal RE. Polymorphonuclear leukocyte inhi-bition by therapeutic concentrations of theophylline is mediated by cyclic-3',5'-aden-osine monophosphate. *Am Rev Respir Dis* 1988;137:25–30.
148. Furth EE, Hurtubise V, Schott MA, Laposata M. The effect of endogenous essential

and nonessential fatty acids on the uptake and subsequent agonist-induced release of arachidonate. *J Biol Chem* 1989;264:18494–18501.

149. Arm JP, Horton CE, Spur BW, Mencia-Huerta JM, Lee TH. The effects of dietary supplementation with fish oil lipids on the airways response to inhaled allergen in bronchial asthma. *Am Rev Respir Dis* 1989;139:1395–1400.

150. Payan DG, Wong MYS, Chernov-Rogan T, et al. Alterations in human leukocyte function induced by ingestion of eicosapentaenoic acid. *J Clin Immunol* 1986;6:402–410.

151. Ferreri NR, Howland WC, Stevenson DD, Spiegelberg HL. Release of leukotrienes, prostaglandins, and histamine into nasal secretions of aspirin-sensitive asthmatics during reaction to aspirin. *Am Rev Respir Dis* 1988;137:847–854.

152. Arm JP, O'Hickey SP, Spur BW, Lee TH. Airway responsiveness to histamine and leukotriene E_4 in subjects with aspirin-induced asthma. *Am Rev Respir Dis* 1989; 140:148–153.

153. Israel E, Dermarkarian R, Rosenberg M, et al. The effects of a 5-lipoxygenase inhibitor on asthma induced by cold, dry air. *N Engl J Med* 1990;323:1740–1744.

154. Ford-Hutchinson AW. Regulation of the Production and Action of Leukotrienes by MK-571 and MK-886. In: Samuelsson B, Paoletti R, Ramwell PW, Folco G, Granstom E, ed. *Advances in Prostaglandin, Thromboxane, and Leukotriene Research* New York: Raven Press, 1990;21A:9–16.

155. Smith LJ, Geller S, Ebright L, Glass M, Thyrum PT. Inhibition of leukotriene D_4-induced bronchoconstriction in normal subjects by the oral LTD_4 receptor antagonist ICI 204,219. *Am Rev Respir Dis* 1990;141:988–992.

156. Kips JC, Joos GF, Lepeleire ID, et al. MK-571, a potent antagonist of leukotriene D_4-induced bronchoconstriction in the human. *Am Rev Respir Dis* 1991;144:617–621.

157. Manning PJ, Watson RM, Margolskee DJ, et al. Inhibition of exercise-induced bronchoconstriction by MK-571, a potent leukotriene D_4-receptor antagonist. *N Engl J Med* 1990;323:1736–1739.

158. Cloud ML, Enas GC, Kemp J, et al. A specific LTD_4/LTE_4-receptor antagonist improves pulmonary function in patients with mild, chronic asthma. *Am Rev Respir Dis* 1989;140:1336–1339.

159. O'Byrne PM, Dolovich J, Hargreave FE. Late asthmatic responses. *Am Rev Respir Dis* 1987;136:740–751.

160. Shephard EG, Malan L, Macfarlane CM, Mouton W, Joubert JR. Lung function and plasma levels of thromboxane B_2, 6-ketoprostaglandin $F_{1\alpha}$ and β-thromboglobulin in antigen-induced asthma before and after indomethacin pretreatment. *Br J Clin Pharmacol* 1985;19:459–470.

161. Lupinetti MD, Sheller JR, Catella F, FitzGerald GA. Thromboxane biosynthesis in allergen-induced bronchospasm: evidence for platelet activation. *Am Rev Respir Dis* 1989;140:932–935.

162. Sladek K, Dworski R, FitzGerald GA, et al. Allergen-stimulated release of thromboxane A_2 and leukotriene E_4 in humans. *Am Rev Respir Dis* 1990;141:1441–1445.

163. Beasley RCW, Featherstone RL, Church MK, et al. Effect of a thromboxane receptor antagonist on PGD_2- and allergen-induced bronchoconstriction. *J Appl Physiol* 1989; 66:1685–1693.

164. Howarth PH, Durham SR, Lee TH, et al. Influence of albuterol, cromolyn sodium, and ipratropium bromide on the airway and circulating mediator response to allergen bronchial provocation in asthma. *Am Rev Respir Dis* 1985;132:986–992.

165. Diaz P, Gonzalez MC, Galleguillos FR, et al. Leukocytes and mediators in bronchoalveolar lavage during allergen-induced late-phase asthmatic reactions. *Am Rev Respir Dis* 1989;139:1383–1389.

166. Richards IM, Griffin RL, Oostveen JA, et al. Effect of leukotriene B_4 antagonist U-75302 on antigen-induced bronchopulmonary eosinophilia in sensitized guinea pigs. *Am Rev Respir Dis* 1989;140:1712–1716.

167. Kirby JG, Hargreave FE, Cockcroft DW, O'Byrne PM. Effect of indomethacin on allergen-induced asthmatic responses. *J Appl Physiol* 1989;66:578–583.

168. Seltzer J, Bigby BG, Stulbarg MJ, et al. Ozone-induced change in bronchial reactivity to methacholine and airway inflammation in humans. *J Appl Physiol* 1986;60:1321–1326.

169. Springer TA. Adhesion receptors of the immune system. Nature 1990;346:425–434.
170. Albelda SM. Endothelial and epithelial cell adhesion molecules. *Am J Respir Cell Mol Biol* 1991;4:195–203.
171. Leff AR, Hamann KJ, Wegner CD. Inflammation and cell-cell interactions in airway inflammation. *Am J Physiol (Lung Cell Mol Physiol)* 1991;260:L189–L206.
172. Barton RW, Rothlein R, Ksiazek J, Kennedy C. The effect of anti-intercellular adhesion molecule-1 on phorbol-ester-induced rabbit lung inflammation. *J Immunol* 1989; 143:1278–1282.
173. Noonan TC, Gundel RH, Desai SN, et al. The effects of an anti-CD18 antibody (R15.7) in antigen-induced airway hyperresponsiveness (AH) and cell influx in guinea pigs. *Agents Actions* 1991;34:211–213.
174. Lo SK, Everitt J, Gu J, Malik AB. Tumor necrosis factor mediates experimental pulmonary edema by ICAM-1 and CD18-dependent mechanisms. *J Clin Invest* 1992; 89:981–988.
175. Mulligan MS, Warren JS, Smith CW, et al. Lung injury after deposition of IgA immune complexes—requirement for CD18 and L-arginine. *J Immunol* 1992;148:3086–3092.
176. Williams TJ, Hellewell PG. Adhesion molecules involved in the microvascular inflammatory response. *Am Rev Respir Dis* 1992;146:S45–S50.
177. Dustin ML, Springer TA. Lymphocyte function-associated antigen (LFA-1) interaction with intercellular adhesion molecule-1 (ICAM-1) is one of at least three mechanisms for lymphocyte adhesion to cultured endothelial cells. *J Cell Biol* 1988;107:321–331.
178. Vedder NB, Harlan JM. Increased surface expression of CD11b/CD18 (Mac-1) is not required for stimulated neutrophil adherence to cultured endothelium. *J Clin Invest* 1988;81:676–682.
179. Tonnesen MG, Anderson DC, Springer TA, et al. Adherence of neutrophils to cultured human microvascular endothelial cells: stimulation by chemotactic peptides and lipid mediators and dependence upon Mac-1, LFA-1, p150,95 glycoprotein family. *J Clin Invest* 1989;83:637–646.
180. Wegner CD, Gundel RH, Reilly P, et al. Intercellular adhesion molecule-1 (ICAM-1) in the pathogenesis of asthma. *Science* 1990;247:456–459.
181. Look DC, Keller BT, Rapp SR, Holtzman MJ. Selective induction of intercellular adhesion molecule-1 by interferon-γ in human airway epithelial cells. *Am J Physiol (Lung Cell Mol Physiol)* 1992;263:L79–L87.
182. Tosi MF, Stark JM, Smith CW, et al. Induction of ICAM-1 expression on human airway epithelial cells by inflammatory cytokines: effects on neutrophil-epithelial cell adhesion. *Am J Respir Cell Mol Biol* 1992;7:214–221.
183. Greve JM, Davis G, Meyer AM, et al. The major human rhinovirus receptor is ICAM-1. *Cell* 1989;56:839–847.
184. Staunton DE, Merluzzi VJ, Rothlein R, et al. A cell adhesion molecule, ICAM-1, is the major surface receptor for rhinoviruses. *Cell* 1989;56:849–853.
185. Ando M, Fukuda T, Nakjima H, Makino S. Expression of intercellular adhesion molecule-1 (ICAM-1) is upregulated in the bronchial mucosa of symptomatic asthmatics. *J Allergy Clin Immunol* 1992;89:215.
186. Wardlaw AJ, Bentley AM, Menz G, et al. Expression of the adhesion molecules ICAM-1 and ELAM-1 in the bronchial mucosa in asthma. *J Allergy Clin Immunol* 1992;89:164.
187. Gundel RH, Wegner CD, Torcellini CA, Letts LG. The role of intercellular adhesion molecule-1 in chronic airway inflammation. *Clin Exp Allergy* 1992;22:569–575.
188. Wegner CD, Gundel RH, Churchill L, et al. Mac-1 (CD11b/CD18) mediates antigen–induced eosinophil activation and airway hyperresponsiveness in monkeys. *Am Rev Respir Dis* 1992;145:A461.
189. Osborn L. Leukocyte adhesion to endothelium in inflammation. *Cell* 1990;62:3–6.
190. Kishimoto TK. A dynamic model for neutrophil localization to inflammatory sites. *J NIH Res* 1991;3:75–77.
191. Lawrence MB, Springer TA. Leukocyte rolling on a selectin at physiologic flow rates: distinction from and prerequisite for adhesion through integrins. *Cell* 1992;65:859–864.
192. Gundel RH, Wegner CD, Torcellini CA, et al. Endothelial leukocyte adhesion molecule-1 mediate antigen-induced acute airway inflammation and late-phase airway obstruction in monkeys. *J Clin Invest* 1991;88:1407–1411.

193. Georas SN, Liu MC, Newman W, et al. Altered adhesion molecule expression and endothelial cell activation accompany the recruitment of human granulocytes to the lung after segmental antigen challenge. *Am J Respir Cell Mol Biol* 1992;7:261–269.
194. Holtzman MJ, Look DC. Cell adhesion molecules as targets for unraveling the genetic regulation of airway inflammation. *Am J Respir Cell Mol Biol* 1992;7:246–247.
195. Haskard DO, Lee TH. The role of leukocyte-endothelial interactions in the accumulation of leukocytes in allergic inflammation. *Am Rev Respir Dis* 1992;145:S10–S13.
196. Bousquet J, Chanez P, Lacoste JY, et al. Eosinophilic inflammation in asthma. *N Engl J Med* 1990;323:1033–1039.
197. Walsh GM, Mermod J, Hartnell A, Kay AB, Wardlaw AJ. Human eosinophil but not neutrophil adherence to IL-1-stimulated human umbilical vein endothelial cells in $\alpha4\beta1$ (very late antigen-4) dependent. *J Immunol* 1991;146:3419–3423.
198. Dobrina A, Menegazzi R, Carlos TM, et al. Mechanisms of eosinophil adherence to cultured vascular endothelial cells. Eosinophils bind to the cytokine-induced endothelial ligand vascular cell adhesion molecule-1 via the very late activation antigen-4 integrin receptor. *J Clin Invest* 1991;88:20–26.
199. Weller PF, Rand TH, Goelz SE, Chi-Rosso G, Lobb RR. Human eosinophil adherence to vascular endothelium mediated by binding to vascular cell adhesion molecule 1 and endothelial leukocyte adhesion molecule 1. *Proc Natl Acad Sci USA* 1991;88:7430–7433.
200. Nakajima S, Look DC, Holtzman MJ. Selective cytokine regulation of T-lymphocyte adherence to epithelial and endothelial cells. *J Cell Biochem* 1993;17A:351.
201. Voraberger G, Schafer R, Stratowa C. Cloning of the human gene for intercellular adhesion molecule 1 and analysis of its 5'-regulatory region. *J Immunol* 1991;147:2777–2786.
202. Look DC, Pelletier M, Holtzman MJ. Selective cytokine control of the ICAM-1 promoter and identification of the interferon-γ response element in cultured epithelial cells. *J Cell Biochem* 1993;17A:334.
203. Iademarco MF, McQuillan JJ, Rosen GD, Dean DC. Characterization of the promoter for vascular cell adhesion molecule-1 (VCAM-1). *J Biol Chem* 1992;268:16323–16329.
204. Anderson DC, Springer TA. Leukocyte adhesion deficiency: an inherited defect in the Mac-1, LFA-1, and p150,95 glycoproteins. *Am Rev Med* 1987;38:175–194.
205. Rothlein R, Czajkowski M, O'Neill MM, et al. Induction of intercellular adhesion molecule 1 on primary and continuous cell lines by pro-inflammatory cytokins. Regulation by pharmacologic agents and neutralizing antibodies. *J Immunol* 1988;141:1665–1669.
206. Baker C, Altman LC. The effects of dexamethasone (D) and cromolyn sodium (CS) on intercellular adhesion molecule-1 (ICAM-1) expression on human nasal epithelial cells (HNE). *J Allergy Clin Immunol* 1992;89:212.
207. Marlin SD, Staunton DE, Springer TA, et al. A soluble form of intercellular adhesion molecule-1 inhibits rhinovirus infection. *Nature* 1990;344:70–72.
208. Lineberger DW, Graham DJ, Tomassini JE, Colonno RJ. Antibodies that block rhinovirus attachment map to domain 1 of the major group receptor. *J Virol* 1990;64:2582–2587.
209. Fecondo JV, Kent SBH, Boyd AW. Inhibition of intercellular adhesion molecule 1-dependent biological activities by a synthetic peptide analog. *Proc Natl Acad Sci USA* 1991;88:2879–2882.
210. Lane TA, Lamkin GE, Wancewicz E. Modulation of endothelial cell expression of intercellular adhesion molecule 1 by protein kinase C activation. *Biochem Biophys Res Commun* 1989;161:945–952.
211. Carpen O, Pallai P, Staunton DE, Springer TA. Association of intercellular adhesion molecule-1 (ICAM-1) with actin-containing cytoskeleton and alpha-actinin. *J Cell Biol* 1992;118:1223–1234.
212. Chiang M, Chan H, Zounes MA, et al. Antisense oligonucleotides inhibit intercellular adhesion molecule 1 expression by two distinct mechanisms. *J Biol Chem* 1991;266:18162–18171.
213. Corrigan CJ, Kay AB. CD4 T-lymphocyte activation in acute severe asthma. Relationship to disease severity and atopic status. *Am Rev Respir Dis* 1990;141:970–977.
214. Street NE, Mosmann TR. Functional diversity of T lymphocytes due to secretion of different cytokine patterns. *FASEB J* 1991;5:171–177.

215. Robinson DS, Hamid Q, Ying S, et al. Predominant T_{H2}-like bronchoalveolar T-lymphocyte population in atopic asthma. *N Engl J Med* 1992;326:298–304.
216. Walker C, Bode E, Boer L, et al. Allergic and nonallergic asthmatics have distinct patterns of T-cell activation and cytokine production in peripheral blood and bronchoalveolar lavage. *Am Rev Respir Dis* 1992;148:109–115.
217. Plaut M, Pierce JH, Watson CJ, et al. Mast cell lines produce lymphokines in response to cross-linkage of FcεRI or to calcium ionophores. *Nature* 1989;339:64–67.
218. Boulay J-L, Paul WE. The interleukin-4-related lymphokines and their binding to hematopoietin receptors. *J Biol Chem* 1992;267:20525–20528.
219. Rothenberg ME, Owen WF Jr, Silberstein DS, et al. Eosinophils cocultured with endothelial cells have increased survival and functional properties. *Science* 1987; 237:645–647.
220. Lopez AF, Sanderson CJ, Gamble JR, et al. Recombinant human interleukin 5 is a selective activator of human eosinophil function. *J Exp Med* 1988;167:219–224.
221. Rothenberg ME, Owen WF Jr, Silberstein DS, et al. Human eosinophils have prolonged survival, enhanced functional properties, and become hypodense when exposed to human interleukin 3. *J Clin Invest* 1988;81:1986–1992.
222. Moser R, Fehr J, Olgiati L, Bruijnzeel PLB. Migration of primed human eosinophils across cytokine-activated endothelial cell monolayers. *Blood* 1992;79:2937–2945.
223. Gulbenkian AR, Egan RW, Fernandez X, et al. Interleukin-5 modulates eosinophil accumulation in allergic guinea pig lung. *Am Rev Respir Dis* 1992;148:263–265.
224. Chand N, Harrison JE, Rooney S, et al. Anti-IL-5 monoclonal antibody inhibits allergic late phase bronchial eosinophilia in guinea pigs: a therapeutic approach. *Eur J Pharmacol* 1992;211:121–123.
225. Walker C, Virchow J-C, Bruijnzeel PLB, Blaser K. T cell subsets and their soluble products regulate eosinophilia in allergic and nonallergic asthma. *J Immunol* 1991; 146:1829–1835.
226. Howard M, Farrar J, Hilfiker M, et al. Identification of a T cell-derived B cell growth factor distinct from interleukin 2. *J Exp Med* 1982;155:914–923.
227. Pene J, Rousset F, Briere F, et al. IgE production by normal human B cells induced by alloreactive T cell clones is mediated by IL-4 and suppressed by IFN-γ. *J Immunol* 1988;141:1218–1224.
228. Hart PH, Vitti GF, Burgess DR, et al. Potential antiinflammatory effects of interleukin 4: suppression of human monocyte tumor necrosis factor α, interleukin 1, and prostaglandin E_2. *Proc Natl Acad Sci USA* 1989;86:3803–3807.
229. Conrad DJ, Kuhn H, Mulkins M, Highland E, Sigal E. Specific inflammatory cytokines regulate the expression of human monocyte 15-lipoxygenase. *Proc Natl Acad Sci USA* 1992;89:217–221.
230. Schleimer RP. Effects of glucocorticosteroids on infammatory cells relevant to their therapeutic application in asthma. *Am Rev Respir Dis* 1990;141:S59–S69.
231. Borish L, Mascali JJ, Dishuck J, et al. Detection of alveolar macrophage-derived IL-1β in asthma. Inhibition with corticosteroids. *J Immunol* 1992;149:3078–3082.
232. Vecchiarelli A, Siracusa A, Cenci E, Puliti M, Abbritti G. Effect of corticosteroid treatment on interleukin-1 and tumour necrosis factor secretion by monocytes from subjects with asthma. *Clin Exp Allergy* 1992;22:365–370.
233. Hultsch T, Albers MW, Schreiber SL, Hohman RJ. Immunophilin ligands demonstrate common features of signal transduction leading to exocytosis or transcription. *Proc Natl Acad Sci USA* 1991;88:6229–6233.
234. Walsh CT, Zydowsky LD, McKeon FD. Cyclosporin A, the cyclophilin class of peptidylprolyl isomerases, and blockade of T cell signal transduction. *J Biol Chem* 1992;267:13115–13118.
235. Calderon E, Lockey RF, Bukantz SC, Coffey RG, Ledford DK. Is there a role for cyclosporin in asthma? *J Allergy Clin Immunol* 1992;89:629–636.
236. Alexander AG, Barnes NC, Kay AB. Trial of cyclosporin in corticosteroid-dependent chronic severe asthma. *Lancet* 1992;339:324–328.

Subject Index

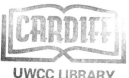